Comprehensive Coronary Care

'One man is as good as another until he has written a book.'
From *The Letters of Benjamin Jowett, Volume 1.* (1899) Abbott and Campbell.

Dedicated to Sheena, Alex and Luci, Rose, Luke and Jack, who continue to support us whilst we are bettering ourselves.

For Baillière Tindall:

Senior Commissioning Editor: Ninette Premdas
Project Development Manager: Mairi McCubbin
Project Manager: Gail Wright
Designer: Judith Wright

Comprehensive Coronary Care

Nigel I Jowett MB BS MRCS LRCP MD FRCP
Director of Clinical Medicine, Consultant Physician and Cardiologist,
Pembrokeshire and Derwen NHS Trust, Haverfordwest; Director, Healthstart, Pembrokeshire, UK

David R Thompson BSc MA PhD MBA RN FRCN FESC
Professor of Nursing, Department of Health Sciences, University of York, York, UK

Foreword by

Roger Boyle
National Director for Heart Disease, Department of Health, London, UK

THIRD EDITION

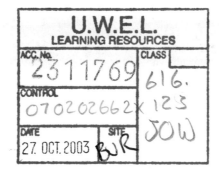

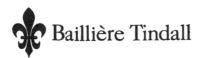

Baillière Tindall

BAILLIÈRE TINDALL
An imprint of Elsevier Science Limited

First edition 1989
Second edition 1995
Third edition 2003

ISBN 0 7020 2662 X

British Library Cataloguing in Publication Data
A catalogue record for this book is available from the British
Library

Library of Congress Cataloging in Publication Data
A catalog record for this book is available from the Library
of Congress

Note
Medical knowledge is constantly changing. As new
information becomes available, changes in treatment,
procedures, equipment and the use of drugs become
necessary. The authors and the publishers have taken
care to ensure that the information given in this text is
accurate and up to date. However, readers are strongly
advised to confirm that the information, especially with
regard to drug usage, complies with the latest legislation
and standards of practice.

ELSEVIER SCIENCE
your source for books,
journals and multimedia
in the health sciences
www.elsevierhealth.com

The
publisher's
policy is to use
**paper manufactured
from sustainable forests**

Printed in China by RDC Group Limited

Contents

Foreword

A quarter of a century ago the only real tools of the trade available in coronary care units (CCUs) were opiates and defibrillators. Now the CCU staff face a much more formidable challenge with a complex array of treatment options that need tailoring to each individual patient.

First, they must keep pace with the burgeoning evidence base of effective interventions. Excellence in care requires not only up-to-date knowledge of the latest technologies and when to apply them correctly but also a systematic approach that ensures simple things are always done correctly. As coronary care staff strive to offer optimal care to every acutely ill patient following the latest clinical trials or guidelines, they still have to ensure that the patient and their carers are fully informed and cared for in a considered, caring and honest fashion.

Excellence also requires teamwork. Success in providing top quality care is dependent on a skilled, informed and professional workforce that can work together as a team spanning all the various disciplines along the patient pathway before, during and after admission to hospital.

Case mix has also changed. Admissions of patients with acute coronary syndromes now outnumber those with ST elevation myocardial infarction. So the daily agenda now extends beyond accurate diagnosis and eligibility for thrombolysis to a more complex decision matrix that includes triage, risk stratification and choice of a much wider range of interventions than would have seemed possible just a decade ago.

Staff have had to accept that audit has become a permanent feature of their work. Nearly every coronary care unit in England now contributes to the national audit of acute myocardial infarction, (Myocardial Infarction National Audit Programme) with the regular publication of process measures reflecting the quality of care.

There have also been a number of national initiatives that have challenged hospitals to modernise and improve.

The White Paper, *Saving Lives: Our Healthier Nation* (DoH 1999) sets the challenging target of a 40% reduction in cardiovascular deaths by 2010. The *National Service Framework for Coronary Heart Disease (NSF for CHD)* published in March 2000 (DoH 2000) mapped out a blueprint as to how this might be achieved, placing coronary heart disease at the forefront of health policy across England. Similar initiatives also exist in Scotland and Wales.

In England, the *NHS Plan* (DoH 2000) prioritised coronary heart disease, at the same time setting out how the NHS should develop to provide the nation with a first-class, patient-centred service and to make the NHS a better place in which to work.

The *NHS Plan* also announced the Coronary Heart Disease Collaborative. This has now been set up and is being rolled out across England to thirty separate sites as part of the Modernisation Agency. The aims of this movement are to co-ordinate the whole journey of the CHD patient through the healthcare system giving them more certainty and choice while improving the experience for them and their carers. The programme is intended to improve quality of care by a process of redesign and service improvement. Of the six key topics included, acute myocardial infarction, angina, secondary prevention and rehabilitation are of particular relevance here.

The *NSF for CHD* has been taken up by NHS staff with considerable enthusiasm. The combination of their hard work together with considerable financial investment has allowed major progress to be made. A plan aimed at producing continuous improvement in care has resulted in more patients being treated more rapidly and with greater consistency than ever before. Therapies known to be effective after heart attack are being taken up more widely and more needy patients are being included in rehabilitation programmes.

In these rapidly changing times, it is imperative that the staff who care for heart patients are kept fully informed and up-to-date. This text, the third edition, makes a major contribution to preparing staff for the major task ahead of them. Written by an experienced team combining medical and nursing expertise with extensive clinical and research experience, this text will make an important addition to every CCU library. It will encourage our industrious and committed staff to learn and further explore the evidence base in the pursuit of excellence and improvement in care.

Dr Roger Boyle

Preface

This new edition of our book coincides with the publication of the National Service Framework for Coronary Heart Disease, and the NHS Plan. Within these documents, the British government has prioritised and pledged more investment in coronary heart disease, with improvements in prevention, diagnosis, treatment and rehabilitation. This third edition of *Comprehensive Coronary Care* has required an extensive rewrite to cover the huge changes in acute cardiac care over the last 6 years. It takes into account the substantial and ever-growing evidence base for cardiac care as well as the radical changes in the design and delivery of services from prevention through to rehabilitation. Myocardial infarction has been redefined, and patients presenting with acute coronary syndromes are now receiving the intensive approach they need. We have also seen rapid advances in percutaneous coronary intervention, and innovative approaches to cardiac surgery. This millennium has also seen the International Liaison Committee on Resuscitation (ILCOR) produce the first truly international guidelines for resuscitation.

The Coronary Heart Disease Partnership Programme, established with the NSF and begun in October 2000, is working with a group of cardiac networks across the country to streamline delivery of high-quality, patient-centred care. We hope that this book continues to help all disciplines involved in acute cardiac care to achieve this goal.

Haverfordwest and
York 2003

Nigel I Jowett
David R Thompson

Preface to the first edition

The role of coronary care has changed markedly since its inception in the early 1960s, and it now has an extended importance for patients with other manifestations of coronary artery disease, and for those with critical cardiac dysfunction who require intensive care and cardiovascular monitoring. This book is intended as an up-to-date guide to this current practice of 'cardiac intensive care', and to provide a basis for further exploration of the subject. Because we believe that such practice is not the sole domain of either nursing or medical staff we have tried to utilise an integrated approach, suitable for all those concerned in patient management on the coronary care unit. Some of our material extends outside the traditional boundaries of coronary care, but we think it important that it is appreciated how the patients come to be there, and what may happen to them after they leave.

Whilst we hope that nurses never lose sight of their primary caring role, in reality much of their work in the area of coronary care involves a high degree of medical and technical expertise, and our book reflects this. We have assumed that nurse-readers have a basic understanding of primary nursing, the nursing process, nursing theories and conceptual models, and only salient features are mentioned in the text.

Leicester 1989

Nigel I Jowett
David R Thompson

Acknowledgements

We would like to thank Roger Boyle, David Hawkins, Tom Quinn and Alison Turner for their contributions. Once again, special thanks to Sheena Jowett for typing the manuscript, and to Val Creese for co-ordinating things.

1

Introduction to coronary care

The coronary heart disease epidemic began in North America, Europe and Australia in the early part of the 20th century, peaking in the 1960s and early 1970s. The World Health Organization MONICA project has been monitoring trends and determinants of cardiovascular disease in 21 countries since the mid-1980s (Tunstall-Pedoe et al, 1994) and has shown that deaths from cardiovascular disease across many populations are falling (Fig. 1.1). Two-thirds of mortality reduction is due to a reduction in coronary event rates, whilst reduced case fatality accounts for about one-third (Tunstall-Pedoe et al, 1999). However, despite an overall reduction in mortality of over a third in the decade 1984–1994, coronary heart disease remains the major cause of morbidity and mortality in nearly all industrialised countries. Explanations as to why mortality is falling in recent years have pointed to a combination of prevention, medical and surgical treatments (Beaglehole, 1999).

Unfortunately, although industrialised countries have made huge advances in the management of cardiovascular disease, the epidemic has moved on to the developing countries, where many new populations are experiencing a substantial increase in coronary heart disease, which is associated with approximately 7.2 million deaths worldwide per year (World Health Organization, 1997a). This escalating global burden of ischaemic heart disease is likely to continue until the year 2020 (Murray and Lopez, 1997).

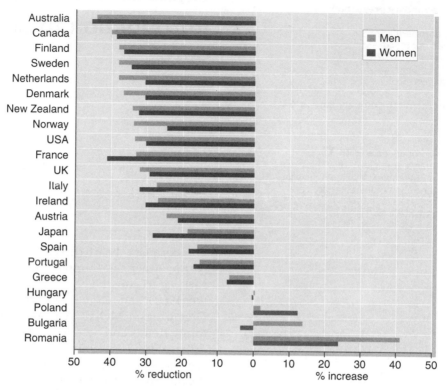

Figure 1.1 Changes in coronary heart disease mortality rates in selected countries (1984–1994) for men and women aged 35–74 years. (Reproduced with permission from the World Health Organization Statistics Annual (1999).)

There are at least three contributory factors that have led to the spread of coronary disease to the developing countries. First, life expectancy in these populations is increasing because of reduced mortality from infectious diseases. Second, genetic factors seem to be conferring susceptibility to coronary disease, particularly in people from South Asia. Finally, and perhaps most importantly, these countries have been adopting the Western life-style, including unhealthy diets, lack of exercise, obesity and, perhaps most importantly, smoking. It is estimated that smoking-related mortality in India will increase from 1% in 1990 to 13% in 2020, and that by then, will also be responsible for over 2 million deaths in China every year (World Health Organization, 1997b).

In the UK, the fall in coronary heart disease mortality of 38% between the early 1970s and the late 1990s has been promising, but mortality has fallen faster in most other developed countries

and death from coronary heart disease in the UK remains amongst the highest in the world (Fig. 1.2). In 2000, 270 000 people in the UK suffered a heart attack, and about 157 000 died from the various manifestations of coronary heart disease (Petersen and Rayner, 2002). This means that one in four men and one in five women die from coronary heart disease and that every 2 min someone in the UK suffers a heart attack. Overall, coronary heart disease is responsible for the deaths of 24% of men and 14% of women before the age of 75 years (Fig. 1.3), thus depriving the country's economy of people in their most productive years and many young families of their parents.

Cardiovascular medicine is a rapidly expanding speciality, and modern therapy for coronary heart disease means that more people are surviving myocardial infarction. The fall in cardiovascular mortality has been most marked in younger patient groups; more than 60% of coro-

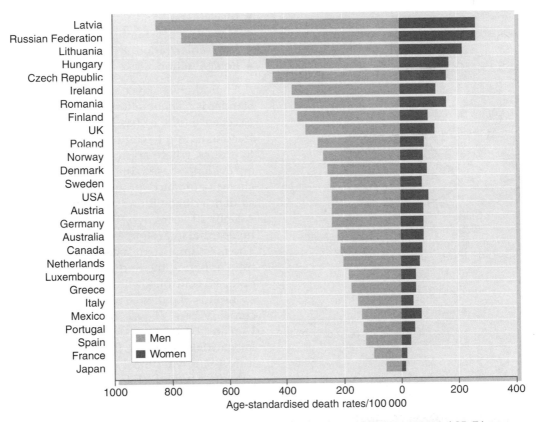

Figure 1.2   Death rates from coronary heart disease in selected countries for men and women aged 35–74 years. (Reproduced with permission from the World Health Organization Statistics Annual (1999).)

nary deaths now occurring in people aged over 75 years (British Heart Foundation, 2002). Since coronary heart disease mortality remains high, it appears that death is being postponed rather than being prevented, and, because more people now survive the initial heart attack, the medical caseload for the consequences of coronary disease will increase dramatically in coming years. In addition, the elderly population is increasing, and this group has the highest incidence of cardiovascular diseases, including the commonest precursors of heart failure, coronary artery disease and hypertension. An estimated 1.4 million people in the UK have angina, and the mean age of patients with heart failure in the community is now 76 years (Cowie et al, 1999).

With increasing morbidity from the complications of acute myocardial infarction, long-term disability and ill health often persist. Many post-infarct patients never feel well again, are unable to work and some remain confined to the house. Production losses cost the UK economy double that of any other single illness. The estimated cost of coronary heart disease to the National Health Service is in excess of £1600 million, over half of which is hospital costs spent in caring for the victims of heart attack, as well as an estimated 2 million cases of angina and heart failure. Coronary heart disease accounts for 3% of all hospital admissions in England.

In 1999, the UK Department of Health set out the national strategy in *Saving Lives: Our Healthier Nation*, which with '*Smoking Kills*' forms an ambitious series of linked complementary health policies (Department of Health, 1999a). The measures included the introduction of the National Service Framework for Coronary Heart Disease which has set national standards of care for coronary heart disease prevention and therapy to improve health, reduce variations in management and

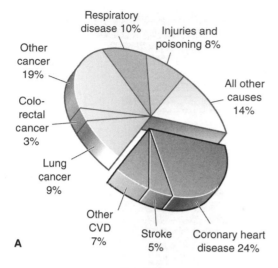

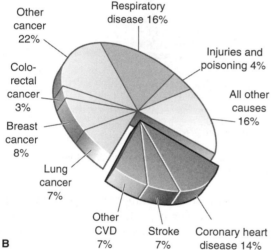

Figure 1.3 (**A**) Deaths by cause in the UK (2000) for men under the age of 75 years. (**B**) Deaths by cause in the UK (2000) for women under the age of 75 years. (Both reproduced with permission from Petersen S, Rayner M (2002) *Coronary Heart Disease Statistics*. London: British Heart Foundation Database.)

promote fast, high-quality services. The document sets out 12 standards of cardiac care, with summaries of how these are to be achieved and within what time period (Department of Health, 2000). The standards cover:

- Reducing heart disease in the population
- Preventing coronary heart disease in high-risk patients
- Treating acute coronary syndromes

- Investigating and treating angina
- Managing heart failure
- Revascularisation
- Rehabilitation.

Clinical governance will help implement these standards. The National Institute for Clinical Excellence (NICE) has been set up to commend treatments and to commission clinical guidelines to ensure, where appropriate, that interventions are evidence-based. Information about NICE, the clinical guidance programmes and sources of evidence can be found at www.nice.org.uk.

Until 20 years ago, the management of acute myocardial infarction was essentially supportive. The most important recent advances have come from applying the findings of multinational randomised controlled clinical trials involving many thousands of patients, which have revolutionised coronary care. It was the Clinical Trial Service Unit in Oxford that started the trend for these 'mega-trials', from the first International Study of Infarct Survival (ISIS-1) in 1988, with over 16 000 patients studied (ISIS-1 Collaborative Group, 1988), to ISIS-4, which recruited a huge total of 58 000 patients (ISIS-4 Collaborative Group, 1995). Modern management of acute coronary syndromes is now much more proactive, and has resulted from the application of improved understanding of the pathophysiology of myocardial infarction, its risk factors and newly acquired evidence-based interventions (Box 1.1).

PRIMARY AND SECONDARY PREVENTION

Coronary heart disease almost always results from atherosclerosis, usually in the form of eccentric plaques, which are variably distributed in the coronary artery tree. The atherosclerotic process starts in early life, and fatty streaks may be found in up to half of children less than 15 years of age and fibrous-plaque lesions in 8% of those aged 2–15 years (Berenson et al, 1998). The estimated prevalence of coronary heart disease in asymptomatic, middle-aged men in the UK is 4%. When symptoms emerge, coronary artery disease

---

Box 1.1 Summary results of the 'mega-trials'

ASPIRIN for ALL suspected acute myocardial infarction or unstable angina (+ LONG-TERM aspirin after leaving hospital)
Benefit: 24 lives per 1000 (+ definite EXTRA from LONG TERM; increased benefits when given early with clopidogrel in unstable angina – 28 fewer coronary events per 1000 patients treated)

FIBRINOLYTICS for patients with bundle branch block or ST elevation that are within 0–12 h of pain onset
Benefit: 30 lives per 1000 in these patients (or more, with aspirin and EARLIER treatment)

BETA-BLOCKERS, STARTED EARLY with intravenous dose (except in shock or persistent hypotension) and continued LONG TERM
Benefit: about 7 lives per 1000 in first month (+ 10–20 EXTRA per year from LONG TERM + 21 fewer re-infarctions)

ACE INHIBITORS, STARTED EARLY (except in shock or persistent hypotension) and continued LONG TERM, especially in those with left ventricular dysfunction
Benefit: about 5–8 lives per 1000 in first month (perhaps 14 lives per 1000 in high-risk groups + EXTRA from LONG TERM in those with left ventricular dysfunction, perhaps 40 cardiac events per 1000 treated)

STATINS, LONG TERM
Benefit: about 7 deaths per 1000 treated (plus 52 fewer cardiovascular events per 1000 treated)

Note: Heparin, magnesium, calcium antagonists and nitrates provide little or no net benefit (and little difference between different fibrinolytic agents).

---

presents as angina in about 50% of cases and as myocardial infarction in 30%. Traditionally, cardiovascular management strategies have focused on treating those with overt disease, but about a half of heart attacks and a third of fatal heart attacks occur in patients with no prior manifestations of atherosclerosis (Deedwania, 2001). Sudden cardiac death is also sometimes the first and final sign of coronary disease.

The detection of coronary artery disease is often delayed because the extent of coronary atheroma may be masked by collateral coronary circulation; coronary insufficiency only becomes obvious when there is disequilibrium between the demand for oxygen by the myocardium and the coronary blood supply. By the time the clinical signs and symptoms of coronary heart disease have developed, atherosclerosis is often found to be in an advanced stage, with multiple stenosed arteries lined by calcified and necrotic atheromatous plaques. Therapy at this stage would seem nothing more than palliative and provides good reason for particular emphasis on preventative measures.

Primary prevention aims to stop heart disease developing in a population. It encompasses all methods used to reduce the risk of asymptomatic individuals developing coronary heart disease, preventing the first heart attack or delaying the

appearance of other symptoms related to myocardial ischaemia, such as dysrhythmias, heart failure and angina. Two strategies have been employed:

1. A *population strategy* attempts to influence the environment and life-style of a whole population (e.g. reducing smoking).
2. A *high-risk strategy* identifies those at highest risk of developing coronary disease and aims to reduce risk in those individuals (e.g. reducing their blood pressure or cholesterol level).

Secondary prevention includes any treatment that reduces the risk of death or a second coronary event in a patient who has already suffered a myocardial infarction, or has demonstrated other signs of cardiovascular disease. It aims to retard the progress of atherosclerosis and preserve left ventricular function. Secondary prevention is needed in far fewer patients to achieve a significant effect on morbidity and mortality.

The distinction between primary and secondary prevention is artificial, because many different factors may lead to damage of the coronary vasculature in different individuals and populations to produce the same result – i.e. accumulation of atheroma and coronary heart disease. Attention is usually focused on certain factors that have been implicated in the accelerated development of atherosclerotic disease (Wood et al, 2000). These include hypertension, hyperlipidaemia, diabetes mellitus, cigarette smoking, obesity, physical inactivity and stress. However, these disorders alone are not implicated in all cases of coronary heart disease, and there may be an additional inherited risk. The presence of early coronary heart disease in a first-degree relative is very common in young patients who present with myocardial infarction and, as such, represents a strong risk factor. This, of course, may simply reflect the similarity of a shared environment and life-style, but it is likely that there is a significant genetic predisposition (Jowett, 1984). In the next decade, gene testing is likely to become an established component of preventing coronary artery disease (Day and Wilson, 2001), with identification of genetic variants that have a predictive value. This will allow a more cost-effective way of risk factor intervention by directing preventive therapy and counselling at those who will benefit most.

The recent decline in cardiovascular mortality appears to be mainly attributable to improvements in secondary prevention (Rosamond et al, 1998; Tunstall-Pedoe et al, 1999). Somewhat surprisingly, the effects of risk factor intervention have been smaller than expected (Kuulasmaa et al, 2000), and it is improved medical management of the post-infarct patient that has mostly been responsible for a continuing reduction in coronary mortality. Improved surgical techniques (bypass surgery and percutaneous intervention) are also significantly enhancing prognosis and are now having a major impact on reducing cardiovascular mortality.

The accomplishments of coronary care units in implementing therapies to limit infarct size and treat potentially fatal dysrhythmias following myocardial infarction should not be underestimated. The incidence of ventricular fibrillation is about 5% of admissions to coronary care, of which over 90% are now reversed.

PRE-HOSPITAL CORONARY CARE

Without doubt, the two most important advances in the management of acute myocar-

dial infarction have been improved methods of resuscitation from cardiac arrest and early restoration of flow in the infarct-related coronary artery by fibrinolytic drugs or primary angioplasty. Currently, thrombolysis saves about 30 lives per thousand patients treated (Fibrinolytic Therapy Trialists' Collaborative Group, 1994), although this benefit is probably doubled for those treated within the first 'golden hour' after the onset of symptoms (Boersma et al, 1996). Reducing delay in providing thrombolytic treatment has been a major goal for hospitals in recent years, and various strategies for 'fast-track' administration either in accident and emergency departments or in coronary care units have been proposed.

The potential benefits of pre-hospital coronary care for patients with acute myocardial infarction are great, but there remain many major training issues (Waine et al, 1993). Even simple interventions such as pain relief and aspirin administration are often omitted (Wyllie and Dunn, 1994; Moher and Johnson, 1994), and pre-hospital thrombolysis on a large scale has so far proved impracticable. At present, emphasis is placed on reducing delays in patients calling for help, and using ambulance paramedics rather than general practitioners in providing early resuscitation and rapid transport to hospital.

SUDDEN CARDIAC DEATH

Most heart attack deaths occur outside hospital and are medically unattended (Volmink et al, 1998). The term 'sudden cardiac death' is used to describe natural death due to a cardiac cause where individuals at one moment appear fit and well and then collapse, to die in less than an hour and often immediately. Sudden cardiac death comprises about two-thirds of all sudden deaths, and most are attributable to coronary artery disease. In the majority of cases it is impossible to determine whether death has been caused by re-entrant ventricular fibrillation starting at the borders of a pre-existing myocardial scar, or whether the death is due to primary ventricular fibrillation following an acute coronary thrombosis. Some of these people will have experienced chest pain or dyspnoea in the preceding few days, and most will have a previous history of cardiovascular disease. The reason for death is often not clear, even if a postmortem examination is carried out, because the probability of finding an acute coronary lesion (plaque rupture with thrombosis) ranges widely and increases with the duration of prodromal symptoms before death. Developing myocardial infarction cannot be recognised in most cases because the earliest histological change (invasion by leucocytes) does not develop until 12–24 h after coronary occlusion. The presence of occlusive thrombus at necropsy is almost pathognomonic of developing infarction (de Wood et al, 1980) and is found in about a third of sudden cardiac deaths (Davies, 1992). An additional 43% of autopsies demonstrate non-occlusive intraluminal thrombus, suggesting that acute coronary thrombosis was the cause of the sudden death. Plaque fissuring is seen in some cases, but, as this is a random and recurrent event, it may be found in people who die from unrelated causes. It thus appears that a quarter of sudden cardiac deaths are not related to myocardial infarction, and are believed to be due to malignant ventricular dysrhythmias. These 'electrical' coronary deaths appear to be a distinct pathological entity, and advances in electrophysiological cardiology have highlighted a group of patients suitable for implantation of automatic implantable cardioverter defibrillators (see Ch. 13).

The proportion of cardiac deaths occurring out of hospital has risen in recent years from about two-thirds to three-quarters because in-hospital mortality has fallen. Those of us working in hospital practice must realise that our view of acute myocardial infarction is based on caring for survivors of a devastating clinical event that has already taken its major toll.

BYSTANDER RESUSCITATION

In the UK Heart Attack Study (Norris, 1998), three-quarters of heart attack deaths in people less than 75 years old occurred outside hospital. The majority occurred in the home and were witnessed. An analysis of the records of out-of-hospital cardiac deaths found that only 16% of witnesses attempted resuscitation, and 91% of people were dead before the call for help was made (Fitzpatrick et al, 1992). This is important because the chances of survival are directly related to the speed with which resuscitative measures can be instituted. The concept of the 'chain of survival' describes the interventions that are needed for optimal survival.

The links in the chain of survival are:

- Recognition of cardiac arrest
- Early activation of appropriate emergency services
- Early basic life support
- Early defibrillation
- Early advanced life support.

'Bystander resuscitation' by members of the public has a major role in saving lives for the 16% of heart attack deaths that occur in public places, usually the street. If there is a prompt call for help with rapid admission to hospital within an hour of onset of symptoms, 140 deaths per thousand calls could be prevented by timely resuscitation and early thrombolysis (Norris, 1998). The next link in the chain is effective basic life support. Unfortunately, it appears that, although members of the general public appreciate the value of bystander resuscitation, they do not take the steps to acquire the necessary skills. Worse still, for those who know what to do, the effectiveness of their resuscitative attempts is doubtful (Wiseman et al, 1989).

In Seattle, USA, up to half the general population are fully trained in bystander-initiated resuscitation. Such a programme of public education has resulted in a doubling of survival rates following witnessed cardiac arrest, and, of those resuscitated, half leave hospital (Thompson et al, 1979). In the UK, the British Heart Foundation has launched the HeartStart project to teach citizen resuscitation, including basic airway management and cardiopulmonary resuscitation. The development of automatic external defibrillators (AEDs) now allows basic-level providers of resuscitation to administer defibrillatory shocks, and the wider availability of these defibrillators could further increase the likelihood of survival from out-of-hospital cardiac arrest (Dickey and Adgey, 1992). At the moment training in the use of AEDs is usually limited to those who may be called upon to provide emergency care, including medical and nursing staff, ambulance service personnel, the police, firefighters and airline cabin crew. Before the introduction of AEDs, only 15% of out-of-hospital cardiac arrest cases had their circulation restored, and of these only half survived to leave hospital. It is worth noting that 80% of all sudden cardiac deaths occur in persons with known cardiovascular disease, usually within 18 months of hospital discharge following acute myocardial infarction. Since two-thirds of episodes of cardiac arrest occur at home, family members could be targeted for instruction in basic life support and defibrillation. At the moment, AED use by lay members is difficult to support, but as part of a medically controlled programme could be of considerable benefit in the future.

PRE-HOSPITAL THROMBOLYSIS

With the recognition that the provision of early and skilled intervention is of major importance, pre-hospital care has taken on a more important role in recent years. Coronary ambulances were first described by Pantridge and Geddes (1967), with the aim to get a defibrillator to the patient, relieve pain and stabilise rhythm before travel to hospital. Since then, the importance of thrombolysis has emerged, and the 'stay-and-stabilise' strategy for immediate care of the cardiac patient is no longer appropriate. Delays in reperfusion strategies are inevitable, and the United Kingdom Heart Attack Study (UKHAS) reported that only 2% of patients were receiving thrombolytic therapy within the first 'golden hour' following onset of symptoms (UKHAS Collaborative Group, 1998). Specialised coronary ambulances were originally staffed by medical and nursing personnel, but now suitably trained paramedics can carry out most of the emergency care, including defibrillation and administration of thrombolytic agents (Lewis et al, 1993; Pantridge, 1994). The European Myocardial Infarction Project Group found that patients

treated by mobile coronary ambulance teams receive thrombolysis up to an hour before those who are taken to hospital (EMIP, 1993).

Since most cases of coronary thrombosis occur at home, there is an opportunity for general practitioners to be very much in the forefront of pre-hospital myocardial salvage (Colquhoun, 1993). Where general practitioners offer a first-response service, the 'call-to-needle' time may be well within the National Service Framework target of 60 min if the patient is more than 30 min from the hospital (Rawles et al, 1998). An overview of the clinical trials of pre-hospital thrombolysis showed a 17% reduction in 30-day mortality (Morrison et al, 2001). Practicability and resources remain a major problem for pre-hospital thrombolysis on a large scale. Practically speaking, pre-hospital treatment should be given at least 1 h sooner if it is going to reduce mortality, and anything less than this probably makes hospital thrombolysis equally effective. Despite extensive training and investment, the European Myocardial Infarction Project saved 55 min and only just demonstrated a positive effect. In most cities, it is likely that rapid transmission to hospital is the best method of management ('scoop-and-run'), and pre-hospital thrombolysis is likely to be of greatest value in rural areas where the journey time is likely to cause the major delay in admission to hospital (Rawles et al, 1998).

PRE-HOSPITAL DELAYS

The most common reason for pre-hospital delay is the patient himself. By the time many patients call for help, the benefits of thrombolysis are limited. Despite public education campaigns and individual education of the post-coronary patient, delays after the onset of symptoms average 2–3 h before presentation to hospital (Kereiakes et al, 1990), and many present more than 12 h after onset of symptoms. This patient group are typically older, female and with a previous history of cardiovascular disease (Table 1.1). The delay in the call for help is usually greatest when symptoms begin at night. About one-quarter of non-fatal infarctions are 'silent', with no or atypical symptoms, and occur particu-

Table 1.1 Time between onset of coronary symptoms and call for medical help in 200 patients admitted to our coronary care, with and without previous myocardial infarction (MI)

Time (hs)	Previous MI	No previous MI
<0.5	28	20
0.5–1	18	15
1–3	42	27
3–24	5	9
>24	7	29
Total	100	100

larly in the elderly and those with diabetes (Kannel and Abbott, 1984).

Reduction of pre-hospital delay is a major challenge for modern coronary care. Although public education on the symptoms of heart attack and what to do about them is important, it is vital that access to emergency services is improved. General practitioners need to develop practice policies for responding rapidly to patients with chest pain, and those patients at high risk of acute myocardial infarction and their family should be informed of the practice policy. These patients also need information about what to do and who to call should they develop symptoms of a heart attack. *NHS Direct* provides advice to people calling about suspected heart attacks and arranges for the ambulance service to send appropriately trained and equipped help immediately. Primary care teams should ensure that an emergency call is made to the ambulance services before attending, and arrange to rendezvous with an emergency ambulance at the patient's home. General practitioners should be prepared to give oxygen, aspirin, nitrates and adequate intravenous analgesia and, if pre-hospital thrombolysis is being contemplated, they need to be fully aware of the indications, contraindications and side-effects of such treatment and should have a defibrillator available. Direct communication between the ambulance and the admitting coronary care unit is desirable, so that there is no delay between arrival at the hospital door, triage and thrombolysis. All patients with chest pain who directly contact the emergency services require an emergency (Category A) response to reach the caller within

8 min in a vehicle containing a defibrillator and staff trained in its use. The transfer of the patient to hospital should be achieved within 30 min (Department of Health, 2000).

Recent enthusiasm for improving the speed of delivery of thrombolytic treatment may hide the true benefits of acute coronary care, including getting a defibrillator to the patient. Early resuscitation may have actually saved more lives than thrombolysis. Indeed, it was the importance of rhythm monitoring and prompt defibrillation that revolutionised the management of coronary patients and led to the establishment of coronary care units when it was first suggested more than 40 years ago (Julian, 1961).

ACUTE AND INTERMEDIATE CORONARY CARE IN HOSPITAL

In-hospital fatality from acute myocardial infarction remains high. Although the clinical trials of thrombolysis suggest that case fatality rates have been reduced to 7%, mortality rates are likely to be more than double this figure, because normal acute coronary care includes all the high-risk groups often excluded by trials. The benefits of thrombolysis to the individual patient may not be as great as trials would suggest, but patients who do not receive, or are ineligible for, thrombolysis are at high risk of death (Brown et al, 1999).

The first priority within hospital is to identify those patients presenting with an acute coronary syndrome who need immediate attention for haemodynamic stabilisation and reperfusion therapy. An estimated 22 600 patients present with first-time exertional angina in the UK every year (Ghandi et al, 1995). Chest pain is a worrying symptom for the patient and medical practitioner alike, since it is often difficult to differentiate between cardiac and non-cardiac pain. Certain subgroups of patients present with unusual symptoms of coronary ischaemia. Women often present with 'atypical' chest pain, whereas the elderly complain of shortness of breath (Then et al, 2001). Rapid-access chest pain clinics may provide swift reassurance or timely intervention (Wood et al, 2001). In 2000, we saw

179 patients in our chest pain clinic, of which only 35% were found to have cardiac or other important chest pain. We were able to discharge 116 patients immediately, with reassurance for both general practitioner and patient. A further 25 required only one more outpatient appointment to sort out their management.

For patients seen with acute chest pain in the accident and emergency department, or admitted directly to an admissions unit, a system for rapid chest pain triage is needed to ensure that the appropriate cases obtain urgent treatment at the earliest opportunity (Burns et al, 1989). Stable angina may progress rapidly to unstable angina, acute myocardial infarction, or even sudden death within days of first presentation. The primary method of screening for an acute coronary syndrome is by determining the presence of chest pain and obtaining a standard resting 12-lead electrocardiogram (ECG). Between 70% and 80% of patients with acute myocardial infarction present with chest pain (Kannel, 1987), but up to half may not have ST elevation at presentation (Goldberg et al, 1988).

Using the ECG, patients presenting with a possible acute coronary syndrome may be classified as:

- *Fast-track*: definite myocardial infarction. ECG shows ST elevation or bundle branch block, and the patient has no contraindications for thrombolysis.
- *Intermediate track*: other coronary syndromes with minor ECG changes, or myocardial infarction with relative contraindications to thrombolysis.
- *Slow track*: possible acute coronary syndrome, or myocardial infarction where thrombolysis is contraindicated.

Fast-track patients should be sent directly to the coronary care unit, and reducing the in-hospital delay in getting these patients to the coronary care unit has been a major task in recent years. The triage system should preferably bypass routine assessment by the on-call general medical team or casualty staff, with direct admission to the coronary care unit or to a chest pain assessment unit.

CHEST PAIN UNITS

Chest pain assessment units are a new development to facilitate a more conclusive cardiac evaluation while avoiding unnecessary hospital admission. Such units may also have an important role in the management of patients with acute coronary syndromes initially triaged as slow or intermediate track (Farkouh et al, 1998). Currently, the design and location of such units differ but will continue to evolve (Brillman et al, 1995). Some key features are that they are readily accessible, have suitably trained physicians and nurses and have adequate monitoring and resuscitation facilities. The use of critical care pathways is particularly suited to these units to allow an early decision about the presence or absence of an acute coronary syndrome.

The most important triage tool is the 12-lead ECG. For patients who present with anginal pain, ST segment elevation on the ECG has a specificity of 91% and a sensitivity of 46% for diagnosing acute myocardial infarction (Rude et al, 1983). Hence, it should take no more than a few minutes to confirm or reject the diagnosis of acute myocardial infarction, obtain a brief history and ensure that there are no contraindications to thrombolysis. The standards laid down by the National Service Framework for Coronary Heart Disease state that patients qualifying for thrombolysis should be able to receive treatment within 60 min of their call for professional help. Permitted delays are:

- Response time by the ambulance: up to 8 min
- Transportation time: up to 30 min
- Arrival at hospital to thrombolysis: up to 20 min.

The call-to-door time should thus be a maximum of 40 min, and the door-to-needle time should be no more than 20 min. The target call-to-needle time should therefore be less than 1 h.

PRIMARY ANGIOPLASTY

Primary angioplasty provides an alternative to thrombolytic therapy for re-establishing coronary patency in acute myocardial infarction. Until 1993, angioplasty was only utilised for patients with easily inducible post-infarction angina, but was not attempted until at least 3 weeks following thrombolysis, because of perceived dangers. The Primary Angioplasty in Myocardial Infarction (PAMI) trial showed the feasibility and safety of the procedure (Grines et al, 1993). A systematic review of randomised controlled trials in which patients were assigned to thrombolysis or angioplasty within 6–12 h of onset of symptoms of myocardial infarction indicates that primary angioplasty may reduce the 30-day death rate from 6.5% to 4.4% (Weaver et al, 1997). This equates to 21 fewer deaths per 1000 patients treated by angioplasty rather than by thrombolysis. Non-fatal re-infarction and stroke were also reduced by 11.9% to 7.2% and by 2% to 0.7%, respectively. These advantages appear to be sustained in the long term (Zijlstra et al, 1999). Implantation of coronary arterial stents further improves clinical outcome, and reduces the need for additional revascularisation procedures (Grines et al, 1999). Guidelines from the American College of Cardiology and American Heart Association state that primary angioplasty should be considered as an alternative to thrombolysis if the time from admission to balloon inflation (door-to-balloon time) is less than 90 min (Ryan et al, 1996). The intervention must be performed by a skilled operator, who performs more than 75 procedures per year, within a centre that carries out more than 200 angioplasties per year. Unfortunately, few UK centres can fulfil these criteria on a 24-h, 365 days per year basis, and for most hospitals thrombolysis will remain the usual first-line therapy.

Despite the known beneficial effects of early reperfusion, only a minority of patients receive timely intervention (Gitt and Senges, 2001). Adherence to current thrombolytic guidelines and improved access to specialist centres for primary angioplasty in patients ineligible for thrombolysis are obvious ways of improving this.

THE ROLE OF THE CORONARY CARE UNIT

Before coronary care units existed, treatment of acute myocardial infarction was directed towards the healing of the infarct and the prevention of cardiac rupture, and usually involved prolonged periods of bedrest. Thromboembolic complications were frequent, and the enthusiasm for positive inotropic agents such as digoxin and noradrenaline (norepinephrine) probably contributed to the mortality in most hospitals of around 25–30%. With the recognition of the importance of rhythm monitoring, cardiopulmonary resuscitation and prompt defibrillation, the management of coronary patients was revolutionised (Julian, 1961). The first purpose-built coronary care unit was opened on 20 May 1962 by Hughes Day in Kansas City; others quickly followed in Toronto, Sydney, New York and Philadelphia (Day, 1972). From then on, medical and public demand led to the development of many similar units so that, by the early 1970s, most large hospitals had facilities for monitoring the acute coronary patient, either as part of a general ward or on a separate intensive care unit. Following establishment of coronary care units, inpatient mortality approximately halved, probably secondary to the recognition and appropriate treatment of serious dysrhythmias (Julian 1961, 1987).

Modern coronary care units now provide:

- A separate area within the hospital for the care and monitoring of patients with acute myocardial infarction and other acute cardiac conditions
- Care by nurses and physicians with specialist training
- An environment for rapid and effective resuscitation
- An environment for rapid and effective restoration of myocardial perfusion
- A place where the complications of acute myocardial infarction can be detected early and treated appropriately
- The start of the rehabilitation process.

Roughly half of the patients admitted to coronary care have a complicated clinical course, and most problems occur soon after admission. In general, patients with larger myocardial infarcts have more complications and a poorer prognosis; much depends upon how much functional myocardium is preserved. Intervention to salvage ischaemic myocardium has become a major goal in the modern management of myocardial infarction, with special attention paid to relieving coronary obstruction and improving myocardial perfusion by coronary thrombolysis or percutaneous coronary intervention. Although the early success of coronary care units was due to better recognition and treatment of dysrhythmias, effective myocardial salvage, improved haemodynamic monitoring methods and effective pharmaceutical agents for the treatment of heart failure have now led to a further reduction in peri-infarction mortality. Routine use of fibrinolytic therapy, aspirin, statins and angiotensin-converting enzyme (ACE) inhibitors has reduced the overall mortality from coronary heart disease in men by 72% and 56% in women (Tunstall-Pedoe et al, 2000).

Apart from the management of acute myocardial infarction, coronary care units now have an extended role in the management of many other cardiac problems. These include other presentations of acute coronary syndromes, congestive heart failure, dysrhythmias and cardiogenic shock. The modern unit is therefore not really a coronary care unit but an acute cardiovascular unit. Since the acronym CCU is likely to remain, perhaps we should refer to these areas as 'cardiac care units'.

STAFFING OF CORONARY CARE UNITS

The staffing and organisation of coronary care units are of great importance. Nursing staff levels usually depend upon local conditions, but should be at least 1.5 times that of general medical wards. Minimum standards for all staff should include the capability of assessing the acutely ill patient, the ability to apply basic and advanced cardiac life support and an understanding of modern cardiac drugs and procedures. Coronary care units have been found to be a practical location for providing high-quality specialised nursing and medical care to patients with acute coronary syndromes and other cardiac conditions. The style of management will vary from unit to unit, but most function better where decisions are democratic rather than autocratic. This is more likely to encourage individual initiative and helps to reduce stress levels in staff members on the unit, which would otherwise be transmitted to the patient. A consultant in cardiovascular medicine usually undertakes administrative duties, but it is desirable that selection and training of staff, unit policy and therapy are discussed by all senior staff on the unit.

Patients are usually investigated and treated by two groups of doctors: trainee physicians and their supervising consultants. Whilst the consultant staff direct the management of the patients, the junior medical staff are responsible for the day- to-day care of the patients on the unit. Since patients on these units require constant supervision, it is usually not possible for this to be undertaken on a 24-h basis by medical staff, and the responsibility has fallen to the nursing staff, thus extending the role of nursing. With the increased duties and responsibility assumed by cardiac care nurses, the traditional doctor–nurse relationship is altered, which often proves awkward to the uninitiated (Jowett, 1986). The nursing staff have a vital role in the smooth running of these units and often provide the key to successful patient management.

CORONARY CARE AND THE CARDIAC NURSE SPECIALIST

Since the introduction of coronary care units, the role of the nurse has had to change. Rather than remain in the sphere of traditional nursing, the profession has had to redefine its function to keep pace with advances in medical treatment and technology (Hatchett and Thompson, 2002). New initiatives such as the National Service Framework for Coronary Heart Disease (Department of Health, 2000) and the NHS Plan (Secretry of State for Health, 2000) have given cardiac care nurses the opportunity to undertake a wider range of clinical tasks to improve patient care. Such innovations may include ordering diagnostic investigations, making and receiving direct referrals, admitting and discharging patients for specified conditions and, within agreed protocols, managing patient caseloads. In cardiac care, there are great opportunities for nurses to test out and develop these roles, as outlined in *Making a Difference* (Department of Health, 1999b) and the *Code of Professional Conduct* (Nursing and Midwifery Council, 2002). Nurses are increasingly directing, leading or coordinating a number of cardiac services, including the early initiation of thrombolysis, cardiac rehabilitation and the management of heart failure clinics (Thompson and Stewart, 2002). New roles, such as the nurse consultant, will help service delivery. However, some roles have been widely criticised as not so much enhancing nursing roles but rather filling gaps left by failure to employ sufficient medical staff. The European Working Hours directive has effectively halved the working hours of junior medical staff, a gap that has not yet been filled by appropriate recruitment. Many nurses will no doubt be eager to undertake extended roles, but should not lose touch with their primary nursing role, or be seduced into inappropriate tasks or areas where there has been insufficient training and supervision.

Cardiac care by the nurse requires that she is skilled at:

- Giving complete nursing care to the patient and family under her care
- Collecting and recording clinical data and taking prompt and appropriate action when necessary
- Communicating with the patient, relatives, colleagues and co-professionals.

The nurse needs to be competent in assessing the various needs of the patient and his family, to ensure the provision of physical comfort and emotional support (Thompson, 1990). The illness itself, hospitalisation and therapy present their own problems, to say nothing of the effect of the alien and technical atmosphere of an intensive care unit, which frequently frightens trained medical and nursing staff on their first visit, let alone patients and their relatives. Liberalised visiting rules for patients in coronary care can be helpful, and no harmful physiological effects have been attributable to unrestricted visiting policies.

Good cardiac care nursing is based upon general nursing principles of maintaining as near normal a life-style as possible and helping the patient to perform daily activities. It is only in addition to this that the nurse needs to be skilled in technological advances, although experience in advanced cardiac life support and defibrillation is obviously indispensable.

Until recently, nurses have tended to rely on others for guidance and direction, rather than assuming the role of decision-maker. The ability to make decisions quickly has become essential within coronary care and can only come with expertise and knowledge. As professionals, nurses have a responsibility to themselves, as well as to their patients and colleagues, for continuing education. This includes frequent updating by reading relevant literature and keeping informed of professional issues and clinical practice. The recent reforms in nurses' education will ensure that this is an obligatory and not an optional part of patient care. The medical profession is now obliged to take compulsory, rather than optional, study leave for continuing professional development. Research and its clinical application is also a normal part of medical training but a relatively new concept in coronary care nursing. It should not be seen to be the sole domain of the medical staff.

DESIGN AND ORGANISATION OF THE CORONARY CARE UNIT

The design and layout of the unit has to be a compromise between desirability and practicality. A separate unit within the hospital complex is desirable, but there are advantages in locating the unit adjacent to other critical care areas, such as high-dependency or intensive care units. Close access to exercise stress testing, echocardiography and a pacing room with catheter laboratory (if available) is useful. Accommodating patients in individual rooms often seems advantageous, so that they are unaware of other patients' problems and are protected from the high drama of cardiac arrests. However, although this design may allow privacy and promote rest, it makes no allowance for direct vision of the patient by the staff. Constant visual observation is a prime consideration in acute coronary care and, apart from its main role of spotting early signs of distress, may contribute towards the patients' overall feeling of well-being. Without this, patients may feel isolated and fearful about not being discovered if they were to collapse. Most units offer a combination of open-plan and side-rooms.

The doorways on coronary care should be wide enough to permit the passage of beds in and out of the unit without the need to transfer from trolley to bed, which causes a great deal of physical effort, especially if the patient is overweight or arthritic. It may also involve involuntary use of the Valsalva manoeuvre, producing potentially adverse vagal stimulation. Forced expiration against a closed glottis causes sudden and intense changes in systolic blood pressure and heart rate, and may predispose the patient to ventricular dysrhythmias. Paradoxically, since age attenuates autonomic cardiovascular responsiveness, avoiding the Valsalva manoeuvre is especially important in persons younger than 45 years.

Bed areas must be large enough to accommodate staff and equipment and should probably be no smaller than 10 m². Each bed should have piped oxygen and suction and must be of suitable design for manoeuvring in case of cardiac arrest. Bed design has improved over the years, and we now use electrical profiling beds ('Evolution', Hill-Rom, Leicestershire). These have many useful features, including adjustability for height, autocontouring controls, rapid Trendelenburg/reverse Trendelenburg controls, easily removable head and foot boards and collapsible built-in side-rails. Two handles under the head section activate a rapid, cushioned release to flatten the bed should cardiac arrest occur, and the sleep surface is rigid enough to enable effective chest compressions.

Equipment should be located on the walls and fixed securely. Bedside monitors need to be connected to the central station to allow constant cardiac monitoring (Jowett, 1997). There should be sufficient natural (and artificial) light, with window views to the outside world, so that the patient does not become unduly disorientated.

The ability to see a clock is particularly helpful in this respect. Noise insulation and air-conditioning are important for comfort and to promote rest. A separate procedure room away from the main unit is desirable for elective cardioversion and temporary pacing. Provision should be made for interviewing relatives in private and should be additional to a normal visitors' waiting room. Staff coffee and rest rooms are useful for periods of relaxation. A lecture room could also be included in coronary care unit design, equipped with projection facilities and audiovisual aids, for continuing medical education and rehabilitation group meetings.

CLINICAL CARE PATHWAYS

The use of clinical or critical care pathways has emerged to improve the quality and consistency of care (Hofman, 1993). Clinical pathways are management plans that display goals for patients and provide the sequence and timing of actions necessary to achieve these goals with optimal efficiency. Critical pathways have been developed for several cardiovascular diseases and procedures including coronary artery bypass surgery, diagnostic cardiac catheterisation, coronary angioplasty, acute myocardial infarction and unstable angina (Cannon et al, 1999). These conditions tend to be more suitable for critical pathway development because of the predictable course of events that occur during hospitalisation. Use of such pathways may help reduce variation in care, decrease resource utilisation, improve guideline compliance and potentially improve quality of care (Every et al, 2000).

The National Service Framework for Coronary Heart Disease has encouraged hospitals to develop such a structured and systematic approach in the generalised care of patients with acute coronary syndromes. This pathway should form part of the clinical record, and could include either a paper or electronic prompt that lists various evidence-based interventions. Such records also facilitate clinical audit. The coronary care unit lends itself to a critical care pathway approach in the management of the various coronary syndromes, heart failure or common rhythm disturbances (Reinhart, 1995) and help with continuity of care when the patient leaves the unit.

STEP-DOWN UNITS

Since the risk of primary ventricular fibrillation is highest in the first few hours following myocardial infarction, there is little need for uncomplicated cases to remain on the coronary care unit for longer than 2 days. Some patients can be transferred within the first 24 h after admission if they do not have risk factors such as a history of previous infarction, persistent ischaemic pain, heart failure, hypotension, or haemodynamically compromising ventricular dysrhythmias. It is unlikely that such patients will require transfer back to the coronary care unit or will die in the hospital. However, those patients who survive to discharge remain at risk of further cardiovascular events, long-term survival being most closely related to the age of the patient and their left ventricular function. Patients with high-risk features such as post-infarction angina or heart failure should be referred for angiography without further investigation. Exercise stress testing helps select other patients who will benefit from elective revascularisation (Beller, 1997).

The provision of an intermediate ('step-down') coronary care unit can form a bridge between more intensive acute coronary care and management in a general medical ward, and allows the more efficient use of high-dependency beds (Bonvissuto, 1994). Staffing of these units by coronary care trained nurses allows patients to benefit from continuity of care as well as uniformity of approach. Such units may ensure that all discharge plans, such as medication plan and risk-factor control, are in place, with arrangements for exercise stress testing and rehabilitation.

Early ambulation following acute myocardial infarction and early discharge from hospital should be encouraged for low-risk patients. In the 1960s, the duration of bedrest was extended to several weeks to limit physical exertion and sympathetic stimulation. Assistance with eating was common, and enforced bedrest was the norm. Now, a short period of bedrest seems prudent for most patients with acute myocardial infarction, with allowances for bedside commode use, and prolonged bedrest is unnecessary except for patients who are haemodynamically unstable. Low-level activities such as toileting, assisted bathing and light ambulation should be used to prevent physiological deconditioning, which may occur in as little as 6 h if the patient is kept in the supine position. Early mobilisation will prevent the complications caused by bedrest, particularly thromboembolic disorders, and will additionally reduce depression and physical weakness. A protocol for encouraging the patient quickly back to normal activity (Table 1.2) may best be undertaken on a step-down unit, where the use of telemetry to monitor cardiac rhythm in the presence of immediate and practised resuscitation facilities is of advantage (Kuchar et al, 1987). An additional benefit of step-down units is that early (phase I) rehabilitation and education can take place with all the patients together, as a form of group therapy, perhaps with the husband or wife being present. Inclusion of spouses in teaching also increases learning and retention over time. In these days of shorter hospital stays, discharge planning needs to be started promptly by a skilled multidisciplinary team as soon as possible after hospital

Table 1.2 Typical physical activity plan following acute myocardial infarction

Time	Activity
Day 1	Bed or chair rest
Day 2	Sit out of bed or chair; discharge from coronary care unit
Day 3	Walk around ward and to toilet
Day 4	Try stairs
Day 5–7	Submaximal exercise stress test Discharge home
Day 7–14	Exercise within home and garden
Day 14–28	Gradual increased walking outside home (20–30 min, once or twice daily) Enrol in rehabilitation programme (phase III)
Day 28	Symptom-limited exercise stress test
Day 42	Outpatient review Return to work Recommence driving (in line with DVLA regulations)

admission and continue through the early discharge period (phase II rehabilitation). Patient education effectively decreases emotional distress, increases knowledge and changes behaviour following a heart attack. Patients often need information about risk factors and self-management techniques (e.g. what to do if they get chest pain) rather than information about the disease itself. The decreasing length of hospital stays has raised concern about adequate opportunity for appropriate patient education, although short educational sequences have been shown to produce outcomes comparable to lengthy sessions. Innovative presentation styles using programmed instruction and audiovisual techniques can produce benefits comparable to individual educational sessions. Not all patients may be ready to learn during hospitalisation, and methods of accommodating them are needed. Use of a single repository for all educational materials (e.g. a binder that travels with the patient) may provide consistency and identify goals achieved and those that remain.

REHABILITATION

A heart attack is usually a devastating experience for most patients, particularly for those who have never been ill before. Like all major illnesses, a myocardial infarction has a physical, psychological and behavioural impact on patients and their families. While most patients make a good cardiological recovery, some degree of chronic invalidism is common, often affecting their vocation, hobbies, social life and sexual activity. Depression occurs in up to a third of post-infarction patients and often impedes recovery. For example, of the 30–50% of patients who fail to return to work following their heart attack, only in a minority of cases are there genuine physical reasons for non-return to their former occupation (Monpere et al, 1988).

Cardiac rehabilitation after myocardial infarction can promote recovery and reduce the chances of death within the next few years by up to 25%. It has also been shown to improve prognosis and function for those with other manifes-

tations of coronary heart disease, including stable angina and heart failure. The quality of life also may be improved for these patients by the relief of stress and anxiety and other measures to prevent cardiac neurosis. Rehabilitation after an acute coronary syndrome should be part of an integrated treatment programme, and should conform to the guidelines and standards laid out by the UK British Association for Cardiac Rehabilitation (BACR UK) in an agreed way across primary, secondary and tertiary care (Thompson et al, 1996). Unfortunately, rehabilitation services are still poorly developed in some areas (Thompson et al, 1997), and health authorities must now include in their health improvement programmes the provision of a comprehensive cardiac rehabilitation programme for all cardiac patients.

Cardiac rehabilitation programmes differ in organisation, but most comprise sections on exercise and relaxation, with discussion and education. Many programmes are now combined with secondary prevention modules, ensuring all interventions are in place. Audits of life-style, risk factors and therapeutic management of patients with established coronary disease show that the majority fail. The EUROASPIRE II survey assessed 5556 patients from 15 countries in the convalescent phase following acute myocardial infarction, and found that 21% were still smoking cigarettes, 31% were obese, 50% had raised blood pressure and 58% had raised serum cholesterol (EUROASPIRE II Group, 2001). Prescription of evidence-based drugs was also sub-optimal, with only 86% taking aspirin, 63% taking beta-blockers, 38% ACE inhibitors and 61% lipid-lowering agents. Hence, there remains considerable potential to reduce recurrent coronary disease through implementation of these simple proven interventions.

The needs of the cardiac patient vary and thus require the expertise of a diverse team rather than doctor and nurse alone. Other team members may involve physiotherapists, pharmacists, dietitians, occupation therapists and social workers. Although the programme may be multidisciplinary, a nurse or physiotherapist usually coordinates activities. Nursing staff with cardiology training can play a significant role in family education and physical rehabilitation of the patient, and their input is increasing in counselling sessions, exercise programmes and relaxation classes (Thompson, 1994). Free discussion is to be encouraged at all times, with particular advice on diet, smoking, exercise, work and sexual activity. Videotapes and pamphlets may be useful in this context, with rehabilitation tailored to individual patient's needs. The formal rehabilitation programme is run on an outpatient basis (phase III) and extended into the long term to maintain health and functional ability (phase IV).

The average general practice has approximately 10–12 cases of myocardial infarction per annum. This is too small a number upon which an individual practice can run an effective rehabilitation programme, so involvement of the rehabilitation team in the community is vital. Also, effective communication between the coronary care team and the primary care members cannot be overemphasised. To this end, the British Heart Foundation developed the cardiac liaison nurse scheme in 1995, as specialists in both the hospital and the community. There are now about 44 posts where the overall aim is to see patients within 1 week of discharge to ensure continuing education and risk factor modification. Their work complements that of the rehabilitation team, impacting on both phase II and phase IV. These posts have an invaluable role in forging links between primary, secondary and tertiary care.

REFERENCES

Beaglehole R (1999) International trends in coronary heart disease mortality and incidence rates. *Journal of Cardiovascular Risk*, **6**: 63–68.

Beller GA (1997) Determining prognosis after acute MI in the thrombolytic era. *BMJ*, **14**: 761–762.

Berenson GS, Srinivasan SR, Bao W et al (1998) Association between multiple cardiovascular risk factors and atherosclerosis in children and young adults. *New England Journal of Medicine*, **338**: 1650–1656.

Boersma E, Maas ACP, Simoons ML (1996) Early thrombolytic treatment in acute myocardial infarction: reappraisal of the Golden Hour. *Lancet*, **348**: 771–775.

Bonvissuto CA (1994) Avoiding unnecessary critical care costs. *Healthcare Financial Management*, **48**: 47–52.

Brillman J, Mathers-Dunbar L, Graff L et al (1995) Management of observation units. *Annals of Emergency Medicine*, **25**: 823–840.

British Heart Foundation (2002) *Coronary Heart Disease Statistics*. London: British Heart Foundation.

Brown N, Melville M, Gray D et al (1999) Relevance of clinical trial results in myocardial infarction to clinical practice: comparison of four years outcome in participants of thrombolytic trials, patients receiving routine thrombolysis and those deemed ineligible for thrombolysis. *Heart*, **81**: 598–602.

Burns JMA, Hogg KJ, Rae AP et al (1989) Impact of a policy of direct admissions to a coronary care unit on use of thrombolytic treatment. *British Heart Journal*, **61**: 322–325.

Cannon CP, Johnson EB, Cermignani M et al (1999) Emergency department thrombolysis critical pathway reduces door-to-drug times in acute myocardial infarction. *Clinical Cardiology*, **22**: 17–20.

Colquhoun MC (1993) General practitioners and the treatment of myocardial infarction: the place of thrombolytic treatment. *British Heart Journal*, **70**: 215–217.

Cowie MR, Wood DA, Coats AJS et al (1999) Incidence and aetiology of heart failure. A population based study. *European Heart Journal*, **20**: 421–428.

Davies MJ (1992) Anatomic features in victims of sudden coronary death. *Circulation*, **85** (suppl 1): 19–24.

Day HW (1972) History of coronary care units. *American Journal of Cardiology*, **30**: 405–407.

Day INM, Wilson DI (2001) Genetics and cardiovascular risk. *BMJ*, **323**: 1409–1412.

Deedwania P (2001) Global risk assessment in the presymptomatic patient. *American Journal of Cardiology*, **88**: 17J–22J.

Department of Health (1999a) *Saving Lives: Our Healthier Nation*. London: The Stationery Office.

Department of Health (1999b) *Making a Difference. Strengthening the Nursing, Midwifery and Health Visiting Contribution to Health and Healthcare*. London: Department of Health.

Department of Health (2000) *National Service Framework for Coronary Heart Disease*. London: The Stationery Office.

de Wood MA, Spores J, Notske LT et al (1980) Prevalence of total coronary occlusion during the early hours of transmural myocardial infarction. *New England Journal of Medicine*, **303**: 897–902.

Dickey W, Adgey AAJ (1992) Mortality within hospital after resuscitation from ventricular fibrillation outside hospital. *British Heart Journal*, **67**: 334–338.

EMIP: The European Myocardial Infarction Project Group (1993) Pre-hospital thrombolytic therapy in patients with suspected acute myocardial infarction. *New England Journal of Medicine*, **329**: 383–389.

EUROASPIRE II Group (2001) Life-style and risk factor management and use of drug therapies in coronary patients from 15 countries. Principle results from EUROASPIRE II. *European Heart Journal*, **22**: 554–572.

Every NR, Hochman J, Becker R et al for the Committee on Acute Cardiac Care, Council on Clinical Cardiology, American Heart Association (2000) Critical pathways. *Circulation*, **101**: 461–464.

Farkouh ME, Smars PA, Reeder GS et al (1998) A clinical trial of a chest pain observation unit for patients with unstable angina. Chest Pain Evaluation in the Emergency Room (CHEER) Investigators. *New England Journal of Medicine*, **339**: 1882–1888.

Fibrinolytic Therapy Trialists' Collaborative Group (1994) Indications for fibrinolytic therapy in suspected acute myocardial infarction: collaborative overview of early and major mortality from all randomised trials of more than 1000 patients. *Lancet*, **343**: 311–322.

Fitzpatrick B, Wall GCM, Tunstall Pedoe H (1992) Potential impact of emergency intervention on sudden deaths from coronary heart disease in Glasgow. *British Heart Journal*, **67**: 250–254.

Ghandi MM (1995) Incidence, clinical characteristics and short-term prognosis of angina pectoris. *British Heart Journal*, **73**: 193–198.

Gitt AK, Senges J (2001) The patient with acute myocardial infarction who does not receive reperfusion treatment. *Heart*, **86**: 243–245.

Goldberg R, Gore J, Alpert J et al (1988) Incidence and case fatality rates of acute myocardial infarction (1975–1984): the Worcester Heart Attack Study. *American Heart Journal*, **115**: 761–767.

Grines CL, Browne KF, Marco J (1993) A comparison of immediate angioplasty with thrombolytic therapy for acute myocardial infarction. *New England Journal of Medicine*, **328**: 673–679.

Grines CL, Cox DA, Stone GW et al (1999) Coronary angioplasty with or without stent implantation for acute myocardial infarction. Stent Primary Angioplasty in Myocardial Infarction Study (Stent-PAMI) Group. *New England Journal of Medicine*, **341**: 1949–1956.

Hatchett R, Thompson DR (2002) *Cardiac Nursing: A Comprehensive Guide*. Edinburgh: Churchill Livingstone.

Hofman PA (1993) Critical path method: an important tool for co-ordinating clinical care. *Journal of Quality Improvement*, **19**: 233–246.

ISIS-1 Collaborative Group (1988) Mechanisms for the early mortality reduction produced by beta-blockade started early in acute myocardial infarction. *Lancet*, **1**: 921–923.

ISIS-4 Collaborative Group (1995) A randomised factorial trial assessing early oral Captopril, oral mononitrate and intravenous magnesium sulphate in 58,050 patients with suspected acute myocardial infarction. *Lancet*, **345**: 669–685.

Jowett NI (1984) *Recombinant DNA Gene-specific Probes and the Genetic Analysis of Diabetes, Hyperlipidaemia and Coronary Heart Disease*. MD Thesis, University of London.

Jowett NI (1986) The junior doctor on the intensive care unit. *Intensive Care Nursing*, **1**: 177–179.

Jowett NI (1997) *Cardiovascular Monitoring*. London: Whurr.

Julian DG (1961) Treatment of cardiac arrest in acute myocardial ischaemia and infarction. *Lancet*, **ii**: 840–844.

Julian D (1987) The history of coronary care units. *British Heart Journal*, **57**: 497–502.

Kannel WB (1987) Prevalence and clinical aspects of unrecognised myocardial infarction and sudden unexpected deaths. *Circulation*, **75** II: II4–II5.

Kannel WB, Abbott RD (1984) Incidence and prognosis of unrecognised myocardial infarction. An update on the Framingham study. *New England Journal of Medicine*, **311**: 1144–1147.

Kereiakes DJ, Weaver WD, Anderson JL et al (1990) Time delays in the diagnosis and treatment of acute myocardial infarction: a tale of 8 cities. Report from the Pre-hospital Study Group and the Cincinnati Heart Project. *American Heart Journal*, **120**: 773–780.

Kuchar DL, Thorburn CW, Sammel NL (1987) Prediction of serious arrhythmic events after myocardial infarction: signal averaged ECG, Holter monitoring and radionuclide ventriculography. *Journal of the American College of Cardiology*, **9**: 531–538.

Kuulasmaa K, Tunstall-Pedoe H, Dobson A et al (2000) Estimation of contribution of changes in classic risk factors to trends in coronary-event rate across the WHO MONICA project populations. *Lancet*, **355**: 675–687.

Lewis SJ, Holmberg S, Quinn E et al (1993) Out-of-hospital resuscitation in East Sussex: 1981–1989. *British Heart Journal*, **70**: 568–573.

Moher M, Johnson N (1994) Use of aspirin by general practitioners in suspected acute myocardial infarction. *BMJ*, **308**: 760.

Monpere C, Francois G, Broudier M (1988) Effect of comprehensive rehabilitation programme in patients with 3-vessel coronary artery disease. *European Heart Journal*, **9**: M28–M31.

Morrison LJ, Verbeek PR, McDonald AC et al (2001) Mortality and pre-hospital thrombolysis for acute myocardial infarction. A meta-analysis. *JAMA*, **283**: 2686–2692.

Murray CJL, Lopez AD (1997) Alternative projections of mortality and disability by cause 1990–2020; global burden of disease study. *Lancet*, **349**: 1498–1504.

Norris RM on behalf of the United Kingdom Heart Attack Study Collaborative Group (1998) Fatality outside hospital from acute coronary events in three British health districts 1994–95. *BMJ*, **316**: 1065–1070.

Nursing and Midwifery Council (2002) *Code of Professional Conduct*. London: Nursing and Midwifery Council.

Pantridge JF, Geddes JS (1967) A mobile intensive care unit in the management of myocardial infarction. *Lancet*, **11**: 271–273.

Pantridge JF (1994) Mobile intensive care in the management of myocardial infarction. *Coronary Artery Disease*, **1**: 294–302.

Petersen S, Rayner M (2002) *Coronary Heart Disease Statistics*. London: British Heart Foundation Database (www.dphpc.ox.ac.uk/bhfhprg).

Rawles J, Sinclair C, Jennings K et al (1998) Audit of pre-hospital thrombolysis by general practitioners in peripheral practices in Grampian. *Heart*, **80**: 231–234.

Reinhart SI (1995) Uncomplicated myocardial infarction: a critical path. *Cardiovascular Nursing*, **31**: 1–7.

Rosamond WD, Chambless LE, Folsom AR et al (1998) Trends in the incidence of myocardial infarction and in mortality due to coronary heart disease 1987 to 1994. *New England Journal of Medicine*, **339**: 861–867.

Rude RE, Poole WK, Muller JE et al (1983) Electrocardiographic and clinical criteria for recognition of acute myocardial infarction based on analysis of 3697 patients. *American Journal of Cardiology*, **52**: 936–942.

Ryan TJ, Anderson JL, Antman EM et al (1996) ACC/AHA guidelines for the management of patients with acute myocardial infarction: executive summary. *Circulation,* **94:** 2341–2350.

Secretary of State for Health (2002) The NHS plan. (Cmnd 4818–1). London: The Stationery Office.

Then KL, Rankin JA, Fofonoff DA (2001) Atypical presentation of acute myocardial infarction in 3 age groups. *Heart and Lung,* **30:** 285–293.

Thompson DR (1990) *Counselling the Coronary Patient and Partner.* London: Scutari Press.

Thompson DR (1994) Cardiac rehabilitation services: the need to develop guidelines. *Quality in Health Care,* **3:** 169–172.

Thompson DR, Stewart S (2002) Nurse-directed services: how can they be made more effective? *European Journal of Cardiovascular Nursing,* **1:** 6–9.

Thompson DR, Bowman GS, Kitson AL et al (1996) Cardiac rehabilitation in the United Kingdom: guidelines and audit standards. *Heart,* **75:** 89–93.

Thompson DR, Bowman GS, Kitson AL et al (1997) Cardiac rehabilitation services in England and Wales: a national survey. *International Journal of Cardiology,* **59:** 299–304.

Thompson RG, Hallstrom AP, Cobb LA (1979) Bystander initiated cardiopulmonary resuscitation in the management of ventricular fibrillation. *Annals of Internal Medicine,* **90:** 737–740.

Tunstall-Pedoe H, Kuulasmaa K, Amouyel P et al (1994) Myocardial infarctions and coronary deaths in the World Health Organization MONICA project. Registration procedures, event rates, and case fatality rates in 38 populations from 21 countries in four continents. *Circulation,* **90:** 583–612.

Tunstall-Pedoe H, Kuulasmaa K, Mahonen M et al (1999) Contribution of trends in survival and coronary event rates to changes in coronary heart disease mortality: 10-year results from 37 WHO MONICA project populations. *Lancet,* **53:** 1547–1557.

Tunstall-Pedoe H, Vanuzzo D, Hobbs M et al (2000) Estimation of contribution of changes in coronary care to improving survival, event rates, and coronary heart disease mortality across the WHO MONICA Project populations. *Lancet,* **335:** 688–700.

United Kingdom Heart Attack Study (UKHAS) Collaborative Group (1998) Effect of time from onset of coming under care on fatality of patients with acute myocardial infarction: effect of resuscitation and thrombolytic treatment. *Heart,* **80:** 114–120.

Volmink JA, Newton JN, Hicks NR et al (1998) Coronary events and case fatality rates in an English population: results of the Oxford myocardial infarction incidence study. *Heart,* **80:** 40–44.

Waine C, Hannaford P, Kay C (1993) Early thrombolysis therapy: some issues facing general practitioners. *British Heart Journal,* **70:** 218–222.

Weaver WD, Simes RJ, Betriu A et al (1997) Comparison of primary coronary angioplasty and intravenous thrombolytic therapy for acute myocardial infarction: a quantitative review. *JAMA,* **278:** 2093–2098.

Wiseman MN, Whimster F, Skinner DV (1989) Resuscitation skills among the general public in London. *BMJ,* **299:** 434.

Wood DA, de Backer G, Faergeman O et al (2000) *Clinician's Manual on Total Risk Management. A Guide to Prevention of Coronary Heart Disease.* London: Science Press.

Wood DA, Timmis A, Halinden M (2001) Rapid assessment of chest pain. *BMJ,* **323:** 596–597.

World Health Organization (1997a) *Conquering Suffering, Enriching Humanity.* Geneva: WHO.

World Health Organization (1997b) *Tobacco or Health. A Global Status Report.* Geneva: WHO.

World Health Organization (1999) *WHO Statistics Annual.* Geneva: WHO.

Wyllie HR, Dunn FG (1994) Pre-hospital opiate and aspirin administration in patients with suspected myocardial infarction. *BMJ,* **308:** 760–761.

Zijlstra F, Hoorntje JCA, de Boer MJ et al (1999) Long-term benefit of primary angioplasty as compared with thrombolytic therapy for acute myocardial infarction. *New England Journal of Medicine,* **314:** 1413–1419.

2

Anatomy, physiology and pathology

THE ANATOMY OF THE HEART

The heart is a hollow muscular organ located behind the costal cartilages in the middle mediastinum. The size of the heart corresponds quite accurately with the size of the patient's clenched fist and weighs about 280–340 g. It lies obliquely in the chest and resembles an inverted cone, with the base facing upwards and the apex pointing downwards, forwards and to the left (Fig. 2.1). About two-thirds of the heart lies to the left, and one-third to the right, of the median plane. The apex lies a little below and medial to the left nipple in the 5th intercostal space and can usually be seen as the apex beat.

At the junction of the upper one-third and lower two-thirds of the heart, a deep oblique *atrioventricular (AV) groove* passes round the heart, separating the atria from the ventricles. From this, two other grooves extend towards the apex, anteriorly (the *anterior interventricular groove*) and posteriorly (the *posterior interventricular groove*). These mark the position of the *interventricular septum*, which separates the right and left ventricles internally. The junction of the posterior interventricular and posterior AV grooves is known as the *crux*. Internally, at this junction, the *interatrial septum* joins the interventricular septum.

The tough, fibrous pericardium encloses the heart and serves to limit any sudden cardiac distension. Within the fibrous pericardium and extending onto the surface of the heart is a thin, delicate membrane, the *serous pericardium*. This

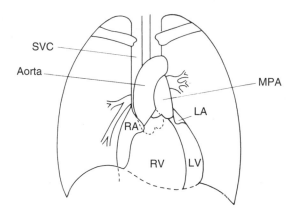

Figure 2.1 Anterior view of the heart. RA, right atrium; LA, left atrium; RV, right ventricle; LV, left ventricle; MPA, main pulmonary artery; SVC, superior vena cava.

and the adjoining portions of the great vessels. Where the great vessels pass through the fibrous pericardium, the two layers of the serous pericardium are reflected back and become continuous with one another. Between the two layers is a potential space, the *pericardial cavity*. This normally contains a small amount of fluid secreted by the serous pericardium, which acts as a lubricant to facilitate movement of the heart within the pericardial cavity.

The fibrous pericardium blends with the tunica adventitia of the great vessels and is firmly attached to the central tendon of the diaphragm below, and to the back of the sternum by the sternopericardial ligaments.

THE CHAMBERS AND VALVES OF THE HEART

The heart consists of four chambers: two *atria* above and two *ventricles* below (Fig. 2.2). The

has been invaginated by the heart during development, to form a two-layered structure. The outer parietal layer lines the inner surface of the fibrous pericardium, and the inner visceral layer (*epicardium*) covers the outer surface of the heart

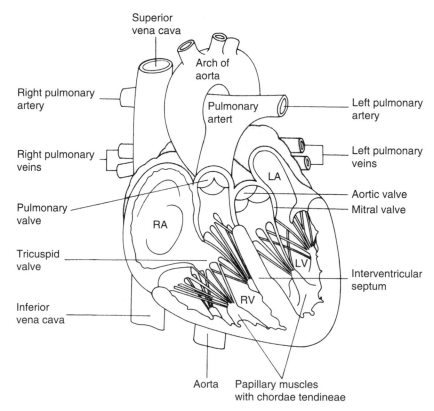

Figure 2.2 The internal anatomy of the heart. RA, right atrium; LA, left atrium; RV, right ventricle; LV, left ventricle.

right and left sides of the heart are separated by the interatrial septum and the interventricular septum. The main valves of the heart are the *mitral* and *aortic* valves on the left side of the heart, and the *tricuspid* and *pulmonary* valves on the right side of the heart. The valves are complex avascular structures and are very strong. During a normal lifetime, they will open and close some 2700 million times.

The right atrium

The right atrium lies to the right of and slightly behind the right ventricle, and anterior and to the right of the left atrium. It forms the lower right lateral heart border on the chest radiograph.

The right atrium is a thin-walled (2 mm) chamber that receives the venous return to the heart from the two largest veins in the body, the *superior and inferior venae cavae*. The right atrium also drains the coronary sinus and the anterior cardiac veins. The opening of the superior vena cava is valveless, but the inferior vena cava and the opening of the coronary sinus have rudimentary valves. The inner surfaces of the posterior and septal walls are smooth, whilst the surfaces of the lateral wall and the right atrial appendage are composed of parallel muscle fibres known as the *pectinate muscles*. Posteriorly, they end on a longitudinal elevation (the *crista terminalis*), which runs from the right side of the opening of the superior vena cava to the right side of the orifice of the inferior vena cava. This is marked externally on the surface of the right atrium by a shallow groove, the *sulcus terminalis*. On the interatrial septum is a depression known as the *fossa ovalis*, which marks the site of the fetal foramen ovale. The right AV orifice and the tricuspid valve perforate the floor of the right atrium. This valve has three triangular cusps: septal, anterior and posterior.

The right ventricle

The right ventricle is located directly beneath the sternum. It is the most anteriorly located chamber, with its inferior border located beneath the xiphoid process. The crescent-shaped chamber has a relatively thin outer wall (5 mm), which is approximately one-third the thickness of the left ventricular wall. The pulmonary trunk rises from a cone-shaped area at the base of the ventricle, the *infundibulum*. Blood entering the infundibulum is ejected superiorly and to the right, through the pulmonary valve and into the pulmonary artery. The pulmonary valve has three semilunar cusps: anterior, right and left. On the inner surface of the right ventricular wall are a number of irregular projections of raised muscle bundles (*trabeculae carneae*). The *papillary muscles* project into the ventricular cavity to become continuous with the *chordae tendineae*, which are attached to the free border of the cusps of the tricuspid valve. Contraction of the ventricle not only opposes the tricuspid valve cusps, but also prevents the valve being pushed back into the atrium, by maintaining tension on the chordae tendineae. A large, rounded muscle bundle, the *moderator band*, crosses the cavity of the right ventricle from the interventricular septum to the anterior wall. This conveys the right bundle branch of conducting tissue to the ventricular muscle. The right ventricle receives venous blood from the right atrium during ventricular diastole and expels it against low resistance (25–32 mmHg pressure) into the pulmonary circulation during ventricular systole.

The left atrium

The left atrium is the most posterior chamber and lies to the midline behind the right ventricle. It is the only cardiac chamber not normally visible on the chest X-ray. The left atrium receives blood from the pulmonary veins. It serves as a reservoir during left ventricular systole and as a conduit during left ventricular filling.

The chamber is roughly cuboidal in shape and somewhat smaller than the right atrium, with slightly thicker walls (about 3 mm). A small conical pouch (the *auricle*) projects from the upper left corner. It receives the four pulmonary veins, arranged in pairs on each side; all four orifices are devoid of valves.

The interior of the left atrium is smooth, except in the auricle, where the ridges of the pectinate muscles occur. The left atrial aspect of the septum is roughened, being the flap valve of the fossa ovalis. In the floor is the circular left AV orifice, guarded by the mitral valve. The latter is so called because it possesses two unequal triangular cusps, arranged like a Bishop's mitre.

The left ventricle

The left ventricle receives blood from the left atrium during ventricular diastole and ejects blood against high resistance into the systemic circulation during ventricular systole. It forms the lower left lateral cardiac border and lies posteriorly and to the left of the right ventricle, and below and to the left of the left atrium.

The chamber is conical, and its apex lies approximately in the 5th intercostal space within the midclavicular line. As it normally expels blood against a much higher resistance than the right ventricle, the walls of the left ventricle are much more muscular than those of the right ventricle (8–15 mm). The interventricular septum is also thick and muscular, except for a small membranous area. The septum separates the two ventricles, and its upper portion additionally separates the right atrium from the left ventricle.

Below and posteriorly, the left ventricle communicates with the left atrium through the left atrioventricular orifice and the mitral valve. The two papillary muscles are much larger than those of the right ventricle, and, from these, chordae tendineae are attached to both cusps of the mitral valve. Above and anteriorly, the left ventricle opens into the aorta. The portion of the ventricular chamber immediately adjoining the aorta is known as the *vestibule*. The aortic valve is in continuity with the mitral valve by a fibrous, double-looped band, shaped like a figure 8. The aortic valve has three semilunar cusps (right, left and posterior), which are stronger than those of the pulmonary valve. At the origin of each cusp, the walls of the aorta show a slight dilatation or *sinus*. The right coronary artery arises from the right aortic sinus and the left coronary artery from the left aortic sinus, the orifice of each artery arising above the level of the cusp. These

three aortic sinuses are known collectively as the *sinuses of Valsalva*.

The atrioventricular junction

There is no muscular continuity between the atria and the ventricles except through the conducting tissue of the *atrioventricular (AV) node* and *AV bundle*. The aortic and mitral valves have strong fibrous rings that prevent the orifices from stretching and rendering the valves incompetent. These rings are continuous with a dense fibrocartilaginous mass, sometimes called the heart skeleton. This framework affords a firm anchorage for the attachment of the atrial and ventricular musculature, as well as the valvular tissue. The pulmonary valve does not have a ring, and that of the tricuspid valve is only partially formed.

THE TISSUES OF THE HEART

The main mass of the heart consists of muscular tissue (the *myocardium*), which is lined by the *endocardium* and covered by the visceral layer of serous pericardium (the *epicardium*). Blood and lymphatic vessels, nerves and specialised conducting tissues lie within the myocardial mass.

The epicardium

The epicardium consists of a single layer of mesothelial cells covering a thin layer of loose connective tissue, which contains elastic fibres, small blood vessels and nerves. It is in places separated from the myocardium by a layer of adipose tissue, which carries the coronary blood vessels.

The myocardium

The myocardium is composed of specialised involuntary cardiac muscle. Individual myocardial cells are grouped in bundles in a connective tissue framework, which carries small blood and lymphatic vessels and autonomic nerve fibres. The density of capillaries in cardiac muscle cells is much greater than in skeletal muscle, because of its higher blood requirements. The myocardium is thickest towards the apex and thins towards the base.

The myocardium consists of a network of muscle fibres that show transverse and longitudinal striation and which branch and connect with each other. The ends of the cells are in very close contact with adjacent cells, and the 'joints' can be seen as thick dark striations called *intercalated discs*. Because of the close relationship of one muscle fibre with the next, once contraction starts in any part it cannot remain localised and spreads throughout the entire network of muscle cells.

The endocardium

The endocardium is in continuity with the lining of the blood vessels (*tunica intima*). It is much thinner than the epicardium and consists of a lining of endothelial cells, a middle layer of dense connective tissue containing many elastic fibres and an outer layer of loose connective tissue in which there are small blood vessels and specialised conducting tissue. The heart valves are formed by folds of endocardium, thickened by a core of fibrous tissue extending in from the tissue

of the sulcus. The endocardium and myocardium are firmly bound together by connective tissue.

THE CONDUCTING SYSTEM

In addition to the purely contractile muscle fibres comprising the atria and ventricles, the heart possesses certain specialised muscle cells that form the conducting system. These cells initiate and conduct electrical impulses within the heart, to produce myocardial contraction. The conducting system comprises:

- The sinus node
- The atrioventricular (AV) node
- The bundle of His
- The right and left bundle branches
- The peripheral ramifications of the bundle branches (Purkinje fibres).

The sinus node

The sinus node is the normal site of initiation of the heart beat. It is situated at the junction of the superior vena cava with the right atrium (Fig. 2.3). The top end of the crista terminalis marks this junction internally. The node is spindle-shaped, about 25 mm long and about 3 mm

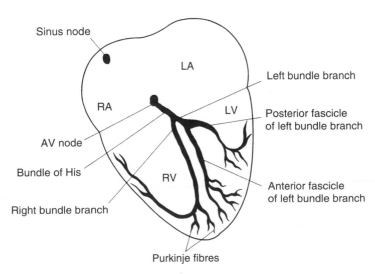

Figure 2.3 The conducting tissues of the heart. RA, right atrium; LA, left atrium; RV, right ventricle; LV, left ventricle; AV, atrioventricular.

wide. The framework of the node is collagenous, interlaced by bundles of small conduction fibres. There are numerous autonomic nerve endings in the node, with parasympathetic fibres derived from the right vagus nerve. The blood supply is via the nodal artery, which in 60% of people arises from the right coronary artery. In the remaining 40%, it arises from the left coronary artery.

Specialised pathways (*internodal tracts*) may exist in the atria, linking the sinus and the AV nodes, but there is no histological evidence of this. Conduction seems to occur preferentially along the thick muscle bundle of the right atrium.

The atrioventricular junction

The AV junction comprises the AV node and AV bundle (of His). The AV node lies between the opening of the coronary sinus and the posterior border of the membranous interventricular septum. The node is divided into a transitional zone and a compact portion. Its function is to cause a delay in transmission of the cardiac impulse from the atria to the ventricles, so that the atria have time to expel their contents into the ventricles before systole.

The AV node has a structure similar to that of the sinus node, but there is much less collagen in the framework, and the conduction fibres are thicker and shorter than those in the sinus node. There is a rich autonomic nerve supply, the parasympathetic fibres being derived from the left vagus nerve. The blood supply is from a specific nodal artery (*ramus septi fibrosi*), which arises from the right coronary artery in 90% of cases and from the left circumflex artery in the remaining 10%. The AV bundle extends from the AV node, along the posterior margin of the membranous portion of the interventricular septum, to the crest of the muscular septum. Here it bifurcates into the *right and left bundle branches*. The AV bundle is oval or triangular in cross-section. The fibres of the bundle run parallel to one another, unlike the fibres of the sinus and AV nodes, which interweave. The AV bundle and the proximal few millimetres of both bundle branches are supplied by the terminal branch of the AV nodal

artery and from the septal branches of the left anterior descending artery.

The bundle branches

The right and left bundle branches extend subendocardially along both sides of the interventricular septum. The right bundle is a cord-like structure that passes down the right side of the interventricular septum towards the apex, lying more deeply beneath the endocardium than does the left main bundle. It then runs in the free edge of the moderator band, to reach the base of the anterior papillary muscle, where it ramifies amongst the right ventricular musculature.

The left bundle branch is an extensive sheet of fibres that passes down the left side of the interventricular septum. The initial part of the left bundle is fan-shaped and breaks up into two interconnecting left and right hemifascicles (see Fig. 2.3). The terminal branches of the bundle branches are the *Purkinje fibres*, which ramify within the ventricular myocardium.

Septal arteries from the left anterior descending artery supply the bundle branches.

THE CORONARY CIRCULATION

The heart and proximal portion of the great vessels receive their blood supply from the two *coronary arteries*, which originate from the sinuses of Valsalva (Fig. 2.4).

The right coronary artery

The right coronary artery arises from the right coronary sinus of the aorta and runs forward to the AV groove, giving off a small branch to the sinus node. It follows the sulcus downwards and round the inferior margin of the heart, giving off a marginal branch to supply the right ventricular wall. It then winds around the heart to the posterior aspect and passes down in the interventricular groove as the *posterior descending coronary artery*, which supplies the ventricles and interventricular septum. Frequently, a transverse branch continues in the posterior AV groove, supplying branches of the left atrium before

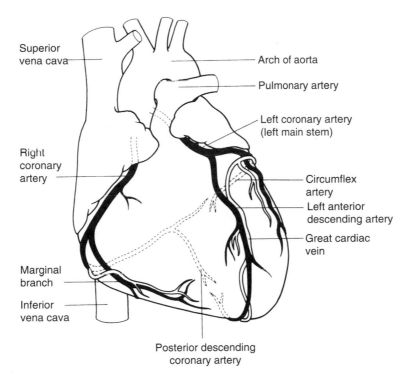

Figure 2.4   The coronary circulation.

anastomosing with the circumflex branch of the left coronary artery. Branches of the right coronary artery supply the conducting tissues, the right ventricle and the inferior (diaphragmatic) surface of the left ventricular wall.

The left coronary artery

The left coronary artery arises from the left posterior sinus of the aorta, runs to the left behind the pulmonary trunk and then runs forwards between it and the left auricle to the AV groove. Here, it divides into two branches: an *anterior descending* branch and a *circumflex* branch.

The left anterior descending artery descends in the anterior interventricular groove to the apex of the heart, where it turns back to ascend a short distance up the posterior interventricular groove, anastomosing with the posterior interventricular branch of the right coronary artery. Diagonal branches supply the anterior ventricular wall; septal branches supply the interventricular septum.

The left circumflex branch passes round the left margin of the heart in the AV groove under the left atrial appendage, supplying branches to the left atrium and the left surface of the heart. In some individuals, the circumflex artery gives rise to the posterior descending artery; this is called a left-dominant coronary artery system. Other coronary artery variants include:

- Single coronary artery
- Circumflex branch arising from the right aortic sinus.

The *left marginal* branch arises from the circumflex artery and runs down the left margin of the left ventricle.

Within the myocardium, there are rich anastomoses between the right and left coronary arteries, but the vessels involved are small. These anastomoses are genetically determined and can enlarge in the event of a gradual coronary artery occlusion, providing collateral circulation to the affected area of muscle. However, if the occlusion is sudden, necrosis of a segment of cardiac muscle will result, since these vessels cannot enlarge acutely.

The coronary veins

Most of the venous drainage of the heart is from veins that run with the coronary arteries and drain directly into the right atrium. The *coronary sinus* occupies the posterior part of the AV groove, between the left atrium and left ventricle. It receives the great, middle and small *cardiac veins* and opens directly into the right atrium. One or two large anterior cardiac veins also open directly into the right atrium, while smaller veins (*venae cordis minimae*) open directly into the heart chambers.

LYMPHATIC DRAINAGE

The heart is rich in lymphatic capillaries. Large vessels form the subendocardial and subepicardial lymphatic plexuses. The main collecting trunks accompany the larger blood vessels in the grooves of the heart. One large trunk ascends on each side of the heart to end in anterior mediastinal lymph nodes below the arch of the aorta and at the bifurcation of the trachea. The final drainage is to the thoracic duct, although there may be a connection with the bronchomediastinal trunk on the right side.

THE NERVE SUPPLY TO THE HEART

Because of 'intrinsic rhythmicity', the heart can beat even if removed completely from the body. However, the heart is well supplied with both sympathetic and parasympathetic nerve fibres, which can modify cardiac function by changing the heart rate and strength of myocardial contraction. Control of the autonomic nerves is via the cardiac centre in the medulla oblongata of the brain.

The sympathetic fibres derive from the cervical and upper thoracic sympathetic ganglia, via the superficial and deep cardiac plexuses. The parasympathetic supply is from the vagus. Sympathetic nerve fibres supply the sino-atrial (SA) node, atrial muscle, AV node, specialised conduction tissue and ventricular muscle. Parasympathetic nerve fibres supply mainly the sinus node and the AV node and, to a lesser extent, the atrial and ventricular muscle.

Vagal stimulation to the heart is mediated by acetylcholine, which decreases heart rate and, probably, strength of ventricular contraction. The main action on the AV node is to slow conduction and lengthen the refractory period. In contrast, stimulation of the sympathetic fibres leads to the release of noradrenaline (norepinephrine), which acts specifically on beta-1 adrenergic receptors in cardiac muscle. Circulating adrenaline (epinephrine) from the adrenal medulla may also elicit cardiac responses. Adrenergic stimulation increases both heart rate and force of contraction. Conduction velocity increases and there is shortening of the refractory period in the AV node.

The vagal and sympathetic nerves are distributed to the heart by the cardiac plexus, which lies between the concavity of the aortic arch and the tracheal bifurcation. Pressure changes in the aorta and carotid arteries can affect cardiac performance. Sensory receptors (*baroreceptors*) can detect increased pressure in the aorta and carotid arteries. Sensory impulses travel via the vagus and glossopharyngeal nerves and pass to the vasomotor centre in the medulla, causing slowing of the heart rate (Marey's reflex). These baroreceptors can be artificially stimulated by carotid sinus massage.

It is thought that most of the cardiac fibres of the right vagus terminate in the sinus node, and the majority of the fibres of the left vagus terminate in the AV node. Some vagal fibres probably terminate in the walls of the great veins near their entrance to the right atrium and are responsible for the cardiac acceleration that accompanies increased venous return to the heart (Bainbridge reflex).

Chemoreceptors

Chemosensitive cells are located in two *carotid bodies* (at the carotid bifurcation) and several *aortic bodies* adjacent to the aortic arch. They detect changes in blood PO_2, PCO_2 and pH. The afferent impulses arising in these fibres alter respiration, heart rate and vasomotor tone. The efferent impulses from the chemoreceptors pass with the afferent fibres from the pressor receptors via the glossopharyngeal and vagus nerves to the vasomotor centre in the medulla.

HISTOLOGY

The heart comprises two major types of cell:

- Myocardial cells specialised for contraction
- Automatic cells specialised for impulse formation.

Myocardial cells

The myocardial cells provide the mechanical pumping action of the heart by shortening in response to electrical stimulation. Each cell is about 100 µm long and 15 µm wide, containing a central nucleus and numerous (about 150) myofibrils aligned along the cell's axis. Each fibril runs the length of the cell and is made up of repeating functional subunits, or *sarcomeres*, containing actin and myosin arranged hexagonally. The thin *actin* filaments are attached to a limiting membrane (*Z-line*) and interdigitate with the thicker central *myosin* fibres. The sarcomeres of adjacent myofibrils are aligned at the Z-line. During contraction, the actin filaments slide together, bringing the Z lines closer together. The forces that generate sliding (i.e. contraction) occur at bridges between the actin and myosin (Fig. 2.5). It is the heads of the myosin molecules that form these bridges and contain the enzyme ATPase which is responsible for breaking down ATP (adenosine triphosphate) to provide the energy for contraction. It is likely that the greater

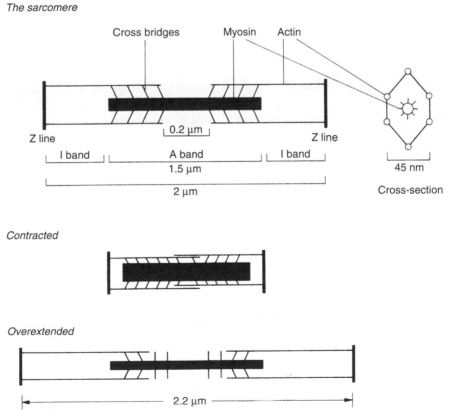

Figure 2.5 The sarcomere.

the number of bridges, the more forceful the contraction. The thicker myosin filaments (seen as the *A band* on microscopy) are 1.5 μm long and have a central portion (0.2 μm) that is devoid of bridges. The thin actin filaments (seen as lateral *I bands*) are shorter (1 μm), so it can be seen that maximum bridging takes place when the overall sarcomere length is between 2.0 and 2.2 μm. If the sarcomere is stretched beyond these limits, some bridges become disengaged, which will limit the force of contraction. Starling's Law of the heart (Starling, 1918) states that, within physiological limits, the greater the diastolic volume of the heart the greater the energy of contraction. This is why the graphs demonstrating Starling's Law fall off at the upper limits of myocardial stretching (Fig. 2.6). However, this simplified concept is modified by the action of another contractile protein, *troponin*. This is attached to the actin filaments and has an inhibitory effect that must be counteracted before actin and myosin can produce contraction. This is mediated by free calcium ions.

A large number of mitochondria are present (one-third of the cell volume); these are responsible for generating the large amount of energy required to maintain cardiac contraction. Energy is produced by the process known as oxidative phosphorylation, in which substrates such as glucose, lactate and free fatty acids are oxidised to replenish the energy sources ATP and creatine phosphate.

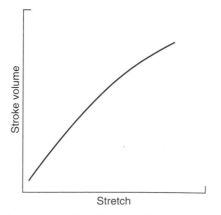

Figure 2.6 Ventricular function (Starling's) curve.

The limiting cell membrane is known as the *sarcolemma*, and adjacent cells are held together by intercalated discs. Electrical resistance through these discs is about 1/400th of the resistance through the outside membrane of the myocardial fibre, allowing virtually free passage of electrical currents from one myocardial cell to the next, without encountering significant resistance. The myocardial cells are so tightly bound together that stimulation of any single cell causes the action potential to spread to all adjacent cells, eventually spreading throughout the entire myocardial network.

Automatic cells

Automaticity describes the ability of specialised cardiac tissue to initiate electrical impulses. The cells responsible are known as *pacemaker* or *automatic* cells. In the sinus node, these will discharge spontaneously about 80 times per minute, although automatic cells elsewhere will have a slower discharge rate. In the AV node, for example, this may be 60 times per minute, and in the ventricles 40 times per minute. This system of 'escape rhythms' exists to prevent rhythm failure should the sinus node fail to discharge. Sometimes the rate of discharge will increase in places other than the sinus node, and these regions then take over the pacemaker function of the heart. This is often seen following acute myocardial infarction (e.g. accelerated idionodal or idioventricular rhythms).

Both myocardial cells and automatic cells can transmit impulses, but the specialised conducting tissues are used preferentially since they allow a more rapid and ordered carriage of impulses through the heart.

CARDIAC ELECTROPHYSIOLOGY

The electrolyte concentrations within cardiac cells and in the extracellular fluid are of major importance for electrical stimulation of the heart. The ions primarily involved in the generation of a cardiac action potential are sodium (Na^+), potassium (K^+) and calcium (Ca^{2+}). The predominant intracellular ion is potassium (K^+), and the predominant extracellular ions are sodium (Na^+) and calcium (Ca^{2+}). There are also negatively charged ions present: protein (Pr^-) within the cell and chloride (Cl^-) and bicarbonate (HCO_3^-) outside.

In the normal resting state, the potential across the myocardial cell membrane is about −90 mV. An active, energy-consuming, 'sodium pump' maintains the relative concentration of Na^+ and K^+, and thus the electrical difference across the cell membrane. The pump transfers K^+ into the cell up to five times more rapidly than it extrudes Na^+. Within the cell, the concentrations of potassium and sodium are 140 and 10 mmol/1, respectively, whereas outside the concentrations are 4 and 140 mmol/1. This ionic imbalance helps to maintain the resting membrane potential at −90 mV, and the cells are then said to be 'polarised'. Should an electrical stimulus reach the cell membrane, permeability is altered, allowing a change in ionic concentrations and depolarisation of the cell.

There are distinct phases of electrical activity in myocardial cells during the generation of an action potential (Fig. 2.7).

1. *Polarisation (phase 4)*. In the resting (inactive) state, the cell has a membrane potential of −90 mV and is said to be polarised. The cell interior is negatively charged with respect to the exterior.

2. *Depolarisation (phase 0)*. When electrical activation of the cell occurs, changes in the permeability of the cell membrane result in marked shifts in ionic concentrations. There is a rapid influx of positively charged Na^+ into the cell (the fast sodium current) until a threshold potential of -60 mV is reached. At this critical potential, membrane permeability is further increased, with a secondary rapid intracellular passage of Na^+, accompanied by a moderate but more sustained influx of Ca^{2+}. Depolarisation is represented by

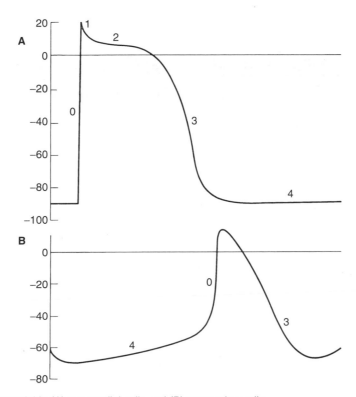

Figure 2.7   The action potential in (A) myocardial cells and (B) pacemaker cells.

the upstroke or spike on the action potential curve.

It can be seen that, after excitation, the polarity of the membrane has been reversed, the membrane potential changing rapidly from –90 mV to a slightly positive value of +20 mV. The cell now has a net positive intracellular charge and negative extracellular charge (Fig. 2.8). Since this is the reverse pattern to that of the surrounding cells, a potential difference exists and an electrical current will flow from one cell to the next, and so on.

3. *Repolarisation (phases 1–3).* Repolarisation is the process whereby the cell is returned to its normal resting state. This has three phases, the first of which is the 'overshoot' when Cl^- re-enters the cell and there is a slow fall in intracellular charge to +10 mV (phase 1 of the action potential). After the initial spike, the membrane remains depolarised (for 0.15 s in atrial muscle and 0.3 s in ventricular muscle), exhibiting a plateau, followed by the abrupt descent that rep-

resents repolarisation. The plateau phase (phase 2) of the action potential reflects a moderate and sustained slow influx of Ca^{2+}, which accompanies the more marked but less sustained influx of Na^+. The entry of calcium into the cell is essential for excitation–contraction coupling (see below). An efflux of K^+ balances the Ca^{2+} and Na^+ influx. Thus, the net effect is a relative balance of positive charges, which gives rise to the plateau.

The downstroke of phase 3 represents the rapid efflux of K^+ from the cell, when membrane permeability to K^+ increases markedly.

Following repolarisation, phase 4 recovery ensues, whereby sodium is actively pumped out again and potassium in so that the cell becomes repolarised. The transmembrane potential returns to its resting level of –90 mV, and the action potential ends.

Once depolarisation has started, it is inevitably transmitted along the length of the cell to the adjacent cells. In this manner, a single electrical stimulus can depolarise the whole heart.

The action potential in automatic cells

The action potential in automatic cells differs from that in myocardial cells. The specialised fibres of the conduction system have the inherent ability to initiate an electrical impulse spontaneously without external influence. Because these cells are responsible for initiating the electrical impulse, phase 4 of the action potential does not properly exist and the cells have an unstable resting phase, with slow spontaneous phase 4 (diastolic) depolarisation (Fig. 2.7). A slow continuous movement of Na^+ into the cells produces this slow depolarisation during diastole, which reduces the intracellular negative charge until a threshold potential is reached and full depolarisation takes place.

THE REFRACTORY PERIOD

The myocardium is normally refractory to restimulation during the initial phase of systole. The

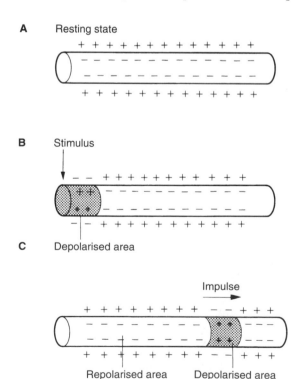

Figure 2.8 Myocardial cell transmembrane potential (**A**) at rest, (**B**) during depolarisation and (**C**) during repolarisation.

normal *effective refractory period* of the ventricle is 0.25–0.3 s and occurs when the potential lies at about –55 mV. Stimulation, no matter how strong, does not produce an action potential. Certain antidysrhythmic agents act by lengthening or shortening this refractory period.

Following the effective refractory period there is a *relative refractory period* of about 0.05 s, during which the muscle can be stimulated but with difficulty. Just after this is a vulnerable period, when even a very weak stimulus can evoke a potential.

The normal refractory period of the atrium is about half that of the ventricles, and the relative refractory period is an additional 0.03 s. As a result, the atria can beat much faster than the ventricles.

MYOCARDIAL CONTRACTION

The mechanism by which the action potential causes the myofibrils to contract is known as *excitation–contraction coupling*. Electrical excitation produces mechanical activation, leading to myocardial contraction.

Electrical excitation

The function of the automatic cells is to regulate the contraction of the myocardial cells by providing the initial electrical stimulation. Their contractile elements are sparse and do not contribute significantly to the cardiac contraction.

Normally, the activating impulse spreads from the sinus node in all directions. It travels at a rate of about 1 m/s, thus reaching the most distant parts of the atrium in only 0.08 s. A delay of approximately 0.04 s in AV transmission occurs during passage through the node, which allows atrial systole to be completed. From the atria, the wave of electrical excitement passes rapidly along the specialised muscle fibres of the AV bundle, bundle branches and peripheral ramifications of these branches. The spread of excitation causes contraction of the ventricular musculature.

Mechanical activation and myocardial contraction

The unit of contraction is the sarcomere, which contains the two contractile proteins: actin and myosin (see above). The contractile process is initiated when the nerve impulse reaches the cardiac cell and travels along the sarcolemma. A series of fine branching T-tubules (the *sarcoplasmic reticulum*) runs from the sarcolemma to the inner contractile elements. These allow any electrical changes occurring at the cell membrane to be rapidly transmitted to the myofibrils and provide the link between the electrical and mechanical activities of the heart.

When an action potential reaches the cardiac muscle membrane, it spreads to the interior of the cell via the sarcoplasmic reticulum. This releases Ca^{2+} from pouches (*cisternae*) in the T-tubules. These diffuse into the myofibrils to catalyse a chemical reaction that activates the sliding of the actin and myosin filaments along each other, to effect contraction. The strength of myocardial contraction is dependent upon the concentration of Ca^{2+}, as well as on the rate of ATP production. At the end of contraction, Ca^{2+} in the sarcoplasm is rapidly pumped back into the cisternae.

CARDIAC PHYSIOLOGY

The heart is a double pump that maintains two circulations: the pulmonary circulation and the systemic circulation. These serve to transport oxygen and other nutrients to the body cells, remove metabolic waste products from them and convey substances (e.g. hormones) from one part of the body to another. At rest, the heart beats at about 70–80 beats/min and pumps about 5 litres of blood. During exercise, the rate may approach 200 beats/min and the cardiac output may increase to as much as 20 litres.

THE CARDIAC CYCLE

The function of the heart is to maintain a constant circulation of blood through the body. It acts as a pump whose cyclical contraction (*systole*) and relaxation (*diastole*) is known as the *cardiac cycle*. This cyclical activity is normally initiated by spontaneous generation of an action potential at the sinus node. The impulse travels at about 1 m/s through the atrial muscle to produce atrial systole. Tissues at the AV groove prevent transmission from atrial to ventricular muscle, and conduction can take place only through specialised tissues in the AV junction. The duration of the cardiac cycle is about 0.8 s, producing an average heart rate of 75 beats/min. Provided the heart receives excitation along the normal pathways, the heart rate remains constant; each successive cardiac cycle follows the same pattern of systole and diastole.

The duration of atrial systole is about 0.1 s and that of ventricular systole 0.3 s. Thus, the combined duration of atrial and ventricular systole is approximately 0.4 s. The timing remains fairly constant at fast heart rates, so that any increase in heart rate decreases diastolic timing. Complete cardiac diastole normally lasts 0.4 s, but, as the pulse rate increases, the diastolic interval decreases. Since coronary perfusion takes place in diastole, fast heart rates may critically impair the myocardial blood supply.

Atrial function

Atrial diastole lasts for 0.3 s, during which venous blood drains into the atria, which act as a reservoir, storing the blood. The AV ring moves upwards at the end of ventricular systole, causing a rise in atrial pressure (the *'v' wave*). The AV valves then open and the ventricles rapidly begin to fill, allowing the valve cusps to float upwards into opposition. The atria then contract (the right usually very slightly before the left), a process taking 0.1 s. Blood is forced through the AV valves into the ventricles, increasing ventricular filling by about 10–20% and priming the ventricles for contraction.

Since there are no valves between the right atrium and the venae cavae, some blood is also expelled backwards during atrial contraction, causing a transient rise in the central venous pressure: the *'a' wave* (Fig. 2.9). The delay of electrical transmission at the AV node allows the atria to empty completely before ventricular contraction starts.

Ventricular function

The pressure of blood in the ventricles begins to rise whilst that in the relaxing atria is falling. The cusps of the AV valves snap shut (causing the first heart sound, S_1) and are held in opposition by the pull of the papillary muscles on the chordae tendineae. After closure of the AV valves, the blood pressure rises because of isometric contraction of the ventricular muscle. During this phase, the ventricles alter their shape (becoming shorter and fatter), although not their volume (this is called isovolumetric contraction). This momentarily causes a backward bulging of the AV valve cusps into the atria and produces a transient increase in atrial pressure (the *'c' wave*).

When the rising ventricular pressure exceeds the pressure in the aorta and pulmonary artery, the semilunar aortic and pulmonary valves open. The isotonic phase of contraction then begins,

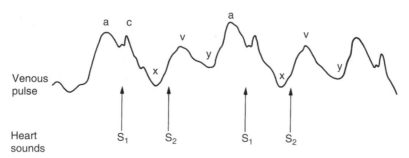

Figure 2.9 The venous pulse waveform.

and the ventricular contents are ejected. Descent of the AV ring during ventricular systole causes a fall in right atrial pressure (the 'x' descent).

As the ventricular muscle relaxes and the pressure falls below that in the aorta and pulmonary artery, the semilunar valves close (the second heart sound, S_2), producing the dicrotic notch on arterial pressure traces. The aortic valve closes slightly before the pulmonary valve. Simultaneously, blood enters the atria and the intra-atrial pressure gradually rises, so that, when the AV valves open, blood flows rapidly from the atria to the ventricles, producing the third heart sound (S_3), heard in some children and young adults.

HAEMODYNAMICS

The circulation is a continuous circuit, although it is often conveniently subdivided into the systemic and pulmonary circuits.

The pulmonary circulation

The pulmonary circuit is a low-pressure system with short, wide, thin-walled vessels and a small capacity (500–900 ml). The mean pressure in the circuit in the adult is approximately 15 mmHg, which is less than one-sixth that in the systemic circulation. It circulates all the blood from the right ventricle to the left atrium. As blood is carried through the pulmonary vascular bed, carbon dioxide diffuses outwards into the lungs and oxygen is absorbed.

The pulmonary trunk carrying deoxygenated blood passes upward from the right ventricle and divides into two main *pulmonary arteries*, one passing to each lung. Within the lungs, the arteries divide and subdivide to form the pulmonary capillary bed where gaseous exchange takes place. Eventually, these capillaries join up to form two main *pulmonary veins*, carrying oxygenated blood to the left atrium.

The systemic circulation

The systemic circulation is a high-pressure system that supplies all the tissues of the body

(except the lungs) with blood. The aorta is elastic in nature, which helps it function both as a reservoir for blood during the rapid ejection phase from the left ventricle and as a compression chamber to help propel the blood forward. As the branches arising from the aorta divide, the total cross-sectional area of the arteries, arterioles and capillaries increases and the average velocity of blood flow decreases. The arterioles offer the largest resistance to flow. In the capillary bed, there is often stasis of flow in some capillaries and an active flow in others. The normal systemic capillary pressure is about 24–25 mmHg, and the normal systemic capillary blood volume at rest is about 5% of the total volume (250 ml).

Coronary blood flow

The primary function of the coronary circulation is to provide an adequate supply of oxygen to support the metabolic demands of the heart. The rate of oxygen consumption is the major factor that determines coronary blood flow. Myocardial oxygen consumption (mVO_2) is related to myocardial work in response to exercise or other stimuli, including drugs such as adrenaline (epinephrine), noradrenaline (norepinephrine), calcium, thyroxine and digitalis.

About 4% of cardiac output passes into the coronary vessels (about 225 ml/min), which fill in diastole. During systole, the coronary vessels are compressed so that the resistance to flow at that time is sharply increased. Coronary blood flow is largely determined by the calibre of the coronary arteries themselves and is regulated almost entirely by the local metabolic needs of the working cardiac muscle.

REGULATION OF MYOCARDIAL FUNCTION

The normal adult blood volume is about 5 litres; about 3.5 litres are in the systemic (predominantly venous) circulation. The volume in the heart is about 0.6 litre, bringing the total central circulation in the heart and lungs to about 1.5 litres. Not all blood is expelled from the left ventricle at the end of systole. The residual volume, the *left ventricular end diastolic volume* (LVEDV), is about 140 ml. The quantity of blood ejected during ventricular systole (the *stroke volume*) is only about 80–100 ml; hence the *ejection fraction* is approximately 80/140 = 60%. If the heart rate is 70 beats/min, then:

Cardiac output = Heart rate (beats/min) ×
Stroke volume (ml/beat)
= about 5.6 litres

The cardiac output may increase up to 20 litres during heavy exertion. To alter cardiac output to meet changing bodily demands for tissue perfusion, the heart rate or stroke volume (or both) must be altered. These mechanisms normally operate together to increase the cardiac output as required.

The main determinants of cardiac output are stroke volume and heart rate. If the stroke volume is constant, cardiac output will linearly follow heart rate. However, stroke volume varies constantly, and thus the heart rate must alter to maintain the cardiac output.

Stroke volume is determined by:

- Preload (filling of the heart during diastole)
- Afterload (resistance against which the heart must pump)
- Contractility of the heart muscle.

Preload

Preload is the tension exerted on cardiac muscle at the end of diastole, usually expressed as the *left ventricular end diastolic pressure*. This is determined by the volume of blood in the left ventricle at the end of diastole (LVEDV). The Frank–Starling Law of 1918 states that, within physiological limits, increases in LVEDV are accompanied by an increase in stroke work. Hence, although the volume of blood passing through the heart may vary considerably, cardiac muscle fibres can contract more forcefully to cope with increased loads. This intrinsic ability of the heart to adapt to changing loads of inflowing blood can be shown graphically (Fig. 2.6) and is approximately linear. Unfortunately, once the load increases beyond physiological limits, the heart begins to fail. Preload can be estimated by

measurement of left and right atrial pressures. Clinically, this is done either by a central venous pressure line in the right atrium or by a Swan–Ganz catheter measuring the pulmonary capillary wedge pressure to approximate the pressure in the left atrium.

Afterload

Afterload is the force opposing ventricular ejection and is a function of both arterial pressure and left ventricular size. Two major determinants of left ventricular afterload are the resistance of the aortic valve and systemic vascular resistance. Conditions that increase afterload include those causing obstruction to ventricular outflow (e.g. aortic stenosis) and those causing high systemic vascular resistance (e.g. hypertension).

Contractility

Contractility is an intrinsic property of the heart and exists independently of loading. Sympathetic nervous stimulation or drugs such as adrenaline (epinephrine), noradrenaline (norepinephrine) or dopamine can increase the speed and force of contraction. These improve the speed and strength of contraction (i.e. they have positive inotropic and chronotropic effects) by increasing ATP production and calcium (Ca^{2+}) fluxes. Myocardial hypoxia, ischaemia and beta-blocking agents have the reverse effect and decrease cardiac contractility (negative inotropic and chronotropic effects). The contractile state can be gauged by the size of the ejection fraction. The normal ejection fraction is 0.60–0.75, i.e. the left ventricle ejects about 60–75% of its contents during systole. This may be estimated by echocardiography or nuclear scanning or at cardiac catheterisation. Using the Frank–Starling graphs, contractility can be represented by different curves; higher degrees of contractility displace the curve upwards and to the left (Fig. 2.10).

BLOOD PRESSURE

Blood pressure can be defined as the force or pressure that the blood exerts upon the vessel

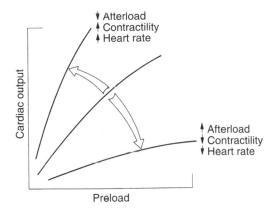

Figure 2.10 Ventricular function (Starling's) curves showing the effects of preload, afterload, contractility and heart rate.

walls. When the ventricle contracts, blood is forced into an already full aorta, and the pressure wave produces a systolic blood pressure of about 120 mmHg (16 kilopascals, kPa). During complete cardiac diastole, the arterial pressure falls to about 80 mmHg (11 kPa).

Blood pressure is maintained through many variables, including:

- Cardiac output
- Blood volume
- Peripheral resistance
- Elasticity of the vessel walls
- Venous return.

Cardiac output is controlled by pulse rate and stroke volume. An increase in cardiac output raises both systolic and diastolic blood pressure, but an increase in stroke volume increases the systolic pressure to a greater degree. Blood volume is obviously important, as can be seen by the fact that blood pressure falls in shock. This may be due to an absolute loss of blood volume (e.g. haemorrhage) or a relative loss of circulating volume when there is widespread vasodilatation (e.g. septicaemic shock).

Peripheral resistance is controlled via sympathetic vasoconstrictor nerves originating in the vasomotor centre of the medulla oblongata. Normally, the artery walls are in a state of mild constriction, giving rise to 'resting tone'. Selective vasoconstriction and vasodilatation can take place around the body, to ensure a constant blood supply to the vital organs, especially the heart and brain.

The elasticity of the arterial walls is important to propel the blood forwards. Distension and recoil occur throughout the arterial system. During diastole, arterial recoil maintains the diastolic blood pressure. As the arterial tree ages, atheromatous deposits cause 'hardening of the arteries'. Elasticity is lost and the systolic blood pressure rises, since the arterial walls are unable to buffer the effect of the ventricular systolic shockwave.

Venous return via the superior and inferior venae cavae also plays an important role in maintenance of the blood pressure. The force of the left ventricle is not sufficient on its own to force blood round the body. It is therefore assisted by muscular contraction and respiration. Contraction of skeletal muscle puts pressure on the veins and squeezes blood forwards. Valves prevent backward flow. The negative intrathoracic pressure caused by inspiration also helps, by sucking blood into the heart. In addition, diaphragmatic movement raises the intra-abdominal pressure, squeezing blood out of the abdominal vessels.

PATHOLOGY

ATHEROSCLEROSIS

The term coronary heart disease is used to describe the effects of impaired or absent blood supply to the myocardium. In the majority of cases, this is caused by atheromatous obstruction of the coronary arteries, and atherosclerotic changes are found in virtually all patients with acute myocardial infarction. It is a complex disorder, characterised by progressive accumulation of cholesterol within the intima of large and medium arteries, with infiltration and proliferation of vascular smooth muscle cells (VSMCs). Until recently, atherosclerosis was considered a slowly progressing degenerative disease, predominantly affecting the elderly. However, the development and progression of atherosclerosis is a dynamic, inflammatory process that is readily modifiable (Weissberg, 2000). An important feature is the focal distribution of atheroma as plaques. There is a predilection for these plaques to occur around branching vessels, or areas of arterial curvature, suggesting that haemodynamic stresses may play an important initiating role. The role of repeated endothelial injury from toxins (e.g. from smoking), vasospasm and other haemodynamic stresses is generally assumed to be central to the initiation and progression of these lesions. The mature atherosclerotic plaque evolves over decades, and has a soft lipid-rich core (*athere*, Greek for gruel or porridge) walled off by a hard fibrous capsule (*skleros*, Greek for hard).

Atherosclerotic plaques can be classified into three general types:

1. *Fatty streaks*. The process of atherosclerosis begins with development of flat, lipid-rich lesions, termed fatty streaks. These may be present from early childhood in countries with high rates of coronary heart disease, and occur where the endothelium has been damaged. Such streaks have been observed in the aorta and coronary arteries in children as young as 2 years old (Berensen et al, 1998). Blood-borne monocytes penetrate the vessel wall, and transform into fat-laden macrophages (foam cells) within the intima by absorbing low-density lipoprotein (LDL)-cholesterol. The lesions are yellowish in appearance and cause little or no obstruction to the affected artery. They are thought to be benign in themselves but are the precursors of advanced atheromatous lesions. Conversion of the fatty streak to atheroma depends upon the proliferation and differentiation of VSMCs to fibroblasts and the elaboration of collagen.

2. *Fibrous plaques*. Fatty streaks become more fibrous with time to produce white plaques that protrude into the lumen of the artery. The number of fibrous plaques increases rapidly between the ages of 15 and 35 years, particularly in those with cardiovascular risk factors (Strong et al, 1999). As the plaque develops, there is proliferation of VSMCs which synthesise and deposit matrix and connective tissue to form a tough

fibrous cap. Lipids released when foam cells die form layers of fat and cell debris (the 'lipid pool') trapped beneath the fibrous cap. The fibrous plaque often progresses, with potential for luminal narrowing, or it may degenerate. Fibrous plaques in the coronary vessels of 204 trauma death patients were found in 69% of those aged 26–39 years and in 8% of those aged 2–15 years (Berenson et al, 1998).

3. *Advanced (complicated) lesions*. These are degenerative lesions composed of fibrous tissue, fibrin and intracellular and extracellular lipid and, often, extravasated blood. The necrotic, lipid-rich core increases in size and often becomes calcified.

Atherosclerosis is a dynamic balance between lipid-driven inflammatory cells within the substance of the plaque that associate with plaque rupture, and the natural stabilising properties of the surrounding VSMCs.

Plaque rupture

Plaque rupture is a common event, and is usually asymptomatic. However, plaque rupture is the initiator of most acute coronary syndromes and sudden cardiac deaths. Most of the adult population have advanced atherosclerotic plaques in their coronary arteries, and, although many will eventually suffer an acute coronary event, most will not; why this is the case is not known. Plaque fissuring is a random and unpredictable event, occurring in response to inflammation, mechanical stresses, coronary artery spasm and other factors acting on the coronary vasculature. The risk of plaque rupture does not seem to depend on plaque size or severity of the stenosis, but primarily on plaque morphology (Falk et al, 1995). Vulnerable plaques are recognised by:

- A large lipid pool (more than 40% of overall plaque volume)
- Low VSMC numbers in the cap
- High numbers of macrophages
- A thin fibrous cap.

High circulating concentrations of LDL-cholesterol in the blood increase foam cell activity and the size of the lipid pool, making plaques more likely to rupture; other risk factors such as diabetes and cigarette smoking increase the likelihood of occlusive thrombus should plaque rupture occur. The risk of an acute coronary syndrome will depend not on the total number of atheromatous plaques in the coronary tree, but on the number of vulnerable plaques. Plaque composition is much more important than size. Plaques that produce mild degrees of stenosis (under 50% diameter occlusion), or which may not even be visualised at coronary angiography, precipitate most episodes of acute coronary thrombosis.

The accumulation of subendothelial lipid exacerbates a local inflammatory reaction that weakens the fibrous cap. The integrity of the fibrous cap is a critical determinant of plaque stability and is at its weakest at the shoulder region, where the fibrous cap meets the normal arterial wall. The lesion grows across the inner surface of the artery, and secretion of collagenases by the foam cells exacerbates weakness at the shoulder. The only cell that can repair the cap and protect against plaque rupture is the VSMC. There is normally a balance between inflammation leading to breakdown of the fibrous cap and VSMC proliferation and collagen synthesis maintaining fibrosis and integrity of the cap. If the 'wound healing' response of the VSMCs is overcome, the plaque breaks down and initiates thrombosis.

Plaque erosion and rupture

Atherosclerosis is not a continuous process, but a disease with phases of stability and instability. Angiographic studies during acute cardiac events show two types of plaque in the coronary artery tree (Davies, 1992).

Type I lesions have smooth, regular edges with evidence of endothelial erosion. Although the integrity of the fibrous cap and lipid pool is unaltered, it is the loss of endothelium that stimulates platelet adhesion and thrombus formation.

Type II lesions are more common and have ragged, irregular edges, often showing a filling defect on angiography. There is a deep plaque fissure in the fibrous cap that allows blood to dissect inwards, forming a platelet-rich thrombus within the intima.

Symptoms of the acute coronary syndromes appear to be related to plaque erosion or rupture – a dynamic process that may occur over a period of hours to days.

Plaque erosion often occurs at the site of a pre-existing severe stenosis, and exposes the underlying connective tissue matrix. A thin layer of platelets forms over the surface of the plaque, and may initiate adherent thrombus. Since the thrombus does not track deep down into the plaque, it may be more vulnerable to fibrinolysis. Plaque erosion is more common in women and underlies up to 50% of cases of sudden death and a quarter of cases of acute myocardial infarction.

Plaque rupture is the major cause of acute coronary thrombosis. Plaque rupture exposes the highly thrombogenic collagenous matrix and cholesterol pool to the circulation, which inevitably triggers platelet accumulation. This results in fibrin deposition and the formation of thrombus with partial or total vessel occlusion. The thrombus tracks down into the plaque itself, and then expands and distorts the plaque from within. The thrombus may cause rapid changes in the severity of stenosis and may result in total or subtotal vessel occlusion (Fig. 2.11). In unstable angina, the thrombus is platelet-rich and appears white. Blood flow may sweep activated platelets into the distal intramyocardial arteries and cause micro-infarcts. Spontaneous thrombolysis may explain short-lived episodes of vessel occlusion and associated symptoms and transient ECG changes, and, as the thrombus fragments, micro-embolisation may occur into the myocardial microvasculature. The platelet-rich thrombus may release vasoconstrictor agents such as serotonin and thromboxane A_2, which may induce vasospasm, either at the site of the thrombosis or within the microcirculation. This is a dominant effect in Prinzmetal angina, which is characterised by transient abrupt vasoconstriction within a segment of coronary artery.

The intermittent attacks of myocardial ischaemia that occur in the unstable coronary syndromes are thus caused by:

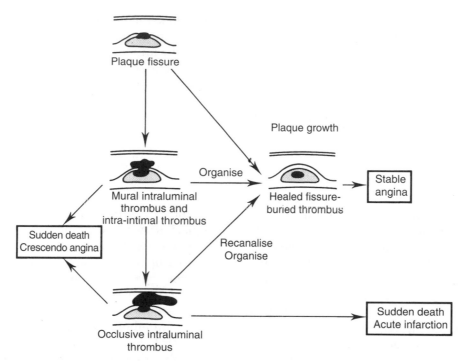

Figure 2.11 Relationship between the clinical expressions of coronary heart disease and the stages of plaque fissuring.

- The thrombus waxing and waning with intermittent occlusion
- Intense vasoconstriction
- Platelet embolisation to the microvasculature.

Depending upon the duration of vessel occlusion, and degree of repeated embolisation from the unstable plaque upstream, there may be varying effects on the myocardium. The myocardium may escape undamaged, or show small areas of necrosis, often not detected by routine cardiac enzyme estimation, such as creatine kinase (CK or CK-MB), but may be so by troponin estimation.

Pacification of the plaque

It is likely that most episodes of plaque disruption are clinically silent but still contribute to the progression of coronary disease. Plaque healing takes place with endogenous fibrinolysis dispersing the thrombus, and smooth muscle cells migrating into the area to 'smooth out' and repair the fibrous cap. The final result becomes a stable lesion that may cause anything from minor irregularities to an important chronic occlusion. Up to 60% of patients with stable angina and 85% of those with previous myocardial infarction and angina have segments of artery in which the original channel is replaced by several small channels, suggesting recanalisation through a previously occlusive thrombus. Those lesions that remain irregular in outline at angiography and do not smooth out after an episode of unstable angina remain vulnerable to further episodes of disruption. As the plaque grows and encroaches on the arterial lumen, blood flow is limited, and shear forces across the lesion may make it more likely to fissure. In the future, cardiovascular magnetic resonance imaging (MRI) may be able to determine plaque vulnerability by assessing both the size of the lipid pool and the integrity of the fibrous cap.

ATHEROMA AND OTHER CAUSES OF MYOCARDIAL ISCHAEMIA

The symptoms of myocardial ischaemia result from an imbalance between myocardial oxygen demand and supply. Oxygen demand depends mainly upon heart rate, strength of myocardial contraction and left ventricular wall tension. When the heart rate increases, systolic timing does not alter by very much, and the increased heart rate occurs at the expense of diastolic timing. As a result, there is a reduction in coronary perfusion time (which takes place in diastole), despite the higher demands placed upon it by the increased heart rate. Additionally, sympathetic stimulation leads to an increase in the force of contraction, which increases myocardial oxygen demand. Increased wall tension will also increase myocardial work and is determined by intracardiac pressures and volumes secondary to changes in preload and afterload.

In general, the delivery of oxygen to the myocardium varies with coronary blood flow, which is in turn determined by perfusion pressure. Abnormalities of the vessel wall, abnormalities in blood flow or abnormalities in the blood itself may compromise perfusion pressure.

1. *Abnormalities of the coronary vessel wall*. Fixed or reversible lesions may impair coronary blood supply. Atheroma is the most common cause of coronary stenosis, although congenital lesions, such as coronary ectasia, may be responsible. Clinically important restriction to ordinary flow occurs when the diameter of the lumen is reduced by more than 50%, usually resulting in angina. An abrupt diminution or total loss of coronary blood supply will ultimately result in acute myocardial infarction. Studies of patients who had suffered a myocardial infarction and had undergone coronary angiography shortly before the event have shown that it is usually the smaller lesions (causing under 50% diameter occlusion) that are responsible for the acute event (Falk et al, 1995). Moreover, many plaques that were responsible for the infarction were actually invisible at angiography. This suggests that it will be medical rather than surgical therapies that will have the major effect on reducing the risk of plaque rupture and its consequences.

Coronary artery spasm gives rise to intermittent, reversible stenoses and is the underlying abnormality in 'variant angina', described by Prinzmetal et al (1959). Both spasm and atheroma are usually present in patients with symptomatic coronary heart disease, although their precise contribution to impairing myocardial perfusion at any given time will differ. Coronary artery spasm occurs in many patients with unstable angina and may also follow the sudden withdrawal of nitrate therapy. The usual situation is for spasm and fixed stenosis to act in combination – i.e. vascular contraction takes place around a fixed obstruction, causing a critical reduction in flow, which leads to regional ischaemia. However, temporary occlusion of coronary flow by spasm, even in the absence of atheroma, can lead to angina or even myocardial infarction.

Rarely, the coronary vessel wall may be involved in inflammatory diseases, such as systemic lupus erythematosus and polyarteritis nodosa, which may cause symptomatic occlusion.

2. *Abnormalities in blood flow*. Valvular heart disease, especially aortic stenosis, will impede blood flow from the left ventricle and reduce perfusion of the coronary arteries. This may provoke angina, even in the absence of coronary atheroma.

3. *Abnormalities in the blood*. Anaemia will prevent adequate oxygen carriage and may provoke angina. Hyperviscosity syndromes, such as polycythaemia and myeloma, may result in myocardial ischaemia by slowing blood flow.

It can be seen that the myocardium can be rendered ischaemic by mechanisms other than fixed atherosclerotic lesions in the coronary arteries. Acute coronary syndromes often occur at rest or during minimal exertion when there is little or no demand placed upon the heart. The precipitating cause would, therefore, seem to be decreased oxygen supply to the heart, rather than increased oxygen demand, and it is now known that several mechanisms – atherosclerosis, platelet adhesion, coronary thrombosis and coronary artery spasm – interact in the clinical manifestations of acute coronary disease.

THE MANIFESTATIONS OF CORONARY ATHEROSCLEROSIS

The main clinical manifestations of atherosclerotic coronary plaques are unstable angina, myocardial infarction and sudden death. These clinical syndromes are dependent on several underlying factors, including the degree and abruptness of obstruction of coronary blood flow, the duration of decreased myocardial perfusion and the oxygen demand at the time of coronary obstruction.

Sudden death

A sudden death is one that occurs from natural causes, in which the patient dies within an hour of developing symptoms, and often immediately. Coronary heart disease is responsible for about 70% of sudden deaths (sudden cardiac death), but about half will have had no previously recognised heart disease. Sudden cardiac death is common, representing an estimated 25–30% of all cardiovascular deaths, and thus responsible for up to 100 000 deaths in the UK each year.

Sudden cardiac death has two major underlying causes: vascular (haemorrhagic or thromboembolic) and dysrhythmic (electrical). These may occur alone or, more commonly, together. Ambulatory electrocardiography in patients dying suddenly suggests that ventricular tachycardia (VT) or ventricular fibrillation (VF) is the usual cause of death (Milner et al, 1985). Most cases are probably initiated by an acute event, such as coronary artery spasm, acute plaque fissuring or perhaps coronary emboli arising from ulcerated plaques, producing distal microinfarcts. The presence of occlusive thrombus at necropsy is almost pathognomonic of developing infarction (de Wood et al, 1980), and is found in about a third of cases of sudden cardiac death (Davies, 1992). An additional 43% demonstrate non-occlusive intraluminal thrombus. The finding of plaque fissuring alone is probably unhelpful in determining the cause of death, as this is a random and recurrent event and may be found in people who die from unrelated causes. It thus appears that a quarter of sudden cardiac deaths are not related to myocardial infarction, and the cause is assumed to be electrical (VT or VF), precipitated by left ventricular dysfunction secondary to myocardial ischaemia. However, many of these patients may have died from myocardial infarction, but, as histological changes of infarction do not occur for 4–6 h, there may be no firm morphological, enzyme or electrocardiographic evidence.

Myocardial infarction and unstable angina

Unstable angina, non-Q wave and Q wave myocardial infarction represent a continuum of the same disease process, presenting clinically as *unstable coronary syndromes*. They are usually characterised by plaque rupture and a stuttering or abrupt reduction in coronary artery blood flow. In unstable angina, occlusion tends to be transient and episodic, and the vessels show type II plaques undergoing fissuring, often with non-occlusive luminal thrombus. Distal micro-embolisation of platelets and thrombus into small myocardial vessels is very common, and alteration in tissue perfusion is present in most cases. Arterial spasm commonly associates with type I atheromatous stenoses.

Myocardial infarction refers to necrosis of myocardial cells, and is usually associated with an occlusive thrombus in one or more of the coronary arteries, superimposed on an advanced and disrupted atherosclerotic plaque. Although occlusive thrombi are found in up to 90% of patients immediately following myocardial infarction, this frequency diminishes as time passes because of spontaneous thrombolysis. The speed with which some arteries re-open suggests that spasm may play an important role. About 1% of patients with acute myocardial infarction have normal coronary arteriograms, and the cause of the infarction remains speculative (Brecker et al, 1993). It is possible that a small atheromatous plaque has ruptured and resolved without any residual obstruction. Typical patients are young, heavy smokers or older women. In general, prognosis is excellent, but risk factor intervention seems appropriate (Da Costa et al, 2001). Whether these patients benefit from other interventions such as statins, beta-blockers (which might provoke spasm) or ACE inhibitors is not known.

LEFT VENTRICULAR REMODELLING

The term 'remodelling' essentially refers to the complex structural changes in the left ventricular myocardium that follows acute myocardial infarction, resulting in the infarcted myocardium being replaced by fibrous scar tissue. Both the infarcted and the non-infarcted myocardium are involved in this remodelling process, which has an important effect on subsequent left ventricular function and, hence, prognosis. Coronary occlusion quickly leads to transmural myocardial ischaemia, and myocardial contraction in the area affected ceases within seconds. Pain is usually experienced within 1 min and changes on the ECG may be produced within 30 s. After about 20–30 min, myocardial necrosis begins, and progresses in a wavefront from endocardium to epicardium. Ischaemia is greater in the subendocardium than in the subepicardium because wall tension is greater (increasing oxygen requirements) and because it relies on the terminal portions of epicardial vessels. Necrosis is centred on a zone most devoid of collateral circulation, and from this a wavefront of necrosis spreads out to involve 80–90% of the ischaemic zone after a period of 4–6 h. At the same time as the wave moves outward, it moves upwards towards the epicardium, so that the evolving infarct will have a large area of endocardial necrosis and a smaller area of epicardial damage. If more than two-thirds of the ventricular wall is involved, the infarction is termed 'transmural'. If it involves less than this, it is termed a non-transmural infarction. In most cases of transmural myocardial infarction, the infarct-related artery is only mildly to moderately stenotic prior to plaque rupture. The infarcted area is first red at because of 'stuffing in' of the red cells (*infarct = stuffed in*). The area later becomes pale as the necrotic muscle swells and squeezes out the extravasated blood. Finally, the infarcted area is replaced by fibrous scar tissue over the course of 1 week to 3 months.

Early left ventricular remodelling starts within the first 24 h of coronary occlusion, and is a long process, generally completed within 4–6 weeks following the acute myocardial infarction. The infarcted area becomes progressively thinner and at the same time expands, resulting in ventricular dilatation. This area of infarct expansion develops within hours of injury and provides a site for the formation left ventricular thrombus. As infarct expansion proceeds over the early weeks, there is the possibility of aneurysm formation and subsequent left ventricular rupture. While these changes are going on, there is progressive lengthening and hypertrophy of the residual non-infarcted myocardium. The lengthening process increases the shape and volume of the left ventricle, and this late phase of remodelling can continue over months or even years, leading to progressive ventricular dilatation. The early effects of left ventricular remodelling are beneficial because ventricular dilatation reduces filling pressures, enabling the heart to generate larger stroke volumes. However, the presence of dilatation and remodelling is associated with later development of left ventricular failure and death. Global ventricular dilatation, with distortion of the cavity, results in an increase in left ventricular volume and defines overall prognosis: the bigger the volume, the greater the mortality (Vannan and Taylor, 1992). Not all infarcts undergo significant remodelling. The site of the infarct does not seem to be important, but it is the small infarcts that tend to heal without any dilatation. Those patients with extensive myocardial infarction and persistent occlusion of the infarct-related artery are most at risk of ventricular remodelling, and dilatation is more likely to occur if the left ventricular ejection fraction is less than 40%. Most of these patients will have signs of significant cardiac failure. Prevention of infarct expansion and remodelling may be effected by early and complete reperfusion of the infarct-related artery. Even late perfusion beyond the stage where there is much change for myocardial salvage seems to protect against dilatation, presumably because the healing process is improved. This perhaps emphasises the importance of opening the infarct-related artery in all large infarcts.

The process of remodelling is probably a physical phenomenon related to the increased loads on various segments of the heart. Reducing these loads should be beneficial, particularly if there is systemic hypertension. Early and long-term use of ACE inhibitors following myocardial infarction helps attenuate ventricular remodelling and its sequelae, mostly by limiting ventricular expansion. This is why ACE inhibitors are of value following acute myocardial infarction, particularly for those with extensive myocardial infarction, overt heart failure, or echocardiographic evidence of left ventricular dysfunction (St John Sutton, 1994).

MYOCARDIAL HIBERNATION AND STUNNING

Hibernating myocardium refers to a situation caused by chronic low-flow ischaemia, with coronary blood flow that is too feeble to allow contraction but just sufficient to prevent necrosis. Thus, the myocytes 'sleep', but remain viable. This may be the situation in the border zone of peri-infarction tissue. The longer hypoperfusion remains, the greater the likelihood of functional and structural abnormalities, and a major focus of revascularisation strategies is to identify viable but non-contractile myocardium that may benefit from reperfusional strategies.

Myocardial stunning refers to the situation in which, following a transient episode of ischaemia, blood flow is restored but myocardial contractility does not return immediately, even though the myocytes appear viable. Typically, this can follow thrombolysis for myocardial infarction, but it may sometimes complicate other coronary syndromes, angioplasty or cardiac surgery (Kluner et al, 2001). Normal function may be restored hours, days or even weeks later, and this explains why left ventricular function takes time to recover after successful reperfusion. Repeated episodes of stunning may lead to a condition known as *chronic contractile dysfunction*, which may be difficult to differentiate from hibernation. Stunned myocardium complicating cardiogenic shock will respond to inotropic stimulation as long as reperfusion has been established so that ischaemic damage is not worsened, which of course will aggravate the effects of stunning.

Hence, impaired left ventricular function following myocardial infarction is not always irreversible. Resting injection of thallium with late re-imaging is a sensitive method for evaluating myocardial viability. If thallium uptake is greater than 50% of normal in the territory of the infarct, revascularisation should improve myocardial performance. Positron emission tomography scanning is more sensitive, but is not widely available.

REFERENCES

Berenson GS, Srinivasan SR, Bao W et al (1998) Association between multiple cardiovascular risk factors and atherosclerosis in children and young adults. *New England Journal of Medicine*, **338:** 1650–1656.

Brecker SJD, Stevenson RN, Roberts R et al (1993) Acute myocardial infarction in patients with normal coronary arteries. *BMJ*, **307:** 1255–1256.

Da Costa A, Isaak K, Faure E et al (2001) Clinical characteristics, aetiological factors and long-term prognosis of myocardial infarction with an absolutely normal coronary angiogram: a 3-year follow up study of 91 patients. *European Heart Journal*, **22:** 1459–1465.

Davies MJ (1992) Anatomic features in victims of sudden coronary death. *Circulation*, **85** (suppl 1): 19–24.

de Wood MA, Spores R, Natske LT et al (1980) Prevalence of total coronary occlusion during the early hours of transmural myocardial infarction. *New England Journal of Medicine*, **303:** 897–902.

Falk E, Shah PK, Fuster V (1995) Coronary plaque disruption. *Circulation*, **92:** 657–671.

Kluner RA, Arimie B, Kay GL et al (2001) Evidence for stunned myocardium in humans: a 2001 update. *Coronary Artery Disease*, **12:** 349–356.

Milner PG, Platia EV, Reid PR et al (1985) Ambulatory electrocardiographic recordings at the time of fatal cardiac arrest. *American Journal of Cardiology*, **56:** 588–592.

Prinzmetal M, Kennamer R, Merliss R et al (1959) Angina pectoris. I. A variant form of angina pectoris: preliminary report. *American Journal of Medicine*, **27:** 375–388.

Starling EH (1918) *The Linacre Lecture on the Law of the Heart*. London: Longmans Green.

St John Sutton M (1994) Should ACE inhibitors be used routinely after infarction? Perspectives from the SAVE trial. *British Heart Journal*, **71:** 115–118.

Strong JP, Malcom GT, McMahan CA et al (1999) Prevalence and extent of atherosclerosis in adolescents and young adults: implication for prevention from the Pathobiological Determinants of Atherosclerosis in Youth Study (PDAY). *JAMA*, **281:** 727–735.

Vannan MA, Taylor DJE (1992) Ventricular modeling after myocardial infarction. *British Heart Journal*, **68:** 257–259.

Weissberg PL (2000) Atherogenesis: current understanding of the causes of atheroma. *Heart*, **83:** 247–252.

3

Coronary heart disease: risk factors and primary prevention

Cardiovascular disease is the single most common cause of morbidity and mortality in both men and women in the UK. Of the quarter of a million cardiovascular deaths in 2000, just over 124 000 were from coronary heart disease (Fig. 3.1). Evidence suggests that coronary heart disease is largely preventable by adopting a healthy life-style and effective management of high blood pressure and cholesterol.

Various epidemiological studies have found associations between the occurrence of coronary heart disease and physical, biochemical and environmental characteristics of populations and individuals, termed *risk factors*:

- *Non-modifiable risk factors* are those that cannot be changed, and include male gender, increasing age, ethnic origin, a low birth weight and a family history of premature coronary heart disease.
- *Modifiable risk factors* are those that can be altered, the most important of which are hypercholesterolaemia, cigarette smoking and hypertension.

Although, by definition, each risk factor associates positively with the risk of coronary heart disease, it does not mean that any of these risk factors actually causes heart disease. Indeed, many patients presenting with coronary heart disease do not have identifiable risk factors. In addition, there is no relationship between particular risk factors and the severity or extent of atheroma.

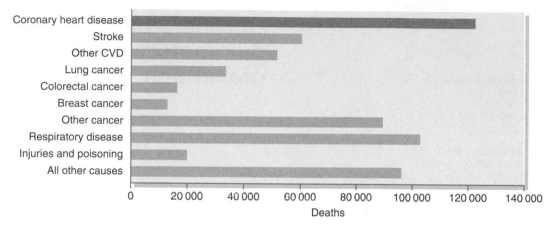

Figure 3.1 Mortality by cause in the UK, 2000. (Reproduced with permission from Petersen S, Rayner M (2002) Coronary Heart Disease Statistics. London: British Heart Foundation Database.)

Modifiable cardiovascular risk factors are very common in the UK adult population (Table 3.1): over half of the population have total serum cholesterol greater than 5.0 mmol/l, more than a quarter smoke cigarettes and most take little or no exercise (Petersen et al, 2000). Because these risk factors are common in the population, they tend to 'cluster' in individuals; this is important because cumulative risk is not just additive but synergistic (Criqui, 1986), with one factor multiplying the risk of another (Fig. 3.2). The Multiple Risk Factor Intervention Trial (MR.FIT) has confirmed that individuals are more at risk of coronary heart disease if they have multiple mild risk factors, rather than if they only have one severe risk factor (Neaton and Wentworth, 1992).

In the 1990s, primary prevention of cardiovascular disease focused on managing individual risk factors, rather than considering risk factor combinations and global risk. Emphasis was placed on the *relative* risk reduction for each risk factor, rather than considering how intervention would reduce *absolute* (overall) risk. It is now accepted that the value of any given intervention depends strongly on how it will affect *overall* rather than *relative* risk. For example, statin therapy for reducing serum cholesterol produces a relative risk reduction of about a third. However, if statin therapy is given to two individuals, one of which is at a 10% level of absolute risk and the other at a 30% absolute risk, intervention with statins will produce a three-fold change for the better in the individual at higher risk.

The importance of assessing overall risk is particularly important in primary prevention, because asymptomatic individuals with a number of slightly abnormal risk factors do not usually attract medical attention. However, such people may be at a much higher level of absolute cardiovascular risk than those with just one high risk factor that brings them under medical care (e.g. a high blood pressure, or very high blood cholesterol). Using absolute risk to inform clinical decision-making allows prioritisation of medical resources to those at highest probability of developing coronary heart disease. Assessment charts are now included in many clinical guidelines to help both clinicians (and patients) assess overall risk, and the need for intervention (Jackson, 2000).

Table 3.1 Proportion of all coronary heart disease attributable to different risk factors in the UK and the USA (data from Britton and McPherson, 2000)

Risk factor	UK estimate	US estimate
Blood cholesterol over 5.2 mol/l	46%	43%
Smoking	19%	22%
Obesity (BMI over 30 kg/m²)	6%	17%
Blood pressure over 140/90 mmHg	13%	25%
Physical inactivity	37%	35%

Note: Totals are over 100% due to multiple risk factors in the same individual. BMI, body mass index.

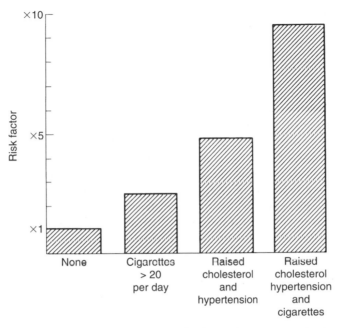

Figure 3.2 The synergistic effect of risk factors on the chances of a first major coronary episode, where blood cholesterol level is greater than 6.5 mmol/1 and blood pressure is greater than 160/95 mmHg.

The British Cardiac Society, the British Hyperlipidaemia Association, the British Hypertension Society and Diabetes UK now recommend that life-style and therapeutic intervention in individuals without clinical evidence of atherosclerotic disease should be strongly influenced by the level of absolute level of risk. Using epidemiological data from the Framingham Study (Dawber 1980; Anderson et al, 1991), their joint guidelines utilise a Cardiac Risk Assessor to calculate a person's absolute 10-year coronary heart disease risk (Wood et al, 1998). Although the data used to construct this assessor were based on a predominantly white, American, middle-class population, the risk equations have been found to be reasonably accurate when applied to North-European populations. Similar risk tables have been published from Sheffield and New Zealand.

Calculation of risk requires knowledge of the individual's age, sex, blood pressure, total and high-density lipoprotein (HDL)-cholesterol, smoking status within the last 5 years, presence of diabetes and evidence of left ventricular hypertrophy on the resting ECG. Blood pressure and cholesterol levels are based on a series of pre-treatment measurements to allow for biological variability. The calculator makes no allowance for ethnic origin, family history, sedentary lifestyle or obesity, all of which may affect absolute risk and should be taken into account.

The joint societies' computer program* calculates the risk of coronary heart disease as the percentage probability of a particular individual sustaining a non-fatal myocardial infarction, or dying from a coronary event within the next 10 years. Patients with established atherosclerotic disease have already declared themselves to be at high risk for recurrent events and do not need to have their risk assessed. These individuals require aggressive secondary preventative risk factor modification (see Ch. 15). Similarly, patients with familial hypercholesterolaemia or malignant hypertension are already at high risk of coronary heart disease, and the assessment charts do not apply. Identification of other

---

*An MS DOS version of the Cardiac Risk Assessor program is available from Professor Paul Durrington, Department of Medicine, Manchester Royal Infirmary, Manchester M13 9WL, UK.

high-risk individuals in the population requires either formal or opportunistic screening.

Those at highest risk (arbitrarily above 30% over the next 10 years) should be offered treatment as a priority. The next step is to offer intervention to those at more than 15% risk, and hopefully it will be possible to turn attention to those with a lesser degree of risk as resources allow. Taking this progressively staged approach to the prevention of coronary heart disease will ensure that delivery of care is balanced with the ability of medical services to identify, investigate and treat patients in the long term.

Although certain pharmacological interventions have been shown to reduce absolute risk at levels of less than 1% per year, managing everyone at this low level of risk, particularly with expensive therapies, would be hugely demanding on NHS resources. There is little point in turning people into patients if we cannot offer appropriate care. If a decision is made not to intervene pharmacologically, this must be reviewed at regular intervals. With advancing age, an individual's risk will increase, and may rise to levels that warrant intervention. Based on figures from the Health Survey for England (Colhoun et al, 1998), it is estimated that about 28% of the male population and 7% of the female population of England are at greater than a 15% 10-year risk of a coronary event.

As most relevant interventions such as smoking cessation, blood pressure control and reducing blood cholesterol reduce both coronary heart disease and stroke, risk factor modification is really about reducing *cardiovascular disease* rather than just coronary heart disease alone. Multiplying the calculated coronary heart disease risk by 4/3 gives a reasonable estimate of overall *cardiovascular* risk (Ramsey et al, 1999).

THE MAJOR CARDIOVASCULAR RISK FACTORS

AGE

Mortality from coronary heart disease rises steeply with increasing age, approximately dou-

bling every 5 years. The incidence of new and recurrent heart attacks also increases with age, and most coronary events occur in the elderly. Although it is assumed that the increase in frequency of heart disease in old age is part of the ageing process, it is probably due to a cumulative effect of exposure to known modifiable risk factors such as smoking, hyperlipidaemia and hypertension over the years, rather than simple degeneration.

Because the absolute risk of cardiovascular disease is higher in the elderly, risk factor modification should have a greater effect than in the same interventions in younger age groups. Hypertension trials consistently confirm benefits in lowering blood pressure in patients up to 80 years of age, and the Medical Research Council/ British Heart Foundation Heart Protection Study (Heart Protection Study Group, 2002) has now shown benefits of cholesterol-lowering with simvastatin in patients up to 80 years of age.

SEX

Coronary heart disease has been thought to be primarily a problem that affects men, and, indeed, the absolute risk is lower at all ages in women until old age, when levels of risk converge with males. The menopause marks an approximate three-fold increase in the risk of coronary heart disease, when it has been assumed that it is the lack of the protective effects of oestrogens that is mostly responsible. However, hormone replacement therapy does not seem to be protective (Hulley et al, 1998), and what is more relevant is that after the age of 55 years many women become obese and have higher blood cholesterol and glucose concentrations than men do. There are also more women than men over the age of 65 years with hypertension. Although male cardiovascular mortality has fallen in the USA since 1980, it has steadily increased in women and now exceeds that in men. This aspect of women's health is often ignored, but half the female population die from heart attack or stroke but less than 4% from breast cancer. Women are poorly represented in risk factor modification trials, but, despite a paucity of supportive evidence, current recommendations make no distinction between men and women.

RACE

Atherosclerosis and coronary heart disease affect all races, but there are marked international differences in the occurrence of coronary heart disease, even allowing for the differences made in disease classification by various countries. The rates of coronary heart disease are very high in those of South Asian origin (India, Bangladesh, Pakistan and Sri Lanka), intermediate in those of European origin (North greater than South) and lowest in those from Africa and China. However, at any given time, different countries are at varying stages of epidemiological transition, with adverse life-style changes that accompany industrialisation and urbanisation. Further, as life expectancy increases, the duration of exposure to risk factors increases. It is thus unclear whether the variation of coronary heart disease in different races is due to environmental or genetic factors. In general, migrants who move from low-risk to high-risk areas change their risk of cardiovascular disease to that of the host country, although, with prolonged exposure to the environment, disease rates tend to return to those of their country of origin. The metabolic response to various risk factors may therefore differ in different populations, and adapt with time.

Risk-assessment tables should be used with caution when assessing patients from ethnic minorities, as the Framingham equation has not been validated in these populations.

GENETIC PREDISPOSITION

Mortality from coronary heart disease in the UK fell by 42% in the years 1987–1997. This large decline can only be explained by changes in prevention and treatment, since alterations in the genetic structure of the population cannot have taken place sufficiently fast to account for such dramatic changes. Nevertheless, it is clear that genetic influences are of importance in the aetiology of coronary heart disease. Coronary heart disease often aggregates in families, especially in those with maternal histories (Rissanen and Nikkila, 1979), and the presence of coronary heart disease in a first-degree relative before the age of 50 years (or 55 years in women) is a strong independent risk factor. Studies of identical and non-identical twins support a genetic influence (Berg, 1983).

Genetic factors affecting susceptibility to coronary heart disease may operate through known modifiable risk factors that run in families, such as dyslipidaemia, diabetes and hypertension, or through as yet undefined genetic mechanisms. Modern recombinant DNA technology has already ascertained the risks of some genetic diseases that increase the risk of coronary heart disease, such as familial hypercholesterolaemia, homocysteinaemia, type III and familial combined hyperlipidaemia (Jowett, 1984). Other suggested 'candidate genes' include those affecting coagulation factors, growth factors, vessel wall proteins, the insulin receptor gene, the ACE gene and the apolipoprotein AI/CIII gene cluster (Jowett et al, 1984; Rees et al, 1985). The Human Genome Project offers the possibility that we will be able to unravel most of the genetic factors that underlie coronary artery disease (Bentley, 2000).

Current cardiovascular risk-assessment tables do not consider family history. Having a family member with coronary disease is common, but for those who have a first-degree male relative with cardiovascular disease before the age of 50 years (or before the age of 55 years in a female relative) the calculated absolute risk should be multiplied by a factor of 1.5.

OBESITY

There are many causes of obesity and, unfortunately, virtually all are environmental. Affluence, familial obesity due to role modelling and eating habits with the Western sedentary life-style all contribute. The instant food market has led to instant obesity, and the increasing consumption of alcohol is also a factor. The diet in industrialised countries has changed dramatically since the 19th century, when most energy was derived from carbohydrate in cereals and potatoes. Fat consumption has increased markedly, particularly from ingestion of meat and dairy produce, and alcohol consumption is much greater. This change in diet has been associated with an increase in the prevalence of obesity. Hormonal imbalance, although a popular excuse, is rarely an underlying cause, and endocrine disorders such as hypothyroidism and Cushing's syndrome usually present with other symptoms.

There are periods of life when weight gain seems more likely. For men, this is between the ages of 35 and 40 years, after marriage, and after retirement. For women, the greatest increases in weight are between the ages of 15 and 19 years, after pregnancy and after the menopause. Asian and African populations are more prone to obesity, particularly the accumulation of abdominal fat. Once weight has been gained, it is difficult to lose; obese children are twice as likely to become obese adults.

A distinction should be made between 'average' weights and 'ideal' weights. *Average weights* are always higher in the West, where we overeat. *Ideal weights* are based on the pooled experience of life assurance companies, who have calculated desirable weight based on excess mortality figures. Subjective assessments of obesity, including the presence of central obesity, are often accurate, but a more precise method of assessment may be made by the body mass index (BMI) that adjusts the weight for height.

$$BMI = \frac{Weight\ (kg)}{Height\ (m)^2}$$

Internationally accepted ranges of BMI used to define degrees of obesity are given in Table 3.2. Since abdominal fat relates more strongly to coronary heart disease than does fat on the limbs or hips, the waist:hip ratio may be a better predictor of cardiovascular mortality than the BMI (Royal College of Physicians of London, 1998). Abdominal obesity is associated with the dysmetabolic syndrome characterised by lipid abnormalities (low HDL-cholesterol and high triglycerides), hypertension, impaired glucose tolerance and cardiovascular disease.

Measuring the waist alone may give the simplest guide to increased risk. An abdominal girth

Table 3.2 BMI ranges defining degrees of obesity (WHO, 1998)

WHO classification	BMI (kg/m²)	Health risk
Underweight	<18.5	Low (but may indicate other health problems)
Normal	18.5–24.9	Average ('ideal' weight)
Overweight	25.0–29.9	Mild increase
Obese	>30.0	
• Class I	30.0–34.9	Moderate
• Class II	35.0–39.9	Severe
• Class III	>40.0	Very severe

of over 102 cm (40 inches) in men and over 88 cm (35 inches) in women should alert the clinician that intervention is required.

Obesity is now recognised as a cardiovascular risk factor in its own right, since there is a progressive increase in the incidence of chronic diseases such as hypertension, diabetes and coronary heart disease with an increasing BMI (World Health Organization, 1998). Overweight individuals also have higher serum cholesterol concentrations and take less exercise.

Other risks of obesity are obstructive sleep apnoea, osteoarthritis of weight-bearing joints, accidental injury and a number of different cancers (e.g. breast, prostatic and colorectal). Respiratory symptoms, varicose veins, depression, hernias and gallstones are all more frequent.

On average, life expectancy is decreased by 15% for every 10% excess of ideal body weight; obesity must therefore be viewed as a serious medical condition rather than a concern surrounding current fashion.

In England, about 46% of men and 32% of women are overweight, and an additional 28% of men and 27% of women are obese. This situation is deteriorating rapidly, and the number of adults who are clinically obese has doubled since 1985. If the 'Health of the Nation' targets set by the Secretary of State for Health in 1992, of reducing the prevalence of obesity down to 6% in men and 8% in women, had been achieved, 2% of the deaths in the UK could have been prevented (Britton and McPherson, 2000).

BLOOD LIPIDS AND LIPOPROTEINS

The major lipids are triglycerides and cholesterol. Cholesterol forms an integral cell membrane component. Triglycerides are stored energy reserves found predominantly in adipose tissue, and are the main vehicles for the transport of fatty acids. Fatty acids are carried from the liver and intestine to the tissues (including the myocardium) for energy, and to the endothelium for prostaglandin synthesis.

Lipids are insoluble in water; thus, in order for them to be transported in blood, they are converted to water-soluble complexes called lipoproteins. The main lipoproteins are:

- *Chylomicrons*: the largest lipoprotein; they consist mainly of dietary triglycerides absorbed by the small intestine.
- *Low-density lipoproteins (LDL)*: the main transport vehicle for cholesterol.
- *Very low-density lipoproteins (VLDL)*: small, triglyceride-rich lipoproteins; they transport lipids synthesised mainly in the liver.
- *High-density lipoproteins (HDL)*: the smallest lipoproteins; they contain cholesterol transported away from cells to the liver.

There is a clear correlation between raised serum cholesterol levels and the risk of coronary heart disease (Law et al, 1994), the relationship being virtually linear with no threshold value (Fig. 3.3). Even in China, a country with very low population levels of serum cholesterol, there is still a linear relationship between coronary heart disease risk at total cholesterol concentrations under 3.5 mmol/l. There is thus no such thing as a 'normal' serum cholesterol level; for every 1% increase in the level of total cholesterol there is a 2–3% increase in the incidence of coronary artery disease.

The average level of serum cholesterol in different populations roughly predicts the risk of coronary heart disease in that population: the higher the average cholesterol, the higher the risk. Furthermore, populations with high numbers of other risk factors but a low serum cholesterol still have a relatively low incidence of coronary heart disease. For example, smoking

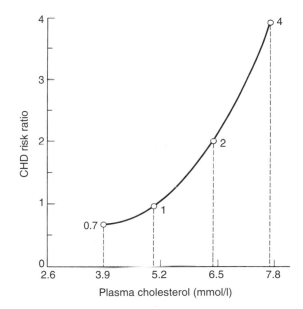

Figure 3.3 Relationship of plasma cholesterol concentrations to mortality, based on a $7\frac{1}{2}$-year follow-up of 17 718 men in the Whitehall study. CHD, coronary heart disease. (Data from Rose and Shipley, 1980.)

and hypertension are frequent in Japan, but serum cholesterol is low, as is the mortality from coronary heart disease. Cholesterol appears to be the permissive factor without which other risk factors have little impact.

The UK population has amongst the highest serum cholesterol concentrations in the world; where the mean serum cholesterol is about 5.5 mmol/l, with over half the population exceeding the 'optimal' level of 5.0 mmol/l (Dong, 1996), including those on treatment!

Although a high total plasma cholesterol concentration is a very strong risk factor for coronary heart disease, the risk actually depends on the concentration of LDL-cholesterol. Low levels of HDL-cholesterol also predict coronary mortality; high levels of HDL-cholesterol (particularly the HDL_2 subfraction) are negatively correlated with atheromatous disease. Low levels of HDL are often associated with other risk factors, such as lack of exercise, diabetes, obesity and cigarette smoking; raised HDL levels are often found in pre-menopausal women, joggers and moderate, regular drinkers of alcohol.

LDL-cholesterol concentrations can be measured in the laboratory, but the assay is expensive. Hence, it is usually estimated by the Friedewald formula:

$$\text{LDL-cholesterol (mmol/l)} = (\text{Total cholesterol} - \text{HDL-cholesterol}) - (\text{Triglyceride} \times 0.45)$$

The Friedewald formula cannot be used if the triglyceride concentration is more than 4.5 mmol/l, and such a finding should lead to a search for an underlying cause, such as excess alcohol, diabetes or obesity. Low HDL-cholesterol and high LDL-cholesterol levels are the major associates of atherosclerotic disease, and a ratio of these two lipoproteins of less than 0.2 appears to be an important predictor of coronary heart disease.

Abnormal concentrations of lipids in the blood are referred to as hyperlipidaemia, and some of them predispose to coronary heart disease (dyslipidaemia). Hyperlipidaemia is often familial and is usually diagnosed by exclusion of known underlying causes of raised serum lipids, the most common of which are diabetes, thyroid disease, renal disease, cholestasis, alcohol and drugs (Jowett and Galton, 1987). Atheromatous plaques progress more quickly in the presence of high serum cholesterol, and successful lipid-lowering may lead to regression of atheroma (Thompson, 1992). In the West of Scotland Coronary Prevention Study (WOSCOPS), healthy adults with blood cholesterol concentrations of between 6.5 and 8.0 mmol/l had reduced cardiovascular mortality when taking pravastatin (Shepherd et al, 1995). The Air Force/Texas Coronary Atherosclerosis Prevention Study (AFCAPS/TEXCAPS) additionally showed that reducing 'normal' cholesterol levels (4.7–6.8 mmol/l) in healthy adults associated with a 37% reduction in non-fatal myocardial infarction and unstable angina as well as in the need for revascularisation (Downs et al, 1998).

The role of hypertriglyceridaemia in the aetiology of coronary heart disease is a little harder to interpret. Although high levels associate with the risk of ischaemic heart disease, this is not an independent risk factor. This is because hypertriglyceridaemia is normally associated with raised LDL-cholesterol and reduced HDL-cholesterol concentrations. Triglyceride levels appear to be more strongly correlated with coronary heart disease risk in women than in men. It is important to detect severe hypertriglyceridaemia, as it may cause acute pancreatitis and can draw attention to other cardiovascular risk factors, such as diabetes and obesity.

Screening for hyperlipidaemia

Hyperlipidaemia is usually asymptomatic and is ordinarily detected by screening, either opportunistically or selectively. There is no evidence to show that routine population screening is cost-effective. Knowledge of one's serum cholesterol concentration may also have unpredictable results. A study of male factory workers found that only half of those who were found to have raised concentrations on routine screening were willing to accept that their result was abnormal. The remainder responded by denial, and refused to make changes to their diet or life-style (Irvine and Logan, 1994).

Selective screening should be offered to those with other cardiovascular risk factors, those with strong family histories of cardiovascular disease, and of course familial hyperlipidaemia. Both the total and HDL-cholesterol concentrations are used to calculate the 10-year risk for coronary heart disease.

Family screening

Many of the primary hyperlipidaemias are familial, and lipoprotein abnormalities may be found in the patient's relations. Measurement of serum lipids should be offered to first-degree relatives of patients with marked hyperlipidaemia, particularly younger males, for whom early therapy will be of most value. This is especially important in monogenic familial hypercholesterolaemia, a dominantly inherited disorder that carries a high risk of early cardiovascular morbidity and death (ten times that of the WOSCOPS population). Familial hypercholesterolaemia affects 1 in 500 of the UK population, and is caused by mutations of the LDL-receptor gene. Typically the patient has a cholesterol concentration over 9 mmol/l, together with cutaneous signs such as an early corneal arcus and tendon xanthomata. Early diagnosis and therapy offer the best hope of improving cardiovascular prognosis.

Screening tests for hyperlipidaemia

The most commonly employed screening test is random serum cholesterol estimation. A non-fasting HDL is sometimes also added, and is needed to assess absolute risk for coronary heart disease. This is particularly true in women, who frequently maintain high HDL-cholesterol levels long after the menopause. In addition, a low HDL-cholesterol is often found in the presence of other risk factors, particularly diabetes, and relying on total cholesterol alone may be misleading. If the total cholesterol is less than 5 mmol/l, there is usually no need for further analysis, unless there is suspicion of another abnormality, such as low HDL-cholesterol or hypertriglyceridaemia. If the random cholesterol is greater than 5 mmol/l, or if there is likely to be another lipid abnormality, total cholesterol, HDL-cholesterol and triglyceride levels should be measured in a sample of venous blood taken, preferably without venous stasis, after an overnight (12-h) fast. Because of the biological and laboratory variability of cholesterol concentrations, a reliable estimate requires at least three separate fasting estimations. Some centres would further explore the index of risk by measuring *apolipoprotein* levels. There are at least ten of these structural parts of the lipoprotein particle. Each is involved with a specific lipoprotein and is concerned with its transport, activation or receptor recognition. Apo A-1 and Apo B are the major apolipoproteins of HDL and LDL, respectively, and increased concentrations may be more predictive of coronary disease than HDL- or LDL-cholesterol levels alone. Lipoprotein(a) is an LDL-like lipoprotein, that has structural similarities to plasminogen, and increased levels may associate with increased cardiovascular risk. Supportive evidence has been conflicting, and no trial has yet looked at the effects of reducing lipoprotein(a) concentrations (Harjai, 1999).

It should be noted that acute illness such as infection, trauma (including surgery) and myocardial infarction might alter serum lipoprotein concentrations so that they are not representative of the patient's baseline values. For example, for about 3 months after acute myocardial infarction, plasma triglycerides may be higher and total cholesterol lower than pre-infarction levels (Brugada et al, 1996).

There is now strong evidence that decreasing serum cholesterol is effective in the primary prevention of coronary heart disease (Shepherd et al, 1995; Downs et al, 1998). As a minimum, treatment should now be offered to those with a coronary heart disease risk of over 3% per year, hopefully being extended to those at a risk of 1.5% per year when resources allow. The recommended threshold for medical intervention is total cholesterol of 5 mmol/l, or LDL-cholesterol of over 3 mmol/l (Wood et al, 1998), marking the level above which there is a marked rise in atherosclerotic cardiovascular events, notably coronary heart disease (Fig. 3.3). An approach to management of blood lipids in primary prevention of

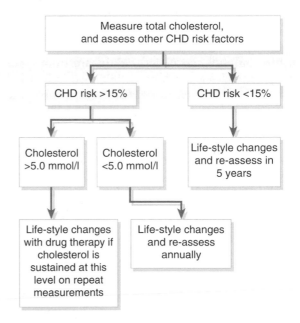

Figure 3.4 Absolute coronary heart disease (CHD) risk and management of blood lipids in primary prevention of CHD and other atherosclerotic disease over 10 years. (Reproduced with permission of BMJ Publishing Group from Wood D, Durrington P, Poulter N et al (1998) Joint British recommendations on prevention of coronary heart disease in clinical practice. *Heart*, **80** (Suppl 2): S15.)

coronary heart disease and other atherosclerotic disease is shown in Fig. 3.4 and is based upon random total cholesterol estimation and the patient's absolute risk.

SMOKING

The human burden of premature morbidity and mortality caused by smoking is immense. No other single avoidable cause of disease accounts for such a high proportion of deaths, hospital admissions or consultations with general practitioners. Cigarette smoking remains the single most important public health issue in the UK, and has been for at least 400 years when, in 1604, King James 1st of England (James VI of Scotland) produced a paper entitled 'Counterblaste to Tobacco'. He noted that smoking was a 'custome loathsome to the eye, hateful to the nose, harmful to the brain and dangerous to the lungs'. Little did the Monarch realise that, four centuries later, more than half of all smoking-related deaths would still be due to respiratory disease, with an additional 7000 deaths from cerebrovascular disease. It was much later that the link with heart disease was made, and we now know that nearly a fifth of smoking-related deaths are from coronary heart disease (Callum, 1998). An individual who smokes 20 cigarettes/day has double the risk of coronary death, and a five-fold increased risk of premature cardiac death (Freund et al, 1993). The risk increases proportionally with the number of cigarettes smoked, and appears to be greater for women (Prescott et al, 1998). A quarter of all smokers will die before the age of 65 years.

Tobacco smoke is a complex aerosol containing two implicated cardiovascular toxins: nicotine and carbon monoxide.

1. *Nicotine*. Nicotine absorption during smoking varies from about 5% to 100%, depending upon smoking patterns; a heavy smoker may absorb about 100 mg of nicotine per day. Nicotine stimulates catecholamine release, and increases myocardial work by raising heart rate, blood pressure and force of myocardial contraction. Additionally, there is a thrombogenic action caused by inhibition of fibrinolysis, and an increase in platelet aggregation and stickiness.

2. *Carbon monoxide*. Carbon monoxide is a cellular poison and makes up about 3–6% of inhaled cigarette smoke. This is eight times the maximum air pollution allowed in industry! It binds 200 times more readily with haemoglobin than does oxygen, which it displaces to form carboxyhaemoglobin. Typically, the haemoglobin of a heavy smoker will be 20% carboxylated, which shifts the oxygen dissociation curve to the left, thereby impairing oxygen release in tissues. Oxygenation is therefore reduced, despite increased myocardial requirements due to nicotinic stimulation. Carbon monoxide may additionally cause endothelial dysfunction, increasing permeability to foam cells and predisposing to atheroma.

The cardiovascular risks of pipe and cigar smoke are variable, but if inhaled is probably not very different to the risks produced by cigarette smoke. The hazards to pipe and cigar smokers who have never smoked cigarettes is thought to be less, because smoking patterns usually differ, with reduced intake of smoke into the lungs. Former cigarette smokers who switch to cigars or a pipe do not reduce their risk of cardiovascular events, presumably because of the tendency to inhale the smoke more like a cigarette. It is also worth noting that self-reports on the depth of inhalation of smoke are extremely inaccurate.

Until recently, the number of adult smokers in the UK has been falling to around 28% of men and 26% of women. Of concern is that smoking in teenagers has increased, and those who start smoking before the age of 20 years increase their cardiovascular risk by 3–5 times (Ball and Turner, 1974). In 1998, 9% of English boys and 11% of girls aged 11–15 years were found to be regular smokers.

About 119 000 men and women die prematurely from smoking-related diseases every year in the UK. Myocardial infarction and sudden death occur 2–4 times more frequently in smokers than in non-smokers (Friedman et al, 1979), and, overall, the risk of death from coronary heart disease is twice that of non-smokers. Apart from cardiovascular causes, smoking contributes to the 24 000 deaths due to bronchitis and to the

30 000 lung cancers. An estimated 21 million working days are also lost due to smoking-related sickness every year.

Passive smoking (also known as involuntary or second-hand smoking) is a term applied to breathing other people's smoke, and is recognised as a significant public health issue since it increases cardiovascular risk by about 20% (Law et al, 1997). About 1% of lung cancer deaths are due to passive smoking. Exposure to cigarette smoke for as little as 30 min can have detrimental effects on the hearts of non-smokers, which is why non-smoking should be considered normal and special provision should be made for smokers, rather than vice versa. Children living in smoking households may 'smoke' up to 150 cigarettes each year, contributing to childhood asthma, chronic chest infections and middle ear infections and probably predisposing them to accelerated atherosclerosis. Treatment of these children costs the NHS an estimated £410 million in England and Wales alone. Passive smoking in the workplace is a major health issue, as well as the effects on lost productivity through sickness-related absences.

Stopping smoking reduces cardiovascular risk by 50% within 2–3 years, and by 10 years the level of risk is similar to that of non-smokers (Doll and Peto, 1976). In England, new targets were announced in the Government's '*Smoking Kills*' document (Department of Health, 1998) aiming to reduce smoking to 26% in adults and to 11% in children by 2005.

HYPERTENSION

Individuals with blood pressure levels at the upper limits of the population distribution of blood pressure have an increased incidence of atherosclerotic, thrombotic and haemorrhagic vascular disease, and an increased morbidity and mortality due to stroke, myocardial infarction and peripheral vascular disease. Overall, hypertension is associated with a two- to three-fold increase in mortality from coronary heart disease. The distribution of blood pressure values in the population is a continuum, and the cut-off point above which patients are considered

hypertensive is arbitrary. Blood pressure levels in the UK are generally high; the mean systolic blood pressure for men in England is about 137 mmHg and for women 133 mmHg. About 41% of men and 33% of women have a blood pressure above 140/90, or are being treated for hypertension. Blood pressure rises with age, and more rapidly after the age of 45 years.

Although rising levels of both systolic and diastolic blood pressure increase the risk of death, the systolic blood pressure is the better predictor of subsequent cardiovascular disease. Isolated systolic hypertension is a particular problem in the elderly, and remains poorly recognised and poorly treated. The importance of isolated systolic hypertension as a risk factor seems to be underestimated, perhaps due to overemphasis on the diastolic pressure in the past (Wilkinson et al, 2000). Ageing is associated with atherosclerotic hardening of the arteries, which causes a raised systolic blood pressure, but a fall in diastolic blood pressure, and hence a widening of the pulse pressure. There is gathering interest in using the pulse pressure as an index of arterial stiffness, which in turn may be a major prognostic indicator of cardiovascular disease.

The risk of hypertension is not uniform: it is higher in those with other risk factors. Once hypertension has induced target organ damage, the risks are greater, and the development of left ventricular hypertrophy associates with a particularly poor prognosis.

The recent British Hypertension Society guidelines support initiation of treatment on the level of overall cardiovascular risk rather than on an arbitrarily designated level of blood pressure (Ramsey et al, 1999). This runs contrary to other international hypertension guidelines (World Health Organization, 1994; Joint National Committee, 1997), which still recommend treatment for all patients if there is sustained elevation of blood pressure of 140–159/90–99 mmHg, regardless of co-existent risk factors. The guidelines from the British Hypertension Society are summarized in Fig. 3.5 and give details of the management of blood pressure in primary prevention of coronary heart disease in relationship

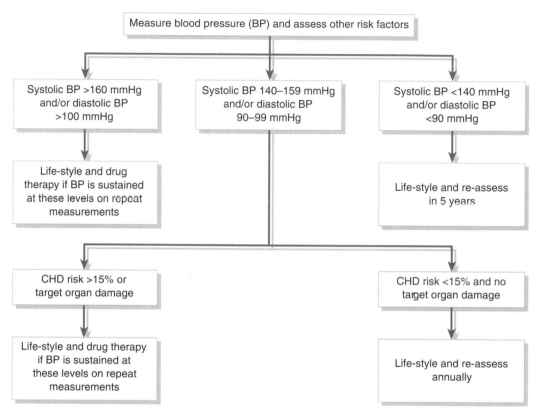

Figure 3.5 Management of blood pressure in primary prevention of cardiovascular disease according to level of absolute coronary heart disease (CHD) risk over 10 years. (Reproduced with permission of BMJ Publishing Group from Wood D, Durrington P, Poulter N et al (1998) Joint British recommendations on prevention of coronary heart disease in clinical practice. *Heart*, **80** (Suppl 2):S18.)

to absolute risk. Mindful of the strong relationship between blood pressure and the risk of stroke, they further suggest that targeting cardiovascular disease rather than just coronary heart disease is preferable, and adjustments can be made by multiplying the coronary heart disease risk by 4/3. The British Hypertension Society also emphasizes that average sustained systolic blood pressures greater than 160 mmHg and diastolic pressures greater than 100 mmHg (90 mmHg in the elderly) are undesirable, regardless of absolute coronary heart disease risk.

Current thresholds and treatment targets for antihypertensive drug treatment may thus be summarized as follows:

- Drug therapy should be started in all patients with sustained systolic blood pressures of over 160 mmHg and/or diastolic blood

pressures over 100 mmHg despite non-pharmacological measures.

- Drug treatment is also indicated in patients with sustained blood pressures of 140–159 mmHg and/or diastolic blood pressures of 90–99 mmHg if target organ damage is present, or if there is established evidence of cardiovascular disease, or diabetes, or the 10-year coronary heart disease risk is more than 15%.

- For most patients, a treatment target of under 140 mmHg systolic and less than 85 mmHg diastolic pressure is recommended. A lower target of under 140/80 is recommended in patients with diabetes (Table 3.3).

National surveys reveal incomplete treatment and control of hypertension. In 1994, it was estimated that approximately half of treated hyper-

Table 3.3 Target blood pressure during antihypertensive treatment (Ramsey et al, 1999)

Blood pressure (mmHg)	Measurement in clinic		Mean daytime ambulatory measurement or home measurement	
	No diabetes	With diabetes	No diabetes	With diabetes
Optimal	<140/85	<140/80	<130/80	<130/75
Audit standard[a]	<150/90	<140/85	<140/85	<140/80

[a]The audit standard reflects the minimum recommended target for blood pressure control.

tensive patients in the UK had inadequately controlled blood pressure (Colhoun et al, 1998), and a major audit in seven other European countries yielded the same results, with a wide divergence of opinions and actual practice of physicians (World Health Organization, 1994). In the USA, the attitude to hypertension is changing, which is reflected in terms of awareness, screening, investigation and management. Over 75% of American patients with hypertension are aware of their diagnosis, and, what is more, the number taking effective antihypertensive treatment has risen from 4 million to 12 million.

DIABETES AND GLUCOSE INTOLERANCE

Patients with diabetes mellitus, particularly type 2 diabetes, are at substantially increased risk of coronary heart disease, being perhaps 2–4 times in men and 3–5 times in women. Importantly, type 2 diabetes should no longer be regarded as 'maturity-onset', as it is now appearing in much younger subjects, and already accounts for one-third of newly diagnosed patients with diabetes under 20 years of age in some parts of the USA (Fagot-Campagna et al, 2000). Around 3% of the adult population in England are known to have diabetes, but numbers are increasing. Since 1991, prevalence has increased by two-thirds in men and a quarter in women. Worldwide, the number of adults with diabetes is predicted to increase to 300 million by 2025 (King et al, 1998).

In the past, the diagnostic criteria for diabetes have been based on predisposition to microvascular complications (e.g. retinopathy, renal disease). However, over 70% of patients with diabetes die from macrovascular disease (mainly coronary heart disease); even asymptomatic hyperglycaemia is an independent risk factor for major coronary events (Shaper et al, 1985). As a consequence, diagnostic criteria for diabetes have been redefined to try and capture all those with impaired glucose tolerance because of their increased risk of macrovascular disease (World Health Organization, 1999). Patients with hyperglycaemia may be broadly classified as having:

- Type 1 diabetes (previously called insulin-dependent diabetes mellitus)
- Type 2 diabetes (previously called non-insulin-dependent diabetes mellitus)
- Impaired glucose tolerance
- Impaired fasting glucose.

Diagnosing diabetes

Diagnosis may be based on a fasting or random blood glucose, but may need a formal 75-g oral glucose-tolerance test (OGTT).

In patients *with symptoms* (polyuria, polydipsia, weight loss, etc.), diabetes is confirmed with:

- A random plasma glucose greater than 11.1 mmol/l *or*
- A fasting plasma glucose greater than 7.0 mmol/l *or*
- 2-h plasma glucose greater than 11.1 mmol/l following a formal OGTT.

In patients *without symptoms*, the tests should be repeated at least once at another time. A random glucose of under 5.5 mmol/l usually excludes glucose intolerance.

- Patients with *impaired glucose tolerance* have twice the risk of developing large vessel atheroma compared to those with normal glucose tolerance. They are identified by having a fasting plasma glucose under 7 mmol/l but a 2-h post-OGTT of more than 7.8 mmol/l (but less than 11.1 mmol/l).

- Patients with *impaired fasting glucose* are not at increased risk of cardiovascular disease, but may develop diabetes, and its risks in the future. They are defined as having a fasting plasma glucose over 6.1 mmol/l but less than 7 mmol/l. These patients need an OGTT to exclude diabetes.

Most diabetic patients are overweight, and the rise in the incidence of type 2 diabetes in the young is largely due to increasing obesity (World Health Organization, 1998). Since weight reduction improves glucose tolerance, diabetes remains one of the strongest modifiable risk factors for cardiovascular disease.

Hypertension is very common in type 2 diabetes, and may be present at diagnosis in nearly 40% of patients. It is highly predictive of cardiovascular complications in this group of patients. Trials such as the United Kingdom Prospective Diabetes Study (UKPDS, 1998) and the HOT trial (Hansson et al, 1998) support reducing blood pressure in patients with diabetes to under 130/80 if there are diabetic complications, or if the calculated annual coronary heart disease risk is over 1.5%. Similarly, cholesterol-lowering agents are indicated for those with total cholesterol concentrations over 5 mmol/l, although the Heart Protection Study now suggests that the threshold may be as low as 3.6 mmol/l. The results of specific cholesterol-lowering trials in patients with diabetes are awaited.

EXERCISE

Whereas, in the past, the manual worker was protected from the effects of a sedentary occupation, the advent of mechanical aids, including the car, conveyor belts, lifts and other devices, has minimized the amount of exercise taken, even by manual workers. The risk of coronary heart disease amongst sedentary people has nearly doubled, and, since 60% of men and 70% of women can be classed as sedentary in the UK,

the attributable risk from physical inactivity to the population is very high.

It is hard to demonstrate the benefits of exercise, since observations may simply reflect a generally healthier life-style in those who take regular exercise. However, those who engage in vigorous sports and keep-fit exercises have half the incidence of fatal and non-fatal coronary events compared with those who do not (Morris et al, 1980). This remains the case regardless of age or the presence of other risk factors. To produce the maximum cardiovascular benefit, the activity needs to be regular and aerobic. The UK government recommends that adults should participate in a minimum of 30 min of accumulated moderate activity on at least 5 days every week (Britton and McPherson, 2000). Moderate intensity is defined as energy expenditure of 5–7.5 kcal/min, and equates to a brisk walk for half an hour. The protective effect of exercise seems to be particularly related to current rather than previous exercise habits.

MINOR RISK FACTORS

PSYCHOSOCIAL WELL-BEING

Four different types of psychosocial factors have been found to be associated with an increased risk of coronary heart disease:

- Stress (especially work-related)
- Anxiety and depression
- Lack of social support
- Personality (especially hostility).

Although many sufferers from coronary heart disease believe that stress must have played a part in their illness, we really do not know its role. The definition and measurement of stress are not easy, although acute mental stress, anger or excitement can precipitate angina. It may be that similar events could lead to transient elevation of blood pressure, which could be the stimulus for producing a dysrhythmia or plaque rupture and hence myocardial infarction, heart failure or sudden death. Stressful life-events often precede admission to coronary care (Solomon et al, 1969).

The influence of personality factors on the incidence of coronary heart disease has become a subject of increasing interest (Hemingway and Marmot, 1999; Whiteman et al, 1997). Amongst the personality traits related to ischaemic heart disease are aggression, hostility and anxiety, or so-called 'type A' behaviour (Friedman and Rosenman, 1959). Type A characteristics include abrupt gestures, hurried speech, impatience, tenseness and rapid, illegible handwriting. There is an intense striving for achievement, competitiveness, time-urgency, being easily provoked and impatient, with over-commitment to vocation or profession and excessive drive. 'Type B' behaviour, in contrast, is characterised by a relaxed, unhurried, satisfied life-style. Neither is a fixed personality trait. Although the type A behaviour pattern may constitute an independent risk factor for coronary heart disease, there is no relation between type A behaviour and the course of coronary heart disease following acute myocardial infarction (Case et al, 1985). In addition, type A behaviour has not been found to relate to new cardiac events in British men, although it is more common in those with ECG or questionnaire evidence of coronary heart disease (Johnston et al, 1987). It might be that type A behaviour confers a risk only in collaboration with other behavioural or psychological factors that result in increased sympathetic (catecholamine) activity that may act as a trigger for plaque rupture.

The 1994 Health Survey for England used a questionnaire to assess levels of depression, anxiety, sleep disturbance and happiness (Colhoun et al, 1998). Higher levels of psychological distress were found in women, and those living in London.

URIC ACID

A high blood uric acid level (with or without gout) is possibly an independent risk factor for coronary heart disease. However, those prone to hyperuricaemia and gout are usually overweight, with co-existent hyperlipidaemia and glucose intolerance.

ALCOHOL

Observational studies consistently show an inverse or U-shaped relationship between alcohol intake and death from coronary heart disease (Thun et al, 1997). Moderate drinking of perhaps 1–2 drinks/day, particularly of wine, is associated with a 20% reduction in coronary events, which is lower than those who do not drink alcohol (Department of Health, 1995). This may be because alcohol ingestion raises HDL-cholesterol levels, inhibits platelets and can ameliorate stress (Steinberg et al, 1991). Alcoholics and heavy drinkers (over 4 units/day) have an increased cardiac mortality, particularly binge-drinkers. This may be due to a hypertensive effect.

HORMONAL FACTORS

An early study from the Royal College of General Practitioners (1974) found that the incidence of myocardial infarction was three times higher in women who used the oral contraceptive pill. Since then, the second- and third-generation contraceptive pills have reduced the hormonal intake, and the risk of myocardial infarction in women taking a modern combined oral contraceptive seems to be increased only in association with additional risk factors. Oral contraception is therefore contraindicated in the presence of severe or multiple cardiovascular risk factors (World Health Organization, 1997). Limited data suggest that progesterone-only pills may be suitable in this group, but will need careful monitoring.

The effect of hormone replacement therapy (HRT) on the course of cardiovascular risk is unclear (Findlay et al, 1994). Work since the 1950s has supported the role of oestrogen in the prevention of atherosclerosis, but more recent trials have been based upon oestrogen given with progesterone, as in most forms of HRT (Stampfer and Colditz, 1992). The results of the Heart and Estrogen/Progestin Replacement Study (HERS) showed no benefit of HRT in secondary prevention of coronary heart disease in postmenopausal women (Hulley et al, 1998). However, the results did suggest that women already taking HRT at the time of their myocardial infarction might benefit from continuation.

THE CARDIOVASCULAR DYSMETABOLIC SYNDROME

The cardiovascular dysmetabolic syndrome (metabolic syndrome, syndrome X or Reaven's syndrome) describes patients with insulin resistance, central obesity, glucose intolerance, hypertension, hypertriglyceridaemia and depressed HDL-cholesterol levels (Fagan and Deedwania, 1998). The common aetiological factor is insulin resistance, which can be present for up to 10 years before glucose intolerance declares itself (Reaven, 1993). Early management of obesity may help prevent diabetes and cardiovascular disease.

HOMOCYSTEINE

Homocysteine is derived from the metabolism of methionine, an essential amino acid that is found primarily in dietary animal protein. Blood concentrations are determined by genetic and nutritional factors, particularly vitamins B_6, B_{12} and folic acid. In 1969, McCulley reported that children with the rare genetic disorder homocysteinuria, who have very high blood levels of homocysteine, developed widespread severe atherosclerosis. Since then, many studies have demonstrated that a high blood concentration of homocysteine is an independent risk factor for atherosclerotic vascular disease and venous thrombosis (Refsum et al, 1998). Homocysteine concentrations rise with age, and are associated with smoking, a sedentary life-style and high intakes of alcohol and caffeine. Blood levels exceeding the upper limit of normal (15 µmol/l) are common, being found in up to a third of patients with vascular disease. What is not known is whether homocysteine has a causal role in the development of atherosclerosis, or whether it is simply a marker for increased vascular risk (Dudman, 1999). Physiological studies show that elevated homocysteine concentrations induce vascular endothelial dysfunction (an early manifestation of atherosclerosis), which lends support to the hypothesis that the relationship between hyperhomocysteinaemia and vascular disease is causal. Plasma homocysteine concentrations can be reduced by 25–30% by oral supplements of vitamin B_6, B_{12} and folate, but it is not known whether reducing homocysteine levels reduces cardiovascular risk and outcome. Large randomised placebo-controlled trials are underway, and are expected to report by 2005. In the meantime, routine measurement of plasma homocysteine is not recommended, but encouraging a healthy diet, rich in B vitamins and folate, for our cardiac patients would seem to be good practice.

REFERENCES

Anderson KM, Wilson PW, Odell PM et al (1991) An updated coronary risk profile: a statement for health professionals. *Circulation*, **83:** 356–362.

Ball K, Turner R (1974) Smoking and the heart. The basis for action. *Lancet*, **ii:** 822–826.

Bentley DR (2000) The Human Genome Project – an overview. *Medicinal Research Reviews*, **20:** 189–196.

Berg K (1983) The genetics of coronary heart disease. In: Steinberg AG, Bearner AG, Motulsky AG et al (eds). *Progress in Medical Genetics*, vol V. Philadelphia: WB Saunders. pp. 52–68.

Britton A, McPherson K (2000) *Monitoring the Progress of the 2010 Target for Coronary Heart Disease Mortality: Estimated Consequences on CHD Incidence and Mortality from Changing Prevalence of Risk Factors*. National Heart Forum: London.

Brugada R, Wenger NK, Jacobson TA et al (1996) Changes in plasma cholesterol levels after hospitalization for acute coronary events. *Cardiology*, **87:** 194–199.

Callum C (1998) *The UK Smoking Epidemic: Deaths in 1995*. London: Health Education Authority.

Case RB, Heller SS, Case NB et al (1985) Type A behavior and survival after acute myocardial infarction. *New England Journal of Medicine*, **312:** 737–741.

Colhoun HM, Dong W, Poulter NR (1998) Blood pressure screening, management and control in England, results from the Health Survey for England 1994. *Journal of Hypertension*, **16:** 747–753.

Criqui MH (1986) Epidemiology of atherosclerosis: an updated overview. *American Journal of Cardiology*, **57:** 18C–23C.

Dawber TR (1980) *The Framingham Study. The Epidemiology of Atherosclerotic Disease*. Cambridge, MA: Harvard International Press.

Department of Health (1995) *Sensible Drinking. The Report of an Inter-Departmental Working Group*. London: The Stationery Office.

Department of Health (1998) *Smoking Kills. A White Paper on Tobacco*. London: The Stationery Office.

Doll R, Peto R (1976) Mortality in relation to smoking. 20 years observations in British male doctors. *BMJ*, **4**: 1525–1536.

Dong W (1996) *Health Survey for England 1994*. London, HMSO.

Downs JR, Clearfield M, Weis S et al (1998) Primary prevention of acute coronary events with lovastatin in men and women with average cholesterol levels: results of the AFCAPS/TexCAPS. Air Force/Texas coronary atherosclerosis prevention study. *JAMA*, **279**: 1615–1622.

Dudman NP (1999) An alternative view of homocysteine. *Lancet*, **254**: 2072–2074.

Fagan TC, Deedwania PC (1998) The cardiovascular dysmetabolic syndrome. *American Journal of Medicine*, **105**: 77S–82S.

Fagot-Campagna A, Petit DJ, Engelgan MM et al (2000) Type 2 diabetes among North American children and adolescents: an epidemiological review and a public health perspective. *Journal of Pediatrics*, **136**: 664–672.

Findlay I, Cunningham D, Dargie H J (1994) Coronary heart disease, the menopause and hormone replacement therapy. *British Heart Journal*, **71**: 213–214.

Freund KM, Belanger AJ, D'Agostino RB et al (1993) The health risks of smoking. The Framingham Study: 34 years of follow up. *Annals of Epidemiology*, **3**: 417–424.

Friedman M, Rosenman RH (1959) Association of specific overt behaviour pattern with blood and cardiovascular findings. *JAMA*, **169**: 1286–1296.

Friedman DG, Dales LG, Ury HK (1979) Mortality in middle aged smokers and non-smokers. *New England Journal of Medicine*, **300**: 213–217.

Hansson L, Zanchetti A, Carruthers SG et al (1998) Effects of intensive blood pressure lowering and low-dose aspirin in patients with hypertension: principal results of the hypertension optimal (HOT) randomised trial. *Lancet*, **351**: 1755–1762.

Harjai KJ (1999) Potential new cardiovascular risk factors: left ventricular hypertrophy, homocysteine, lipoprotein(a), triglycerides, oxidative stress and fibrinogen. *Annals of Internal Medicine*, **131**: 376–386.

Heart Protection Study Group (2002) MRC/BHF heart protection study of cholesterol lowering with simvastatin in 20 536 high-risk individuals: a randomised placebo-controlled trial. *Lancet*, **360**: 7–22.

Hemmingway H, Marmot M (1999) Psychosocial factors in the aetiology and prognosis of coronary heart disease. *BMJ*, **31**: 1460–1467.

Hulley SB, Grady D, Bush T et al (1998) Randomised trial of estrogen plus progestin for secondary prevention of coronary heart disease in post-menopausal women. *JAMA*, **280**: 605–613.

Irvine MJ, Logan AG (1994) Is knowing your cholesterol number harmful? *Journal of Clinical Epidemiology*, **47**: 131–145.

Jackson R (2000) Guidelines on preventing cardiovascular disease in clinical practice. *BMJ*, **320**: 659–661.

Johnston DW, Cook DG, Shaper AG (1987) Type A behaviour and ischaemic heart disease in middle aged British men. *BMJ*, **295**: 86–89.

Joint National Committee (1997) Sixth Report of the Joint National Committee on Prevention, Detection, Evaluation and Treatment of High Blood Pressure. *Annals of Internal Medicine*, **157**: 2413–2446.

Jowett NI (1984) *Recombinant DNA Gene-specific Probes and the Genetic Analysis of Diabetes, Hyperlipidaemia and Coronary Heart Disease*. MD Thesis, University of London.

Jowett NI, Galton DJ (1987) The management of the hyperlipidaemias. In: Hamer J (ed) *Drugs for Heart Disease*, 2nd edn. London: Chapman and Hall.

Jowett NI, Rees A, Caplin J et al (1984) DNA polymorphisms flanking the insulin gene and atherosclerosis. *Lancet*, **2**: 348.

King H, Aubert RE, Herman WH (1998) Global burden of diabetes, 1995–2025: prevalence, numerical estimates and projections. *Diabetes Care*, **21**: 1414–1431.

Law MR, Wald NJ, Wu T et al (1994) Systematic underestimation of association between serum cholesterol and ischaemic heart disease in observational studies: data from the BUPA study. *BMJ*, **308**: 363–366.

Law MR, Morris JK, Wald N (1997) Environmental tobacco smoke exposure and ischaemic heart disease: an evaluation of the evidence. *BMJ*, **315**: 937–980.

McCully KS (1969) Vascular pathology of homocysteinemia: implications for the development of atherosclerosis. *American Journal of Pathology*, **56**: 111–128.

Morris JN, Everitt MG, Pollard R et al (1980) Vigorous exercise in leisure time: protection against coronary heart disease. *Lancet*, **ii**: 1207–1210.

Neaton JD, Wentworth D (1992) Serum cholesterol, blood pressure, cigarette smoking and death from coronary heart disease. Overall findings and differences by age for 316,099 white men. Multiple Risk Factor Intervention Trial Research Group. *Archives of Internal Medicine*, **152**: 56–64.

Petersen S, Rayner M, Press V (2000) *Coronary Heart Disease Statistics*, 2000 edn. London: British Heart Foundation Database.

Prescott E, Hippe M, Schnohr P et al (1998) Smoking and risk of myocardial infarction in women and men: longitudinal population study. *BMJ*, **316**: 1043–1047.

Ramsey LE, Williams B, Johnston GD et al (1999) Guidelines for management of hypertension: report of the third working party of the British Hypertension Society. *Journal of Human Hypertension*, **13**: 569–592.

Reaven GM (1993) Role of insulin resistance in human disease (syndrome X): an expanded definition. *Annual Review of Medicine*, **44**: 121–131.

Rees A, Stocks J, Williams LG et al (1985) DNA polymorphism in the apolipoprotein C-III and insulin genes and atherosclerosis. *Atherosclerosis*, **58**: 269–275.

Refsum H, Ueland PM, Nygard O et al (1998) Homocysteine and cardiovascular disease. *Annual Review of Medicine*, **49**: 31–62.

Rissanen AM, Nikkila EA (1979) Aggregation of coronary risk factors in families of young men with fatal and non-fatal coronary heart disease. *British Heart Journal*, **42**: 373–380.

Rose G, Shipley MJ (1980) Plasma lipids and mortality: a source of error. *Lancet*, **i**: 523–526.

Royal College of General Practitioners (1974) *Oral Contraceptives and Health*. London: Pitman.

Royal College of Physicians of London (1998) *Clinical Management of Overweight and Obese Patients*. London: Royal College of Physicians of London.

Shaper AG, Pocock SJ, Walker M et al (1985) Risk factors for ischaemic heart disease: the prospective phase of the British Regional Heart Study. *Journal of Epidemiology and Community Health*, **39**: 197–209.

Shepherd J, Cobbe SM, Ford I for the West of Scotland Coronary Prevention Study Group (1995) Prevention of coronary heart disease with pravastatin in men with hypercholesterolaemia. *New England Journal of Medicine*, **333**: 1301–1307.

Solomon HA, Edwards AL, Killip T (1969) Prodromata in acute myocardial infarction. *Circulation*, **40**: 463–471.

Stampfer MJ, Colditz GA (1992) Estrogen replacement therapy and coronary disease: a quantitative assessment of epidemiological evidence. *Preventive Medicine*, **20**: 47–63.

Steinberg D, Pearson TA, Kuller LH (1991) Alcohol and atherosclerosis. *Annals of Internal Medicine*, **114**: 967–976.

Thompson GR (1992) Progression and regression of coronary artery disease. *Current Opinions in Lipidology*, **3**: 263–267.

Thun MJ, Peto R, Lopez AD et al (1997) Alcohol consumption and mortality amongst middle aged and elderly US adults. *New England Journal of Medicine*, **337**: 1705–1714.

UKPDS (1998) The United Kingdom Prospective Diabetes Study Group 38. Tight blood pressure control and risk of macrovascular and microvascular complications in type 2 diabetes. *BMJ*, **317**: 703–713.

Whiteman MC, Fowkes FGR, Deary IJ (1997) Hostility and the heart. *BMJ*, **315**: 379–380.

Wilkinson IB, Webb DJ, Cockcroft JR (2000) Isolated systolic hypertension: a radical rethink. *BMJ*, **320**: 1685–1686.

Wood D, Durrington P, Poulter N et al (1998) Joint British recommendations on prevention of coronary heart disease in clinical practice. *Heart*, **80** (suppl 2): S1–S29.

World Health Organization (1994) *Assessing Hypertension Control and Management*. WHO European Series No. 47. Geneva: WHO.

World Health Organization (1997) WHO Collaborative Study of Cardiovascular Disease and Steroid Hormone Contraception. Acute myocardial infarction and combined oral contraceptives: results of an international multi-centre case-control study. *Lancet* **349**: 1202–1209.

World Health Organization (1998) *Obesity: Preventing and Managing the Global Epidemic*. Geneva: WHO.

World Health Organization Expert Committee on Diabetes Mellitus (1999) *Diagnosis and Classification of Diabetes Mellitus and its Complications*. Geneva: WHO.

4

Assessing the patient

Initial contact with patients suspected of having coronary heart disease may be either in a surgery, the cardiology clinic, or following an acute admission to hospital. Patient assessment may be divided into:

- Defining the symptoms
- Demonstration of clinical signs
- Organising appropriate investigations.

The initial assessment usually gives significant clues to the diagnosis, and rapid triage is essential to ensure that those qualifying for thrombolysis receive it as quickly as possible. As it is often a nurse who is the first point of contact, they are in a unique position to utilise their clinical skills to help to identify patients suitable for immediate therapy (Albarran and Kapeluch, 1994). Details of the presenting history may need to be succinct, but can be supplemented later with information from the family, the referral letter, or previous medical and nursing notes.

Apart from the management of acute myocardial infarction, coronary care units now have an extended role in the management of many other cardiac problems. These include heart failure, dysrhythmias and cardiogenic shock. However, approximately one-third of patients admitted to coronary care do not have a cardiological problem (Table 4.1), and the immediate decision is whether or not the patient has a cardiovascular illness and, if so, what needs to be done.

Table 4.1 Primary discharge diagnosis for all patients admitted to the coronary care unit in Withybush General Hospital during 2001

Diagnosis	Percentage
Cardiac (68.8%)	
Myocardial infarction	20.2
Dysrhythmias	13.7
Stable angina	12.5
Unstable angina	9.5
Left ventricular failure	7.0
DC cardioversion	2.9
Other cardiac (e.g. post-cardiac arrest, pericarditis)	3.2
Non-cardiac (31.2%)	
Chest pain of uncertain origin	10.4
Gastrointestinal causes	4.7
Respiratory tract infection	4.3
Musculoskeletal	4.3
Pulmonary embolus	1.5
Syncope	1.1
Anxiety/hyperventilation	0.3
Cerebrovascular accident	0.3
Aortic dissection	0.1
Others (carcinoma of lung, anaemia, gastrointestinal haemorrhage, constipation, spondylitis, diabetic ketosis, renal failure, hypothermia, pleurisy, etc.)	

SYMPTOMS OF CORONARY HEART DISEASE

Chest pain and breathlessness are two of the most common complaints that lead to a patient seeking medical advice. Patients suspected of having an acute coronary syndrome should be assessed on a chest pain or coronary care unit, so that prognosis may be improved by early intensive care. Patients admitted to medical wards are often not considered soon enough for thrombolytic therapy, or for secondary interventions later on (Lawson-Matthew et al, 1994).

Unfortunately, the coronary care unit may be a dangerous place for patients who do not have a cardiovascular disease. All too often it is assumed that ill patients attached to cardiac monitors have had a heart attack, and it is important to consider both alternative and concomitant diagnoses. The frequency with which non-cardiac pain appears on coronary care units demonstrates how difficult it is to determine the origin of chest pain (Table 4.1).

Chest pain can originate from most tissues in the chest (Box 4.1). Diagnosis is often difficult, because the pain may be coming from more than one of these. For example, many patients presenting with angina often have concurrent oesophageal reflux, or chest wall tenderness. Even those with a cardiovascular disease may present with atypical symptoms, particularly the elderly (Then et al, 2001). Obtaining the history may also be difficult if the patient is in pain, distressed or simply frightened.

CHEST PAIN

Many people in the community suffer episodes of chest pain, and the cause is usually benign (Hannay, 1987).

Myocardial ischaemia

Anginal pain is usually described as a constricting ache in the chest, frequently radiating to the jaw, the neck, the back and one or both arms. Patients will often use descriptive phrases like 'a steel band around my chest', or 'like a vice'. The pain is precipitated by exercise, particularly after meals, or in the wind and cold. Rest and glyceryl

Box 4.1 Some causes of chest pain

Cardiovascular causes
Myocardial ischaemia
Coronary artery spasm
Myocardial infarction
Pericarditis
Dissecting aortic aneurysm
Pulmonary embolism
Mitral valve prolapse

Non-cardiac causes
Herpes zoster
Oesophageal reflux
Oesophageal spasm
Hiatus hernia
Pneumonia
Pneumothorax
Pleurisy
Peptic ulceration
Gallbladder disease
Musculoskeletal pain
Da Costa's syndrome (cardioneurosis)

trinitrate (GTN) relieve it quickly. About half the patients presenting with myocardial infarction will have had a previous heart attack or suffer from angina. This is helpful diagnostically, since the patient is often able to identify the cause of his pain.

The origin of anginal pain is probably the myocardium itself. Pain impulses travel via sympathetic fibres to the thoracic sympathetic ganglia, and to nerve roots T1–5. For that reason, the pain is felt in the anterior chest wall and the ulnar aspect of the arm and hand. Even in atypical presentations, ischaemic pain rarely extends beyond the region bordered by the lower jaw and the epigastrium. The location is never so sharply localised that it can be identified with a pointing finger. *Decubitus angina* is induced by lying down, or during sleep. It may be caused by increased wall stress produced by increased cardiac preload, or by coronary spasm induced by dreaming during REM (rapid eye movement) sleep.

Chest pain is a common symptom in women, but nearly half do not have coronary heart disease. The clinical, investigative and prognostic features in men with chest pain are not necessarily applicable to women (Sullivan et al, 1994). Patients with diabetes often have atypical symptoms of myocardial ischaemia, and sometimes do not get chest pain at all (Airaksinen, 2001).

Pericardial pain

Pain is the usual presenting feature of pericarditis. The visceral pericardium is insensitive, and the pain arises from the parietal pericardium. Pericardial pain is sharp, aching and usually made worse by lying back or swallowing. Diaphragmatic pericarditis causes pain to radiate to the left shoulder. The diagnosis is sometimes confirmed by the presence of a pericardial friction rub. Apart from acute myocardial infarction, the most frequent cause of pericarditis is a viral infection. The patient is usually young and fit, and there is often a history of a recent flu-like illness. Other causes of pericarditis include connective tissue disorders (e.g. systemic lupus erythematosus, rheumatoid arthritis or sarcoido-

sis), tuberculosis and renal failure. The ECG classically shows widespread concave ST-segment elevation, but may show T wave changes or be normal.

Aortic dissection

The chest pain of aortic dissection is described as tearing, and classically radiates through to the back, particularly between the shoulder blades. Radiation depends on the vessels involved by the dissection. The condition is associated with shock and loss of peripheral pulses. Myocardial infarction may result if blood tracks round to occlude the coronary arteries, and pericarditis as well if blood leaks through to produce a haemopericardium. The mixture of pains coming from these different tissues can make diagnosis difficult. A history of hypertension, or a family history of Marfan's syndrome or aortic dissection makes the diagnosis more likely, and the diagnosis of aortic dissection should always be considered prior to thrombolysis.

Pain from the lungs

Pleuritic pain is localised and associated with deep respiration. A pleural rub will confirm the diagnosis. Causes include respiratory infections and pulmonary embolism. The latter usually causes dyspnoea and haemoptysis, but large emboli may mimic myocardial infarction, presenting with shock and central chest pain.

A left-sided pneumothorax can be confused with myocardial pain, particularly in tension pneumothorax when shock is present.

Oesophageal pain

Oesophageal pain (heartburn) is the most common cause of chest discomfort in the general population, but, because it is so frequent, a confident diagnosis of oesophageal reflux does not rule out the presence of other pathologies. Differentiating cardiac from oesophageal pain can be difficult, and both sources of pain may coexist (Table 4.2). The denial response makes sufferers more likely to self-diagnose indigestion,

Table 4.2 Site of chest pain and radiation in 200 consecutive medical patients with cardiac and oesophageal pain (Withybush General Hospital, 1991)

Radiation	Primary source of pain	
	Cardiac (%)	Oesophageal (%)
Chest	100	100
Left arm		
All	55	20
To elbow	60	25
Right arm		
All	33	4
To elbow	40	12
Throat/jaw	33	8
Epigastrium	7	35

rather than heart attack. Postmortem examinations of patients who have died from an acute myocardial infarction sometimes reveal antacid tablets in the stomach taken shortly before death.

Oesophageal spasm may associate with gastro-oesophageal reflux and can produce severe and distressing substernal pain. It is responsive to sublingual GTN. Mucosal (Mallory–Weiss) tears may occur after bouts of vomiting, as may oesophageal rupture. Both present with chest pain, and the latter with shock. Other gastrointestinal disorders, such as peptic ulceration and gallbladder disease, often cause difficulty with differential diagnosis. An upper gastrointestinal bleed may present with lower chest pain and shock.

Musculoskeletal pain

Fractures of the ribs, vertebral collapse and other muscular strains can cause chest pain. Pain from Bornholm's disease (intercostal myalgia) and Tietze's syndrome (sternal costochondritis) may be severe, and is usually associated with a flu-like illness in the younger patient.

Skin

Herpes zoster often presents with pain a day or two before the rash appears. If this affects a thoracic nerve root, chest pain may be so severe that it may be indistinguishable from the pain of myocardial infarction.

Chest pain of unknown origin

This is a proper diagnosis, which may be applied to patients presenting with chest pain in whom myocardial ischaemia seems unlikely, and no other cause can be found. The typical patient is a middle-aged man presenting with chronic, intermittent stabbing pain in the left breast, lasting for a few seconds, often radiating down the left arm. GTN has usually been tried and, although claimed to be useful, only works after 30 min.

The problem is how far to investigate these patients. Most have multiple (normal) tests, including coronary angiography. A large number have psychological problems, and are not reassured by normal investigation. About a half of sufferers remain on cardiac medication, most continue to experience pain and 50% remain or become unemployed (Chambers and Bass, 1998). Providing an alternative non-cardiac diagnosis can be difficult, but addressing the patient's concerns may be more important than providing a medical diagnosis.

DYSPNOEA

Dyspnoea means difficulty with breathing, and it is entirely subjective. Many patients who are obviously short of breath at rest will not complain of respiratory difficulties, yet others claim to be short of breath on exertion but are able to complete exercise stress tests with apparent ease. Breathlessness is usually due to cardiorespiratory disorders, obesity or anaemia. Left ventricular failure is the classical cardiac cause of acute breathlessness, with pulmonary oedema causing increased lung rigidity and decreased oxygen transfer. Respiration will, therefore, require greater effort, which is not helped by oedematous narrowing of the larger airways. Dyspnoea may also be caused by a raised left atrial pressure alone, which causes pulmonary venous congestion with few physical signs. The venous congestion reduces vital capacity and stimulates pulmonary stretch receptors, which causes the shortness of breath.

Effort tolerance has been graded by the Criteria Committee of the New York Heart

Association based on symptoms and exercise capacity to classify the severity of heart failure (see Table 14.1; page 294).

Orthopnoea is difficulty with breathing when lying flat. It is often an early symptom of left ventricular failure, but may not be volunteered by the patient who learns to sleep propped up with three or four pillows. The increase in venous return in the recumbent patient reduces vital capacity and lung compliance. In patients with right ventricular failure, an enlarged liver and ascites may contribute to orthopnoea, by diaphragmatic splinting.

Orthopnoea does not automatically indicate heart failure. Patients with chronic obstructive airways disease often complain of waking with dyspnoea and wheezing, which is due to the loss of the diaphragmatic component of their respiratory pattern, corrected by sitting up.

Paroxysmal nocturnal dyspnoea may be viewed as a delayed form of orthopnoea. Dyspnoea is precipitated by the patient sliding down the bed into a horizontal position. The increase in pulmonary congestion leads to dyspnoea, which is reversed by the patient sitting up or standing. Typically, the patient jumps out of bed to an open window, gasping for breath.

Cheyne–Stokes breathing was described independently by John Cheyne in 1818, and William Stokes in 1846. It describes a respiratory pattern that begins with a hardly perceptible respiratory effort that gradually increases in depth until it is very much exaggerated. The effort then dies away, until breathing ceases for a period of about 20–30 s. The whole cycle is then repeated, each cycle lasting for between 1 and 3 min. The mechanism is complex, but essentially the pauses in respiration allow the levels of arterial carbon dioxide to rise, which stimulates the respiratory centre to set off a fresh cycle of breathing. Cheyne–Stokes breathing is common in the elderly, especially during sleep. It is also found in those with chronic chest disease or following a stroke. In cardiac patients, it is common in heart failure, when patients are aware of breathlessness in the fast phase of respiration. Cheyne–Stokes breathing may also be associated with heart rhythm disturbances, such as junctional rhythms and heart block.

SYNCOPE

Syncope is a transient loss of consciousness resulting from inadequate cerebral blood flow, leading to cerebral ischaemia.

Vasovagal attacks are the most common cause of syncope and originate from a combination of vasodilatation and vagally induced bradycardia. Attacks may occur following prolonged standing, or in response to emotion or pain. *Postural hypotension* may be induced by drugs. The face is pale, the pupils are dilated and the pulse and respiration are slow. Peripheral pulses are often impalpable, leading to the frequent diagnosis of cardiac arrest.

Carotid sinus syncope may result from stimulation of the carotid sinus, either during carotid massage or if the patient's neckwear is too tight.

Micturition syncope occurs in older men with nocturia who lose consciousness while voiding urine. This is either because straining reduces venous return and subsequently cardiac output (Valsalva manoeuvre) or because sudden decompression of an over-full bladder causes reflex vasodilatation.

Exertion syncope is a characteristic feature of aortic stenosis, when the cardiac output through the narrow valve cannot meet the demands of increased activity. Similar obstructive lesions are pulmonary stenosis and hypertrophic cardiomyopathy.

Dysrhythmia-induced syncope may result from heart rates that are too slow or too fast to maintain cerebral blood flow. Paroxysmal tachycardias often lead to a marked fall in cardiac output, with resulting syncope. Stokes–Adams attacks may be missed if the ECG is normal between attacks, and associate with complete heart block or sinus arrest. The attack may terminate in a convulsion, leading to an erroneous diagnosis of epilepsy. However, there is no aura, and recovery is prompt and accompanied by flushing, as the blood flows again through vessels dilated by hypoxia. The desire to sleep does not occur, and headache is not as common.

OEDEMA

Oedema is an abnormal accumulation of fluid in the interstitial tissues, and is usually preceded by weight gain from 3–5 kg of extracellular fluid. It is a relatively late manifestation of heart failure. Normally, fluid is exuded into the tissues because arterial capillary pressure (30 mmHg) exceeds plasma oncotic pressure (25 mmHg). However, the fluid is forced back into circulation at the venous end of the capillaries because the pressure here (12 mmHg) is exceeded by the oncotic pressure (25 mmHg). If the venous pressure rises, as in heart failure, the resorption of fluid is impaired and oedema results (Fig. 4.1).

Oedema will preferentially collect in loose tissues, so the distribution of fluid is determined by both gravity and the degree of ambulation. In most patients, the legs and feet are affected, but in those who are confined to bed the fluid accumulates over the sacrum. The oedema characteristically pits when pressure is applied (*pitting oedema*). Greater degrees of oedema will gradually affect the whole of the lower extremities, extending to the torso and eventually the face (*anasarca*). Effusions into the chest and abdomen (*ascites*) occur later in the course of heart failure, for the same reasons.

HAEMOPTYSIS

Coughing up blood is an unusual indicator of cardiac disease. When related to circulatory pathology, the volume of blood is small, and the sputum is usually only streaked. When haemoptysis is related to exercise or is heavy, it usually indicates mitral stenosis, with pulmonary veins rupturing under high pressure. However, frank haemoptysis usually indicates important pulmonary disease such as bronchial carcinoma, tuberculosis, or pulmonary infarction.

PALPITATIONS

Palpitation is an awareness of the heart beat, familiar to those awaiting examinations! Most people are aware of their heart beat at some time, especially at night when lying on the left side. As such, palpitation is a common symptom, regardless of any underlying heart disease. It may be felt and described in many different ways. Some complain of a racing heart, others of thumping or feeling a missed beat, but the description does not always help with diagnosis.

A thumping or pounding heart is the most common complaint and is usually the awareness of normal beats, sometimes exaggerated in strength and speed by sympathetic overactivity (e.g. stress and anxiety). This frequently occurs for prolonged periods and on a daily basis.

Dropped beats are probably the next most common complaint, and these are more frequent if basic sinus rhythm is slow. Ectopic activity and sinus thumping are more frequent when the heart is overstimulated by anxiety or by drugs, including tobacco, caffeine, alcohol, bronchodilators and nasal decongestant sprays.

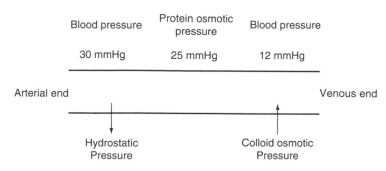

Figure 4.1 Changing pressures within a capillary.

Racing of the heart is usually abnormal if the pulse rate exceeds 130 beats/min. The history may go back for many years if attacks are usually infrequent. If the heart is giving irregular flutters, it is usually due to paroxysmal atrial fibrillation. Frequent ectopic beats may produce the same feeling, and both are common in the elderly.

IMPORTANT CARDIAC SIGNS

CYANOSIS

Cyanosis describes the blue discoloration (cyan) imparted to the skin and mucous membranes when there is more than 5 g of oxygen-depleted haemoglobin in the vessels being considered. Cyanosis is described as either peripheral or central.

Peripheral cyanosis occurs in the fingers and toes. It usually indicates a slowing of peripheral circulation, allowing more oxygen to be extracted as the blood passes through the constricted capillaries. It occurs most commonly in cold weather. In hospital practice, it may be seen in patients with low cardiac output or shock.

Central cyanosis is observed in the lips and tongue, and should be visible at arterial oxygen saturations of less than 85%. Central cyanosis is produced by inadequate oxygenation of the blood as it passes through the lungs (as in pulmonary disease) or sometimes when the lungs are bypassed all together (as in right-to-left intracardiac shunts). Pulmonary cyanosis should respond to increased oxygen concentrations (FiO_2), but there will be little effect if there is an intracardiac right-to-left shunt.

THE ARTERIAL PULSE

Arterial pulses should be examined for rate, rhythm and character of the waveform. Although the rate and rhythm are usually assessed by palpation of the radial artery, an artery closer to the heart is usually better for appreciating pulse waveform. In clinical practice, all features may be best assessed by palpation of the right brachial artery.

Rate

The pulse should be counted over 30 s, unless irregular, when it should not be assessed for less than 1 min. The normal adult pulse rate varies between 60 and 100 beats/min. Slower rates are found in patients taking beta-adrenergic blocking agents, but otherwise usually indicate a bradydysrhythmia. Pulse rates in excess of 100 are often associated with anxiety or pain, and those above 130 beats/min at rest usually indicate an abnormal tachycardia.

Rhythm

The normal pulse is regular, or very slightly irregular if there is a sinus arrhythmia, when the heart quickens on inspiration. An occasional irregularity indicates an ectopic beat, and an irregularly irregular pulse indicates either multifocal ectopic beats or atrial fibrillation. Gently exercising the patient will produce a regular pulse in the former cases, when the resulting rise in heart rate will abolish the ectopics. This will have no effect on the irregularity produced by atrial fibrillation.

Waveform character

The character of the pulse waveform is not often easily appreciated, but can help with diagnosis. Examples include:

- *Pulsus alternans*: alternate high- and low-volume beats as found in left ventricular failure; it indicates poor left ventricular function.
- *Pulsus paradoxus*: an excessive reduction in pulse pressure (over 10 mmHg) on inspiration; it may be found in asthma, pericardial tamponade or pericardial constriction.
- *Collapsing pulse*: large volume with rapid rise and fall, as may occur in thyrotoxicosis or aortic incompetence.
- *Plateau pulse*: low volume, slow rise and slow fall, as found in aortic stenosis.
- *Absent pulse*: due to atherosclerosis, aortic dissection or peripheral embolisation.

JUGULAR VENOUS PRESSURE

The pulsation and level of the internal jugular vein are used to assess the central venous pressure (CVP) and may be seen in front of the sternomastoid muscle. With a normal CVP, pulsation of the internal jugular vein is usually only visible when the patient lies flat. When observing for elevation, the height above the sternal angle should be measured with the patient lying at 45°. Confirmation of the level may be made by pressing on the liver, which transiently increases the CVP by increasing venous return to the heart (*hepatojugular reflux*). Tender liver enlargement may occur in congestive cardiac heart failure, and pulsation may be felt in severe tricuspid incompetence. An elevated jugular venous pressure (JVP) indicates high right-sided cardiac pressures, as in heart failure, pulmonary embolism or cor pulmonale. An elevated JVP early after acute myocardial infarction may signify involvement of the right ventricle, but may be seen if there was congestive cardiac failure preceding the infarct.

Much has been written about the pulsation in the jugular vein, but clinical interpretation is often difficult. Sometimes 'a' and 'v' waves may be seen, which correspond to right atrial and right ventricular contractions. Very large 'a' waves (cannon waves) may be seen when the right atrium contracts against a closed tricuspid valve, as may occur in complete heart block, when atrial and ventricular contraction are not synchronised. There will be no 'a' waves if the heart is in atrial fibrillation, since the atria do not contract.

BLOOD PRESSURE

The first recorded measurement of blood pressure was in 1730, by the Reverend Stephen Hales, who measured the height to which a column of blood reached when he inserted a glass tube into the neck veins of a horse. The tube had to be more than 8 feet long! Fortunately, Scipione Riva-Rocci devised the sphygmomanometer in 1896, which greatly cleaned up and simplified blood pressure estimation. Blood pressure is still most commonly measured indirectly with a sphygmo-

manometer, although precise measurement of arterial blood pressure requires a return to 'old-fashioned' invasive monitoring.

The Riva-Rocci or auscultatory method of blood pressure estimation employs a sphygmomanometer to occlude the brachial artery and a stethoscope to detect sounds of turbulent blood flow within the artery following the release of arterial compression. These sounds are known as the Korotkoff sounds, named after Nicholi Korotkoff, a Russian army surgeon who described them in 1905. Mercury sphygmomanometers are gradually being withdrawn because of potential toxicity, and over the coming years we are likely to see a move away from the Riva-Rocci techniques and associated equipment (O'Brien, 2001). Blood pressure estimation has already been superseded in many areas by automated machinery that can remove observer error, but has not been without problems, mostly surrounding inaccuracy. The British Hypertension Society (BHS) has published standards for the evaluation of blood pressure measuring devices (O'Brien et al, 1993), and those not certified by the BHS or the American National Standards for Electronic or Automated Sphygmomanometers (ANSI/AAMI) should not be used (Jowett, 1997).

Automated machines can also permit prolonged ambulatory blood pressure monitoring (ABPM), which in turn is increasing reliance being placed upon the 24-h ABPM machines for the diagnosis of hypertension. ABPM permits non-invasive measurement of blood pressure over prolonged periods, and provides a more reproducible estimate of the blood pressure (O'Brien et al, 2000). ABPMs is of most value in those suspected of having 'white coat hypertension', which affects up to 30% of the population, particularly the elderly.

Blood pressure continues to be measured in the original units introduced by Poiseuille for the mercury manometer: millimetres of mercury (mmHg). However, the international system of units (SI units), adopted by many countries (including the UK), should have led to replacement of millimetres of mercury by kiloPascals (kPa), where 1 mmHg = 0.13 kPa, or 1 kPa = 7.52 mmHg. Although the kilopascal is used in reporting blood gases, replacing the millimetre of mercury by the kilopascal has been postponed until a suitable replacement has been found to the mercury sphygmomanometer.

Measuring the blood pressure

It is important to realise that considerable variability of blood pressure occurs through the day, and may be affected by such factors as emotion, pain, full bladder or circadian rhythm. Anxiety may raise the blood pressure by as much as 30 mmHg. As far as is practicable, it is therefore important for the patient to be both relaxed and rested.

Most devices for measuring blood pressure are dependent on occlusion of an artery with a cuff to measure the blood pressure, either by detection of the Korotkoff sounds or oscillometrically. The correct selection and application of the pressure cuff is important, especially in small women and obese patients. The choice of cuff size should be based upon the arm circumference, which should be measured at the midpoint between the shoulder and elbow. The width of the cuff bladder should be not less than 40% of the mid-arm circumference (range 40–50%), and should encircle 80% of the circumference of the arm. Terms such as 'paediatric' or 'small adult' are misleading; the correct size is solely dependent upon arm circumference. A simple guide can be employed to show the best available cuff width based upon arm size (Fig. 4.2). The cuff size selected should be recorded, and the same size should always be used for serial measurements in the same patient. Having an adjustable cuff applicable to all adult arms has been proposed.

The cuff should be applied firmly so that the lower edge is 2.5 cm above the antecubital fossa, with the bladder overlying the brachial artery. It must not be twisted or in contact with the patient's clothing. The patient should be comfortable and the forearm supported, slightly extended and externally rotated. The mid-point of the cuff is often marked and should rest over the artery. If the arm is small, it may be easier to put the cuff on upside down so that the tubing is well away from the artery and pointing towards the patient's shoulder.

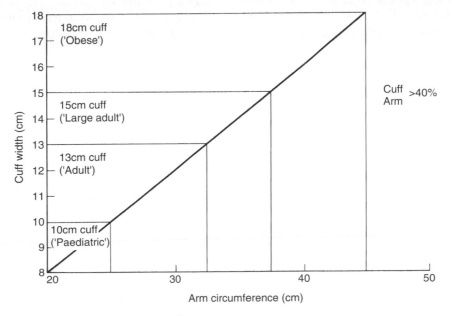

Figure 4.2   Selecting the correct blood pressure cuff.

Correct positioning of the arm is required for accurate blood pressure measurement. The blood pressure rises as the arm is lowered below the level of the heart, and vice versa. Additionally, if the arm is unsupported, isometric muscle contraction needed to hold the arm up against gravity will raise the blood pressure. Hence, the arm should be supported horizontally on a level with the heart. Automatic machines will determine pulse rate and systolic and diastolic blood pressure, although there are some cases in which oscillometric methods are difficult.

If an auscultatory method is being used to determine the blood pressure, the cuff should first be inflated to 70 mmHg, and then in 10-mmHg increments while the brachial pulse is palpated to determine the systolic pressure. The cuff should then be fully deflated and re-inflated to 20–30 mmHg above the previously determined systolic blood pressure. The bladder should then be slowly deflated at 2 mm/s until a faint tapping sound is heard through the bell of the stethoscope, which is applied firmly over the brachial artery. This is phase I of the Korotkoff sounds and is equivalent to the systolic blood pressure. It should be recorded to the nearest 2 mmHg. As the pressure continues to fall, there is often a silent gap (phase II) until the sounds are heard again (phase III). The sounds then become faint again (phase IV) until they disappear com-

pletely (phase V). Both phase IV and phase V have been used in the past as an indication of diastolic blood pressure. Phase IV usually differs by less than 5 mmHg from phase V, but the latter correlates best with intra-arterial pressure. Although accepting that, in certain patient groups (children, pregnant women, elderly, anaemia), there may be a large discrepancy between phase IV and phase V, the general consensus is that phase V should always be used to indicate diastolic blood pressure, unless sounds are heard down to zero. In this instance, both the phase IV and phase V blood pressure should be recorded (e.g. 140/80/0).

Normally, the diastolic blood pressure rises a little on standing, with a slight fall in the systolic blood pressure. In patients with autonomic failure, taking vasodilator medication or in shock, this fall may be very marked (postural or orthostatic hypotension). There is little difference between sitting and lying blood pressure. It is usual to record the blood pressure twice, using the second recording only. The arm used for recording should be noted, although, initially, the pressure in both arms should be recorded, so that a subclavian arterial stenosis is not missed.

There may be several occasions on which blood pressure estimation is difficult (Table 4.3). This is particularly so in hypotensive patients or those with unstable blood pressure; the record-

Table 4.3 Problems in measuring blood pressure

Problem	Cause	Reasons
False high reading	Cuff too small	Small cuff does not adequately disperse the pressure over the arterial surface
	Bladder not centred over the brachial artery	More external pressure is needed to compress the artery
	Cuff not applied snugly	Uneven and slow inflation results in varying tissue compression
	Arm positioned below heart level	Hydrostatic pressure imposed by weight of blood column above site of auscultation additive to arterial pressure: reposition arm to appropriate level
	Very obese arm	Cuff too small for a large arm will cause too little compression of the artery at the suitable pressure level: apply a large thigh cuff to the upper arm if necessary
False low reading	Cuff too large	Pressure is spread over too large an area and produces a damping effect on the Korotkoff sounds
	Arm positioned above heart level	Hydrostatic pressure in the elevated arm causes resistance to pressure generated by the heart

ings may not be completely accurate, and invasive blood pressure monitoring is then recommended (see Ch. 5).

THE APEX BEAT AND CARDIAC IMPULSE

The apex beat marks the maximal thrust of the left ventricle, and is normally seen and felt just inside the midclavicular line in the 5th left intercostal space. The left ventricle produces a sustained heaving or thrusting apex beat if hypertrophied, but, when enlargement is due to dilatation, it is weak and diffuse. It has a 'tapping' quality in mitral stenosis. If there is a left ventricular aneurysm, there may be a double or rocking apical beat. The right ventricular impulse is usually not palpable in health. In pulmonary hypertension or right-sided valve disease, the right ventricle gives rise to a parasternal heave. More usually this is due to mitral incompetence.

The apex may also be displaced by abnormalities of the lungs or rib cage. Collapse of the right lung, for example, will pull the heart to the right, and a thoracic scoliosis may displace the mediastinum either way.

Seeing, or even feeling, the apex beat is probably only possible in 50% of cases (O'Neill et al, 1989), and it is particularly difficult in the obese or in those with hyperinflated chests.

THE HEART SOUNDS

The heart sounds are produced by closure of the valves. Mitral and aortic valve closure precede that of the tricuspid and pulmonary valve, and are louder.

The first sound

The first sound (S_1) is related to closure of the mitral and tricuspid valves and is best heard at the apex. The mitral component is louder, and occurs fractionally before closure of the tricuspid valve. At the onset of ventricular systole, the valve cusps have been forced downwards into the ventricle by atrial contraction, and the sound

relates to snapping back-up again, the movement being checked by the chordae tendineae.

Loud first heart sounds will occur if the left atrial pressure is abnormally high (e.g. mitral stenosis), during fast heart rates or if the atrium contracts very close to ventricular systole (i.e. with a short PR interval). A soft first heart sound occurs if the mitral valve is calcified, or does not move well, or if left ventricular contraction is poor.

When there is dissociated contraction of the atria and ventricles as in complete heart block or ventricular tachycardia, the first sound varies in intensity, depending on the position of the valve at the onset of ventricular systole.

The second sound

The second sound (S_2) is related to closure of the pulmonary and aortic valves and is best heard in the 2nd left intercostal space. It is louder in pulmonary or systemic hypertension. The sound is normally split because the aortic valve closes before the pulmonary valve on inspiration when the right ventricle takes longer to expel the increased venous return. A loud S_2 may be a feature of acute pulmonary embolism.

Wide splitting is caused when the right ventricle is overloaded and the valve is unable to close quickly as in pulmonary stenosis or cor pulmonale. It also occurs in right bundle branch block, when there is delayed right ventricular activation.

Reversed splitting means that the splitting is best heard on expiration, and occurs if the left ventricle is overloaded, as in left ventricular failure. It may also occur in left bundle branch block, because the right ventricle is prematurely activated.

Fixed splitting means that S_2 does not vary with respiration, and occurs when increased venous return affects both ventricles (e.g. atrioseptal defect).

The third sound

The third sound (S_3) is low-pitched and best heard at the apex. It may be normal in the young and in pregnancy, but is usually abnormal in patients over the age of 40 years. In the first phase of diastole, 80% of the blood stored in the atria during systole is transferred to the ventricles. If the volume transferred is abnormally large, the ventricles tense during this rapid filling and produce this added heart sound. S_3 implies heart failure or a widely open mitral valve (mitral regurgitation). A third heart sound is an important indicator of left ventricular dysfunction and poor outcome. It is found in 5–10% of patients admitted with myocardial infarction.

The fourth sound

The fourth sound (S_4) is heard just before S_1, at the apex of the heart. It is probably produced by the atrial kick associated with emptying of the remaining 20% of atrial blood into a nondistending ventricle, as may be caused by left ventricular hypertrophy or hypertrophic obstructive cardiomyopathy. A prominent fourth heart sound is common in patients admitted to the coronary care unit, but probably has no prognostic significance.

Gallop rhythm is often heard in heart failure. The addition of a third heart sound with a tachycardia makes the heart sounds resemble a galloping horse. If both third and fourth heart sounds are present, it is called a *summation gallop*. Gallop rhythm may be normal in young adults and children.

OTHER HEART SOUNDS

Ejection clicks occur immediately after the first heart sound at the time of aortic and pulmonary valve opening, and are usually associated with stenosis of the valves. They are sometimes confused with a fourth heart sound. A midsystolic click may be heard with mitral valve prolapse. An opening snap of the mitral valve is heard in mitral stenosis, but disappears if the valve becomes calcific. The opening snap may be confused with a third heart sound but is much more widely conducted.

A *pericardial friction rub* causes a scratchy sound (like sandpaper) produced by the inflamed visceral and parietal pericardia rubbing against each other. It may be localised, generalised, long-lasting or transient. It is best heard with the patient sitting forward.

HEART MURMURS

Murmurs are sounds caused by turbulent blood flow. This may be either because the blood flow is more rapid, or because it is running a turbulent course.

Murmurs are heard during either systole or diastole, and their intensity is sometimes classed as grades 1–6 for systolic murmurs and 1–4 for diastolic murmurs. Such practice is seldom helpful nor necessary. Clues to the origin of the murmur may be found by determining when the murmur occurs in the cardiac cycle, where and how it is best heard, how loud it is and, finally, where it radiates to.

Innocent or functional murmurs are due to minor turbulence unassociated with any structural abnormality. Functional murmurs are very common in children, and most disappear around puberty. Most are pulmonary flow murmurs. A continuous *venous hum* may be heard over the right clavicle, radiating into the neck. It is reduced by ipsilateral internal jugular vein compression, or lying down.

Pathological murmurs are indicative of a structural or functional cardiac abnormality. Patients on the coronary care unit may develop murmurs related to an acute coronary syndrome, but may have pre-existing murmurs unrelated to their acute problem. It is therefore very important that murmurs are precisely documented to distinguish them from newly developed complications.

Systolic murmurs

These are either pansystolic (i.e. heard throughout systole) or midsystolic (loudest in midsystole). The latter are sometimes called ejection systolic murmurs, as they are usually associated with outflow through a stenosed pulmonary or aortic valve. Innocent and physiological murmurs are virtually always systolic. An apical systolic murmur is common following acute myocardial infarction, and is usually due to papillary muscle dysfunction or prior mitral valve disease. The sudden development of a harsh pansystolic murmur may indicate severe mitral regurgitation due to papillary muscle rupture. Alternatively, it may represent a post-infarction ventriculoseptal defect. It is difficult to differentiate the two clinically, and echocardiography should be carried out urgently.

Diastolic murmurs

These are either early diastolic, mid-diastolic or late diastolic (pre-systolic). They are always low pitched. Early diastolic murmurs are common in the elderly due to mild aortic regurgitation. A loud aortic diastolic murmur in patients presenting with severe chest pain usually indicates aortic dissection.

COMMON MURMURS HEARD IN THE CORONARY CARE UNIT
Pulmonary systolic murmur

This short, 'blowing' murmur is often found in younger patients, and may be heard down the left sternal edge and apex. Some patients will be noted to have a sternal depression or an abnormally straight back ('straight back syndrome'). The mediastinum presumably squashes the heart from front to back, altering blood flow patterns (Davies et al, 1980).

Aortic ejection murmur

This is heard in middle-aged and elderly patients, especially those with hypertension. Aortic valve thickening and dilatation of the ascending aorta are very common. Differentiation from significant aortic stenosis is difficult, and patients should have an echocardiogram.

Mitral systolic murmur

Fibrosis and calcification of the mitral ring are common in the elderly and produce a murmur identical to that of mitral incompetence. Mitral regurgitant murmurs are common following myocardial infarction, either caused by dilatation of the mitral ring, or damage to the mitral apparatus.

A short, late systolic murmur may be due to prolapse of a mitral leaflet into the left atrium at the end of ventricular systole. *Mitral valve prolapse* is the most common valvular abnormality in the UK, with a prevalence of up to 17% in women and 12% in men. Patients are younger, and may be admitted with dysrhythmias. Most cases are asymptomatic, and benign (Alpert, 1993).

SIGNS OF HYPERLIPIDAEMIA
(Fig. 4.3)

A *corneal arcus* is a white ring surrounding the cornea. It is very common in the elderly, owing to degenerative changes (arcus senilis). However, in patients under the age of 45 years, it is frequently associated with high blood cholesterol levels (arcus lipidis).

Xanthelasma are small, raised, yellow plaques on the eyelids, which contain cholesterol. *Tendon xanthomata* are hard nodules found over the knuckles, in the patella and Achilles tendon. These are important signs of familial hypercholesterolaemia, a condition associated with a very high incidence of early and severe coronary heart disease.

Eruptive xanthomata are papules with yellow centres that appear over extensor surfaces and are a clinical clue to severe hypertriglyceridaemia (Jowett, 2002). This often associates with acute pancreatitis, sometimes resulting in admission to the coronary care unit with lower chest pain and shock.

THE DIAGONAL EARLOBE CREASE
(Fig. 4.4)

There is high correlation between severe coronary atherosclerosis and the presence of the earlobe crease (Patel et al, 1992), although the cause is not known.

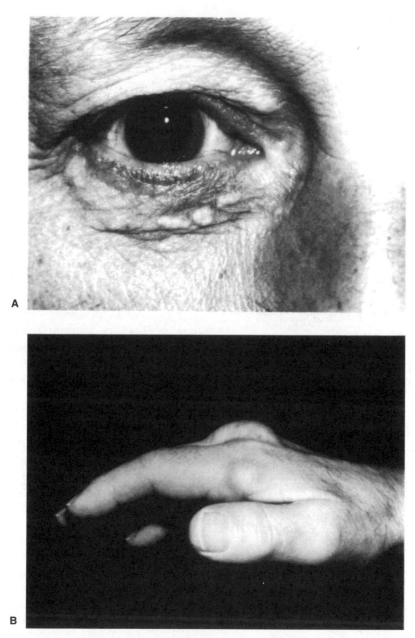

Figure 4.3   Cutaneous signs of high blood lipids. (A) Xanthelasma. (B) Tendon xanthoma.

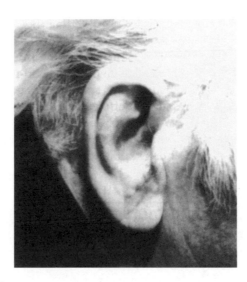

Figure 4.4 Diagonal earlobe crease.

REFERENCES

Airaksinen KE (2001) Silent coronary artery disease in diabetes – a feature of autonomic neuropathy or accelerated atherosclerosis? *Diabetologia,* **44:** 259–266.

Albarran J, Kapeluch H (1994) Role of the nurse in thrombolytic therapy. *British Journal of Nursing,* **3:** 104–109.

Alpert MA (1993) Mitral valve prolapse. *BMJ,* **306:** 943–944.

Chambers J, Bass C (1998) Atypical chest pain: looking beyond the heart. *Quarterly Journal of Medicine,* **91:** 239–244.

Davies MK, Mackintosh P, Clayton RM et al (1980) The straight back syndrome. *Quarterly Journal of Medicine,* **49:** 443–460.

Hannay DR (1987) Symptom prevalence in the community. *Journal of the Royal College of General Practitioners,* **28:** 492–498.

Jowett NI (1997) Monitoring the central venous and arterial blood pressure. *Cardiovascular Monitoring.* London: Whurr. pp: 122–144.

Jowett NI (2002) Milky serum. *Practical Diabetes International,* **19:** 90.

Lawson-Matthew PJ, Wilson AT, Woodmansey PA et al (1994) Unsatisfactory management of patients with acute myocardial infarction admitted to general medical wards.

Journal of the Royal College of Physicians of London, **28:** 49–51.

O'Brien E (2001) Blood pressure measurement is changing! *Heart,* **85:** 3–5.

O'Brien E, Petrie J, Littler WA et al (1993) The British Hypertension Society protocol for the evaluation of blood pressure measurement devices. *Journal of Hypertension,* **11:** S43–S63.

O'Brien E, Coats A, Owens J et al (2000) Use and interpretation of ambulatory blood pressure monitoring: recommendations of the British Hypertension Society. *BMJ,* **320:** 1128–1134.

O'Neill TW, Barry M, Smith M et al (1989) Diagnostic value of the apex beat. *Lancet,* **1:** 410–411.

Patel V, Champ C, Andrews PS et al (1992) Diagonal earlobe creases and atheromatous disease: a postmortem study. *Journal of the Royal College of Physicians of London,* **26:** 274–277.

Sullivan AK, Holdright DR, Wright CA et al (1994) Chest pain in women: clinical, investigative and prognostic features. *BMJ,* **308:** 883–886.

Then KL, Rankin JA, Fofonoff DA (2001) Atypical presentation of acute myocardial infarction in 3 age groups. *Heart and Lung,* **30:** 285–293.

5

Investigation and monitoring of patients with coronary heart disease

Investigation of patients with coronary heart disease may be needed for diagnostic, therapeutic or prognostic reasons. The screening of asymptomatic patients is generally unrewarding, and time is better spent on those with cardiac symptoms, particularly chest pain and dyspnoea. Apart from the very elderly and infirm, all patients with symptoms suggestive of myocardial ischaemia should be referred to hospital for confirmation of the diagnosis and objective assessment by stress testing or perfusion imaging. Prognosis can be favourably influenced by intervention in most cases, and those without coronary heart disease can be reassured. Adequate diagnostic facilities should be available for patients of all ages, especially the elderly in view of the ageing population. Over 80% of all coronary deaths occur in patients over the age of 65 years, and cardiac disease is a major contributory factor to loss of independence of elderly people living at home.

The management sequence may be:

1. *Preliminary (general practice).* The role of the general practitioner is vital in assessing symptoms, as he has knowledge of the patient, his family and home circumstances. Cardiovascular risk assessment often aids diagnosis, and physical examination may identify other causes of cardiac symptoms. Initial investigations by the

primary care team should include a resting electrocardiogram (ECG), chest X-ray and blood testing for haemoglobin, erythrocyte sedimentation rate, renal function tests, fasting blood glucose and lipid profile. All newly diagnosed cases of angina should be referred for objective assessment of myocardial ischaemia, unless contraindicated (de Bono, 1999). Further management may be appropriate in primary care, but referral to secondary care is indicated for those with symptoms despite initial treatment, and those being considered for revascularisation.

2. *Intermediate (district general hospital).* Secondary care should be provided by a physician accredited in cardiovascular medicine. Most district general hospitals should be able to perform exercise stress testing, dynamic (Holter) ECG, ambulatory blood pressure monitoring and echocardiography. Nuclear scanning and radionuclide ventriculography may be available in many of the larger hospitals, and cardiac catheterisation laboratories are being established within some district general hospitals.

3. *Specialist (regional cardiac centre).* Specialist investigation facilities and personnel are needed for transoesophageal echocardiography, electrophysiology and pacing, cardiac catheterisation, coronary angiography, percutaneous coronary intervention and cardiac surgery.

THE ELECTROCARDIOGRAM

The normal electrical impulse originates in the sinus node and is conducted as a wave over the atrium to initiate atrial systole. An electrical barrier exists between the atrial and ventricular myocardium, and further electrical activation can only take place via the atrioventricular (AV) node. This is a group of specialised cells situated on the right side of the interatrial septum, just below the entrance of the coronary sinus. The atrial depolarisation wave activates the AV node, and is then transmitted to the ventricles by the *bundles of His*. The left bundle perforates the intraventricular septum, and both bundles carry the impulse onwards, the septum being activated from left to right. The impulse then spreads over the endocardial surface of the ventricles via the *Purkinje fibres* and through the ventricular myocardium, in a wave passing from the endocardium outwards to the epicardium.

The electrical forces generated by the heart travel in multiple directions simultaneously. The ECG is designed to record these electrical impulses by the placement of electrodes on the body surface; the waveform generated is divided into P, Q, R, S, T and U waves. The *P wave* represents atrial activation, and the *QRS complex* ventricular activation. The *T wave* represents ventricular repolarisation. The atrial repolarisation wave (T_a) is usually not seen, being buried in the QRS complex.

The signals are amplified, and, by convention, the display is arranged so that impulses moving towards a surface electrode give rise to an upward (positive) deflection, whereas impulses moving away from the electrode give a downward (negative) one. To help interpret the patterns of electrical movement, electrocardiography is carried out in different planes. The three major planes are recorded via electrodes on the right arm, left arm and left leg. A fourth electrode is traditionally placed on the right leg, but this is not used for recording and serves as a ground (earth) electrode. The three planes form an electrical triangle, with the heart in the centre (Fig. 5.1). These three bipolar limb leads record the potential difference between a specified pair of electrodes designated standard leads I, II and III.

The normal ECG consists of recordings from 12 leads. In addition to the three standard limb leads (I, II III), there are three unipolar leads (VR, VL and VF), which measure the potential difference between one 'exploring' electrode attached to the limb with respect to a reference potential derived by joining the other two limb lead electrodes. Modern equipment records and augments this signal automatically to produced 'augmented' unipolar leads aVR, aVL and aVF. Six additional unipolar chest (V) leads complete the standard 12-lead ECG and view the heart electrically from the front, as shown in Fig. 5.2. These leads record the potential difference between set points on the chest wall and the average potential obtained from the three limb leads.

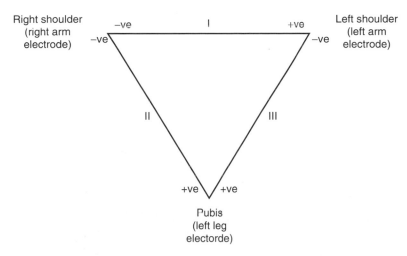

Figure 5.1 The Einthoven triangle (named after Willem Einthoven, 1860–1927, Professor of Physiology, University of Leiden).

POSITIONING OF THE LEADS

The standard (limb) leads are not often confused as they are usually clearly marked on the electrodes. However, exact placement is important (inner aspect of ankles and wrists). Changes in the cardiac axis may occur if the limb leads are taken by placing electrodes proximally on the trunk instead of on the wrists and ankles. Positioning of the chest leads can also vary between serial recordings, and it is important that the correct surface marking is used to prevent artefactual ECG changes between recordings:

- V1: 4th intercostal space, immediately to the right of the sternum
- V2: 4th intercostal space, immediately to the left of the sternum
- V3: midway between V2 and V4
- V4: 5th intercostal space, midclavicular line
- V5: left anterior axillary line, on the same horizontal line as V4
- V6: left mid-axillary line, horizontal with V4 and V5.

Many other additional electrode placements can be used to demonstrate particular aspects of the heart (Jowett, 1997), such as V7 and V8 (further laterally) or $V3_R$ and $V4_R$ (V3 and V4 positions on the right side of the chest).

ASSESSING THE QUALITY OF THE RECORDING

Before analysing an ECG, it is essential to ensure that the recording was obtained correctly. Errors in lead placement or connection, paper speed selection, standardisation and lead labelling are very common. Hence, the technical quality of the recording should always be assessed first:

1. *Standardisation.* A potential of 1 mV should be represented by a 10-mm vertical deflection. A standard test deflection should be recorded at the start and finish of a 12-lead recording.
2. *Speed.* Recordings are usually made at 25 mm/s.
3. *Clear tracings.* Mains interference may produce a fuzzy trace, as also may patient movement caused by cold, shock or fear.
4. *Correct lead placement and labelling.* The net electrical movement in the heart is from lead aVR towards lead II. Hence, in the normal ECG, the complex should be totally positive in lead II (upright P, QRS and T waves) and totally negative in aVR. If the ECG shows very abnormal changes, check the leads and repeat the ECG.

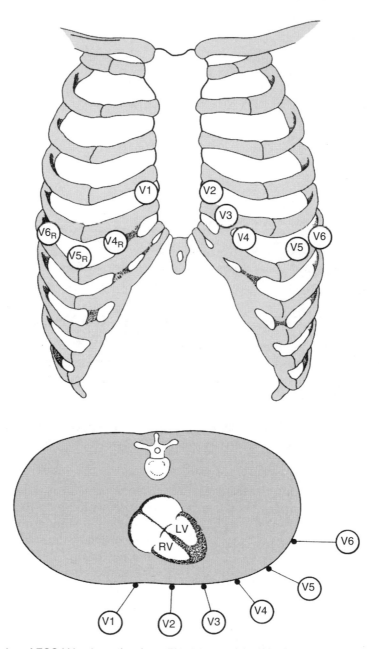

Figure 5.2 The positioning of ECG V leads on the chest. RV, right ventricle; LV, left ventricle.

ANALYSING THE ECG

If a standard approach is made towards an ECG, important changes will not be missed. The sequence should be rate, rhythm, axis and waveform.

Rate

The ECG is recorded at 25 mm/s on standard ECG paper, which has fine lines at 1-mm intervals and heavier divisions every 5 mm. Each millimetre, therefore, represents 0.04 s and each large division is 0.2 s.

To calculate the rate, the number of large squares between two successive complexes should be measured and divided into 300. If the heart rhythm is irregular, a greater number of complexes should be assessed. Special ECG 'rate rulers' can simplify the calculation of rate and also give anticipated values for the QT interval. A pair of dividers is also useful.

Rhythm

Normal sinus rhythm shows a normal P wave preceding each QRS complex, with a constant PR interval. If this is not the case, a dysrhythmia is present.

Axis

The cardiac axis represents the net electrical direction the impulse takes as it spreads through the myocardium. It does not represent the anatomical position of the heart; for example, right axis deviation does not mean that the heart has swivelled around such that it is pointing over the right shoulder! Axis is usually assessed in the frontal plane, with lead I designated 0°, and the 360° circle surrounding the heart divided into +180° (clockwise) and −180° (anticlockwise). Normally the cardiac axis lies between −30° and +90° and can be quickly determined in the following manner:

- *Which lead has equal positive and negative QRS components?* This will be at right angles (90°) to the cardiac axis. However, the impulse could be in either direction, which leads to a further question.
- *Which lead has the predominant QRS vector?* The net electrical movement must be in this direction, as movement towards a surface electrode gives a positive deflection.

Determining the cardiac axis may help in the diagnosis of broad-complex tachycardias, pre-excitation syndromes (e.g. Wolff–Parkinson–White syndrome), pulmonary embolism, conduction defects (hemiblocks), ventricular enlargement (e.g. left ventricular hypertrophy) and congenital heart disease (e.g. atrial septal defects).

Waveform

The size of the different waves, and the intervals between them are subject to biological variability, such as heart rate, age and sex. Values are shown in Fig. 5.3.

P wave

The normal P wave results from the spread of activity from the sinus node across the atria. Right atrial depolarisation occurs first, and causes the initial P wave deflection. Left atrial depolarisation causes the terminal deflection. The net electrical movement is from right to left, so the P wave will be upright in leads I, II and aVF and inverted in aVR. The normal P wave axis lies between +30° and +80°. The P wave should not be greater than 0.12 s in duration and should not be taller than 3 mm in the standard leads or 2.5 mm in the V leads.

Abnormalities may be:

- *Inversion.* This means that the atria are being depolarised from an unusual site, rather than the sinus node (unless there is dextrocardia). The origin may be elsewhere in the atrium, in the AV node or even below this.
- *Excessive height.* A tall, peaked P wave results from right atrial enlargement. Because this is often secondary to pulmonary hypertension, the wave is sometimes referred to as *P pulmonale.*
- *Excessive width.* With left atrial enlargement, the P wave becomes broad and notched, like the letter M. The bifid appearance arises because of slight asynchrony between right and left atrial depolarisation. This is normal, but a pronounced notch often results from mitral valve disease, thus the appearance is known as *P mitrale.*
- *Absent.* The P wave is missing during junctional rhythm or may be replaced by flutter or fibrillation waves.

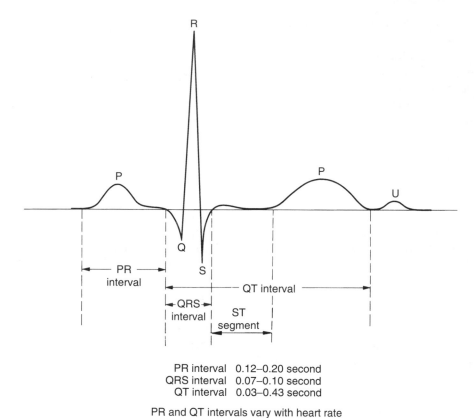

PR interval   0.12–0.20 second
QRS interval   0.07–0.10 second
QT interval   0.03–0.43 second

PR and QT intervals vary with heart rate

Figure 5.3 The ECG cycle showing nomenclature and time intervals.

PR interval

This represents the time taken for atrial activation and AV nodal delay, and increases with age. It is measured from the start of the P wave to the first deflection of the QRS complex. This may be a Q wave, but the term PR interval is still used. It is normally 0.12–0.20 s long (three to five small ECG strip squares). A shortened PR interval is seen when the impulse originates in junctional tissue, or when there are accessory conduction pathways (e.g. Wolff–Parkinson–White syndrome). An increased PR interval indicates AV block.

QRS interval

This represents the total time taken by ventricular depolarisation, and is measured from the first deflection of the QRS complex (whether a Q or R wave) to the end of the S wave. A value greater than 0.12 s (three small squares) is abnormal, and usually indicates an intraventricular conduction disorder (e.g. bundle branch block).

As the depolarisation wave travels through the conduction tissues to the ventricles, the left side of the interventricular septum is depolarised first, spreading to the right, and reflected as a small initial positive R wave in lead V1. Small septal Q waves register simultaneously in leads I, aVL, V5 and V6. These non-pathological Q waves are less than two small squares deep, and less than one small square wide. The shape of the QRS complex varies, and depolarising of the left ventricle predominates (the largest muscle mass). Hence, as the R wave increases steadily from V1 to V6, the S wave diminishes. In general, S waves and R waves should not be greater than 30 mm high.

QT interval

This represents the complete electrical activity time of ventricular stimulation and recovery (depolarisation and repolarisation). It is measured from the beginning of the QRS complex to the end of the T wave and varies with heart rate (the QT interval shortens as the heart rate increases). The corrected QT interval (QT_c) can be calculated by the formula:

$$QT_c = \frac{QT}{\sqrt{RR}}$$

where QT is the QT interval and RR is the RR interval. Practically, the QT interval should be less than 50% of the preceding cycle length and seldom exceeds 0.46 s. A long QT interval may predispose to ventricular tachycardia, typically torsade de pointes.

The QT interval lengthens in heart failure, following myocardial infarction, with hypocalcaemia and with some drugs (antidysrhythmic agents, antibiotics, psychiatric drugs, etc). It is shortened in hypercalcaemia and hyperkalaemia.

T wave

The *T wave results* from repolarisation of the ventricles and might, therefore, be assumed to produce a negative deflection. However, because repolarisation takes place in the opposite direction to depolarisation – i.e. from epicardium to endocardium – the T wave is usually positive and has the same axis as the QRS complex. The T wave may be inverted in leads V1 and V2 in healthy individuals and in V3 in Negroes. T wave inversion in two or more of the right precordial leads is termed *persistent juvenile pattern.*

T waves are normally no greater than 5 mm tall in the standard leads (10 mm in the chest leads), but may be taller in hyperkalaemia, myocardial infarction or ischaemia. Flattening or asymmetrical T wave inversion is a non-specific abnormality but may reflect hypothyroidism or low serum potassium. T wave inversion may be found in myocardial infarction, ventricular hypertrophy or bundle branch block.

ST interval

The *ST segment* is measured from the *J point* (at the junction of the S wave and the ST segment) to the start of the T wave, and should be level with the subsequent TP segment. The ST segment is very slightly curved upwards, but isoelectric. ST displacement or changes in shape are of major importance in electrocardiographic interpretation. Horizontal displacement beyond 1–2 mm upwards or 0.5 mm downwards is abnormal. ST elevation typically occurs in myocardial infarction (when the segment is convex upwards) and pericarditis (when the segment is concave upwards). ST depression is found in myocardial ischaemia and with digoxin therapy.

Frequent mistakes in interpretation of ST morphology are:

- *High ST take-off.* This frequently occurs in young patients, particularly Negroes, and can be up to 2 mm in leads V1–V3 where the rapid ascending S wave merges with the T wave, making the J point difficult to see. A slight notch often accompanies it on the downstroke of the preceding R wave. Benign early repolarisation may also produce ST elevation.
- *ST depression*
  a. ST sag during digoxin therapy.
  b. Downward sloping from the J point during sinus tachycardia. Erroneous diagnoses of myocardial ischaemia may be made during exercise stress tests if the ST shift is not measured 40 ms from the J point.
  c. Ventricular hypertrophy leads to ST depression over the relevant ventricle.

U wave

These are low-voltage, broad waves following the T wave and are probably caused by repolarisation of the mid-myocardium (between epicardium and endocardium), and the His–Purkinje system. They may be seen in healthy individuals, particularly athletes, and may be prominent in hypokalaemia and hypocalcaemia.

INTRAVENTRICULAR CONDUCTION BLOCKS

Intraventricular conduction blocks are often found in patients with or without cardiac disease. The term refers to an impairment or block of conduction in one or more of the fascicles of the conducting tissue distal to the bundle of His. Conduction disturbance may also occur within the ventricles.

BUNDLE BRANCH BLOCK

The main bundle of His divides into two main bundle branches (left and right), which depolarise the ventricles, the left ventricle slightly before the right. Either of these bundles may fail to convey the conduction of electrical activity, resulting in asynchronous ventricular depolarisation and contraction. This abnormal activation will alter the shape and duration of the QRS complex, which will lengthen to more than 0.12 s. Bundle branch block may complicate 10–20% of cases of acute myocardial infarction and is more common with anterior myocardial infarction.

Left bundle branch block

When the left bundle branch is blocked, septal depolarisation commences from right to left, instead of left to right as normally occurs. Hence, the initial Q wave in the left ventricular leads is lost and is replaced by a small, upright R wave. The right ventricle is depolarised before the left (in contrast to normal), which produces an initial R wave in chest lead V1 and an S wave in lead V6. The left ventricle then depolarises, producing an S wave in V1 and a secondary R wave (R′) in V6. The delay in biventricular activation prolongs the QRS duration to more than 0.12 s and alters the QRS morphology, such that a W-shaped complex appears in V1 and an M-shaped complex in V6 (Fig. 5.4).

Right bundle branch block

Because of right bundle branch block, right ventricular depolarisation is delayed and follows that of the left ventricle. This late depolarisation produces a secondary R wave (R′) in the right chest leads and a deep S wave in the left chest leads. The QRS complex is again prolonged to greater than 0.12 s, and the morphology is reversed, such that in V1 there is an M-shaped complex and in V6 a W-shaped complex (Fig. 5.5). Right bundle branch block (RBBB) complicates about 2% of myocardial infarcts and is associated with the later development of complete heart block.

Hemiblocks

The left bundle divides into two hemifascicles, an anterior one running superolaterally and a posterior one running inferomedially. Each of these may become blocked, either on its own or in addition to the main right and left bundles.

Although hemiblock associates with a slight prolongation of the QRS duration, this is usually not appreciated because the duration is still less than 0.12 s. It is recognised by a change in the frontal QRS axis that cannot be explained by any other cause. Left anterior hemiblock (LAHB) is manifest by left axis deviation to less than −30°, whereas left posterior hemiblock (LPHB) produces right axis deviation in excess of +90°. Additionally, QRS morphology may alter to show an RS pattern in lead I and a QR in lead III if there is left posterior hemiblock, whereas the reverse is seen in left anterior hemiblock.

LAHB complicating myocardial infarction is considered benign, but LPHB is usually only seen with extensive myocardial infarction, and is, therefore, associated with a high mortality.

Bifasicular block is a block affecting any two hemifascicles, such as RBBB + LAHB/LPHB or LAHB + LPHB. Bifascicular block after myocardial infarction commonly leads to complete heart block, and prophylactic temporary pacing is sometimes carried out.

Incomplete bundle branch block

This term is used when the morphology of the QRS complex is similar to that observed in

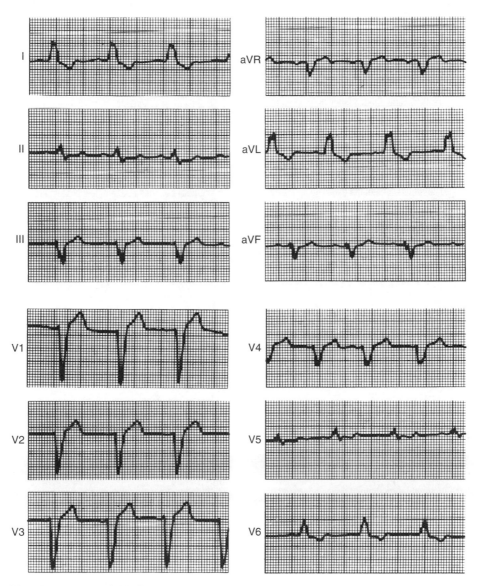

Figure 5.4 ECG: left bundle branch block.

established bundle branch block, but the QRS duration is within normal limits (i.e. under 0.12 s). The changes are not thought to be due to actual conduction block but are indicative of delays caused by prolonged depolarisation of enlarged ventricles.

VENTRICULAR HYPERTROPHY

Ventricular hypertrophy increases the amplitude of the QRS complex. Hypertrophy of the left ventricle increases the height of the R waves in chest leads, whereas hypertrophy of the right ventricle increases the height of the R waves in the right ventricular leads. Septal hypertrophy produces a large, narrow Q wave in the left chest leads.

Unfortunately, many factors can influence the magnitude of the QRS complex, including age, thickness of the chest wall, hyperexpanded chests (as in chronic obstructive airways disease), hypothyroidism and pericardial effusions.

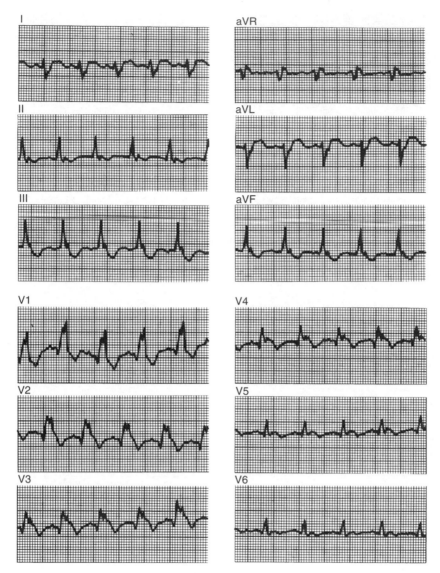

Figure 5.5 ECG: right bundle branch block.

However, the following measurements are useful for the diagnosis of ventricular hypertrophy on voltage criteria:

1. *Left ventricular hypertrophy*
   a. The R wave in V5 or V6 is greater than 27 mm
   b. The S wave in V1 or V2 is greater than 25 mm

   c. The R wave in V5 or V6 plus the S wave in V1 is greater than 35 mm (40 mm in the young)
   d. The R wave in aVF is greater than 20 mm when the QRS axis is vertical.

Confirmatory evidence may be provided by finding left axis deviation less than –30°, ST depression and T wave inversion in V4–V6 and possible P mitrale. The more of these features that are present, the greater the diagnostic value. However, a normal ECG does not exclude significant left ventricular hypertrophy.

2. *Right ventricular hypertrophy*
   a. The R wave is greater than the S wave in V1, and measures more than 5 mm
   b. The R wave in V1 plus the S wave in V5 or V6 is greater than 11 mm

Confirmatory evidence is right axis deviation (over +90°), ST depression and T wave inversion in V1–V3, and possibly P pulmonale.

ATRIAL HYPERTROPHY

1. *Left atrial hypertrophy*. Because of conduction delay through the atrial muscle, the P wave duration is increased to greater than 120 ms, seen best in V1. The different voltage component made by the left atrium may give rise to an M-shaped P wave, the hypertrophied left atrium making a second and delayed peak (P mitrale).

2. *Right atrial hypertrophy*. Even when hypertrophied, depolarisation of the right atrium is usually completed before depolarisation of the left atrium, and the P wave duration does not change. However, the additional voltage makes the P wave peak (P pulmonale) to greater than 2.5 mm, seen best in lead II.

NORMAL FINDINGS

Normal resting ECG findings in healthy adults include:

- Sinus bradycardia or sinus tachycardia
- Sinus arrhythmia
- Prominent U waves
- Wandering atrial pacemaker
- First-degree heart block
- Second-degree heart block (Wenckebach)
- Junctional rhythm
- High ST take-off (benign early repolarisation)
- Tall R waves in the chest leads.

STATIC ECG MONITORING

Monitoring cardiac rhythm forms a vital part of assessment of patients in coronary care and other high-dependency units, and the major impact on the mortality from acute myocardial infarction has resulted from the detection and treatment of dysrhythmias. Static monitoring has provided the opportunity for prompt treatment of changes in rhythm that are likely to have adverse haemodynamic consequences.

The results of such monitoring vary according to whether all potentially serious dysrhythmias are recognised. Fatigue, boredom or distraction limits much 'manual' recording, but computer-linked monitors can detect almost all significant dysrhythmias. Personnel from all specialities often care for patients attached to cardiac monitors, and should be familiar with electrode placement and monitor operation, as well as being able to recognise and distinguish normal and abnormal rhythms.

ELECTRODES

Electrodes are small sensors that can be fixed to the skin to allow the electrical activity of the heart to be detected and transmitted to the monitor for amplification and display. Great advances have been made in the design of these electrodes, and modern disposable, self-adhesive electrodes usually obtain excellent skin contact with minimal or no skin preparation. If the signal is poor:

- The skin should be shaved, particularly if the patient is very hairy. Not only will skin contact be enhanced, but the patient will also be grateful during electrode removal.
- Rubbing the skin with dry gauze or a wooden spatula will remove loose, dry skin (the stratum corneum) and aid electrode contact.
- Wiping the skin with alcohol will remove excess tissue debris, body oil and sweat.

The electrode site should be examined daily for allergic skin reactions, but otherwise there is no need to change the electrodes routinely, unless the signal becomes poor. Non-allergenic electrodes may be used if the patient is sensitive to the adhesive, and any inflammation may be treated with a small quantity of 1% hydrocortisone cream.

The admitting nurse usually selects the appropriate lead placement for the individual patient. The monitor wires either clip or snap onto the chest wires, although it is preferable to do this before the electrodes are placed on the chest, so that the patient is not hurt if pressure is required to push them on.

THE MONITOR CABLE

The signals detected by the electrodes are transmitted to the monitor by a cable. At the distal end, this comprises thin wires about 12 inches long, which connect directly to the surface electrodes. These may be of different colours or labelled 'right', 'left' and 'ground' (or 'earth'). These correspond to the right arm electrode, the left arm electrode and the right leg electrode, respectively. Multichannel cables may allow for full 12-lead ECGs to be recorded. The contacts with the electrodes should be clean and compatible with the surface electrodes being used. The wires should be inspected regularly for breaks in the insulation and any bends or knots. It is useful to form a 'stress loop' with this part of the cable to prevent traction on the electrodes and monitor connections, with consequent electrode separation and movement artefact.

THE BEDSIDE MONITOR

The monitor displays the patient's ECG tracing on a continuous basis. Where there is a central monitoring system with a central console, the ECG pattern is duplicated for all monitored beds and occasionally for telemetry units as well.

The monitor measures the interval between the tallest component of the complexes (usually the R waves), and calculates the heart rate. False heart rates may be registered if, for example, the T wave is of an amplitude equal to that of the R wave, since this will be read as another QRS complex. The amplitude of these complexes may be adjusted by using the gain control, or, if this is insufficient, another lead can be selected by the lead selector control. This control allows the ECG complexes to be recorded in different selected patterns without moving the chest electrodes. A three-electrode system allows the standard limb leads I, II and III to be selected. Five-electrode systems allow leads aVR, aVL and aVF to be selected as well, and 10 leads will allow a full 12-lead ECG to be displayed. Alarms are set to sound when predetermined parameters are met or exceeded.

Most bedside units have a secondary trace under the actual 'real-time' trace. Depending on the degree of sophistication, this holds a memory loop of a few seconds to several minutes. It may allow specific rhythm retrieval and a 'hard copy' rhythm strip to be obtained for more detailed examination or to provide a permanent copy for the patient's records.

MONITORING

Standard ECG limb leads (I, II and III) are normally used for basic ECG monitoring. Chest electrodes are placed in the two infraclavicular spaces (right, negative; left, positive) and at the right sternal edge (earth), which are areas free from underlying muscular masses, thus minimising muscle potential artefact. In this configuration, a tracing similar to standard limb lead I is obtained, but leads II and III may be achieved by lead selection on the monitor. Dysrhythmias may be recognised in any lead, but chest lead V1 is often the best, because it clearly demonstrates the P wave and usually allows clear differentiation between ventricular ectopic beats and those arising from the supraventricular region but being conducted aberrantly. Recording chest lead V1 is contrived by modifying the chest leads, as shown in Fig. 5.6. The positive (+) electrode is placed in the normal V1 intercostal space (4th right); the negative (–) and the earth (G) electrodes are located near the left shoulder and right shoulder, respectively. Modern coronary care practice utilises continuous 12-lead ECG, which allows both rhythm interpretation and ST segment monitoring.

Computerised monitoring

Although visual observation of the monitor by a trained observer was originally used on many

MCL$_1$ (modified CL$_1$)

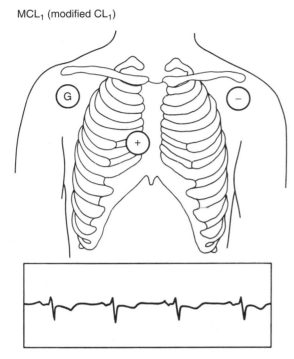

Figure 5.6 Modified chest lead 1 (MCL-1). +, positive electrode; –, negative electrode; G, ground electrode. (From Jowett et al, 1985; reproduced by kind permission of Churchill Livingstone.)

units (and is still usual on general medical wards), many dysrhythmias were missed. The use of computers for the detection of dysrhythmias in acute care units and for the review of rhythms over an extended period is now usual. Computer technology has led to the development of an enormous number of monitors that are able to recognise many dysrhythmias and sound alarms appropriately. Analysis can be performed at various levels of sophistication, from simple dysrhythmia recognition to full reporting of standard 12-lead ECGs. Using a storage mode, display of premature ventricular beat counts and trend analysis is possible for a 24-h period.

AMBULATORY ECG MONITORING

Abnormalities of cardiac rhythm are common and may affect individuals with or without cardiac disease. Such abnormalities may be detected by static monitoring, but if the dysrhythmia is infrequent or transient, extended monitoring techniques are required (Crawford et al, 1999). The standard 12-lead ECG provides little information about cardiac rhythm. The average ECG records about 50 complexes, typically taken with the patient lying down and at rest. Static monitoring techniques also have their limitations and are unsuitable for the detection of short rhythm disturbances, especially if induced by exertion or other factors in the daily life of the patient (Jowett and Thompson, 1985; Jowett et al, 1985). Documentation of abnormal electrical activity may require prolonged continuous recording during exercise.

Ambulatory ECG monitoring was initially designed to document transient disturbances in heart rhythm and conduction, with the aim of establishing a relationship between symptoms and accompanying disturbances in cardiac rhythm. The role of ambulatory monitoring has now expanded to assessing antidysrhythmic therapy, detecting ischaemia and determining prognosis (Mickley, 1994).

Norman 'Jeff' Holter, an American, put forward ideas for a portable ECG recorder in the late 1940s; hence these recording machines are often known as 'Holter recorders'. From the initial bulky, short-duration recorders, these monitors have been refined to light, small, strong machines capable of recording the heart rhythm continuously for several days, often with multiple channels of ECG data being recorded simultaneously. Improvements in solid-state digital technology have enhanced the accuracy of computer analysis, and allow electronic or telephonic transmission of ECG data. These advances, in addition to better signal quality and greater computer arrhythmia interpretation capabilities, have opened up new potential uses for ambulatory ECG.

There are two main types of recorders:

- *Event recorders* store only a brief period of ECG activity when activated by the patient in response to symptoms.
- *Loop recorders* record the ECG in a continuous manner, but store only a brief period of ECG

recording in the memory when the event marker is activated by the patient at the time of symptoms. These recorders can be used for prolonged periods of time to identify infrequently occurring arrhythmias or symptoms that would not be detected by conventional 24-h continuous recorders. Loop recorders can even be implanted for longer-term monitoring. Under local anaesthesia, these small devices are inserted under the skin and function as a single-lead event recorder that may be interrogated through the skin, and removed when no longer needed (Seidl et al, 2000). They may be left in indefinitely, and are suitable for patient with syncopal episodes every 3–12 months. The patient uses a hand-held activator to store information permanently.

The patient is told to carry on normal daily activities, and keep a detailed diary for the day's activities (e.g. sleeping, working and watching television), with clear descriptions and timing of any symptoms, especially faintness, palpitations and dizziness. This diary of timed symptoms and the referral note are of major value during tape analysis and interpretation.

High-speed electrocardioscanners (Fig. 5.7) are able to download information rapidly, although selection of rhythm strips and print-out make full processing a little longer. Presentation of the contents depends upon the clinical circumstances. A full disclosure presentation can print all the complexes in miniature, which is particularly useful for identifying periods of interest. If the patient has experienced symptoms, these periods may be selectively recalled, with a normal-size ECG print-out, including the periods before and after the event. Precise timing is noted on the strips, to allow comparison with the patient's diary, to correlate symptoms and dysrhythmias.

TELEMETRY UNITS

Telemetry is often used for extended peri-infarction cardiac monitoring. The patient is fitted with standard chest electrodes attached to a small transmitter, which is carried in a chest harness or pyjama pocket. The cardiac rhythm is transmitted continuously to a receiver (normally situated on the coronary care unit), where it is displayed, observed and analysed in the same way as for patients on static monitors. The advantage of this system is that patients may be mobilised in the early period following myocardial infarction, while still having the benefits of dysrhythmia monitoring. The transmission range of these

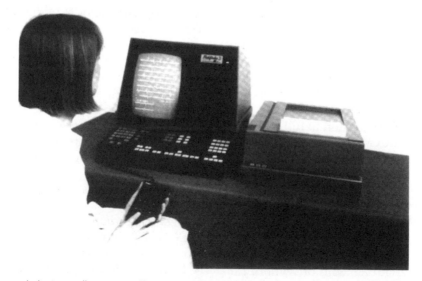

Figure 5.7 High-speed electrocardioscanner. (Reproduced by kind permission of Reynolds Medical Limited.)

units is usually short and thus relatively free from extrinsic radio-interference. Longer-range units have been developed for use by cardiac arrest teams, who may be further away from the receiver units, and by ambulance and paramedic teams outside the hospital. In both cases, the cardiac rhythm may be monitored and advice on drug therapy given by more experienced physicians 'back at base'.

NORMAL LIMITS AND RECORDING ARTEFACTS

Confirmation of a dysrhythmia-induced symptom requires the coincidence of the symptom and a recorded rhythm disturbance. Asymptomatic recordings do not usually help, although evidence of asymptomatic abnormalities, such as short runs of ventricular tachycardia or ischaemic episodes, may help further management. Up to a third of recordings will be normal despite the presence of symptoms during the recording period.

On the other hand, ambulatory monitoring may disclose many dysrhythmias in apparently normal individuals. These are not necessarily pathological, but currently there are no consistent ways of separating normality from abnormality. Most of the general population have isolated ventricular ectopic beats, two-thirds have sinus bradycardia and about one-fifth have very brief episodes of atrial fibrillation. About 0.2% of apparently healthy adults have ventricular bigeminy. Pauses of 2–3 s are very common in athletes, who have high vagal tone. In general, rhythm disturbances are more important and tolerated less well in the elderly than in younger adults.

The interpretation of the pathological significance of rhythm abnormalities is very much dependent on the circumstances. This view may be entirely different in patients recovering from myocardial infarction.

PULSE OXIMETRY

Pulse oximetry is a simple non-invasive method of monitoring the percentage of haemoglobin that is saturated with oxygen ($SaO_2\%$). Oxygen saturation tells us how much of the oxygen-carrying capacity of the haemoglobin is being utilised. Hence:

$$\text{Oxygen saturation} (SaO_2\%) = \frac{\text{Amount of oxygen being carried by the haemoglobin}}{\text{Amount that can be carried by the haemoglobin}}$$

The pulse oximeter consists of a probe attached to the patient's finger or ear lobe, which is linked to a computerised unit that displays the percentage of haemoglobin saturated with oxygen.

HOW OXIMETRY WORKS

The principle of oximetry was developed following the simple observation that oxygenated blood and deoxygenated blood differ in colour: arterial blood appears red, whereas venous blood appears blue. When the two are mixed, the ratio of their concentrations can be determined from the amount of light absorbed at two different wavelengths. Oximetry calculates the ratio of oxygenated to deoxygenated arterial blood in pulsatile capillaries by measuring the amount of red and infrared light absorbed as light sources shine through the capillary beds in the extremities; the result are expressed as a percentage.

The oximeter probe contains the two light-emitting diodes (one red and one infrared), which shine towards a detector located opposite. The diodes are rapidly switched on and off, and the detector records how much of the light has been absorbed on its passage through the tissues. To eliminate the light-absorbing effects of other tissues, the resulting signal registers only the readings from blood pulsating in the capillaries (hence 'pulse' oximetry). The corresponding arterial oxygen saturation is calculated as an average based on the previous few seconds of recording that is constantly being updated.

When haemoglobin carries oxygen, it is converted to oxyhaemoglobin, and the amount of oxygen that can be carried is closely related to the PaO_2 of the blood. This relationship is shown by the oxyhaemoglobin dissociation curve (Fig. 5.8). This relationship is not linear, but

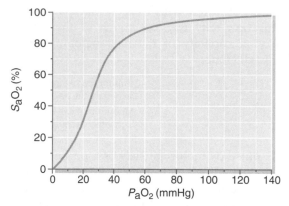

Figure 5.8   The oxyhaemoglobin dissociation curve.

'S' shaped. A saturation of over 97% equates with a normal PaO_2 of over 97 mmHg, but an apparently minor fall in saturation to 90% actually equates to a fall in the PaO_2 to 60 mmHg. This is because of the rapid descent at the end of the plateau, where saturation falls quite rapidly as the PaO_2 declines. If the SaO_2 is found to be less than 80%, there is usually severe hypoxia ($PaO_2 <$ 45 mmHg), and arterial blood gases should be taken to obtain an accurate view. Target saturation during oxygen therapy will vary with such changes as $PaCO_2$, pH and body temperature. These factors cause lateral shifts of the oxygen dissociation curve, either to the left or to the right. Oxygen should be given to keep the SaO_2 at least 90%.

PROBLEMS WITH OXIMETRY

Poor tissue perfusion

The pulse oximeter can only function if enough pulsatile blood passes between the light source and the detector. If tissue perfusion is poor or the pulse is weak, the generated signal will be liable to error.

Abnormal haemoglobins

Compounds that absorb light at the same wavelengths as haemoglobin and oxyhaemoglobin will introduce errors (e.g. nail varnish!). The microprocessor in the oximeter is programmed to parameters derived from the normal oxyhaemoglobin dissociation curve, and abnormal haemoglobins may produce errors. In most cases, the oximeter will underestimate the true saturation, but of far more concern are situations where the oximeter may overestimate saturation, particularly from carboxyhaemoglobin, which can form 5–10% of the total haemoglobin in heavy smokers.

Excessive ambient light

Excessive ambient light may saturate the detector and cause erroneous readings. This is particularly so if there is strong sunlight shining on the probe, or flickering fluorescent lights. Ambient light is a particular problem if the finger is not fully inserted into the finger probe, thereby allowing external light sources to fall on the detector. A lop-sided probe will allow light from the two light emitters to pass directly into the detector, and not through the tissues of the finger.

Motion artefact

Most movement artefact occurs from the probe slipping across the skin whenever the hand is moved; thus the probe and cable should be adequately secured to the patient. The cable should be sufficiently long to permit the patient to move, and it is sometimes useful to fix a 'stress loop' in the cable to the skin, so that traction does not occur directly on the probe. Using the toes is sometimes possible, but poor perfusion at this site is more likely to make readings unreliable. Persistent limb tremor is an occasional problem best circumvented by application of the ear probe. The probe is clipped to the ear lobe or pinna, ensuring that the clip does not pinch the skin and thus impair perfusion.

Other blood gases

Oximeters give no information about the level of $PaCO_2$, and cannot give warning of respiratory failure due to carbon dioxide retention.

HAEMODYNAMIC MONITORING

The ability to recognise and assess serious circulatory changes in patients recovering from acute myocardial infarction is of major importance, both diagnostically and for assessing therapy and prognosis. Although clinical examination of the patient remains of major importance, it may be difficult to assess many patients without invasive monitoring. For example, infarction of the right ventricle may complicate one-third of inferior myocardial infarctions and is associated with a low left atrial pressure, despite elevation of the jugular venous pressure. In patients with long-standing cardiac failure, selective peripheral vasoconstriction may maintain blood pressure while masking a low cardiac output. This group of patients may also develop thickening of the pulmonary vessel walls, allowing a substantial rise in pulmonary capillary pressures before the clinical signs of pulmonary congestion develop. So, while the patient may be judged to have mild left ventricular failure on clinical grounds, haemodynamically there may be pulmonary hypertension, with a substantial reduction in cardiac output.

The term 'haemodynamic monitoring' describes methods of monitoring blood pressure, volume and circulation, usually by indwelling catheters inserted into the heart or major blood vessels. The catheters are connected by fluid-filled tubing to pressure transducers and recording systems. The most frequently measured parameters on coronary care units are the pulse, arterial blood pressure, central venous pressure, intracardiac pressures and cardiac output. In recent years, many techniques have become available that permit easy bedside analysis of the patient's haemodynamic status and cardiac function. The precise method of obtaining and recording these haemodynamic data varies from hospital to hospital and is usually dependent upon the expertise of the staff and available equipment. Typical indications for invasive monitoring are shown in Box 5.1.

Once the catheter has been inserted, it is usually the responsibility of the nursing staff to ensure

Box 5.1 Some indications for invasive haemodynamic monitoring

• Cardiogenic shock
• Unexplained hypotension
• Haemodynamic instability with suspicion or presence of:
  – Pulmonary embolism
  – Right ventricular infarction
  – Aortic dissection
  – Mechanical heart defects (e.g. ruptured interventricular septum or mitral valve)

the patient's comfort and safety and the maintenance of the system, and to obtain and record data. Since the patient's treatment will often rely heavily on the results of monitoring, it is essential that such data are accurate. The nurse should be aware of problems inherent in data acquisition, including common technical and physiological variables that may affect the data. In addition, they should be aware of the effect that specific nursing interventions (e.g. feeding, bathing and positioning) may have on haemodynamic measurements.

PRESSURE TRANSDUCER SYSTEMS

Pressure transducers are electromechanical devices that detect energy changes (e.g. those in pressure and temperature) and convert them to electrical signals. In most forms of haemodynamic monitoring, they detect intravascular pressure changes and convert them into electrical charges for amplification and digital read-out. Usually, pressure changes are transmitted via fluid-filled tubing connected to a supple diaphragm located in a transducer dome. Changes in the intravascular pressure are transmitted from the indwelling cannula to fluid that passes through the transducer dome. Pressure waves are directly transmitted to a diaphragm within the dome, which is connected to a strain gauge. The more the diaphragm is moved by the pressure waves, the greater is the electrical charge generated and the higher the pressure reading on the monitor.

MEASURING THE CENTRAL VENOUS PRESSURE

Central venous pressure (CVP) monitoring is used to measure pressure of blood in the right atrium or superior vena cava. The CVP reflects right ventricular end diastolic pressure (filling pressure or preload) and is determined by blood volume, vascular tone and cardiac performance. Elevation of the CVP is common following acute myocardial infarction, usually reflecting raised right-sided pressures secondary to left ventricular failure. Other causes are right ventricular infarction and cardiac tamponade. Low CVP readings are usually due to hypovolaemia, when infusion of fluid may improve cardiac performance.

CVP catheters are inserted percutaneously, usually into the subclavian or jugular veins, and are advanced to lie in the superior vena cava or right atrium. During central venous catheterisation, it is important that the patient is placed in the Trendelenburg position (i.e. head down). This distends the central veins, which not only reduces the risk of air embolism, but also makes cannulation easier. The right side of the patient is chosen preferentially to prevent damage to the thoracic duct. Placement of the catheter is confirmed by chest X-ray, which will also exclude a pneumothorax.

The CVP is normally measured using manometry, although, because of the sluggish response, a pressure transducer may be preferred, particularly if continuous display of the CVP is required.

Manometry

The manometer (Fig. 5.9) should be placed with the baseline at the level of the right atrium. The baseline may be at zero on the scale, but it is preferable to set it at a higher value (e.g. 10 cm), so that negative pressures can be recorded. A spirit level should be used to ensure that the zero reference point on both the patient and the manometer coincide. The line should be well flushed, by opening up the intravenous fluid

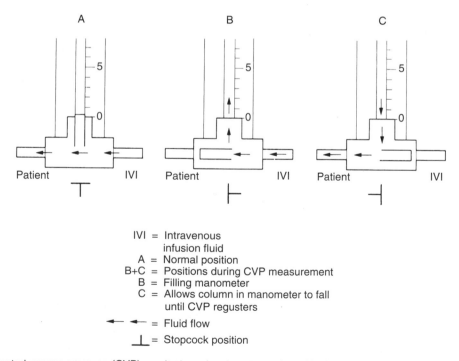

IVI = Intravenous
     infusion fluid
A = Normal position
B+C = Positions during CVP measurement
B = Filling manometer
C = Allows column in manometer to fall
    until CVP regusters

← ← = Fluid flow
⊥ = Stopcock position

Figure 5.9 Central venous pressure (CVP) monitoring, showing stopcock positioning.

line. Free passage of fluid through the system should occur when the infusion rate is turned up, and blood should be freely aspirated if required. Respiratory oscillations should be visible.

Turning the stopcock from the normal position A to position B (Fig. 5.9) should fill the manometer column. The stopcock is then turned to position C, and the fluid is allowed to run down and equilibrate through the CVP line. Normally, the fluid falls freely, although it fluctuates with venous pulsation and respiration. Once the column has settled, the CVP should be measured at the end of expiration and expressed in cmH_2O (normal = 0–10 cmH_2O).

Following CVP measurement, the stopcock should be returned to position A and the infusion rate adjusted as required.

Electrical pressure transducers

This method is most frequently used when measurements are made via the right atrial port of a 4-channel Swan–Ganz catheter. The reading recorded by the transducer is displayed in mmHg (normal = 0–8 mmHg). Correlation of CVP in mmHg and cmH_2O is shown in Table 5.1.

Positioning the patient is extremely important during measurement of the CVP. Ideally, the patient should be lying flat, without a pillow, but, if the patient's condition does not permit this, he can be positioned at 45° or less. During normal respiration, the intrathoracic pressure falls on inspiration. Measuring haemodynamic pressures at end expiration is considered to be the most valid, because the intrathoracic pressure is closest to zero at this point.

INTRA-ARTERIAL BLOOD PRESSURE MONITORING

In haemodynamically unstable patients, measurement of the blood pressure is often difficult, and indirect readings may differ from the actual arterial blood pressure by over 30 mmHg. The insertion of an arterial pressure line is then useful for directly and continuously measuring systolic, diastolic and mean arterial blood pressures, as well as for giving easy access for repeated blood gas sampling. Sites commonly employed are the radial, brachial and dorsalis pedis arteries. However, the closer the cannula is to the heart, the more accurate the waveform and pressure reading; the radial artery is the most commonly utilised site.

Cannulation is performed under local anaesthesia, using a 20-gauge Teflon catheter, which is attached to a T-connector and a pressurised heparin–saline flushing system. This runs continuously at 3–5 ml/h to minimise clotting, vasospasm and intimal damage. A transducer converts the pressures into a digital read-out and displays the arterial waveform. The readings displayed are systolic blood pressure, diastolic blood pressure and mean blood pressure. The mean arterial pressure is, however, not half the sum of the systolic and the diastolic pressure, but is a measurement that integrates the area under the arterial waveform curve to obtain a true mean.

Complications of intra-arterial monitoring are not common but include:

- Arterial occlusion
- Arterial spasm
- Haemorrhage
- Air embolism
- Sepsis
- Ecchymoses.

When the line is removed, pressure over the insertion site should be maintained for at least 5 min, or longer if thrombolytic agents or anticoagulants have been used.

Table 5.1 Conversion of mmHg to cmH_2O (approximate)

($mmHg \times 1.36 = cmH_2O$)	
1 = 1	11 = 15
2 = 3	12 = 16
3 = 4	13 = 18
4 = 5	14 = 19
5 = 7	15 = 20
6 = 8	16 = 22
7 = 10	17 = 23
8 = 11	18 = 24
9 = 12	19 = 26
10 = 14	20 = 27
($cmH_2O/1.36 = mmHg$)	

PULMONARY ARTERY AND PULMONARY ARTERY WEDGE PRESSURES

The value of CVP measurement is often limited, because it reflects the functional state of the right ventricle, which does not always parallel that of the left ventricle. Information about left ventricular function is often essential for complete evaluation.

Monitoring pulmonary artery and pulmonary artery wedge pressures may be useful following myocardial infarction, since they provide data to guide and evaluate therapy. This may be achieved by using a pulmonary artery flotation (Swan–Ganz) catheter (Swan et al, 1970). The Swan–Ganz catheter (Fig. 5.10) is about 80–110 cm long, marked at 10-cm intervals, and is available in three sizes: 5 FG (for children), 6 FG and 7 FG (for adults). The basic model has two lumina.

The larger lumen terminates at the tip of the catheter and is used for recording intracardiac pressures, infusion of fluids and sampling of mixed venous blood. A smaller lumen serves to inflate the latex balloon, which not only helps the catheter to float through the right heart, but also allows repeated, reversible, pulmonary artery occlusion for recording wedge pressures. In some models, there is a third lumen, terminating 30 cm proximal to the catheter tip, which enables simultaneous measurement of right atrial pressures, and a fourth channel that leads to a thermistor located close to the tip. These latter two channels are used together for calculation of right ventricular cardiac output by thermodilution. Other types of catheter are available for pulmonary angiography and pacing, and all can be floated into the pulmonary artery by observing pressure tracings made during passage through the right heart, without requiring fluoroscopy.

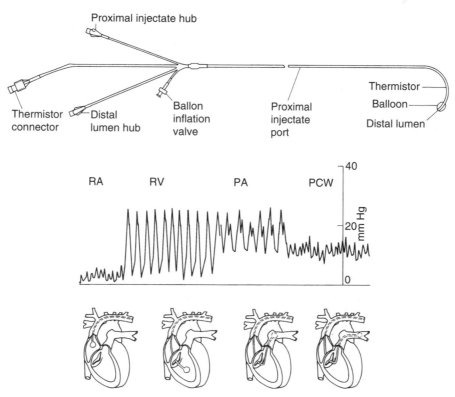

Figure 5.10   The Swan–Ganz thermodilution catheter and typical pressures recorded during its passage through the heart. (From Stokes and Jowett, 1985; reproduced by kind permission of Churchill Livingstone.)

The catheter is normally inserted at the bedside under local anaesthesia.

USES OF SWAN–GANZ CATHETERS

The balloon flotation catheter is particularly helpful in those patients with low cardiac output, hypotension, severe pulmonary oedema and cardiogenic shock (Stokes and Jowett, 1985). It allows quick and easy differentiation of inadequate intravascular volume with a resultant low left-sided filling pressure, and adequate intravascular volume and a high left-sided filling pressure due to extensive left ventricular dysfunction. In the latter patients, the catheter can be used to monitor therapeutic efforts to adjust the left-sided filling pressure so as to maximise cardiac output at the lowest possible filling pressure.

Measurement of pulmonary artery wedge pressure and pulmonary artery pressure

Pulmonary artery wedge pressure is the pressure recorded when the Swan–Ganz catheter has been floated through the right heart and wedged into a peripheral pulmonary artery. The pulmonary arteries are end arteries, and the pulmonary veins contain no valves. The catheter therefore registers the pressure transmitted retrogradely from the left atrium. The pulmonary artery wedge pressure closely relates to the left atrial pressure and provides an indirect method of assessing left atrial pressure. Normal intracardiac pressures recorded by Swan–Ganz catheter are shown in Table 5.2.

Table 5.2 Intracardiac pressures measured by the Swan–Ganz catheter

	Pressure (mmHg)
Right atrium	0–8
Pulmonary artery	
Systolic	15–30
Diastolic	5–12
Pulmonary artery wedge pressure	5–12

Cardiac output

The measurement of cardiac output provides useful information about cardiac performance and response to therapy. Cardiac output may be measured at the bedside using the 4-channel Swan–Ganz catheter by injecting 10 ml of 5% dextrose at 4°C or room temperature into the right atrium via the 30-cm port. A temperature drop of the blood is recorded by the thermistor at the tip of the catheter, which lies in the pulmonary artery. From the recorded changes in temperature, a bedside computer can calculate the cardiac output. A mean of three serial readings is usually taken for the value of cardiac output.

Blood gas analysis

Blood gas analysis can be made on mixed venous blood slowly aspirated via the tip port. Another type of pulmonary artery flotation catheter is fitted with an oximeter, so that continuous measurement of the SaO_2 is possible.

Complications

Complications arising from the use of Swan–Ganz catheters are infrequent. *Dysrhythmias* may be caused by mechanical irritation of the endocardium or valves and are usually noted at the time of catheter insertion, manipulation or removal. Continuous ECG monitoring is therefore desirable, with special attention paid to the rhythm during catheter manipulation. *Pulmonary infarction* may be caused by frequent, prolonged or over-inflation of the balloon, or by thrombus formation around the catheter tip. With time, the catheter tends to migrate through the heart and to wedge spontaneously. If unnoticed, pulmonary infarction can result. If pressures are displayed continuously, any pressure damping (indicating thrombus formation) or spontaneous wedging can be immediately recognised. Rapid inflation of the balloon not only increases the risk of balloon rupture, but may also rupture the pulmonary capillary. This is rare, but patients with pulmonary hypertension are at risk. Balloon inflation should always be slow.

Although the Swan–Ganz catheter is a valuable tool in the management of many conditions, inappropriate use may have lead to increased mortality and morbidity associated with its use (Soni, 1996). It is invasive, and may be particularly hazardous in patients who have recently been thrombolysed. As with all investigations, it is important that the information it acquires justifies its use.

THE CHEST RADIOGRAPH

The standard posteroanterior (PA) chest X-ray is taken at full inspiration, with the patient standing facing the film, which is 1.5 m from the X-ray tube focus. In the standard PA view, the right border of the heart consists (from top to bottom) of the superior vena cava, the ascending aorta and the right atrium. The left border is formed by the aortic arch, the descending aorta, the pulmonary artery and its left main branch, and the left ventricle (Fig. 5.11). A standard PA chest film is preferred because:

- The diaphragm is flattened and allows the bases of the lungs to be seen

- The erect position lowers hydrostatic pressure in the low-pressure pulmonary vascular tree
- The scapulae are slid away from the lung fields
- The PA projection reduces magnification of the heart shadow.

The radiograph should be assessed in a routine method so that nothing is missed.

TECHNICAL QUALITY

All films should be correctly identified and dated. Right and left markers will avoid a misdiagnosis of dextrocardia. If the film is taken straight, the medial ends of the clavicles should be equidistant from the midline, marked by the spinous processes of the vertebrae. A rotated film may suggest cardiomegaly, or hilar tumours. An underpenetrated film will enhance lung markings, often leading to an erroneous diagnosis of pulmonary congestion; this is particularly common in obese patients. It is sometimes worthwhile to note what kilovoltage has been employed, particularly in coronary care, where interpretation of pulmonary congestion is important. A change to a higher kilovoltage on a subsequent chest film will show the apparent clearing of pulmonary oedema.

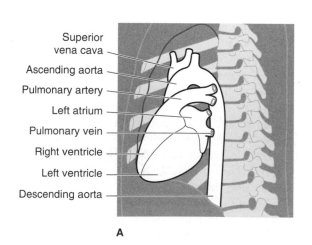

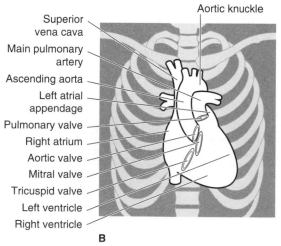

Figure 5.11 A & B Cardiac anatomy (A) on a lateral chest X-ray; (B) on an anteroposterior chest X-ray.

THE HEART

Although a good knowledge of radiographic anatomy is useful to distinguish which part of the heart is responsible for the cardiac enlargement, different underlying processes can produce the same final picture. Enlargement of the left atrium is the most easy to recognise; it gives a projection of 2 cm below the left pulmonary artery shadow and causes a convex bulge immediately below the left main bronchus. In extreme enlargement, the left atrium will protrude above the right atrium, causing a double density at the right border of the heart. Right atrial enlargement simply makes the right border look more prominent, and it produces a long continuous convexity of the right heart border.

Enlargement of the ventricles may be difficult to distinguish on the conventional chest X-ray. Left ventricular enlargement pushes the cardiac shadow downwards and outwards and is found in association with hypertension, aortic valve disease and mitral incompetence. The right ventricle enlarges also forwards, reducing the retrosternal air space on a lateral chest X-ray. A normal left ventricle is sometimes pushed posteriorly by right ventricular enlargement (due to pulmonary hypertension or pulmonary stenosis), and the cardiac apex is rounded and lifted up above the left diaphragm.

The cardiac size is assessed radiologically by determining the cardiothoracic ratio. This is the ratio of the widest part of the heart shadow to the widest transverse thoracic diameter (measured from the inner surface of the ribs). It should be less than 0.5 in adults. The most frequent cause of cardiac enlargement is dilatation due to volume overload. Assessing cardiac size by X-ray is not infallible. Enlargement of the cardiac shadow may be due to pericardial effusion, cardiac dilatation or hypertrophy. Cardiomegaly is common in athletes and does not necessarily indicate dilatation or hypertrophy. Hypertrophy normally leads to a volume reduction within the heart chambers, so that the overall cardiac diameters are only very slightly increased.

The diagnosis of pericardial effusion is not always easy on the standard chest film, because it cannot readily be distinguished from other causes of cardiac enlargement. Large effusions make the heart outline globular; small effusions are hard to detect radiologically and are best detected by echocardiography. If the effusion has formed rapidly, cardiac dilatation may be seen on consecutive films.

THE LUNG FIELDS

The normal divisions of the pulmonary artery can be traced to within about 1 cm of the lung edge. The pulmonary veins are large and horizontal in the lower lung fields, but are seen as smaller linear opacities draining towards the left atrium in the upper lung fields.

Increased pulmonary capillary pressures and diminished cardiac output are the final common pathways for the production of pulmonary oedema. As pressure in the pulmonary veins rises, increasing congestion is seen in the pulmonary vessels until a critical pressure of about 30 mmHg is reached, which marks the onset of pulmonary oedema. Pulmonary congestion occurs first in the lower pulmonary veins, where perivascular interstitial oedema develops. This results in local hypoxia and reflex vasoconstriction in the affected vessels. The blood is then diverted to the upper lung vessels (upper lobe diversion), producing the characteristic radiological picture. The interstitial oedema collects around hilar vessels to produce the 'bat wing' sign, and collection in and around the pulmonary lymphatics gives rise to thin linear opacities called Kerley lines. The *Kerley A lines* (engorged intralobular lymphatics) run from the periphery to the hilum; the more common *Kerley B lines* of interstitial oedema are short parallel lines that run horizontally at the lung peripheries, particularly in the costophrenic angles. As the pulmonary oedema worsens, fluid collects in the alveoli of the lower zones, producing opacities, and later outside the lung to produce pleural effusions.

In patients with long-standing pulmonary hypertension and heart failure, there may be thickening of the pulmonary vessel walls, allowing substantial elevation of pulmonary capillary pressures without clinical congestion. In addition, there may be a lag of up to 48 h between haemodynamic stabilisation and resolution of radiological signs.

THE DIAPHRAGM

The diaphragm should expand to the level of the 5th rib anteriorly on full inspiration. If the patient has not fully expanded his lungs, the heart shadow may suggest cardiomegaly. A fat pad is sometimes seen adjacent to the cardiac border in the obese, and a slight hump of the right diaphragm is frequent in the elderly.

THE MEDIASTINUM

The position and size of the aorta should be noted. Unfolding is common in the elderly and hypertensive patient, and calcification of the aortic knuckle may be seen. An increase in the size of the aortic outline with widening of the mediastinal shadow may indicate aortic dissection, particularly in the presence of a small left pleural effusion.

BONES

Sternal depression (pectus excavatum) may displace the heart and is the cause of a systolic murmur with apparent cardiac enlargement (the 'straight back' syndrome). This may only be visible with a lateral chest film. The heart shadow will also be displaced if there is a thoracic scoliosis. Rib lesions such as fractures or metastases may be a cause of the presenting chest pain.

THE NECK AND UPPER ABDOMEN

A retrosternal goitre may be misdiagnosed as an aortic aneurysm. The presence of intraperitoneal air (air under the diaphragm) should be excluded, since peritonitis may present with chest and shoulder tip pain.

ECHOCARDIOGRAPHY

Echocardiography allows the heart to be studied non-invasively, and is a powerful tool for assessing cardiac anatomy, pathology and function. A transducer generates high-frequency pulses of short duration, which travel through the body at differing velocities, depending upon the tissues encountered, and are echoed back, to be recorded by the same transducer. Cardiac ultrasound uses frequencies of 2.0–5.0 MHz, and, the higher the frequency, the better the resolution (although the worse the tissue penetration).

The two main techniques used are M-mode and two-dimensional (real-time) echocardiography. The Doppler shift effect during ultrasound can be combined with these techniques to provide information on the velocity and direction of blood flow. Colour flow mapping uses a multigated, pulsed Doppler technique to estimate the mean velocity of blood cells within the heart and can identify patterns of blood flow and abnormal jets.

Transthoracic echocardiography is the usual method of obtaining cardiac images by ultrasound. The transducer is placed on the chest wall to obtain different views of the heart through anatomical 'windows'. The technique is limited by the size of these windows, which are found between the ribs and lungs since ultrasound does not travel through bone or air. Technical difficulties may be encountered in up to one-quarter of recordings.

Transoesophageal echocardiography uses a miniature transducer mounted on a modified endoscope, which may be swallowed and positioned directly behind the heart. The image quality is much better because of the proximity of the structures as well as the absence of bone. Biplane probes incorporate two transducers at right-angles to each other, and multiplane probes can permit a 180° view of the heart. The probe frequency is extended up to 7.5 MHz (since depth is not so important), which allows very high resolution.

Indications for transoesophageal echocardiography include assessment and diagnosis of infective endocarditis and aortic dissection. The technique is of major value in assessing prosthetic heart valves, and the detection of left atrial thrombus prior to elective cardioversion.

CROSS-SECTIONAL ECHOCARDIOGRAPHY

Two-dimensional images are built up by the ultrasound beam being swept through a 90° sector of the heart, producing up to 50 cross-sections per second, and generating a recognisable moving image of the heart. Multiple views from different sites on the chest can be used to build up a complete picture of the heart. The images are usually recorded on super-VHS videotape or digitally on optical discs. Photographs can be obtained as a hard copy to file with the notes. On-line computers can be used to measure cardiac dimensions and calculate various parameters, such as ejection fraction and cardiac output. Fall-off in signal can sometimes produce poor images and often makes exact measurement of cardiac function inaccurate.

M-MODE ECHOCARDIOGRAPHY

M-mode echocardiography is a technique that essentially produces a graph of depth of tissues against time. A single 1-cm ultrasound beam is directed through the heart using a scan line selected from the two-dimensional image. The graph is recorded on rapidly moving paper, which allows measurement of intracardiac structures (e.g. wall thickness and cavity dimensions) with timing of events. The M-mode trace does not demonstrate cardiac anatomy and probably should not be interpreted without reference to the cross-sectional image.

DOPPLER ECHOCARDIOGRAPHY

Blood velocity can be calculated by using the Doppler effect on red cells, either by pulsed or continuous wave ultrasound. Pulsed-wave Doppler assesses the velocity of blood at one site, selected by a cursor superimposed on the two-dimensional image. Continuous-wave Doppler emits a constant stream of ultrasound along a single line and superimposes all velocities along that line. Continuous-wave Doppler can resolve very high velocities (e.g. through stenosed valves), whereas pulsed-wave Doppler can measure flow at precise depths in conjunction with the two-dimensional image. The machine software is able to display calculated flow velocities and is very useful in assessing obstructive lesions and septal defects.

COLOUR FLOW ECHOCARDIOGRAPHY

Colour Doppler flow mapping has been one of the most important developments in cardiac ultrasound since cross-sectional echocardiography, and has allowed a better understanding of flow physiology in health and disease. As red blood cells move through the heart at relatively high velocities, the Doppler shift can be detected and assigned a colour depending upon the direction and velocity of blood flow. The blood flow information is displayed over the two-dimensional or M-mode image; by convention, flow towards the transducer is displayed in red, flow away from the transducer is coloured blue and turbulence produces a mosaic of different colours. Maps of different colours can be used, depending upon operator preferences. The technique is very sensitive and can detect the trivial regurgitation that occurs through normal valves when they close. Overinterpretation of the images is a common mistake. For example, we now know that 90% of the normal population have physiological tricuspid and pulmonary regurgitation and one-third have mitral regurgitation (Houston, 1993).

Colour flow imaging is invaluable in the detection of abnormal flows within the heart and great arteries. It may be combined with M-mode echocardiography for timing flow events and distinguishing between systolic and diastolic abnormalities.

STRESS ECHOCARDIOGRAPHY

Stress echocardiography involves the imaging of areas of altered myocardial contractility during exercise or pharmacological stress. It may be used to:

- Diagnose coronary artery disease
- Detect myocardial viability

• Assess prognosis.

Acute myocardial ischaemia is accompanied by the development of regional left ventricular wall motion abnormalities due to the so-called 'ischaemic cascade' (Fig. 5.12). These wall motion abnormalities serve as a marker of the presence and location of flow-limiting coronary arterial stenoses and may be determined by echocardiography. Stress may be induced either by treadmill/bicycle exercise or pharmacologically if the patient cannot exercise. Drugs utilised include dobutamine and arbutamine, or coronary vasodilators such as adenosine and dipyridamole. Two-dimensional echocardiograms are recorded at baseline and immediately after maximal stress. Motion abnormalities are recorded in different segments of the left ventricle, allowing correlation with the expected coronary anatomy. The sensitivity and specificity of stress echocardiography is much better than exercise stress testing, and comparable with nuclear stress testing. The technique can also be used for detecting myocardial viability, and may be used to differentiate areas of infarcted tissue from hibernating myocardium when considering patients for revascularisation.

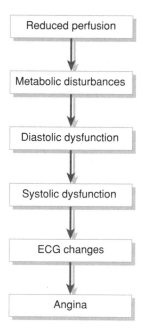

Figure 5.12 The ischaemic cascade.

Hibernating myocardium is characterised by response to inotropic stimulation.

Stress echocardiography is undoubtedly a very useful technique, but is very operator-dependent, as well as being time-consuming. Not all patients are good echo subjects, which may also limit its application.

ECHOCARDIOGRAPHY AND CORONARY CARE

A modern, two-dimensional ultrasound machine is an essential piece of equipment for the coronary care unit, because it is non-invasive, has rapid acquisition time and can be brought to the bedside. In patients with cardiovascular collapse of unknown cause, echocardiography can differentiate between hypovolaemia, severe left ventricular dysfunction, pulmonary embolism and pericardial effusion with tamponade. The intimal flap of an aortic dissection can be seen in many cases of aortic dissection, particularly with transoesophageal echocardiography, and critical aortic stenosis can also be demonstrated and quantified.

Other frequent applications of echocardiography in patients on coronary care include:

1. *Defining the aetiology of cardiomegaly.* Clinical and radiological cardiomegaly may be due to ventricular dilatation, ventricular hypertrophy or pericardial effusion. Echocardiography allows the correct interpretation.

2. *Supporting the diagnosis of ischaemic chest pain.* Regional left ventricular wall dyskinesia is a feature of myocardial ischaemia and may occur before there are any ECG changes. Stress echocardiography, using dynamic exercise or pharmacological stress, may be used to detect wall motion abnormalities.

3. *Assessing complications of myocardial infarction.* Echocardiography is essential for the prompt diagnosis of the complications of acute myocardial infarction. It can quickly distinguish between acute mitral incompetence and an acquired ventriculoseptal defect. It is an essential investigation in patients with cardiogenic shock, to distinguish severe left ventricular damage

from right ventricular infarction or cardiac rupture with tamponade.

4. *Assessment of cardiac failure*. Echocardiography should be carried out in all patients presenting with heart failure to establish the aetiology (Cheesman et al, 1998). Echocardiography may also demonstrate asymptomatic left ventricular dysfunction in post-infarct patients, who will benefit from early administration of ACE inhibitors (St John Sutton, 1994).

5. *Assessing prognosis*. Stress echocardiography has been used to assess residual ischaemia and define prognosis following acute myocardial infarction. Those with negative tests had a 1-year mortality of 2%, but 4–8% if the test was positive (Picano et al, 1993).

6. *Miscellaneous problems*

- *Vegetations* over 3 mm in size may be demonstrable in over half the patients with infective endocarditis. They are seen as rapidly moving masses attached to, or replacing, normal cardiac tissue. Transoesophageal echocardiography is vital for confirmation of the diagnosis and to show complications, such as mycotic abscesses.
- *Mitral valve prolapse* is common (depending upon precise definitions) and is easily identifiable with echocardiography. It may present with dysrhythmias or atypical chest pain.
- *Hypertrophic obstructive cardiomyopathy* may present with chest pain and dysrhythmias. The diagnosis may be established with echocardiography.
- *Prosthetic valve function* may need to be assessed in coronary care admissions to ascertain whether valvular dysfunction is the source of symptoms. Transoesophageal echocardiography is the best way to assess valve dysfunction because of artefactual signals from the prosthesis.

NEW APPLICATIONS FOR ECHOCARDIOGRAPHY

Contrast echocardiography

A variety of echo contrast agents that contain micro-bubbles have been developed. When injected into the blood stream, they produce a cloud of echoes as they pass through the heart that is easily detectable at echocardiography. The technique has been used to detect right to left shunts (e.g. through septal defects), and may be used to define the endocardial border of the left ventricle, to better assess wall motion artefacts.

Acoustic quantification

This is an automatic on-line computerised technique for detecting the interface between the left ventricular endocardial surface and the blood displayed on the two-dimensional image. It enables beat-to-beat estimation of the ejection fraction, and utilising colour enables regional wall abnormalities to be highlighted.

Doppler tissue imaging

This technique uses Doppler pulses on the valves and myocardium, which move at much slower velocities than the red blood cells and can therefore be filtered out. Colour assignment is determined by both velocity and direction of tissue movement, and thus is a powerful tool for assessing regional wall abnormalities. Another potential use of tissue Doppler is localisation of accessory conduction pathways prior to radiofrequency ablation (e.g. in the Wolff–Parkinson–White syndrome). Premature ventricular activation through the accessory pathway is accompanied by earlier contraction in that area.

EXERCISE STRESS TESTING

Many patients with cardiac disease have no signs, symptoms or abnormal investigations at rest, but exercise stress testing may reveal hitherto undocumented abnormalities. The main aims of stress testing are:

- To provoke symptoms, such as chest pain and dyspnoea
- To demonstrate ECG changes with progressive workload

- To determine maximum workload
- To assess prognosis.

The procedure has a low complication rate, although any investigation of patients with myocardial disease carries a risk of cardiac arrest or myocardial infarction. It is usual, therefore, for exercise stress tests to be carried out with a doctor in attendance and with resuscitation facilities available. However, in a series of 20 000 tests in Seattle, there were only six cases of ventricular fibrillation, which occurred in the first 5 min following cessation of the test (Irving et al, 1977). All these patients had myocardial disease, were hypotensive during exercise and were resuscitated. Care is therefore required in high-risk patients, and close monitoring by observation after exercise of those with highly abnormal tests is required, with overnight admission to hospital if there is any concern about delayed response to exercise. The British Cardiac Society (1993) has drawn up guidelines for performing exercise tests in the absence of direct medical supervision.

Despite a wealth of experience, and a great deal of published work on the investigation, controversy still surrounds the interpretation of the test. Although ECG changes are important, they should be interpreted in the context of symptoms, pulse and blood pressure response and recovery time following exercise. In general, early onset of angina, marked and widespread ST depression, slow recovery and a poor blood pressure response are indicative of severe ischaemic heart disease.

METHODS OF STRESS TESTING

Stress testing is usually performed with a treadmill or bicycle, the choice being largely determined by available space. Exercise testing for patients on coronary care is best performed close to the unit for safety reasons. There are several contraindications to stress testing; these are listed in Box 5.2.

Recommended lead systems for detecting regional myocardial ischaemia employ 2–20 electrodes. The simplest and most useful lead for recording is MCL5 (the positive lead in the V5

Box 5.2 Contraindications to ECG stress testing

Cardiac (absolute)
- Within 2 days of acute myocardial infarction
- Unstable angina (not stabilised)
- Uncontrolled symptomatic heart failure
- Acute myocarditis or pericarditis
- Severe aortic stenosis
- Serious uncontrolled dysrhythmias

Cardiac (relative)
- Moderate stenotic valve disease
- Severe hypertension
- Hypertrophic obstructive cardiomyopathy
- Heart block (advanced)

Non-cardiac considerations
- Anaemia
- Elderly or infirm patient
- Gross obesity
- Severe respiratory disease
- Digoxin toxicity
- Electrolyte imbalance

---

interspace and the negative on the manubrium), which will demonstrate up to 90% of detectable abnormalities. However, the most common lead system uses the normal 12-lead recording positions. The torso rather than the limbs are used for the limb leads, to prevent entanglement and to reduce movement artefact.

There are many different protocols designed for different circumstances and available equipment (ACC/AHA, 1997). The protocol should offer:

- An appropriate workload for the patient that will not cause excessive stress
- A gradually increasing workload, with enough time at each level to attain steady-state
- Continuous ECG, heart rate and blood pressure recording
- Resuscitation facilities.

The most common test in the UK is the Bruce protocol (Bruce et al, 1963), which produces a fast increase in progressive workload (Table 5.3). The modified Bruce protocol is much slower, taking 24 min to reach the 12-min equivalent of the Bruce protocol (Table 5.4), but is more suited to older patients, those with recent myocardial

Table 5.3 Bruce protocol for exercise (treadmill) ECG test

Stage	Speed (mph)	Gradient (%)	Duration (min)	METs (units)	Total time (min)
1	1.7	10	3	4	3
2	2.5	12	3	6–7	6
3	3.4	14	3	8–9	9
4	4.2	16	3	15–16	12
5	5.0	18	3	21	15
6	5.5	20	3	>21	18
7	6.0	22	3	>21	21

METs, metabolic equivalents.

Table 5.4 Modified Bruce protocol for exercise (treadmill) ECG test

Stage	Speed (mph)	Gradient (%)	Duration (min)	METs (units)	Total time (min)
0	1.7	0	3	2	3
0.5	1.7	5	3	3	6
1	1.7	10	3	4	12
2	2.5	12	3	6–7	15
3	3.4	14	3	8–9	18
4	4.2	16	3	15–16	21
5	5.0	18	3	21	24
6	5.5	20	3	>21	27
7	6.0	22	3	>21	30

METs, metabolic equivalents.

infarction, or with a stabilised acute coronary syndrome.

OXYGEN UPTAKE AND METABOLIC EQUIVALENTS

The rate of oxygen uptake (VO_2) by the body relates to the ability to achieve a given workload. At rest, the VO_2 is about 3.5 ml/kg/min, which is described as 1 MET (1 metabolic equivalent). Average peak VO_2 in cardiac patients is about 21 ml/kg/min (6 METs); those who can achieve 10 METs have a prognosis with medical therapy as good as those with operative intervention, and those who can achieve 13 METs have an excellent prognosis regardless of other exercise responses. Since exercise protocols differ, effort capacity should be expressed in METs.

There are various parameters that can be observed and assessed during an exercise test. These may be:

- *Symptomatic*: onset of symptoms and relationship to exercise

- *Haemodynamic*: changes in blood pressure and heart rate
- *Electrocardiographic*: changes in the ST segment and cardiac rhythm.

A standard resting ECG should be obtained before the test and current medication needs to be recorded. During the test, the patient should be encouraged to exercise for as long as possible, but signs of fatigue, pain and dyspnoea should be noted, especially in the stoic patient. The blood pressure should be recorded at the termination of each stage.

Automatic ECG recorders will usually record a full 12-lead ECG at predetermined time intervals, and the test is continued until completion or another end-point has been reached (Box 5.3). At the end of testing, the level of the test achieved (with timing and MET) should be recorded, with the reason for stopping. All symptoms and blood pressure readings should be recorded. Maximal ST depression should be noted, although it is best to report only on planar or down-sloping ST segments as indicative of possible myocardial ischaemia.

Box 5.3 End-points of the exercise stress test

Absolute

- Fall in systolic blood pressure >10 mmHg with ischaemia
- Signs of poor perfusion (pallor, cyanosis)
- Patient request
- Sustained VT
- ST elevation in leads without Q waves
- Moderate or severe angina

Relative indications

- Attainment of target heart rate (220 – age; 210 in women)
- Fall in systolic blood pressure >10 mmHg
- Increasing chest pains
- Exaggerated hypertensive response
- Marked ST–T wave changes
- Dysrhythmias

INDICATIONS FOR STRESS TESTING

There are three main reasons for exercise stress testing:

- Assessing patients with chest pain
- Assessing prognosis
- Assessing other exercise-related symptoms.

Assessing patients with chest pain

The major indication for exercise stress testing is the diagnosis of chest pain. Unfortunately, ST changes are not always present during exercise in patients with angiographically defined coronary artery disease, especially if lesions are limited to the circumflex and distal right coronary arteries. False negative tests may also be obtained if the patient is taking beta-blockers, which limit cardiac work, or if exercise has been submaximal. False positive results may be obtained in up to 10% of men and more than 25% of women who have normal resting ECGs. Diagnostic stress testing is therefore of limited value in women (Sullivan et al, 1994). There have been many explanations for false positivity, including ST changes due to hyperventilation or increased sympathetic tone. In some young women without heart disease, multiple resting ST/T wave changes are found on the resting ECG, which worsen (often dramatically) on exercise.

Another peculiar syndrome describes angina in patients with angiographically normal coronary arteries (syndrome X). Invasive studies often show abnormal myocardial contractility, and the condition probably reflects an early form of cardiomyopathy.

Assessing prognosis

Exercise testing has become routine in most hospitals to determine prognosis in patients with ischaemic heart disease. The greater the degree of ST segment shift on exercise, the greater the chance of significant multivessel disease. The exercise time is very important and is often used for risk stratification and to determine mortality (Table 5.5).

The prognosis of patients following myocardial infarction is mostly dependent on left ventricular function, which may be reflected by workload and blood pressure response to formal exercise, as well as circulation to the unaffected myocardium. Although ST changes may reflect poor coronary perfusion, it is the exercise time and blood pressure response that matter most. Inability to perform the test and/or a rise of less than 30 mmHg in the systolic blood pressure seem to identify the high-risk patients and are predictive of future cardiac events. Symptom-limited exercise stress testing may be safely carried out before discharge in selected patients. Typically these are patients under 65 years of age, without dysrhythmias, recurrent ischaemic pain or cardiac failure. The usual recommendation is that pre-discharge tests should be limited to 5 METS (about 9 min of the modified Bruce protocol). Information on functional capacity is

Table 5.5 Mortality for patients with coronary heart disease assessed by the Bruce exercise test (Coronary Artery Surgery Study, 1983)

Stage completed	Mortality (%) at:		Risk
	12 months	24 months	
III	1	5	Low
II	2	11	Intermediate
I	5	19	High

not only useful for prognostic reasons, but may also help in advising future activities and the appropriateness of rehabilitation. For logistic reasons, exercise testing often has to be carried out following discharge from hospital. Those patients who were unable to have a pre-discharge stress test should have a symptom-limited test performed prior to their first outpatient appointment. There is some evidence that late stress testing provides additional information to a submaximal pre-discharge test (Stone et al, 1986). In general, those with normal exercise tests have a good prognosis, as opposed to those with poor exercise tests. Patients without post-infarct angina, and without ST changes during exercise stress testing, do not need coronary angiography (Cross et al, 1993). Those with abnormal tests should be examined further by stress echocardiography, radionuclide studies or coronary angiography.

Since thrombolysis has become routine, there is some concern that dynamic stress testing may have limited value in assessing the prognosis in post-infarct patients, given that diagnostic data were previously defined before the thrombolytic era (Stevenson et al, 1993). By recanalising the infarct-related artery, thrombolytic treatment exposes the patient to the risk of re-occlusion. Conventional stress testing will not reveal this risk, which has been designed to detect reversible ischaemia and left ventricular performance. A study of patients in the TIMI II trial found that an abnormal pre-discharge exercise test did not predict coronary events within 6 months of myocardial infarction (Chaitman et al, 1993). It may be that other non-invasive techniques will become necessary to investigate post-infarct patients who have been thrombolysed.

Assessing other exercise-related symptoms

The aetiology of atypical anginal pain, dyspnoea, palpitations and dizziness may all be clarified by an exercise test. Functional capacity can be gauged by an objective assessment of the severity of symptoms and the degree of limitation imposed by cardiac or other disease. Occasionally, intermittent dysrhythmias may be recorded, and an exercise test may form part of the evaluation of patients with suspected cardiac rhythm abnormalities.

In patients with cardiac failure, an exercise capacity of less than 6 METs is associated with decreased survival; a capacity below 4 METs provides a strong reason for considering heart transplantation.

NUCLEAR SCANS AND NUCLEAR ANGIOGRAPHY

In recent years, there has been a rapid development of radioisotope techniques for the assessment of myocardial disease. Nuclear scans can be used to assess:

- Myocardial perfusion
- Ventricular function
- Myocardial viability
- Prognosis.

Myocardial perfusion imaging is the only non-invasive method of assessing myocardial perfusion, and relies on the radiotracer being distributed throughout the myocardium in proportion to regional blood flow. This has mainly been assessed using thallium and technetium, which are injected intravenously and taken up by the heart, which is then visualised in planar or tomographic modes by a gamma-camera. Radiolabelled agents identify and delineate areas of myocardial hypoperfusion, either by being preferentially taken up by damaged or necrosed myocardium (hot spot detection) or by demonstrating areas of hypoperfusion (cold spot detection). Technetium-99m-labelled pyrophosphate is most commonly used for the former and thallium-201 for the latter.

Thallium-201 is a potassium analogue, which concentrates in normal myocardial cells and can be used to demonstrate myocardial ischaemia and infarction. It is not fixed in the tissues, but washes in and out according to regional blood flow. Abnormal tissue does not take up the tracer and therefore appears as a cold spot on the scan. Poorly perfused areas wash out thallium much more slowly than normal myocardium does.

For dynamic testing, the patient exercises on a bicycle until he becomes symptomatic. Thallium is then injected and the image is obtained in separate views with a gamma-camera. Cold spots may disappear as the myocardium reperfuses, and fixed cold spots indicate old infarct. Patients with significant triple-vessel disease often take up thallium very poorly, with a very slow washout. In those unable to exercise, dipyridamole or adenosine is injected to promote coronary blood flow, and then thallium scanning can be used to detect differential flow through normal and stenosed arteries. Alternatively, dobutamine may be given to precipitate myocardial ischaemia without exercise. Overall image quality is not good with thallium, and image interpretation is often hampered by tissue attenuation artefact from the breasts and diaphragm.

Technetium-99m pyrophosphate is taken up by damaged myocardial cells and is imaged as a hot spot. This may be useful in the diagnosis of recent myocardial infarction, when traditional investigations (enzymes, ECG, etc.) have not been of help.

These multiple planar techniques have been superseded by SPECT (single photon emission computed tomography) imaging, a three-dimensional imaging technique that allows accurate localisation of perfusion defects. This is particularly of value in identifying the coronary vessel involved. Technetium-labelled methoxyisobutyl isonitrile is the usual agent employed, although technetium-labelled tetrofosmin is now being used to produce superior imaging. Myocardial perfusion imaging is of major value for defining prognosis. A normal stress perfusion study predicts a risk of cardiac death or myocardial infarction at less than 1% per year, even where there is angiographically proven coronary artery disease (Zaret and Wackers, 1993a,b).

RADIONUCLIDE VENTRICULOGRAPHY

Radionuclide ventriculography is helpful in defining those patients with poor left ventricular

function whose prognosis may be improved with surgery. More recently, the importance of right ventricular dysfunction in low-output states has been recognised, particularly following inferior and right ventricular infarction. Nuclear scanning may be invaluable for examining these difficult areas of the heart. Ischaemic dysfunction that may only develop during exercise can also be easily visualised by nuclear angiography; it is usually seen as a fall in cardiac output, with the development of regional contraction abnormalities.

There are two main techniques of radionuclide ventriculography: first-pass scanning and multigated acquisition (MUGA) scanning:

1. *First-pass scanning* involves a radiotracer (usually technetium-99m) being injected as a bolus into a peripheral vein and its radioactivity counted on its first passage through the heart. The chambers can be visually separated by its time of passage through the right and left heart, so that images of the right and left heart can be constructed. Wall motion of the anterolateral and inferior aspects of the left ventricle can also be demonstrated.

2. *MUGA scanning* uses technetium to label the patient's red cells. A period of equilibration is allowed; then radioactivity is measured within the heart as it beats and recorded frame by frame in either two or three dimensions by the gamma-camera, which is activated by the ECG (one frame per cycle). Multiple cardiac cycles are averaged and this enables regional wall motion to be visualised (for defining dyskinetic segments and ventricular aneurysms) and can provide information on ventricular volumes, ejection fraction and cardiac output.

In patients recovering from myocardial infarction, radionuclide ventriculography is an excellent way to identify poor left ventricular anatomy and function, which is important prognostically.

Radionuclide ventriculography is mostly used in patients where an echocardiographic window cannot be achieved, and for serial monitoring of patients in cardiac failure or undergoing chemotherapy.

NUCLEAR IMAGING IN ACUTE MYOCARDIAL INFARCTION

In most cases of myocardial infarction, there is adequate diagnostic evidence from the history, ECG and cardiac enzymes. In more difficult cases, nuclear imaging may then complement other investigations, as, for example, in the:

- Diagnosis and localisation of a myocardial infarction in the presence of left bundle branch block or subendocardial necrosis
- Diagnosis of right ventricular infarction
- Detection of new areas of infarction close to old areas of fibrosis
- Diagnosis of peri-operative myocardial infarction.

Thallium-201 cold spot scans are nearly always positive in the first 6 h following myocardial infarction, but are less reliable thereafter. Unfortunately, reversible defects may be found in patients with coronary artery spasm or crescendo angina, and fixed defects may be found if there is myocardial infiltration or old infarction. Technetium-99m scanning is of particular value in right ventricular infarction (Rodrigues et al, 1986) and, in combination with thallium scanning, may be used to separate areas of recent and previous myocardial infarction. Exercise stress testing with thallium is about twice as good at detecting residual ischaemia following myocardial infarction as traditional ECG treadmill testing. It therefore provides a more accurate way of assessing prognosis in post-infarct patients.

SPECT scanning may be used to detect indium-111-radiolabelled monoclonal Fab fragments of specific antibody to cardiac myosin. When myocardial cell membranes rupture soon after infarction, they expose structural myosin, to which these monoclonal antibodies attach. This technique allows very early confirmation of myocardial infarction, but it is very expensive and SPECT scanning facilities are currently limited in the UK.

Magnetic resonance imaging (MRI) is a safe, non-invasive imaging technique that utilises a strong magnetic field to generate a three-dimensional image of the body, including the heart. Cardiac MRI is an evolving technology, with potential to provide information on cardiac morphology, perfusion and left ventricular function. Using specific contrast agents, myocardial perfusion studies can differentiate between infarcted and ischaemic myocardium and can be used in quantification of infarct size. MRI is also useful for assessing left ventricular function (using ECG-gated cine-MRI), assessing the severity of valvular lesions and demonstrating the complications of acute myocardial infarction, including left ventricular aneurysm, intraventricular clot and ventriculoseptal defects. Rapid sequence cine-MRI is being used to assess graft patency following bypass surgery, and flow-contrast techniques allow the estimation of coronary blood flow through vein grafts. MRI is an excellent way of assessing aortic dissection, but transoesophageal echocardiography is more practicable in most units. For less urgent cases, MRI is superior at visualising the descending aorta and arch.

Three-dimensional magnetic resonance coronary angiography (MR-CA) has been shown to be an accurate non-invasive method for identifying disease in the proximal and middle coronary artery segments in some patients, particularly those with three-vessel and left main stem disease. Although conventional angiography remains the standard owing to its high image quality, it is invasive with complications such as myocardial infarction, stroke and sudden death. MR-CA is limited by cardiac and respiratory motion artefacts, but is faster to perform than angiography, and does avoid hospital admission.

Two other techniques are emerging for non-invasive coronary lumen imaging. These are electron beam computed tomography and multi-slice computed tomography, but so far image quality is not good enough for these techniques to replace conventional angiography (de Feyter and Nieman, 2002).

DETECTING MYOCARDIAL VIABILITY

Many patients with poor left ventricular function can benefit from revascularisation procedures if their cardiac muscle is shown not to be irreversibly damaged by fibrosis, but affected by hibernating or stunned myocardium. *Positron emission tomography (PET)* is the most accurate non-invasive imaging technique for detecting myocardial viability, and employs short-lived tracers of blood flow and metabolism. The commonest method employs N-13 ammonia with metabolic imaging using the fluorine-18-labelled glucose analogue fluorodeoxyglucose (FDG). Normally functioning myocardium takes up this glucose analogue, and PET scanning can differentiate between normal myocardium (preserved contractility and positive FDG uptake), infarcted myocardium (impaired contractility and no FDG uptake) and hibernating myocardium (impaired contractility and positive FDG uptake). Patients with a PET mismatch have been shown in small studies to have improvements in mortality and functional capacity following revascularisation (Di Carli, 1998). SPECT imaging is also being developed using conventional gamma-cameras; this will be of great value if shown to be equivalent to conventional PET scanning because of the limited availability of the latter.

CARDIAC CATHETERISATION AND CORONARY ANGIOGRAPHY

Coronary angiography defines the anatomy of the main coronary arteries, and provides assessment of stenoses responsible for clinical symptoms. In addition to coronary angiography, cardiac catheterisation may need to be carried out:

- To record intracardiac pressures and demonstrate pressure gradients
- To measure cardiac output and detect shunting (by measuring blood gases) at different levels
- To identify anatomical and functional anomalies, such as ventricular aneurysms and valvular disease.

There has been a change in the interface between district general hospital cardiology and the major cardiac centres (Brooks, 1997), and the establishment of cardiac catheterisation laborato-

ries in district general hospitals is being encouraged. The laboratory should handle between 1500 and 2000 diagnostic cases per year to ensure efficient use of the facility, and competence of the staff.

CORONARY ANGIOGRAPHY

Selective coronary angiography was introduced in 1959 and is considered the gold standard for defining coronary anatomy. The procedure involves the passage of catheters, under X-ray control, from a peripheral artery (usually femoral or brachial) via the aorta to the coronary arteries. Contrast medium is injected by selective catheterisation of the left and right coronary arteries. The images are then stored on high-speed cine-film or now more commonly by digital image storing techniques to provide a dynamic record of ventricular wall movement, blood flow and intravascular anatomy. Typically, right and left anterior oblique views are taken to allow visualisation of the arterial system, although special views are sometimes required. The extent and severity of the lesions, with assessment of left ventricular function, can be used to determine the patient's prognosis. The procedure takes about half an hour and is performed under local anaesthesia. Better vascular protection by sheaths, improved catheters and new non-ionic low osmolar contrast media have improved the technique considerably in recent years. There is a small morbidity and mortality rate (due to myocardial infarction and dysrhythmias), but this is so low these days (less than 0.1%) as to allow day-case investigation in low-risk cases. Procedure-related complications usually involve trauma at the arterial access site, although some patients react to the contrast medium. Serious complications arise in about 1%.

Angiography is usually recommended:

- For patients with stable angina whose symptoms are significantly affecting their lifestyle, to decide whether surgery is indicated
- For patients with unstable angina following stabilisation

- In selected patients following acute myocardial infarction.

The need for angiography is usually not urgent, and it is probably better to await resolution of the atheromatous plaques and endogenous remodelling of the coronary vasculature following acute myocardial infarction (Davies et al, 1990). Up to 10% of patients will have a left main stem stenosis, and 30% will have triple-artery disease. The remainder do not have severe coronary artery disease, and will not need surgery to improve their symptoms or prognosis. At-risk groups can usually be identified non-invasively (Cross et al, 1993).

Early angiography (immediately or within a few hours of admission) may be performed as a prelude to primary percutaneous transluminal coronary angioplasty, or for failed thrombolysis ('rescue angioplasty'). Angiography is made more difficult then because of the effects of aspirin, glycoprotein inhibitors and thrombolytic agents, particularly at the site of arterial access. Most patients will be returned to the coronary care unit with the sheath left in, and the incidence of bleeding and false aneurysm is higher in this group. In the GUSTO study (GUSTO Angiographic Investigators, 1993), in which patients underwent angiography within 24 h of thrombolysis, 6% had major bleeds requiring transfusion and 1.4% required vascular repair.

Patients with cardiogenic shock, and those who develop mechanical complications of myocardial infarction (ruptured papillary muscle or acquired ventricular septal defect), should undergo angiography with a view to revascularisation and surgical repair. Prior stabilisation with an intra-aortic balloon pump is needed.

REFERENCES

ACC/AHA (1997) American College of Cardiology/American Heart Association guidelines for exercise stress testing. *Circulation*, **96:** 345–354.

British Cardiac Society (1993) Guidelines on exercise testing when there is not a doctor present. *British Heart Journal*, **70:** 488.

Brooks NH (1997) The changing interface between district hospital cardiology and the major cardiac centres. *Heart*, **78:** 519–523.

Bruce RA, Blackman JR, Jones JW et al (1963) Exercise tests in adult normal subjects and cardiac patients. *Pediatrics*, **32:** 742–756.

Chaitman BR, McMahon RP, Terria M for the TIMI Investigators (1993) Impact of treatment strategy on pre-discharge exercise test in the TIMI II trial. *American Journal of Cardiology*, **71:** 131–138.

Cheesman MG, Leech G, Chambers J et al for the British Society of Echocardiography (1998) Central role of echocardiography in the diagnosis and assessment of heart failure. *Heart*, **80:** S1–S5.

Coronary Artery Surgery Study (CASS) Principal Investigators and Associates (1983) A randomised trial of coronary artery bypass surgery: survival data. *Circulation*, **68:** 939–950.

Crawford MH, Bernstein SJ, Deedwania PC et al (1999) ACC/AHA guidelines for ambulatory electrocardiography: executive summary and recommendations: a report of the American College of Cardiology/American Heart Association Task Force on Practice Guidelines (Committee to Revise the Guidelines for Ambulatory Electrocardiography). *Circulation*, **100:** 886–893.

Cross SJ, Lee HS, Kenmure A et al (1993) First myocardial infarction in patients under 60 years old: the role of exercise tests and symptoms in deciding who to catheterise. *British Heart Journal*, **70:** 428–432.

Davies SW, Marchant B, Lyons JP et al (1990) Coronary lesion morphology in acute myocardial infarction: demonstration of early remodeling after streptokinase treatment. *Journal of the American College of Cardiology*, **16:** 1079–1086.

de Bono D for the Joint Working Party of the British Cardiac Society and the Royal College of Physicians of London (1999) Investigation and management of stable angina: revised guidelines 1998. *Heart*, **81:** 546–555.

de Feyter PJ, Nieman K (2002) New coronary imaging techniques: what to expect? *Heart*, **87:** 195–197.

Di Carli MF (1998) Positron emission tomography for assessment of myocardial perfusion and viability. *Cardiology Reviews*, **6:** 290–301.

GUSTO Angiographic Investigators (1993) The effect of tissue plasminogen activator, streptokinase, or both on coronary artery patency, ventricular function and survival after acute myocardial infarction. *New England Journal of Medicine*, **329:** 1615–1622.

Houston AB (1993) Doppler ultrasound and the apparently normal heart. *British Heart Journal*, **69:** 99–100.

Irving JB, Bruce RA, de Rouen T (1977) Variations in and significance of systolic pressure during maximal exercise (treadmill) testing. *American Journal of Cardiology,* **39:** 841–848.

Jowett NI (1997) *Cardiovascular Monitoring.* London: Whurr.

Jowett NI, Thompson DR (1985) Electrocardiographic monitoring. II. Ambulatory monitoring. *Intensive Care Nursing,* **1:** 123–129.

Jowett NI, Thompson DR, Bailey SW (1985) Electrocardiographic monitoring. I. Static monitoring. *Intensive Care Nursing,* **1:** 71–76.

Mickley H (1994) Ambulatory ST segment monitoring after myocardial infarction. *British Heart Journal,* **71:** 113–114.

Picano E, Landi P, Bolognese L et al on behalf of the EPIC Study Group (1993) Prognostic value of dipyridamole echocardiographic study early after uncomplicated myocardial infarction: a large multicenter trial. *American Journal of Medicine,* **11:** 608–618.

Rodrigues EA, Dewhurst NG, Smart LM et al (1986) Diagnosis and prognosis of right ventricular infarction. *British Heart Journal,* **56:** 19–26.

Seidl K, Rameken M, Breunung S et al (2000) Diagnostic assessment of recurrent unexplained syncope with a new subcutaneously implantable loop recorder. Reveal Investigators. *Europace,* **2:** 256–262.

Soni N (1996) Swan song for the Swan–Ganz catheter? *BMJ,* **313:** 763–764.

St John Sutton M (1994) Should ACE inhibitors be used routinely after infarction? Perspectives from the SAVE trial. *British Heart Journal,* **71:** 115–118.

Stevenson R, Umachandran V, Ranjadayalan K et al (1993) Reassessment of treadmill stress testing for risk stratification in patients with acute myocardial infarction treated by thrombolysis. *British Heart Journal,* **70:** 415–420.

Stokes PH, Jowett NI (1985) Haemodynamic monitoring with the Swan–Ganz catheter. *Intensive Care Nursing,* **1:** 9–17.

Stone PH, Turi ZG, Muller J for the MILLIS 5 Study Group (1986) Prognostic significance of the treadmill exercise test performed 6 months after myocardial infarction. *Journal of the American College of Cardiology,* **8:** 1007–1017.

Sullivan AK, Holdright DR, Wright CA et al (1994) Chest pain in women: clinical, investigative and prognostic features. *BMJ,* **308:** 883–886.

Swan HJC, Ganz W, Forrester JS et al (1970) Catheterisation of the heart in man with the use of a flow-directed balloon catheter. *New England Journal of Medicine,* **283:** 447–451.

Zaret BL, Wackers FJ (1993a) Nuclear cardiology, Part 1. *New England Journal of Medicine,* **329:** 775–783.

Zaret BL, Wackers FJ (1993b) Nuclear cardiology. Part 2. *New England Journal of Medicine,* **329:** 855–863.

6

An introduction to the acute coronary syndromes

The term 'acute coronary syndrome' defines a collection of the clinical expressions of acute coronary artery disease classified by the appearance of the presenting 12-lead electrocardiogram (ECG) and concentrations of cardiac markers detected in the blood (Fox, 2000). It includes all cases of acute myocardial infarction and unstable angina, whether accompanied by ST elevation or ST depression, or resulting in Q wave or non-Q wave patterns on the ECG. At one end of this continuum is unstable angina; at the other is acute transmural myocardial infarction.

The syndromes result from the abrupt, total or subtotal obstruction of a coronary artery. Occlusion may be transient (and typically recurrent), or may be permanent, and in most cases is initiated by rupture or erosion of an atheromatous plaque, with later contributions by thrombus, platelet emboli and coronary arterial spasm. Clinical presentation of the syndromes mostly depends upon the site of the occlusion, whether the obstruction is abrupt, or stuttering in onset, whether the coronary occlusion is total, or subtotal, and whether a collateral circulation is present. Spontaneous thrombolysis with fragmentation of the thrombus, or the relief of spasm, sometimes allows reperfusion, and relief from the effects of myocardial ischaemia. However, even if the occlusion is temporary, repetitive embolisation from the unstable plaque may result in focal myocardial necrosis, which is often too small to be detected by electrocardiography, or traditional cardiac enzymes, but which is now detectable by sensitive cardiac markers (Gerhardt et al, 1991). After coronary occlusion, cell death is not immediate, and the size of the infarct may be limited if there is recanalisation of the vessel by spontaneous thrombolysis or therapeutic intervention.

Myocardial infarction may thus be classed as:

- Microscopic (focal)
- Small (<10% of the left ventricle)
- Medium (10–30% of the left ventricle)
- Large (>30% of the left ventricle).

In the absence of an effective collateral blood supply, persistence of an occlusive thrombus in a major epicardial coronary artery results in a fully developed transmural myocardial infarction, which later associates with pathological Q waves on the ECG. The presence and degree of myocardial damage following prolonged ischaemia can be assessed in different ways, including electrocardiography, concentration of cardiac markers, echocardiography or nuclear scanning. Individually, and collectively, these methods will give an indication of the extent of myocardial necrosis, and hence prognosis.

In the past, myocardial infarction was defined by a combination of two of the three classical characteristics: symptoms, cardiac enzymes, ECG changes (Tunstall-Pedoe et al, 1994). However, current technology can now quantify as little as 1 g of myocardial necrosis, and patients formerly diagnosed as having unstable angina may now be found to have evidence of myocardial infarction (McKenna and Forfar, 2002). The current definition of acute myocardial infarction is thus based primarily on the typical rise and fall of serum cardiac markers, but requires supportive evidence that there has been an acute ischaemic event, such as typical cardiac symptoms, ECG changes (ST elevation or depression), or late development of pathological Q waves in the ECG (ESC/ACC, 2000).

Since diagnosis of acute myocardial infarction is now based upon troponin (or other marker) concentrations, there is no threshold below which troponin positivity is without implication.

There is continuity from minor cardiac damage ('infarct-let') detected by minimal troponin positivity (but negativity of cardiac enzymes), to the classical transmural infarct associated with Q waves on the ECG, large rises in cardiac enzyme concentrations, and important complications such as heart failure and dysrhythmias. For contemporary clinicians, the term 'acute myocardial infarction' is now insufficient, and the primary diagnosis should be 'coronary heart disease presenting with myocardial infarction'. Management strategies must now go beyond immediate care, and should seek to determine the extent of the underlying coronary heart disease, and what needs to be done to optimise prognosis.

Troponin positivity will also have many implications for the individual patient. All patients will need advice on life-style modification, and risk-factor modification. In addition, the diagnosis of myocardial infarction might affect work, life insurance, vocational driving and, of course, the psychological status of the patient. The increased number of patients now diagnosed as acute myocardial infarction may also cause spurious changes in epidemiological data over the next few years. Healthcare systems will need to expand to allow appropriate investigation, treatment and rehabilitation for the increased number of patients that are likely to come to medical attention. On the other hand, increasing the sensitivity of diagnosis will identify many more patients who will benefit from intervention, which should reduce future morbidity and mortality. Patients with non-cardiological ailments may also be reassured, and will not need inappropriate medication and follow-up.

CLASSIFICATION OF THE ACUTE CORONARY SYNDROMES

Broadly speaking, the acute coronary syndromes are divided into two main groups:

1. *ST elevation myocardial infarction (STEMI)*. This is acute myocardial infarction presenting with ST elevation, or new bundle branch block

on the presenting ECG, and defines those patients who require urgent reperfusion by thrombolysis or primary angioplasty. Initial diagnosis is based on the clinical history and the standard resting 12-lead ECG alone, although confirmatory evidence may be obtained later by measurement of troponin or other cardiac marker concentrations.

2. *Unstable angina (UA) and non-ST elevation myocardial infarction (NSTEMI).* Patients with UA/NSTEMI present with symptoms of myocardial ischaemia, but have an admission 12-lead ECG that does not show ST segment elevation or bundle branch block. If there is no elevation of cardiac markers, the patient is said to have unstable angina, but if there is positivity of the markers, the patient will have sustained myocardial damage (NSTEMI). UA and NSEMI are referred to as the *unstable coronary syndromes*, and are serious. Patients with confirmed or suspected myocardial ischaemia have a 50% 10-year mortality, and those with NSTEMI have a 10-year mortality of 70% (Herlitz et al, 2001).

Differentiation of the acute coronary syndromes by the presenting 12-lead ECG and troponin concentrations is shown in Table 6.1.

CHEST PAIN UNITS

To help evaluate patients presenting with possible acute coronary syndromes, specialist areas called *chest pain units* have been developed. Such units may permit the early diagnosis of acute myocardial ischaemia and facilitate early therapy. They also have a role in excluding cardiac disease, preventing unnecessary hospital admission. Such units are cost-effective compared with usual in-hospital evaluation (Graff et al, 1997).

Chest pain units may form part of the coronary care unit, the medical admissions unit or be located in the accident and emergency department (Graff et al, 1995). Adequate staffing is critical, both in numbers and experience. Clinical pathways may allow staff to arrive at management decisions as early as possible. Continuous 12-lead ECG recording is very helpful, so that transient ECG changes are not missed. Immediate access to cardiac marker assays is particularly valuable. Nearly all cases of myocardial infarction can be identified within 90 min by measuring troponin, creatine kinase MB (CK-MB) and myoglobin (Ng et al, 2001).

TRIAGE

Patients presenting with symptoms consistent with an acute coronary syndrome should be referred to hospital urgently for further assessment. When such symptoms develop within the first 2 weeks following acute myocardial infarction, there is a high risk of re-infarction, and these patients should be sent directly to coronary care.

Table 6.1 Differentiation of the acute coronary syndromes

Clinical syndrome	ECG features	Troponin
Acute myocardial infarction (STEMI, eligible for thrombolysis)	ST elevation (± Q waves) New bundle branch block Posterior infarction	Positive
Non ST-elevation myocardial infarction (NSTEMI)	ST depression T wave inversion Transient or aborted ST elevation Non-specific changes	Positive
Unstable angina (UA)	Any of the above or a normal ECG	Negative

NB: Troponin positivity depends upon local assay values, and details should be obtained from the biochemistry laboratory. Blood samples should usually be assayed within 2 h.

Patients usually present with one of three symptom patterns:

- New onset of severe angina (less than 2 months)
- Abrupt worsening of previous angina (symptoms becoming more frequent, more severe, more prolonged and less responsive to glyceryl trinitrate)
- Angina occurring at rest (often lasting more than 15 min).

The most important investigation is the 12-lead ECG, preferably carried out during an episode of pain. New ischaemic changes on the ECG confirm the diagnosis of an acute coronary syndrome. Patients with ST-segment elevation need immediate consideration for reperfusional therapy; management is detailed in Ch. 7.

Patients presenting with symptoms suggesting an acute coronary syndrome, but without ST elevation or bundle branch block on the presenting ECG will need troponin estimation, which, if positive, confirms an acute coronary syndrome. If the troponin is not elevated, it should be repeated 12 h after the onset of symptoms. If this is then positive, the diagnosis of an acute coronary syndrome is confirmed; management is covered in detail in Ch. 8.

If the troponin remains negative, patients have an *unconfirmed acute coronary syndrome*, and an alternative diagnosis should be sought and managed appropriately. Further investigations to confirm or refute myocardial ischaemia are appropriate in patients who have recurrent admissions with unconfirmed coronary syndromes. Treadmill stress tests, stress echocardiography and perfusion scanning are often used,

but many patients may need to undergo coronary angiography (Keavney et al, 1996).

RISK ASSESSMENT

Patients presenting with unstable coronary syndromes will be at differing levels of risk for progression to major adverse cardiovascular events, such as myocardial infarction or death. Risk stratification provides important prognostic information, and also determines the treatment strategy. The hazards of acute coronary syndromes have been underestimated in the past, and patients should no longer be discharged with a diagnosis of 'chest pain – MI (myocardial infarction) ruled out'. The PRAIS-UK Registry (Prospective Registry of Acute Ischaemic Syndromes) has shown that acute myocardial infarction or death will affect 12.2% of patients within 6 months (Collinson et al, 2000). Two-thirds of these events occur in the first 30 days following presentation, so risk assessment cannot wait for the usual 6-week follow-up visit in outpatients.

Risk assessment may be complex, and risk score-cards are available (Antman et al, 2000). In general, risk is defined by the severity of the presentation, as well as prior risk factors, but risk may change with time (Table 6.2). Although there are multiple determinants of risk, many are self-evident or easily defined, such as age and other co-morbidities, especially diabetes. Acute risk is signalled by recurrent episodes of chest pain with ST segment changes on the ECG and positivity of cardiac markers. Clues to the extent of underlying cardiac disease, such as residual

Table 6.2 Some features that define risk in acute coronary syndromes

High risk	Medium risk	Low risk
Age over 70 years	History of myocardial infarction and/or left ventricular fibrillation	No high-risk features
ST depression on first ECG	Diabetes	Normal ECG
Refractory angina	Recurrent ischaemia	Clinically stable
Haemodynamic instability	Already on aspirin	No past history of coronary artery disease
Markedly raised troponin	Mildly raised troponin	Troponin not raised

ischaemia or left ventricular function, are major determinants of prognosis, and can be assessed easily in most hospitals. Factors such as increasing age, diabetes, hypertension, smoking, heart failure or previous myocardial infarction positively associate with the extent and severity of underlying coronary disease. Minor ischaemic events may have serious consequences in those with prior extensive coronary disease.

Elevated cardiac troponin (cTn) concentrations identify patients at high risk of complications; in general, the higher the cTn concentration the greater the risk of death (Fig. 6.1). However, cTn elevation should not be viewed in isolation. A rise in cTn could simply reflect a sustained episode of ischaemia to a small area of myocardium, and as such probably represents low risk. However, a similar concentration of troponin might be produced by a brief episode of ischaemia to a large (but perhaps vulnerable) area of myocardium, or perhaps episodes of recurrent ischaemia. These latter situations are more likely to associate with high risk. cTn ele-

vation should therefore be viewed in perspective, with knowledge of the patient, the ECG appearances, and an assessment of left ventricular function.

RISK ASSESSMENT FOLLOWING TREATMENT

Risk assessment is a continuous process. After initial assessment and treatment, increased risk is indicated by:

- A raised cTn concentration
- Recurrent ischaemic symptoms
- Recurrent ischaemic ST segment changes (with or without symptoms)
- A positive exercise stress test
- Poor left ventricular function.

Patients with the worst prognosis are those with continuing or recurrent symptoms, and ischaemic ST segment changes despite anti-ischaemic medical treatment (refractory acute coronary syndrome). This is particularly so if the symptoms occur soon after a myocardial infarction, or where there is evidence of pre-existing coronary heart disease.

Most high-risk patients can be identified in the acute phase, but there are some that respond readily to treatment, but remain at high risk. It is important to identify this group before discharge from hospital (Table 6.3).

A symptom-limited exercise stress test (using the modified Bruce protocol) is the simplest way to define residual ischaemia. Increased risk is associated with poor exercise tolerance (less than 7 METS), poor blood pressure response, or induced dysrhythmias during the stress test (Stevenson et al, 1994). Perfusion scanning is helpful in those unable to use the treadmill, although

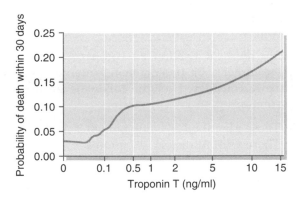

Figure 6.1 Probability of death within 30 days according to troponin T level on admission to hospital. (Adapted with permission from Ohman et al, 1996. Copyright © 1996 Massachusetts Medical Society. All rights reserved.)

Table 6.3 Methods of risk stratification for patients with unstable coronary syndromes

Time of assessment	Method of assessment		
At presentation	Clinical history	Baseline ECG	Cardiac markers
At 6–8 h	Recurrent ischaemia	ST instability	Cardiac markers
At 24 h	Recurrent ischaemia	Response to therapy	Cardiac markers
Pre-discharge	Left ventricular function (echo)	Stress test	Angiographic findings

these patients automatically identify themselves as a high-risk group. Inducible ischaemia alone has a low predictive value for death and myocardial infarction in the first year (Shaw et al, 1996), but results may be combined with the troponin T concentration to stratify risk (Table 6.4)

Apart from troponin concentrations, the other main determinant of long-term risk is left ventricular function. Those patients with an ejection fraction of less than 40% represent a high-risk group requiring treatment with an ACE inhibitor, and usually coronary angiography. For many patients, clinical criteria may be sufficient to exclude or confirm significant left ventricular dysfunction, but, for the rest, echocardiography or radionuclide ventriculography is indicated.

MANAGEMENT ACCORDING TO RISK

Guidelines for the management of UA/NSTEMI have been published in the UK, Europe and America (ACC/AHA, 2000; Bertrand et al, 2000; British Cardiac Society, 2001). There are many similarities, and all guidelines present an 'ideal' framework for management, based upon evidence from clinical trials. However, many of these trials focused on selected populations, and subgroups such as the elderly and women are not well represented. Nevertheless, the conclusions essentially remain the same, and should be applied to all patients until there is evidence to the contrary. A contemporary overview of management of the acute coronary syndromes is shown in Figure: 6.2, and may be summarised as:

1. *Low risk.* If the cTn result is negative, and the stress test result indicates a low-risk category, the patient can be discharged from hospital. The diagnosis may remain uncertain, and other non-cardiological investigations may be appropriate. Patients are at low risk of a cardiac event whatever the diagnosis, and subsequent outpatient review is appropriate for further investigations, and adjustment or cessation of drug treatment.

2. *Intermediate risk.* This includes patients without high-risk features but with a stress test that indicates intermediate risk, or those with a mildly elevated cTn but with a stress test result indicating a low risk. Early coronary angiography cannot be considered mandatory, since there is currently no evidence that routine investigation improves outcome. A 'wait-and-see' policy may be adopted, with a low threshold for angiography.

3. *High risk.* High-risk patients require intensive therapy with beta-blockers, aspirin, clopidogrel, low molecular weight heparin and glycoprotein IIb/IIIa inhibitors. Coronary angiography should be arranged and performed before discharge from hospital. Myocardial revascularisation is usually required.

MYOCARDIAL REVASCULARISATION

Early revascularisation by coronary artery bypass surgery, or percutaneous intervention, is usually considered for the following groups of patients:

- Those identified as being at high risk
- Those with refractory symptoms
- Those identified not to be at immediate high risk, but thought to have significant residual ischaemia
- Patients awaiting coronary artery bypass surgery.

Table 6.4 Risk of cardiac death or myocardial infarction at 5 months after an episode of unstable angina (adapted from Lindahl et al, 1997)

Exercise tolerance test risk category	Troponin T concentration (µg/l)		
	< 0.06	0.06–0.2	>0.2
High	22%	19%	34%
Medium	7%	9%	16%
Low	1%	7%	5%
Unable to exercise	3%	16%	27%

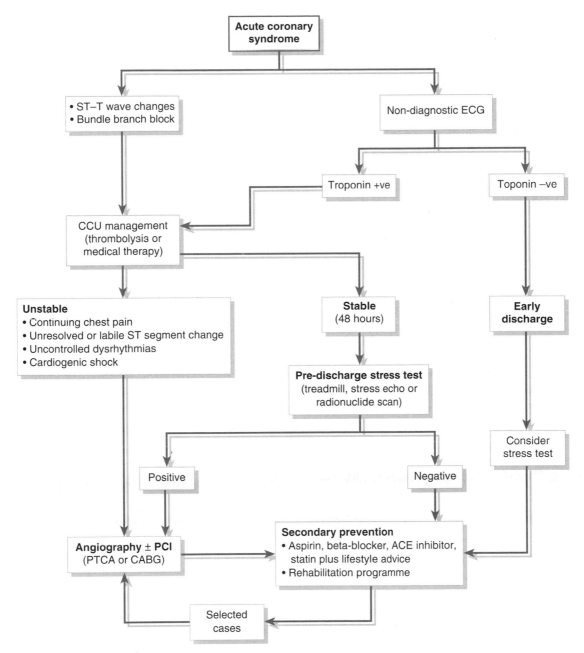

Figure 6.2 Overview of management of the acute coronary syndromes. CCU, coronary care unit; ACE, angiotensin-converting enzyme; PCI, percutaneous coronary intervention; PTCA; percutaneous transluminal coronary angioplasty; CABG, coronary artery bypass graft.

Percutaneous coronary intervention (PCI) refers to various percutaneous techniques, including percutaneous transluminal coronary angioplasty (PTCA), intracoronary stenting and athero-ablative techniques (e.g. atherectomy, laser, etc). Most interventions involve PTCA, with direct or adjunctive stenting to reduce acute vessel closure and late vessel stenosis.

There is wide variation in the number and type of patients presenting with acute coronary syndromes who are referred for revascularisation. The frequency differs widely between, and often within, countries, but those hospitals with high revascularisation rates do not necessarily have better outcomes compared with those with lower revascularisation rates (Fox, 2000). Previous studies of routine coronary angiography and myocardial revascularisation in patients with unstable angina or non-Q wave myocardial infarction recruited highly selected groups of patients, and overall outcomes and risks of procedures do not reflect the usual coronary care patients. There is thus some uncertainty about the precise threshold of risk for coronary angiography or intervention, but routine early myocardial revascularisation with angioplasty or bypass surgery is certainly not appropriate for all (McCullough et al, 1998). Since resources are limited, it is most appropriate to reserve invasive investigations and interventions for those patients with recurrent symptoms or ischaemia, or who are otherwise judged to be at high risk. Local guidelines between secondary and tertiary centres are highly desirable.

CARE OF PATIENTS AFTER LEAVING HOSPITAL

The risk of progression to myocardial infarction or death is highest within the first 8 weeks, after which patients resume a clinical course similar to those who have chronic stable angina. Evaluation in-hospital gives an opportunity to assess long-term care and prepare the patient for returning to normal activities. Aggressive risk-factor modification is the mainstay of long-term treatment. (Gibbons et al, 1999). The ABCDE checklist may be helpful:

- A: aspirin, ACE inhibitors and anti-angina agents
- B: beta-blockers and blood pressure
- C: cholesterol, clopidogrel and cigarettes
- D: diet and diabetes
- E: education and exercise.

The blood pressure should be maintained below 140/85 mmHg, and statins with dietary advice will be needed to lower total serum cholesterol concentrations to less than 5 mmol/l (LDL-cholesterol to below 3 mmol/l) or by a factor of 30%, whichever results in the lower cholesterol (National Service Framework, 2000). ACE inhibitors should be used in those who also have left ventricular dysfunction (ejection fraction under 40%). Meticulous control of blood pressure and glucose is vital in those who also have diabetes. Hormone replacement therapy may continue, but should not be initiated for secondary prevention (Hulley et al, 1998).

A cardiac rehabilitation course should be available to all those recovering from an acute coronary syndrome, and may enhance patient education and compliance with medication. The healthcare team should work with the patient and their family to instruct on specific targets for cholesterol, blood pressure, weight and exercise levels. Discharge instructions should include a written instruction sheet; both the patient and family should know what to do if symptoms return. Formal or informal telephone follow-up may provide reassurance.

THE FUTURE

For patients with STEMI, a number of new thrombolytic agents are in development, such as polyethylene-glycolated staphylokinase and amideplase (a hybrid of tissue plasminogen activator and pro-urokinase). Centres for primary angioplasty are still few and far between, but hopefully will increase. *Facilitated percutaneous revascularisation* involves use of pharmacological reperfusion before transfer to a tertiary centre for angiography and PCI if required, and may be advantageous if the receiving hospital does not have appropriate angiography services. Full-dose thrombolysis followed by early PCI has not been helpful, but half-dose thrombolytics with glycoprotein IIb/IIIa inhibitors followed by PCI may be beneficial for those who fail to reperfuse. However, bleeding complications are frequent, and the risk:benefits of these interventions have yet to be determined (Brodie and Stuckey, 2002).

For those who present with UA/NSTEMI, glycoprotein IIb/IIIa inhibitors have been shown to have maximal benefit on those undergoing PCI (Simoons, 2001). The FRISC II and Tactics/TIMI 18 trials using stents and periprocedural glycoprotein IIb/IIIa antagonists suggest that there are many more patients who would benefit from early PCI than are currently being referred (Wallentin et al, 2000). Second-generation oral IIb/IIIa inhibitors with longer half-lives and greater stability may offer beneficial effects to a wider group of patients.

Aggressive acute lipid-lowering could also be important, and it is hoped that data from the Global Registry of Acute Coronary Events (GRACE) will identify this (Fox and Gore, 2001). Although there has been conflict over whether early statin treatment might stabilise or destabilise vulnerable plaques, the MIRACL study confirmed that acute administration of high-dose potent statins was safe (Schwartz et al, 2001), and reduced recurrent ischaemic events over the next 16 weeks.

SOME DEFINITIONS

Acute coronary syndromes

Clinical presentations of coronary heart disease caused by permanent, temporary, complete or partial coronary arterial occlusion, including UA (unstable angina), STEMI and NSTEMI (ST and non-ST elevation myocardial infarction).

Acute myocardial infarction

A positive troponin or typical rise and fall of other biochemical cardiac markers, with at least one of the following:

- Symptoms of ischaemia
- ECG changes of ischaemia (ST elevation or depression)
- Development of Q waves
- Recent PCI
- Postmortem findings.

From a practical point of view, patients with acute myocardial infarction may be classified as:

1. *ST elevation myocardial infarction (STEMI)*. Patients presenting with symptoms of myocardial ischaemia, accompanied by ST elevation on the ECG. These patients usually release high levels of cardiac enzymes into the circulation and subsequently develop Q waves on the ECG. This group includes those with new bundle branch block or posterior ECG changes.

2. *Non-ST elevation myocardial infarction (NSTEMI)*. Patients presenting with symptoms of myocardial ischaemia, but without ST elevation on the presenting ECG. The ECG is usually abnormal, but may be normal. Cardiac markers will be positive.

Unstable coronary syndromes

Patients presenting with anginal chest pain at rest or on minimal exertion who have evidence of underlying coronary disease as indicated by one or all of the following:

- ST segment depression, T wave inversion or transient ST elevation on the ECG
- Raised cardiac markers
- Evidence of coronary artery disease at angiography or on perfusion scanning.

These patients will be classified as *unstable angina* (UA) or *non-ST elevation myocardial infarction* (NSTEMI), based on detection of cardiac markers (Table 6.1).

Suspected acute coronary syndrome

Patients presenting with symptoms suggestive of UA, but with a normal initial ECG, and no previous history of coronary artery disease.

Stabilised acute coronary syndrome

Patients with an unstable coronary syndrome (UA or NSTEMI), whose condition has become stable with initial treatment, and who have non-invasive investigations that indicate low risk. There is no evidence that routine angiography or

PCI affects outcome for these patients (Scanlon et al, 1999). Risk stratification is required.

Refractory acute coronary syndrome

Recurrence of anginal symptoms with ischaemic ECG changes despite adequate treatment with aspirin, clopidogrel, low molecular weight heparin and anti-ischaemic drugs.

Recurrent acute coronary syndrome

Recurrence of symptoms or ischaemic ECG changes despite treatment with aspirin, clopido-grel and anti-ischaemic drugs within 2 months of the diagnosis of a confirmed acute coronary syndrome.

Non-Q wave myocardial infarction/ subendocardial myocardial infarction

These terms imply a non-transmural myocardial infarction, but are retrospective diagnoses based on late ECG changes, or postmortem findings. They do not help in acute management. Patients will have presented with STEMI or NSTEMI.

REFERENCES

ACC/AHA (2000) Guidelines for the management of patients with unstable angina and non-ST elevation myocardial infarction. Executive summary and recommendations. *Circulation*, **102:** 1193–1209.

Antman EM, Cohen M, Bernink PJ et al (2000) The TIMI risk score for unstable angina/non-ST elevation MI: a method for prognostication and therapeutic decision making. *JAMA*, **284:** 835–842.

Bertrand ME, Simoons ML, Fox KAA et al (2000) Management of acute coronary syndromes without persistent ST segment elevation. Recommendations of the Task Force of the European Society of Cardiology. *European Heart Journal*, **21:** 1406–1432.

British Cardiac Society (2001) Guidelines for the management of patients with acute coronary syndromes without ECG ST segment elevation. *Heart*, **85:** 133–142.

Brodie BR, Stuckey TD (2002) Mechanical reperfusion therapy for acute myocardial infarction: stent PAMI, ADMIRAL, CADILLAC and beyond. *Heart*, **87:** 191–192.

Collinson J, Flather M, Fox KA et al (2000) Clinical outcomes, risk stratification and practice patterns of unstable angina and myocardial infarction without ST elevation: Prospective Registry of Acute Ischaemic Syndromes in the UK (PRAIS-UK). *European Heart Journal*, **21:** 1450–1457.

Department of Health (2000) *National Service Framework for Coronary Heart Disease*. London: The Stationery Office. Ch. 2.

ESC/ACC (2000) Myocardial infarction re-defined: consensus document of the joint European Society of Cardiology/American College of Cardiology. *European Heart Journal*, **21:** 1502–1513.

Fox KAA (2000) Acute coronary syndromes: presentation, clinical spectrum and management. *Heart*, **84:** 93–100.

Fox KAA, Gore JM (2001) Rationale and design of GRACE: a multinational registry of patients hospitalised with acute coronary syndromes. *American Heart Journal*, **141:** 190–199.

Gerhardt W, Katus H, Ravkilde J et al (1991) Troponin T in suspected ischaemic myocardial injury compared with mass and catalytic concentrations of S-creatine kinase isoenzyme MB. *Clinical Chemistry*, **37:** 1405–1411.

Gibbons RJ, Chattergee K, Daley J et al (1999) ACC/AHA/ACP-ASIM guidelines for the management of patients with chronic stable angina. *Journal of the American College of Cardiology*, **33:** 2092–2197.

Graff L, Joseph T, Andelman R et al (1995) American College of Emergency Physicians information paper. Chest pain units in emergency departments: a report from the short-term observation services section. *American Journal of Cardiology*, **76:** 1063–1069.

Graff LG, Dallara J, Ross MA et al (1997) Impact on the care of the emergency department chest pain patient from the Chest Pain Evaluation Registry study. *American Journal of Cardiology*, **80:** 563–568.

Herlitz J, Karlson BW, Sjölin M et al (2001) Ten year mortality in subsets of patients with an acute coronary syndrome. *Heart*, **86:** 391–396

Hulley S, Grady D, Bush T et al (1998) Randomised trial of estrogen plus progestin for secondary prevention of coronary heart disease in post-menopausal women. Heart and Estrogen/progestin Replacement Study (HERS) research group. *JAMA*, **280:** 605–613.

Keavney B, Haider YM, McCance AJ et al JD (1996) Normal coronary angiograms: financial victory from the brink of clinical defeat? *Heart*, **75:** 623–625.

Lindahl B, Andren B, Ohlsson J and the FRISC study group (1997) Risk stratification in unstable coronary artery disease. Additive value of troponin T determinations and pre-discharge exercise tests. *European Heart Journal*, **18:** 762–770.

McCullough PA, O'Neill WW, Graham M et al (1998) A prospective randomised trial of triage angiography in acute coronary syndromes illegible for thrombolytic therapy. Results of the Medicine versus Angiography in

Thrombolytic Exclusion (MATE) trial. *Journal of the American College of Cardiology,* **32:** 596–605.

McKenna CJ, Forfar JC (2002) Was it a heart attack? *BMJ,* **324:** 377–378.

Ng SM, Krishnaswamy P, Morissey R et al (2001) Ninety-minute accelerated critical pathway for chest pain evaluation. *American Journal of Cardiology,* **88:** 611–617.

Ohman EM, Armstrong PW, Christenson RH et al (1996) Cardiac troponin T levels and risk stratification in acute myocardial ischemia. *New England Journal of Medicine,* **335:** 1333–1341.

Scanlon PJ, Faxon DP, Audet AM et al (1999) ACC/AHA guidelines for coronary angiography. *Journal of the American College of Cardiology,* **33:** 1756–1824.

Schwartz GG, Olsson AG, Ezekowitz MD et al (2001) Effects of atorvastatin on early recurrent ischemic events in acute coronary syndromes: the Myocardial Ischemia Reduction with Aggressive Cholesterol Lowering (MIRACL) study; a randomised controlled trial. *JAMA,* **285:** 1711–1718.

Shaw LJ, Peterson ED, Kesler K et al (1996) A meta-analysis of pre-discharge risk stratification after acute myocardial infarction with stress electrocardiography, myocardial perfusion and ventricular function imaging. *American Journal of Cardiology,* **78:** 1327–1337.

Simoons ML (2001) Effect of glycoprotein IIb/IIIa receptor blocker abciximab on outcome in patients with acute coronary syndromes without early coronary revascularisation: the GUSTO IV-ACS randomised trial. *Lancet,* **357:** 1915–1924.

Stevenson R, Wilkinson P, Marchant B (1994) Relative value of clinical variables, treadmill stress testing and Holter ST monitoring for post-infarction risk stratification. *American Journal of Cardiology,* **70:** 233–240.

Tunstall-Pedoe H, Kuulasmaa K, Amouyel P et al (1994) Myocardial infarctions and coronary deaths in the World Health Organization MONICA project. Registration procedures, event rates, and case fatality rates in 38 populations from 21 countries in four continents. *Circulation,* **90:** 583–612.

Wallentin L, Lagerqvist B, Husted S et al (2000) Outcome at 1 year after an invasive compared with a non-invasive strategy in unstable angina coronary artery disease: the FRISC II invasive randomised trial. Fast Revascularisation during Instability in Coronary Artery Disease Investigators. *Lancet,* **356:** 9–16.

7

Management of ST elevation myocardial infarction

Despite improvements in the primary prevention and treatment of established coronary heart disease, acute myocardial infarction is responsible for between one-third and one-half of all cardiovascular deaths, and is the major cause of death in most developed countries. In 2000, 270 000 people in the UK suffered a heart attack, and about 157 000 died from the various manifestations of coronary heart disease (Petersen and Rayner, 2002). Most cardiac deaths occur out of hospital (Norris, 1998), so our experience of acute myocardial infarction on the coronary care unit is based on caring for survivors of a devastating clinical event that has already taken a major toll (Table 7.1). Thrombolytic therapy, aspirin, beta-blockers, statins and angiotensin-converting enzyme (ACE) inhibitors may favourably influence the prognosis of these patients, but many do not receive these evidence-based interventions, and 10–15% of the patients who reach hospital will die before discharge. Another 15–20% will die during the following year (Gandhi, 1997).

Table 7.1 Percentage distribution of 28-day fatalities, expressed as median (range), for patients 35–64 years in the MONICA Project, 1985–1990 (Chambless et al, 1997)

Time	Men (%)	Women (%)
Pre-hospital	70 (58–80)	64 (42–75)
Hospital < 24 h	22 (15–36)	27 (19–46)
1–28 days	14 (8–21)	16 (11–30)

Minimising the delay in coming under medical care for those with an evolving myocardial infarction reduces the chance of death from ventricular fibrillation, and maximises the potential benefit from reperfusional strategies to salvage myocardium at risk. Once in hospital, patients are best managed on coronary care units rather than on general medical wards, because the chances of resuscitation are two to three times higher. Inpatient mortality fell by about 10% following the introduction of coronary care units in the 1960s, mainly due to the prompt recognition and treatment of potentially fatal dysrhythmias. Patients admitted to medical wards are also not considered soon enough for thrombolytic therapy, or for other secondary interventions (Lawson-Matthew et al, 1994). Reductions in hospital mortality have mainly been achieved by faster admission procedures, infarct limitation strategies (thrombolysis and primary angioplasty) and enhanced therapy for cardiogenic shock and heart failure.

LIMITING THE EXTENT OF INFARCTION

Although it has been recognised for over 60 years that the extent of myocardial infarction is related to the duration of coronary occlusion (Blumgart et al, 1941), the clinical importance of opening the infarct-related artery to re-establish normal myocardial perfusion has only recently been realised (Braunwald, 1993). Necrosis of viable myocardial tissue mainly occurs during the first 30–90 min following coronary occlusion, and early and complete opening of the artery limits infarct size, preserves left ventricular function and increases survival (GUSTO Angiographic Investigators, 1993). The zone of potentially salvageable myocardium lies between the irreversibly damaged central core and normal myocardial tissues at the periphery. The severity and location of the coronary artery occlusion, the patency of other coronary arteries, and the presence of collateral vessels affect the size of this 'border zone'.

Primary angioplasty (percutaneous transluminal coronary angioplasty, PTCA) is the most efficient way of restoring coronary patency, and should be utilised if it can take place within 90 min of admission by experienced catheter laboratory staff, in a centre with surgical back-up (Ryan et al, 1996; Weaver et al, 1997). Access to such facilities for most patients is currently not possible, and attempts to restore coronary patency is usually by thrombolysis. *Thrombolytic therapy* during the first hour results in a 50% mortality reduction – or 50–60 patients' lives saved per 1000 treated (Boersma et al, 1996).

There are several cardiac drugs that may be used early to help maintain myocardial viability while reperfusion is attempted:

- *Aspirin* should be given as soon as possible. It calms the ruptured plaque by reducing inflammation, and helps prevent coronary platelet emboli causing distal micro-infarcts (Antiplatelet Trialists' Collaboration, 1994). Clopidogrel is an alternative for aspirin-intolerant patients, and should be given in combination with aspirin when treating unstable coronary syndromes (CURE, 2001).
- *Intravenous beta-adrenergic blocking agents* will reduce heart rate and contractility, limit myocardial damage, and perhaps inhibit ventricular fibrillation.
- *Nitrates* decrease cardiac preload, and thus reduce myocardial work and augment endocardial perfusion. The reduction in myocardial stretch reduces compression on the collateral coronary arteries, which enhances collateral circulation. Since coronary arterial spasm in the presence of a fixed atheromatous lesion complicates over one-third of cases of myocardial infarction, the early use of nitrates may help re-establish coronary blood flow.
- *Supplemental oxygen therapy* increases the oxygen gradient between the normal myocardium and border zone myocardium. Most patients with acute myocardial infarction have mild arterial hypoxaemia. This is caused by impaired pump function, leading to high pulmonary venous pressures, varying degrees of pulmonary interstitial oedema, ventilation/

perfusion mismatches and impaired gas diffusion. Diamorphine-induced hypoventilation may also contribute. Oxygen therapy may thus limit the size of the final infarcted area (Maroko et al, 1975).

PRE-HOSPITAL MANAGEMENT

The first evidence of myocardial infarction may be sudden death, and most fatalities occur before a call for help is made (Fitzpatrick et al, 1992). Three-quarters of these heart attack deaths occur in the home (Norris, 1998; Volmink et al, 1998), and the remainder in public places (16%), nursing homes (3%), in the ambulance (3%), at work (2%) or in the doctor's surgery (1%). Warning symptoms are common, although their significance may go unrecognised by the patient or by those from whom he may seek advice. Intermittent chest pain is the most common prodromal symptom in the majority of patients (Table 7.2).

Recognising that most deaths occur before arrival in hospital, the concept of pre-hospital coronary care was popularised in the 1960s (Pantridge and Adgey, 1969), using 'coronary ambulances' to carry trained staff, with equipment for resuscitation, haemodynamic stabilisation and rhythm monitoring to the patient. Initially, medical practitioners and specialist nurses manned these ambulances, but now paramedical personnel provide primary emergency care in most areas. The most important part of

Table 7.2 Premonitory symptoms in 100 sequential cases of myocardial infarction admitted to our coronary care unit

Symptoms[a]	Percentage
Angina	
New	11
Old	17
Chest pain	26
Emotional stress	19
Dyspnoea	13
Lethargy	10
Palpitations	4
None	46

[a]Note that some symptoms were multiple.

coronary ambulance training is the application of early cardiac defibrillation, which has had a major impact on the reduction of out-of-hospital coronary mortality. The effectiveness of such a system has been shown in many cities around the world, including Brighton, Belfast, Seattle and Melbourne, where pre-hospital care may have decreased coronary mortality by about 14% (Goldman and Cook, 1984). However, these services cannot function satisfactorily unless there has been community education in the recognition of the presenting symptoms of myocardial infarction, with basic training in cardiopulmonary resuscitation, allowing emergency services to reach the patient. Bystander-initiated resuscitation is associated with improved survival to discharge from hospital to home (Gallagher et al, 1995).

Apart from effective resuscitation, there are other first-line measures that ambulance services can provide. The insertion of intravenous cannulae and the administration of aspirin, nitrates, analgesics and oxygen may help limit the infarction, and pre-hospital thrombolysis has been used and evaluated in different settings. The GREAT and EMIP studies demonstrated that resuscitation with thrombolysis could be given in the community, and may be of particular value in rural populations (GREAT Study Group, 1992; EMIP, 1993). The standard 12-lead electrocardiogram (ECG) is vital to assess eligibility for thrombolysis (Boersma et al, 1998), and may be interpreted on site by computerised ECG, or transmitted by cellular phone or fax to the cardiac unit to receive guidance if there is doubt. False positive diagnoses are then limited to less than 1% (Grijseels et al, 1995). An overview of clinical trials has shown that pre-hospital thrombolysis is associated with a 17% reduction in 30-day mortality (Weaver, 1995), although a similar reduction in mortality might be achieved by getting the patient to hospital faster ('scoop and run' policy). Despite extensive training and investment, the European Myocardial Infarction Project saved just 55 min, and only just demonstrated a beneficial effect. Practically speaking, pre-hospital treatment should be given at least 1 h sooner if it is going to reduce mortality, and anything less than this probably makes hospital thrombolysis equally effective. Hence, if local circumstances make it impossible to reduce the 'call-to-needle time' to less than 60 min, pre-hospital thrombolysis must be considered (National Service Framework, 2000). The logistics of this are complicated, and unless general practitioners have been specially trained and supported (Waine et al, 1993), or there is provision of a well-equipped, well-trained mobile emergency unit, ensuring rapid transmission of the patient to a coronary care unit is preferred.

The European Society of Cardiology has issued guidelines for the pre-hospital management of acute heart attacks (Arntz et al, 1998).

DELAYS IN THE TREATMENT OF CORONARY THROMBOSIS

There are several, usually unavoidable, delays that can occur between the onset of symptoms and admission to the coronary care unit:

- Between the onset of symptoms and the call for help
- Between the call for assistance and the arrival of medical help
- During transport to hospital
- Within the hospital.

Many patients delay seeking medical attention after the onset of symptoms; this has been our experience (Table 7.3). Older patients and women wait longer before calling for help, perhaps because their symptoms are atypical and unrecognised (Burnett et al, 1995). The advice of the patient's family may be sought before any

contact is made with a medical practitioner, and such patterns of behaviour may not be modifiable by education (Bergin-Blohm et al, 1996). Further time is wasted in waiting for the emergency doctor to visit, formulate a diagnosis, arrange hospital admission and organise transport. General practitioners should be prepared to make a diagnosis on the basis of information over the telephone, and, unless they can reach the patient within 15 min, they should send an ambulance rather than attend the patient first.

IMMEDIATE MANAGEMENT IN HOSPITAL

The journey to hospital is usually brief, but delays can occur during admission procedures and in the X-ray and emergency departments. Direct admission to coronary care and/or rapid triage policies must exist if cardiac mortality and morbidity are to be minimised. Despite worries, such arrangements do not usually lead to congestion of the coronary care unit or to a significant number of inappropriate admissions. Our experience shows that the majority of cases are correctly directed to coronary care (Table 7.4).

A 'fast-track' admission system can reduce in-hospital delay if patients present to the accident and emergency or other departments. Targeted clinical examination, with a 12-lead ECG, within 10 min of arrival helps select patients for thrombolytic therapy, and routine evaluation by the admitting medical team is bypassed (Pell et al, 1992). Patients can be classified as:

- *Fast-track*: myocardial infarction, qualifying ECG (ST elevation or bundle branch block) and no contraindications for thrombolysis.

Table 7.3 Time between onset of coronary symptoms and call for medical help in 200 patients admitted to our coronary care unit with and without previous myocardial infarction (MI)

Time (h)	Previous MI	No previous MI
<0.5	28	20
0.5–1	18	15
1–3	42	27
3–24	5	9
>24	7	29
Total	100	100

Table 7.4 Analysis of a year's admissions to the coronary care unit at Withybush General Hospital, 2001

Diagnosis	Men	Women	Number	Percentage
Myocardial infarction	146	87	233	20
Other cardiac	336	226	562	49
Non-cardiac	227	133	360	31
Total	709	446	1155	100

- *Slow-track*: probable myocardial infarction with dubious ECG changes or relative contraindications to thrombolysis.
- *No track*: myocardial infarction unlikely or thrombolysis is contraindicated.

Such a system should not require any additional staff or resources and may halve the in-hospital delay to thrombolysis.

ADMISSION TO CORONARY CARE

There are several interventions that need immediate consideration following admission to the coronary care unit. Many of these will happen simultaneously, and the usual medical sequence of history, examination, investigation and treatment is generally not the most effective way of patient management. If fast-tracking/triage has not already been carried out, a rapid clinical appraisal is the first step to assess the likelihood of myocardial infarction and the need for thrombolysis.

HISTORY AND EXAMINATION OF THE PATIENT

Taking a history from patients on a coronary care unit is often easy; somebody somewhere must have thought the history was suggestive of an acute coronary syndrome. The initial enquiry should be brief, and serve to answer two questions:

- Does the patient need thrombolysis?
- Are there any contraindications to receiving thrombolysis?

Taking a more complete clinical history will still be needed, but this can usually wait until treatment is commenced. Obtaining essential information in the acute phase of the illness, when the patient is in pain and feeling faint or nauseated, is not ideal, and the complete story often becomes clearer when the patient has been settled with analgesia and anti-emetics. Although it is essential that there is no delay in instigating treatment, it is important to appreciate the psy-chological stress placed upon the patient who has been rushed into hospital via an emergency ambulance, to be delivered to the high-technology world of the coronary care unit. Autonomic imbalance or impaired left ventricular function may result in nausea, vomiting, sweating, peripheral vasoconstriction and varying degrees of dyspnoea. The typical patient will therefore be cool, clammy, in pain and frightened. Both verbal and tactile communication are important.

The physical appearance and clinical findings in patients suffering from acute myocardial infarction are extremely variable and alter with time and the presence of any co-existent complications. There are often no physical abnormalities. The general appearance of the coronary patient is dependent upon the physical and psychological impact that the illness has upon the particular individual. Hence, although some patients will appear quiet and anxious, others may appear excessively agitated and restless. The situation will be ameliorated or aggravated if the patient has had a previous hospital admission or myocardial infarction, depending upon his clinical and social course in-hospital.

Pulse and blood pressure

Variations in pulse rate and blood pressure usually depend on the amount of pain, the size of the infarct and the degree of left ventricular dysfunction, but may be influenced by overactivity of the autonomic nervous system. Inferior and true posterior myocardial infarctions are usually associated with parasympathetic overactivity (bradycardia, hypotension and heart block), whereas anterior and lateral infarction myocardial infarctions are associated with sympathetic stimulation (tachycardia and hypertension). In some patients, profound hypotension may follow the administration of nitrates.

The jugular venous pressure

The jugular venous pressure is usually normal unless there is pre-existing congestive heart failure or pulmonary disease, or there has been right ventricular infarction.

The heart sounds

The first heart sound is often diminished and muffled as a result of left ventricular dysfunction, and reversed splitting of the second sound is common, reflecting conduction delay within the ischaemic left ventricle. Fourth heart sounds are usual, thus their absence makes a large myocardial infarction unlikely. Third heart sounds are less common, and reflect left ventricular failure. As such, it implies a poorer prognosis. Detecting these low-pitched sounds is often difficult in patients who are obese or have hyperinflated chests, such as those with emphysema. Auscultation over the carotid or subclavian vessels may then amplify the heart sounds.

Cardiac murmurs

The murmur of mitral incompetence is present in many patients in the early stages of myocardial infarction because of papillary muscle dysfunction or dilatation of the mitral ring in association with left ventricular failure. Other murmurs may indicate pre-existing valvular disease, which may or may not have predisposed the individual to myocardial infarction. For example, aortic stenosis may cause myocardial infarction in the presence of little or no coronary atherosclerosis.

INTRAVENOUS ACCESS AND BLOOD SAMPLING

Insertion of an intravenous line will allow administration of an analgesic and an anti-emetic by injection. Intramuscular routes are inadequate, since drug absorption from vasoconstricted muscle capillary beds in the 'shut-down' patient is erratic. In addition, this route is contraindicated if thrombolysis is being considered because of the risk of intramuscular haematomas. The use of topical antiseptics such as Betadine (povidone–iodine) does not reduce the risk of cannula-related infection, and cleaning the skin with an alcohol wipe is sufficient (Thompson et al, 1989). This has the added advantage of removing skin oils and allowing the cannula to be fixed more securely to the skin with adhesive

tape. The cannula needs to be flushed every 8–12 h with normal saline and before and after every intravenous drug. The use of a heparin solution does not prolong cannula patency or reduce infection (Jowett et al, 1986).

Baseline blood tests are often taken at the same time as cannula insertion, but care is required if blood samples are withdrawn through the cannula: too small a cannula or too rapid an aspiration can cause haemolysis of the blood sample, with misleading results. Blood should be sent for analysis of the following.

Full blood count

This will detect anaemia or polycythaemia. The white cell count (WBC) and erythrocyte sedimentation rate (ESR) are initially normal but rise in response to muscle necrosis. The WBC peaks at about 15 000 cells/mm^3 after 2–4 days; higher levels suggest complications, such as infection or pericarditis. The ESR often remains elevated for 2–3 weeks.

Urea and electrolytes

Assessment of renal function and the potassium concentration are particularly important in patients taking digoxin or diuretics. Hypokalaemia appears to be associated with high levels of circulating catecholamines, and reduces the threshold for ventricular fibrillation. Maintaining a serum potassium of over 4 mmol/l is recommended. Measuring the magnesium level is useful if patients have been on high doses of diuretics.

Serum cardiac markers

When myocytes are damaged, they lose membrane integrity and large intracellular protein molecules leak out and may be detected in the blood. Although measuring 'cardiac enzymes' has been routine in coronary care units for many years, recently introduced tests are not for enzymes, so the preferred term is *serum cardiac markers*. The cardiac troponins are currently the best markers for the definitive detection of myocardial damage, and are proving highly effective in the risk stratification of patients with chest pain, reducing unnecessary admissions, and in targeting drug therapy in high-risk patients. If troponin estimation is not available, other markers may be used, such as total creatine kinase, CK-MB and myoglobin (Fig. 7.1).

Creatine kinase

Creatine kinase (CK) is found in high concentrations in both skeletal and cardiac muscle, as well as the brain, but the MB subfraction (CK-MB) is almost exclusively found in the human heart. CK-MB activity rises within 4–8 h of myocardial infarction to reach a peak between 12 and 24 h and disappear again by about 72 h. The CK-MB isoform $CK-MB_2$ occurs in one form in the heart, but occurs in other forms in the plasma. Raised levels of $CK-MB_2$ have improved sensitivity and specificity for detecting myocardial damage

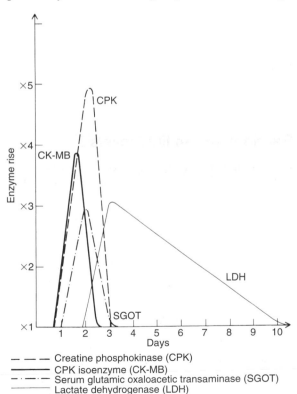

Figure 7.1 Serum enzyme release following acute myocardial infarction.

within 6 h of myocardial infarction. Levels are first detectable in the blood at 2–4 h and peak at 6 12 h.

Myoglobin

Myoglobin is a small haem protein found in skeletal and cardiac muscle. It is released 1–3 h following myocardial infarction, peaking at 4–8 h, and returning to normal within 24 h. It has been found to be more sensitive than CK-MB, but is not specific for cardiac damage. Results can be obtained in less than 2 min, and bedside estimation in the emergency room or on the coronary care unit may allow early exclusion of myocardial infarction.

Cardiac troponins

The troponins are proteins that are bound to the thin filaments of the contractile apparatus of the myocyte in both skeletal and cardiac muscle. There are three troponin proteins (troponins T, I and C), and assays are now available for both cardiac troponin T (cTnT) and cardiac troponin I (cTnI). cTnT and cTnI are released into the blood within 3 h of injury to the heart, peaking at 12–24 h, and remain elevated for up to 14 days. Unlike other cardiac markers, cTn is not detectable in healthy subjects, so even minor elevations indicate myocardial damage. Troponin estimation in acute coronary syndromes is of prognostic value (Fig. 6.1); a positive cTnT predicts mortality of 11.9% at 30 days in patients presenting with chest pain and an abnormal ECG, compared with a 30-day mortality of 3.9% in those with a negative cTnT. A raised cTn also identifies those patients who are most likely to benefit from specific treatments (Collinson, 1998). cTnI and cTnT are equivalent in diagnostic and prognostic efficacy (Maynard et al, 2000).

The profile of troponin release is initially similar to that of creatine kinase, as a small proportion of troponin is cytosolic. The remainder of troponin is protein-bound and will be released slowly for many days after myocardial infarction, although it may be accelerated by reperfusion (Fig. 7.2). The diagnostic time window is

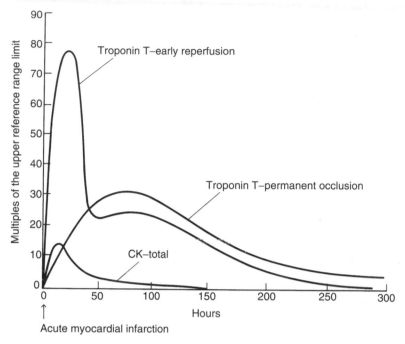

Figure 7.2 Pattern of troponin T release following early perfusion of the myocardium.

generally 72 h, with 100% sensitivity for diagnosing myocardial damage 12 h after presentation to hospital. There is no better way of making a late diagnosis of myocardial infarction as levels may remain elevated for as long as 14 days.

Practical use of biochemical markers

The different cardiac markers may be of value in different clinical situations, but using multiple tests both together and at different times may enhance diagnosis. For example, nearly all cases of myocardial infarction can be identified within 90 min by measuring troponin I, CK-MB and myoglobin (Ng et al, 2001). Positivity of any of these three indicates myocardial infarction, but negativity of all three excludes myocardial infarction. These combination tests may help with early triage of patients presenting with chest pain, but are likely to be very expensive.

The diagnostic values of total CK-MB, CK-MB isoforms, myoglobin, cTnI and cTnT were compared in patients presenting to emergency department with chest pain (Fromm et al, 2001).

The CK-MB isoforms were the most useful marker for triage. Troponin estimation was best for late diagnosis. All markers tested provided similar prognostic information.

Random serum lipid levels

Early assessment of random serum lipid concentrations will give an indication of pre-existing hyperlipidaemia (Brugada et al, 1996). If not carried out within 24 h, a formal lipid profile assessment will not be possible for many weeks, since cholesterol concentrations are suppressed and triglyceride concentrations elevated for about 3 months following acute myocardial infarction.

Blood glucose level

Patients with diabetes presenting with acute coronary syndromes have a hospital and long-term mortality nearly twice that of non-diabetics (Mak et al, 1997; McGuire et al, 2000). Up to 10% of admissions to coronary care are found to have previously undiagnosed diabetes, and share this excess mortality (Tenerz et al, 2001). A random blood glucose measurement is also of prognostic importance (Capes et al, 2000). Those with an admission blood sugar of less than 7 mmol/l usually have uncomplicated courses, whereas those with concentrations over 9 mmol/l are much more likely to develop complications.

Much of the excess mortality in patients with diabetes is due to the high incidence of cardiac failure that is not explained by infarct size, or the extent of coronary arterial disease, and has been attributed to a specific diabetic cardiomyopathy (Francis, 2001). Myocardial function may also be impaired by metabolic changes that occur in the early stages of acute myocardial infarction. The release of stress hormones (cortisol, catecholamines, growth hormone and glucagon) produce insulin resistance with hyperglycaemia, and endogenous insulin release is suppressed. The combination of low insulin levels with high catecholamine concentrations is associated with the release of free fatty acids that increase myocardial oxygen requirements and depress mechanical performance. Controlling the plasma glucose and fatty acid concentrations by insulin infusion could help preserve myocardial function and reduce morbidity and mortality.

The DIGAMI trial (Malmberg, 1997) randomised patients with acute myocardial infarction and a blood glucose of over 11 mmol/l to either continued normal treatment or blood glucose control (7–10.9 mmol/l) by insulin infusion. Insulin was continued for at least 24 h after admission, followed by four subcutaneous insulin injections daily for 3 months. Mortality at 1 year was reduced by 29% in those treated with insulin infusions.

Conventional post-infarction treatment with beta-blockers, ACE inhibitors and statins reduces mortality in patients with diabetes, but remains underutilised (Chowdhury et al, 1999; Rutherford, 2001).

ASPIRIN

Aspirin should be given at the earliest opportunity, unless there is a clear history of a major bleeding risk, or aspirin hypersensitivity. Aspirin enhances the benefits of thrombolysis, and reduces early and late morbidity (ISIS-2 Collaborative Group, 1988). The initial dose should be at least 150 mg, being chewed and held in the mouth rather than being swallowed; this enhances absorption and prevents the aspirin being regurgitated. Although the timing of aspirin ingestion is not thought to be critical, administration *prior* to thrombolysis may be associated with greater reduction in mortality compared with later treatment (Friemark et al, 1998). Treatment should continue for life (75–325 mg daily). The CAPRIE trial (1996) has confirmed that clopidogrel is a useful alternative to aspirin.

NITRATES

Coronary arterial spasm is a common associate of acute coronary thrombosis, and nitrates should be of benefit. The findings of the ISIS-4 (ISIS-4 Collaborative Group, 1995) and GISSI-3 (1994) trials have thrown some doubt on routine use, but the high cross-over rate to nitrates for post-infarction angina in the trials may have diluted the true value. Most would still recommend early administration of sublingual or buccal nitrates in those with ST segment elevation on the ECG to relieve vasospasm and anginal pain. Intravenous nitrates may be of particular value in patients with large anterior infarcts, hypertension, peri-infarction heart failure or recurrent pain (ACC/AHA, 1999). The intravenous route allows minute-to-minute titration, depending upon heart rate and blood pressure. Caution is required if the patient is hypotensive or is already taking nitrate therapy.

ANALGESIA

The provision of early and adequate pain relief is of major importance. Intravenous diamorphine is the drug of choice, and is well tolerated following myocardial infarction. Diamorphine relieves pain and anxiety that may stimulate catecholamine release. An initial intravenous dose of diamorphine, 2.5–5.0 mg, should be given at 1 mg/min, followed by further 2.5-mg doses until pain is relieved.

The most common side-effects of opiate therapy are nausea and vomiting, which can be reduced by simultaneous administration of an anti-emetic such as metoclopramide. Cyclizine causes vasoconstriction, and prochlorperazine can only be given by mouth or intramuscularly, so cannot be recommended. Opiates must be used with care in patients with chronic obstructive pulmonary disease, as respiratory depression may occur within minutes and last for up to 6 h. Opiate therapy also reduces gastric and intestinal motility, so oral absorption of important drugs such as diuretics may be impaired.

Intravenous beta-blockers, thrombolysis and nitrates all reduce pain, and decrease the need for analgesic drugs, probably by limiting ischaemic damage. The rapid and complete relief pain that accompanies early reperfusion suggests that the pain that accompanies acute myocardial infarction is due to continuing ischaemia in threatened, but still viable, myocardium, rather than from already infarcted cardiac muscle.

OXYGEN

Oxygen is a drug and should be administered in a dose just sufficient to produce the desired effect; additional oxygen is probably innocuous but wasteful. Repetitive hypoxaemia is probably worse that a single episode, and intermittent oxygen therapy has been likened to intermittent drowning. It is usual practice to administer continuous low-flow oxygen for 24–48 h (100% oxygen at 2–4 litres/min) for the relief of known or presumed hypoxaemia.

Nasal cannulae are preferred to face masks, which spend most of their time oxygenating the forehead. Oximetry can be used to regulate oxygen to achieve an oxyhaemoglobin saturation of about 95%, although it should not be used as the sole means of assessing adequacy of ventilation; oximetry only gives information about oxygenation, not about oxygen carriage (Davidson and Hosie, 1993). Assessment of arterial blood gases is indicated if there is any doubt as to the accuracy of pulse oximetry. The concentration of inspired oxygen may need to be altered according to arterial blood gas estimation (Table 7.5).

CHEST RADIOGRAPHY

It is still common practice for a portable antero-posterior (AP) chest film to be taken on admission to the coronary care unit. The clinical value of this in most cases is dubious, as most are performed under suboptimal conditions and have inherent limitations caused by the AP projection and the inability to position the patient properly.

Although it may serve to exclude other causes of chest pain, such as aortic aneurysm, pneumonia and pneumothorax, the chest X-ray is most often requested to detect heart failure. However, this indication is also limited. There may be a 12-h lag between haemodynamic dysfunction and the radiographic appearances of cardiac failure. Furthermore, radiological heart failure may take up to 4 days to resolve following haemodynamic stabilisation (Kostuk et al, 1973). A normal chest X-ray usually excludes significant heart failure.

A chest film should be carried out following prolonged resuscitation or after central catheterisation to exclude pneumothorax, and/or check to the catheter position.

Table 7.5 Oxygen masks, flow rates and approximate concentrations of delivered oxygen

Mask oxygen flow (litres/min)	Approximate concentration of delivered oxygen (%)			
	Edinburgh	MC	Nasal cannulae	Hudson
1	25–30	–	25–30	–
2	30–35	30–50	30–35	25–38
4	35–40	40–70	32–40	35–45
6	–	55–75	–	50–60
8	–	60–75	–	55–65
10	–	65–80	–	60–75

ECG MONITORING

Careful monitoring of cardiac rhythm and the prompt treatment of dysrhythmias has sharply reduced hospital deaths from myocardial infarction, and all patients should be connected to a suitable cardiac monitor as soon as possible (Jowett et al, 1985). If the patient is being transferred from the accident and emergency department, a portable monitor must accompany the patient to the coronary care unit.

THE ECG IN ACUTE MYOCARDIAL INFARCTION

A standard 12-lead ECG should be carried out within 10 min of the patient's arrival to confirm the diagnosis and assess suitability for thrombolysis. The ECG can change within seconds of coronary occlusion, and over 80% of patients with acute myocardial infarction will have an abnormal ECG on presentation (Goldberg et al, 1988).

There is no single ECG change produced by myocardial ischaemia and infarction; the findings depend upon the duration and location of the ischaemic insult. The initial ECG is sometimes normal, and even pre-existing abnormalities are not helpful if they do not change with time. In typical transmural myocardial infarction, there is an evolving sequence of ST–T changes with Q wave formation (Fig. 7.3). Infarction limited to the inner part of the ventricular wall (subendocardial infarction) interferes with repolarisation rather than depolarisation, and produces ST depression and deep symmetrical T wave inversion (Fig. 7.4).

ACUTE TRANSMURAL MYOCARDIAL INFARCTION

The hallmark of transmural myocardial infarction is the Q wave. Transmural necrosis produces an electrical 'window' in the ventricle, so that an overlying recording skin electrode will record a cavity potential, as if the electrode were inside the heart. Because the ventricles are depolarised

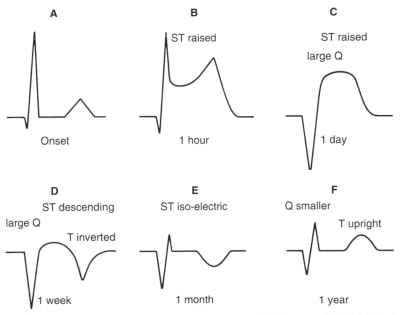

Figure 7.3 Evolution of ECG changes following acute transmural myocardial infarction: (A) ECG may be normal or show non-specific changes; (B) development of Q wave and concave ST segment elevation; (C) fully developed Q wave and convex ST elevation; (D) ST segment descends and T wave inverts; (E) ST segment now isoelectric, T wave often still inverted; (F) Q wave permanent but smaller. In 10% of patients the ECG is normal.

06-Mar-2002 06:13:40

Coronary Care Pembs And Derwen NHS Trust

Routine report

```
Rate    65    . AGE NOT ENTERED, ASSUMED TO BE 50 YEARS FOR PURPOSE OF ECG INTERPRETATION
PR     163    . NORMAL SINUS RHYTHM, RATE  65.................normal P axis, PR, rate & rhythm
QRSD    95    . REPOL ABN, PROBABLE ISCHEMIA, ANTEROLAT LEADS.........ST dep, T neg, I aVL V2-V6
QT     416
QTc    432

--Axis--
P       45
QRS     70
T      111
```

- ABNORMAL ECG -   Unconfirmed diagnosis.

MedGRAPHICS LTD

Figure 7.4 ECG: non-transmural (sub-endocardial) myocardial infarction.

from the inside outwards, an electrode placed inside the heart would record a large negative deflection (a Q wave), as the impulse travels outwards from within.

Normally, small ('septal') Q waves are seen in the left ventricular leads, caused by depolarisation of the septum from left to right. Pathological Q waves are greater than 0.04 s in duration and greater than 2 mm in depth (but not less than 25% of the R wave) in the standard leads. The Q wave in standard lead III should only be considered abnormal if it exceeds 0.03 s and is accompanied by Q waves in leads II and aVF. The 'normal' Q wave in lead III usually diminishes or disappears on deep inspiration, but a pathological Q wave will remain. In the left ventricular leads, pathological Q waves are greater than 4 mm in depth in V4 and V5, and greater than 2 mm in V6. Q waves associate with negative or biphasic T waves, and may be produced by any process that forms a myocardial window (e.g. cardiomyopathies, amyloidosis and cardiac tumours). Q waves are sometimes seen in left ventricular hypertrophy.

DETERMINING THE SITE OF INFARCTION

Infarction Q waves usually develop within the first 24–48 h in the leads that face the area of necrosis, although they may sometimes be found within 2 h of the onset of chest pain (Adams et al, 1993). Correlating the ECG findings with knowledge of the coronary circulation may help determine the site of the infarction, although normal coronary vasculature varies widely from person to person, and it is thus only possible to make generalisations (Box 7.1).

The three major coronary vessels are:

- The right coronary artery (RCA)
- The left anterior descending artery (LAD)
- The left circumflex artery (LCx).

The RCA supplies the right atrium, the right ventricle and the inferior left ventricle. Blood is

---

Box 7.1   Major coronary arteries and the structures supplied by each

Right coronary artery (RCA)
  Right atrium
  Right ventricle
  Inferior left ventricle
  Sinus node
  Atrioventricular node
  Posterior interventricular septum

Left anterior descending (LAD) coronary artery
  Anterior wall of left ventricle
  Anterior interventricular septum
  Apex of left ventricle
  Bundle of His and bundle branches

Left circumflex (LCx) coronary artery
  Left atrium
  Lateral and posterior left ventricle
  Posterior interventricular septum

---

also conveyed to the sinus node, the atrioventricular (AV) node and the posterior portion of the ventricular septum. Hence, occlusion of the RCA can produce infarction of the inferior and posterior left ventricle and, sometimes, the right atrium and ventricle. Ischaemia or oedema of the sinus and AV nodes may produce bradycardia and heart block (Fig. 7.5).

The left main stem of the left coronary artery divides into its two main branches, the left anterior descending (LAD) artery and the left circumflex (LCx) artery. The former supplies the anterior left ventricular wall, the apex and the interventricular septum. There are septal perforating branches, which additionally supply blood to the bundle of His and bundle branches. Occlusion of the LAD leads to infarction of the anterior left ventricular wall, the cardiac apex and the interventricular septum. The LCx supplies the remainder of the left ventricle and, sometimes, the posterior part of the interventricular septum; in some people, it additionally supplies the sinus and AV nodes. Occlusion of the LCx leads to leads to lateral infarction, sometimes associated with conduction problems. Left main stem occlusion effectively leads to infarction of the entire left ventricle, and is often rapidly fatal unless relieved.

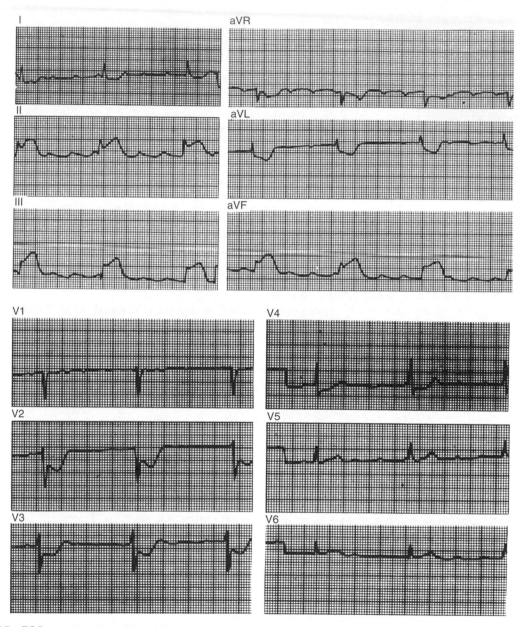

Figure 7.5 ECG: complete heart block following occlusion of the right coronary artery.

COMMON ECG PATTERNS OF INFARCTION

The following ECG patterns of infarction may be seen in the standard 12-lead ECG:

- *Anterior myocardial infarction* (Fig. 7.6) gives rise to changes in leads V1–V4 (anteroseptal infarction), standard leads I and aVL and V4–V6 (anterolateral infarction)
- *Inferior myocardial infarction* produces changes in the inferior leads II, III and aVF (Fig. 7.7)
- *High lateral myocardial infarction* may be seen only in leads I and aVL

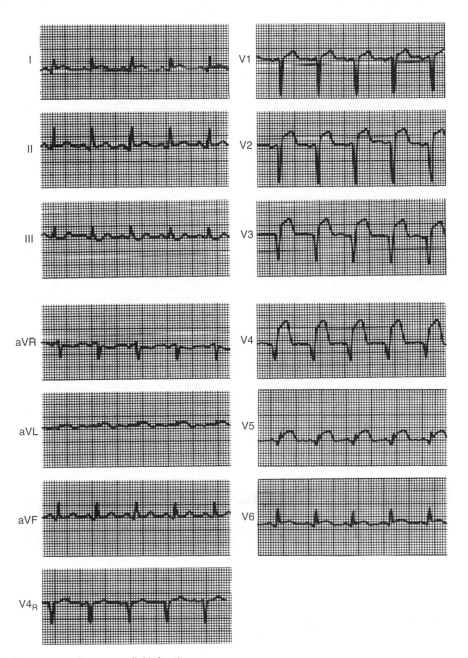

Figure 7.6   ECG: acute anterior myocardial infarction.

- *Apical infarction* can be seen in leads V5 and V6
- *Posterior myocardial infarction* does not produce Q waves in the standard 12-lead ECG, since no lead directly overlies the area of necrosis. Instead, the diagnosis must be implied on the basis of reciprocal tall R waves in leads opposite the area (V1–V3), with ST depression (Fig. 7.5). Right ventricular hypertrophy and right bundle branch block should be excluded.

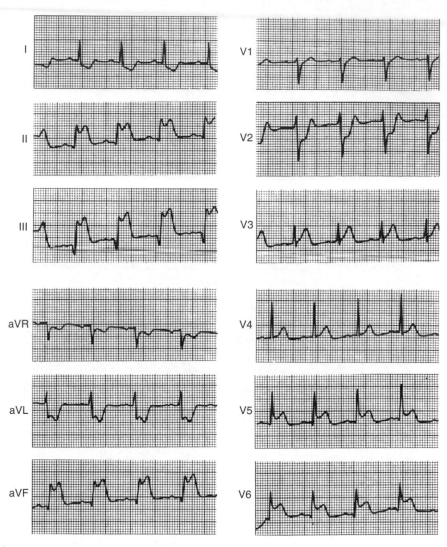

Figure 7.7   ECG: acute inferolateral myocardial infarction.

ECG changes do not always appear in the 'classical' leads, and additional leads may be required to locate infarcts at unusual sites. For example, V7 and V8 (placed further round the chest) are useful for diagnosing lateral infarcts, and leads in the 2nd and 3rd intercostal spaces may locate high lateral infarcts.

With the passage of time following myocardial infarction, the Q waves may regress or even disappear because the scar contracts away from the surface electrode, or because small intraventricu-lar conduction pathways are established in relation to the infarct.

ST SEGMENT AND T WAVE CHANGES

The earliest ECG sign of acute transmural myocardial ischaemia is elevation of the ST segment, sometimes accompanied by very tall, hyperacute T waves. The ST segments are usually convex upwards, although are sometimes concave or flattened. Without reperfusion, these acute ST–T wave changes may take hours or days to resolve. ST segment depression is often seen in leads facing away from the affected area. Originally, these 'reciprocal' changes were thought to be artefactual, but are more likely to indicate ischaemic myocardial tissue away from the infarction site. Patients showing 'reciprocal' ST depression have a worse long-term prognosis than those without (Krone et al, 1993).

The ST–T wave changes usually resolve over the following weeks, although T wave inversion often persists. Transient ST elevation occurs in Prinzmetal angina. Persistent ST elevation in the chest leads often indicates formation of a ventricular aneurysm.

Patients with acute myocardial infarction presenting with ST depression alone do not appear to benefit from thrombolysis and have a bad prognosis (Gheorghiade et al, 1993).

RIGHT VENTRICULAR AND ATRIAL INFARCTION

Isolated or additional infarction of the atria and right ventricle are probably more common than realised, and are often difficult to recognise.

Isolated right ventricular infarction is found at between 5% and 10% of autopsies (Rodrigues et al, 1986). About one-third to one-half of patients with inferior infarction sustain some damage to the right ventricle, and most regain normal right ventricular function over a period of weeks to months, suggesting right ventricular stunning rather than necrosis. Failure to recognise right ventricular infarction may lead to inappropriate management. Demonstration of 1-mm ST segment elevation in lead V_{4R} is the single most important ECG sign of right ventricular ischaemia (Klein et al, 1983). Changes may also be seen in V_{5R} and V_{6R}, but may be transient, with resolution in over half of cases within 10 h of onset of chest pain. All patients with inferior changes on their presenting ECG should have V_{4R} checked as routine.

Atrial infarction occurs in about 10% of cases of myocardial infarction and may be recognised by altered P wave morphology and deviation of the PR segment. Atrial dysrhythmias are a common complication, particularly atrial fibrillation.

NON-TRANSMURAL (SUBENDOCARDIAL) MYOCARDIAL INFARCTION

The subendocardium is especially prone to ischaemia, because the high intraventricular pressure limits its blood supply. Q wave development usually requires more than 50% of the wall thickness to be involved, so myocardial infarction limited to the subendocardium will not give rise to Q waves, but is accompanied by deep, symmetrical T wave inversion, sometimes with permanent ST depression (see Fig. 7.4).

ECG CHANGES THAT MIMIC MYOCARDIAL INFARCTION (PSEUDO-INFARCTION)

There are many circumstances in which ECG appearances may be confused with those of myocardial infarction. It is important to recognise these, since misdiagnosis may lead to inappropriate thrombolysis.

1. *Normal ECG variants*. High ST take-off is often seen in young adults, especially in the septal leads, and ST changes can also be produced by changes in posture or by hyperventilation. T wave inversion may be normal in leads V1 and V2 (and V3 in Negroes). Poor R wave progression across the chest leads, or QS complexes, occasionally occurs in V1 and V2 as a normal variant in tall, thin individuals or those with chest wall deformities (e.g. pectus excavatum), because of positional changes of the electrodes relative to the heart.

2. *Myocarditis and pericarditis*. Q waves may occur in myocarditis or with myocardial infiltrates. Concave ST elevation with widespread T wave inversion occurs with pericarditis; reciprocal ST depression does not occur.

3. *Metabolic influences*. Transient Q wave formation may follow metabolic insults such as hyperkalaemia or hypoglycaemia. ST–T wave changes are characteristic of hypo- and hyperkalaemia.

4. *Left ventricular hypertrophy*. Left ventricular hypertrophy secondary to hypertension or aortic stenosis may produce poor R wave progression in leads V1–V3. These may be confused with pathological Q waves, particularly if there are co-existent ST–T wave changes of left ventricular strain.

5. *Pulmonary embolism*. QR waves in leads V1–V3 are seen in right ventricular hypertrophy or strain. The classic $S_1/Q_3/T_3$ pattern described in acute pulmonary embolism is associated with non-infarction Q waves in standard leads III and aVF. Widespread T wave inversion and a sinus tachycardia are more usual.

6. *Miscellaneous conditions*. Very deep inverted T waves are sometimes found after intracerebral bleeds, probably due to altered autonomic tone, and may be confused with the changes of subendocardial infarction. Similar T wave changes are often seen after tachydysrhythmias or Stokes–Adams attacks. T wave inversion, caused by catecholamine stimulation, sometimes occurs in normal hearts and can be reversed with beta-blockade. Hyperventilation may also produce transient ST–T wave changes.

TREATMENT OF CORONARY THROMBOSIS

Myocardial infarction is associated with the presence of fresh thrombus in the affected coronary artery, in a dynamic interaction involving coronary artery spasm, platelet aggregation and a fissured atheromatous plaque (Davies and Thomas, 1985). Complete absence of blood flow in the infarct-related artery is usual. Small platelet emboli are shed before the artery becomes occluded, causing multiple, small, distal occlusions in the area supplied by the coronary vessel ('micro-infarcts'). Spontaneous thrombolysis may take place to a varying degree in about 30% of patients within the first 12–24 h (de Wood et al, 1980). Hence, there may be varying consequences of acute coronary thrombosis, ranging from micro-infarcts to full transmural infarction.

Thrombolysis was one of the most significant advances in the treatment of acute myocardial infarction in the 20th century. Ironically, the observation in the 1930s that streptokinase, a breakdown product of some streptococcus strains, could liquefy clotted blood came long before coronary care units, bedside monitors and defibrillators existed. It was another 25 years before attempts to re-open coronary arteries with streptokinase were reported in the treatment of acute myocardial infarction (Fletcher et al, 1958; Dewar et al, 1963).

Thrombolytic agents are actually *fibrinolytic* agents that activate plasminogen to form plasmin, which degrades fibrin and breaks down fresh thrombus. Intracoronary administration of streptokinase in acute myocardial infarction was used in the late 1970s, but it was the exceptionally important GISSI study that showed thrombolysis was equally effective when given systemically (GISSI Study Group, 1987). The beneficial effects of thrombolysis were confirmed by the second International Study of Infarct Survival (ISIS-2 Collaborative Group, 1988), and over 200 000 patients have since been randomised in thrombolytic trials, making it one of the most extensively researched medical therapies.

THROMBOLYTIC GUIDELINES

Before therapeutic intervention with thrombolytic agents, there are certain considerations, including:

- Who should be treated
- When and how to administer the drug
- The choice of thrombolytic agent
- What to do after thrombolysis.

Who should be treated?

It must be remembered that not all patients derive the same benefit from thrombolysis, and, in some, the benefits may be marginal, so the risk/benefits must be considered. Those likely to derive most benefit are patients with anterior infarcts, diabetics, the elderly and those in cardiogenic shock. The overview from the Fibrinolytic Therapy Trialists' Collaborative

Group (1994) has helped clarify who should be treated; our current coronary care guidelines for thrombolysis are shown in Box 7.2.

The main contraindications to administration of thrombolytic drugs are:

- Previous haemorrhagic stroke or other stroke within 1 year
- Active bleeding, but not menstruation
- Suspected aortic dissection
- Following traumatic cardiopulmonary resuscitation
- Intracranial neoplasm.

Relative contraindications include:

- Uncontrolled hypertension (blood pressure more than 180/110 mmHg)
- Recent trauma or surgery (under 4 weeks)
- Cerebrovascular surgery
- Previous stroke
- Anticoagulant therapy
- Aortic aneurysm
- Advanced liver disease
- Intracardiac thrombus
- Active peptic ulceration
- Pregnancy.

Box 7.2 Guidelines for thrombolysis in acute myocardial infarction

Pain

- Chest pain consistent with acute myocardial infarction

ECG changes

- ST elevation of > 0.1 mV (1 mm) in at least two contiguous leads
- New, or presumed new, bundle branch block (Note: Posterior infarction may present with ST depression with prominent R wave in leads V1–V2)

Time since onset of symptoms

- 0–6 h: greatest benefit
- 6–12 h: probable benefit
- > 12 h: diminishing benefit unless continuing or stuttering pain

Age

- Age is not an important consideration
- Biological age is probably more important
- Clear-cut benefits are seen in patients less than 75 years old
- Very elderly patients have few clear-cut benefits

Genuine contraindications to thrombolysis exist in 7–10% of patients (French et al, 1996), but many more patients are denied therapy, particularly those with diabetes and the elderly (Weaver et al, 1991; Lynch et al, 1993) – two subgroups who may benefit most.

The concerns in the elderly are mainly of inducing stroke. However, the GUSTO-1 trial showed that thrombolysis reduced mortality in all but the oldest patients (over 85 years). Long-term data from the ISIS-2 trial also show that the absolute survival advantage following thrombolysis is as least as good for older as for younger patients (Baigent et al, 1998).

Patients with diabetes are often not treated with fibrinolytic agents, perhaps because of fear of inducing intra-ocular bleeding (Shotliff et al, 1998). However, patients with diabetes derive greater benefit from thrombolysis than those without diabetes (Fibrinolytic Therapy Trialists' Collaborative Group, 1994), and none of the 300 patients with proliferate retinopathy in the GUSTO-1 trial suffered retinal bleeding (Mahaffey et al, 1997).

Complications of thrombolysis

The major risks of thrombolysis are intracranial haemorrhage, systemic haemorrhage, immunological complications, dysrhythmias and hypotension.

Intracranial haemorrhage complicates between 0.2% and 1% of cases, and is fatal in over 50%. The risk is greater with tissue plasminogen activator (tPA) and reteplase than for streptokinase, especially in elderly patients. Overall, there are about four additional strokes (mostly cerebral haemorrhage) per 1000 patients treated.

Major systemic haemorrhage affects about 7 cases per 1000 patients treated. Haemorrhagic complications may be treated by direct pressure on the source of bleeding, intravenous tranexamic acid or fresh frozen plasma. Temporary pacemakers and Swan–Ganz catheters should be inserted via the antecubital fossa or femoral vein to prevent possible occult bleeding following central catheterisation.

Fever and allergic reactions are frequent with streptokinase, and may be reduced by pre-treatment with hydrocortisone and chlorpheniramine. Anaphylaxis is a rare complication, although the accompanying hypotension may be mistaken for cardiogenic shock. Hypotension is a frequent accompaniment of thrombolytic therapy with streptokinase.

Dysrhythmias may accompany reperfusion of the ischaemic myocardium. These 'reperfusion dysrhythmias' are usually without clinical significance. Idioventricular rhythm is the most frequent abnormality, although some cases will develop ventricular tachycardia or ventricular fibrillation. Intravenous beta-blockade may help to protect the myocardium during thrombolysis and could reduce the incidence of reperfusion dysrhythmias.

When and how to administer the drug

For myocardial salvage to be optimised, thrombolysis must be attempted as early as possible. The Fibrinolytic Therapy Trialists' Collaborative Group (1994) analysis shows a gradual reduction in benefit with delay in administration of thrombolytic therapy, with each hour of delay translating into 1.6 additional lives lost per 1000 patients treated. However, survival benefits are not linear, and are twice as great in those treated in the first 2 h than in those treated after 2 h (Boersma et al, 1996). The usual time limit for thrombolysis is 12 h from the onset of symptoms (Cobbe, 1994), and too few patients presenting more than 12 h after the onset of symptoms have been studied to allow benefits to be determined (Collins et al, 1997).

The choice of thrombolytic agent

The two most common thrombolytic agents used in the UK remain streptokinase and tissue plasminogen activator (tPA). Anisoylated plasminogen–streptokinase activator complex (APSAC) has now been withdrawn, probably because the antigenicity, adverse effects and reperfusion rates were no different from those of streptokinase.

One of the world's largest therapeutic trials randomised streptokinase, APSAC and tPA blindly against each other in 41 299 patients with suspected acute myocardial infarction (ISIS-3 Collaborative Group, 1992). There was no difference in mortality between the treatment groups, but there were fewer cerebral bleeds with streptokinase, and, overall, this was found to be the safest drug. Thus streptokinase is generally used as the agent of first choice based on results of the ISIS-3 trial, as well as cost. This practice changed slightly in favour of tPA following the GUSTO trial (GUSTO, 1993), which suggested that front-loaded tPA is more beneficial in younger patients treated within 4 h of onset of symptoms, especially if the infarct is large and involves the anterior wall. With the exception of this group, the choice of fibrinolytic regimen appears to make little difference to overall survival, because the regimens that resolve coronary thrombi more rapidly produce greater risks of cerebral and systemic haemorrhage (Collins et al, 1997).

Streptokinase

Streptokinase is a metabolic product of the group C beta-haemolytic streptococcus, which causes activation of plasminogen, leading to lysis of the fibrin within the fresh thrombus. Unfortunately it is not clot-specific and causes a systemic thrombolytic state by depleting fibrinogen and alpha-2 antiplasmin concentrations. Streptokinase is also antigenic and may produce allergic side-effects, such as fever, rash and even anaphylactic shock. Previous streptococcal infections may induce antibodies to streptokinase, and predispose the patient to allergic reactions and reduced clinical efficacy. Antistreptolysin titres begin to develop from the third day following administration of streptokinase and persist for years (Squire et al, 1999). Up to 20% of patients presenting with myocardial infarction will have had a previous infarct, are likely to have been exposed to streptokinase and should not be re-challenged (Cross, 1993).

Tissue plasminogen activator

Tissue plasminogen activator (tPA) is a naturally occurring protein with greater clot specificity than streptokinase; thus fibrinogen and alpha-2 antiplasmin concentrations are less likely to become depleted. Cloning of the tPA gene has provided large quantities of the drug for clinical use, but despite price reductions it remains relatively expensive. The drug is normally given as a 10-mg intravenous bolus, followed by 50 mg over 1 h and the remainder over 2 h. Accelerated or front-loaded tPA, as used in the GUSTO-1 study, is given as a 15-mg bolus, followed by 50 mg over 30 min and the remainder over 60 min.

New thrombolytic agents

A number of new thrombolytic agents are in different stages of clinical development with the aim of being easier to deliver, less antigenic, not so expensive and more effective. The new plasminogen activators are bioengineered mutants of wild-type tPA. They have enhanced fibrin (clot) specificity, with resistance to natural inhibitors such as plasminogen activator inhibitor-1. These drugs have longer half-lives, allowing single or double bolus injection rather than infusions.

Reteplase is administered in two 10-IU boluses 30 min apart, and produces similar benefits to accelerated tPA (Bode et al, 1996), with only a marginal benefit over streptokinase, although there were fewer complications such as atrial fibrillation and cardiogenic shock.

Tenecteplase was compared with front-loaded tPA in the ASSENT-2 trial, and was found to be equivalent for 30-day mortality (ASSENT-2 Investigators, 1999), but with a wider safety margin. The ease of administration of tenecteplase by a single bolus injection may make it easier to use both in and out of hospital.

Lanoteplase and *saruplase* (a recombinant urokinase plasminogen activator) have not shown superiority over tPA.

Staphylokinase is produced by *Staphylococcus aureus* and has fibrinolytic properties. A dose of 10–20 mg given over 30 min resulted in coronary artery patency similar to that achieved with accelerated tPA. Unfortunately, neutralising antibodies are produced, as with streptokinase, which may limit re-challenge. This may also be a problem with *Desmodus salivary plasminogen activator*, which is secreted by the vampire bat (*Desmodus*), because the molecules are not derived from humans and may be antigenic.

What to do after thrombolysis

To achieve the best outcome of thrombolysis, the infarct-related artery must:

- Be opened early
- Be opened completely
- Have maintained patency.

Although new plasminogen activators have been shown to achieve more rapid or complete infarct vessel patency than tPA, this has not resulted in an improvement in survival, suggesting that the relationship between coronary artery patency and survival is not direct. A possible explanation lies in microvascular obstruction, since patency of the infarct-related epicardial artery does not assure microvascular flow, or normal myocardial perfusion. Platelet microemboli from the unstable plaque produces transient micro-vascular occlusion, or micro-infarcts, and are likely to be responsible for the 'no flow' phenomenon often seen at coronary angiography following successful recanalisation. Anterior infarcts are more prone to this than inferior infarcts. Microvascular obstruction carried a four-fold increase in adverse events, including death, re-infarction, or the development of congestive heart failure in a group of patients after myocardial reperfusion treatment (Wu et al, 1998).

Underlying the coronary thrombotic event is a fissured atherosclerotic plaque, which initially leads to the formation of a platelet thrombus seen angioscopically as 'white' thrombus (van Belle et al, 1998). Surrounding this area of platelet aggregation is the 'red' thrombus, which is fibrin rich. Current thrombolytic agents do not actually attack thrombin, but the fibrin in the red thrombus. Thrombin, previously enmeshed in the red thrombus, is exposed, and exerts potent platelet pro-aggregatory effects, promoting microvascular embolisation. So, rather than aiming to achieve complete dissolution of the thrombus alone, approaches to prevent embolisation of part of the thrombus into the microcirculation should be considered.

Heparin is of value in maintaining vessel patency (de Bono, 1987); low molecular weight heparin offers practical and potential pharmacological advantages over unfractionated heparin, not least because of its more predictable bioavailability. Subcutaneous enoxaparin has been shown to be at least as effective as infusions of unfractionated heparin when given for 3 days following thrombolysis with tPA, with a trend towards higher recanalisation and lower re-occlusion rates (Ross et al, 2001). In practice, enoxaparin is given at a dose of 30 mg intravenously, followed by 1 mg/kg subcutaneously for 3 or more days (ASSENT-3 Investigators, 2001).

Utilising a more aggressive antiplatelet approach may also allow a reduced fibrinolytic dose, thereby minimising the prothrombotic state and the risk of intracerebral haemorrhage (Gurbel et al, 1998). Combined low-dose tPA or rPA (reteplase) with full-dose platelet glycoprotein IIb/IIIa inhibitors, such as abciximab or eptifibatide, yielded a 50% improvement in early infarct vessel patency (Topol, 2000).

Residual atheromatous stenoses may be found by angiography in 80–90% of cases following thrombolysis. Re-accumulation of thrombus may occur in up to 40% within the first week, although this is not usually totally obstructive, or accompanied by symptoms. Symptomatic re-occlusion of the infarct-related artery occurs in about 5–8% of patients, mostly within the first 3 days. These patients have a more complicated clinical course and a higher mortality if further attempts to achieve patency are not made or fail (Ohman et al, 1990).

FAILED THROMBOLYSIS

Coronary artery patency and flow are important and independent prognostic predictors in patients following thrombolysis, and the prognosis in patients who do not reperfuse is worse than in those who do. Epicardial coronary flow may be classified by the TIMI (thrombolysis in myocardial infarction) flow grade (Table 7.6).

Table 7.6 Classification of coronary artery flow and myocardial perfusion seen at angiography (TIMI and TMP grading system)

Grade	
TIMI flow	
0	No penetration of contrast past the clot in the infarct-related artery
1	Contrast flows past vessel occlusion, but does not fill to the end of the vessel
2	Infarct-related vessel fills to full length, but flow is slower than that down normal adjacent vessels
3	Normal filling of infarct-related artery in comparison to adjacent vessels
TMP perfusion	
0	No or minimal blush
1	Dye does not leave myocardium; blush persists to next injection
2	Dye strongly persists at end of washout, but gone by next injection
3	Normal myocardial blush; mildly persistent at the end of washout

This semiquantitative tool has shown that early failure of thrombolytic treatment is associated with a 30-day mortality of over 15%. At least 30% of patients fail to recanalise by 2 h following treatment, although only a minority show signs of continuing ischaemia. Why thrombolysis fails in some cases is not clear. Those at risk are generally older, non-smokers, those with a previous infarct and of course those for whom there has been a delay in treatment. Mechanical problems, such as a large thrombus, or a large degree of fixed stenosis, may reduce the efficacy of thrombolysis.

Vessel patency means there is some flow down the vessel however effective, and the term *recanalisation* is used when a previously occluded vessel has been re-opened. Unfortunately, demonstrating an open vessel does not necessarily imply that flow is occurring down to tissue level. Patients with TIMI-2 and -3 flow both have open arteries, but those with TIMI-2 flow have a worse prognosis, probably because of impaired microvascular circulation. It has become clear that it is actually tissue perfusion, and not just an open artery, that is critical to myocardial salvage. The term *reperfusion* refers to re-establishing circulation at capillary level, which cannot be easily determined. Full reperfusion following thrombolysis fails in 60–75% of cases and is associated with a mortality of 16–20% (de Belder, 2001). The *no-flow phenomenon* arises because of platelet emboli and other atheromatous debris occluding flow in the microvasculature, with ischaemia-induced endothelial swelling and distal vessel vasoconstriction also playing a part. Perfusion defects following acute myocardial infarction may be visualised by contrast echocardiography, and closely relate to lack of contractile recovery and irreversible myocyte damage (Reffelmann and Kloner, 2002). Fortunately, collateral flow may help restore tissue perfusion despite poor flow in the infarct-related artery.

Just as TIMI flow grades are important in assessing epicardial artery flow, so the TIMI myocardial perfusion (TMP) grading system may be used to define myocardial perfusion (Appleby, 2001). Like TIMI flow, perfusion is graded TMP-0 to TMP-3, based on myocardial 'blushing' as angiographic dye passes in and out of the myocardium (Table 7.6). This provides independent risk stratification among patients with normal TIMI-3 epicardial flow.

Diagnosing failed thrombolysis

It is not known how best to determine failed thrombolysis (Kovlack and Gershlick, 2001). Helpful clues may be the following:

1. *Clinically.* Cessation of chest pain may indicate success in reperfusion, although analgesia may mask this, so it is not of value on its own. Other factors may also raise the pain threshold, such as age and diabetes. Conversely, continuing chest pain does not imply failure to achieve TIMI-3 epicardial flow, possibly because of poor tissue perfusion. Chest pain may also occur during reperfusion, especially in those with large infarcts.

2. *Reperfusion dysrhythmias.* Although frequent, the appearance of so-called reperfusional dysrhythmias does not necessarily indicate success. Idioventricular rhythm is perhaps the most common marker of reperfusion, but the relief of chest pain, resolution of ST segments and

appearance of dysrhythmias only occur in 15% of patients.

3. *The 12-lead ECG.* Patients whose ECG returns to normal in the early period following thrombolysis have preserved left ventricular function and a low mortality, but non-resolution of ST segment elevation associates with a poor outcome. The best ECG marker of reperfusion is a greater than 50% decrease in ST segment elevation at 60 min in the single lead with the maximum ST elevation at presentation (Oldroyd, 2000; Sutton et al, 2000). Repeated 12-lead ECGs may be helpful in identifying these patients, although continuous ST monitoring allows this to be done more easily (Klootwijk et al, 1996).

4. *Biochemical markers.* A rapid peak in myoglobin concentration is a marker of recanalisation, and can be used at bedside. There are no cardiac markers that can differentiate between TIMI-2 and TIMI-3 flow. Detection of reperfusion by biochemical markers may be too late to allow a change in therapy.

What to do if thrombolysis fails

It is difficult to know when to decide that thrombolysis has failed. Premature decisions may lead to unnecessary further interventions, but waiting too long may allow further myocardial damage.

Further thrombolysis is probably the most often tried intervention, particularly in hospitals without catheter facilities. Unfortunately, evidence that it works is limited (Drenth et al, 1998). Potential benefits may be offset by increased bleeding risks, particularly when performed more than 6 h after initial fibrinolysis.

Rescue angioplasty is an increasingly utilised intervention, although optimal timing is not known. A Dutch study in a hospital without catheterisation facilities showed that transferring patients to a regional centre for rescue angioplasty in patients with extensive myocardial infarction is safe and feasible (Vermeer et al, 1999). Delays are of course inevitable because of the time taken to administer and judge the efficacy of fibrinolysis. Salvage angioplasty rates are about 85% compared with rates of 95% or primary angioplasty, and the patient still has the risk of systemic haemorrhage. In-hospital mortality in this group is over 25% (Ross et al, 1998). Hypotension and bleeding associated with thrombolysis make invasive procedures more difficult, and, if attempts at rescue angioplasty fail, there is a high mortality of up to 40%. Rescue angioplasty is most beneficial in patients presenting with a first infarct, particularly if it is anterior and intervention is delivered within 6–8 h of onset of chest pain (de Belder, 2001).

Emergency bypass surgery (coronary artery bypass graft) seems unlikely to emerge as a form of treatment for failed thrombolysis. There are no trials in this group of patients, and angioplasty is less risky and easier to deliver.

Antiplatelet therapy with agents other than routine aspirin might have a role, since it is predominantly platelet micro-emboli that are responsible in part for the no-flow phenomenon that sometimes follows successful recanalisation with fibrinolytics. Clopidogrel and the glycoprotein IIb/IIIa inhibitors may prove useful in this respect.

INAPPROPRIATE ADMINISTRATION OF THROMBOLYTIC THERAPY

Although thrombolysis has become standard care for myocardial infarction, apprehension over complications often limits its use. The risk of bleeding and stroke are well appreciated, and reports of the disastrous consequences in patients with aortic dissection and pericarditis strengthen this concern (Blankenship and Almquist, 1989). Serious consequences of misdiagnosis were observed in the ASSET trial, in which patients with non-coronary chest pain who underwent thrombolysis had a mortality of 9.5%, against a mortality of 1.2% in those treated with placebo (Wilcox et al, 1988). Given the high incidence and multiple aetiologies of chest pain, one needs to guard against inappropriate administration of thrombolytic agents. For example, misdiagnosis rates of 41% have been reported if ECG criteria are not used (TEAHAT Study Group, 1990). Use of simple guidelines, as in Box 7.2, is associated with a low rate of inappropriate thrombolysis (Chapman et al, 1993).

THROMBOLYSIS AND COMPLETE HEART BLOCK

Complete heart block is a common complication of acute inferior myocardial infarction. Provided there are no contraindications, thrombolysis should be given immediately, as for other cases of myocardial infarction, along with atropine. Atrioventricular conduction usually improves, and many cases of complete heart block may be tolerated without the need to insert a temporary pacemaker (Jowett et al, 1989).

INTRAVENOUS BETA-BLOCKADE

Intravenous beta-blockade reduces pain, recurrent ischaemia and mortality in patients with acute myocardial infarction, with a 2–3-fold reduction in the risk of cardiac rupture (Freemantle et al, 1999). Despite these benefits, intravenous beta-blockade is not often given acutely in the UK, perhaps because of unwarranted fear of inducing bradycardia, hypotension and heart failure. In the ISIS-4 trial, only 5% of UK patients received intravenous beta-blockade compared to about 30% of those enrolled in the USA.

Beta-blockade is particularly valuable in those with persistent sinus tachycardia and associated hypertension. Metoprolol and atenolol may be given by slow intravenous injection of 5 mg, followed by a further 5 mg after 5 min while monitoring the patient. The pulse rate should remain above 50 beats/min and the blood pressure above 100 mmHg systolic. If tolerated, oral treatment should be continued for at least 2–3 years to achieve maximum benefit.

ANGIOTENSIN-CONVERTING ENZYME INHIBITORS

Routine use of ACE inhibitors in unselected patients following acute myocardial infarction was determined in the GISSI-3 (1994) and ISIS-4 (1995) studies. Broadly speaking, these trials showed some benefit, but most gain occurred in those patients with overt cardiac failure or an ejection fraction of less than 40%. The SAVE (Pfeffer et al, 1992) and AIRE (AIRE Investigators, 1993) studies both looked specifically at patients with heart failure following recent myocardial infarction, and showed that ACE inhibitors commenced within the first week significantly reduced mortality and serious cardiovascular events (St John Sutton, 1994). The ACE inhibitor should be introduced at a low dose once the patient is haemodynamically stable, with titration over the next few days if tolerated. The duration of therapy is unknown, but should continue in the presence of ongoing left ventricular dysfunction.

The benefit of ACE inhibition following myocardial infarction is not necessarily a class effect (Furberg et al, 1999). The ACE inhibitors employed in post-infarction trials, and the doses used, are given in Table 7.7.

In the HOPE study (Heart Outcomes Prevention Study Investigators, 2000), ramipril 10 mg was used in patients with significant risk for cardiovascular disease, but not necessarily in those with left ventricular dysfunction. The drug reduced a broad range of cardiovascular outcomes by a fifth, and reduced the overall mortality by 16%. However, the definition of normal left ventricular function in this study was an ejection fraction of greater than 40%. This certainly is not normal, so some of the beneficial effect may have particularly affected those with mildly impaired left ventricular function. Nevertheless, the benefits of ACE inhibition were additive and had similar magnitude to other proven strategies such as aspirin and beta-blockers.

MAGNESIUM

Despite early reports of benefits of intravenous magnesium sulphate (Woods et al, 1992), the ISIS-4 study showed a non-significant mortality excess. Routine use is not recommended, but there may be a role in patients with hypokalaemia since low serum potassium concentrations are often associated with low serum magnesium concentrations.

ANTICOAGULANTS

The routine use of anticoagulants in acute myocardial infarction is controversial, but should be of benefit in:

- Preventing deep vein thrombosis and pulmonary emboli
- Preventing left ventricular thrombi and peripheral embolisation
- Possibly limiting infarct size.

Venous thromboembolism and fatal pulmonary emboli are common in all medical patients, and many do not receive prophylaxis. For patients with myocardial infarction, the risk is at least moderate, with a 10–40% risk of a deep vein thrombosis, and an approximate 1% risk of fatal pulmonary embolism (THRIFT II Consensus Group, 1998). Low-dose unfractionated heparin or low molecular weight heparin should be given to all patients from admission until they are fully ambulant. We currently use enoxaparin 40 mg once daily for those not receiving post-thrombolysis heparin.

Full-dose anticoagulant therapy (heparin followed by warfarin, or prolonged subcutaneous high-dose calcium heparin) is recommended in those at increased risk of thromboembolic complications, including those with:

- Active thromboembolic phenomena
- Prolonged cardiac failure

Table 7.7 ACE inhibitors used in post-infarction trials

Drug	Dose	Trial	Reference
Captopril	50 mg three times a day	SAVE	Pfeffer et al, 1992
Lisinopril	10 mg daily	GISSI-3	GISSI-3, 1994
Enalapril	20 mg twice daily	CONSENSUS	Swedberg et al, 1992
Ramipril	5 mg twice daily	AIRE	Hall et al, 1997
Trandolapril	4 mg daily	TRACE	Kober et al, 1995

- Atrial fibrillation
- Left ventricular aneurysm
- Cardiogenic shock
- Severe obesity
- An inability to ambulate
- Extensive anterior myocardial infarction.

The duration of therapy is not clear, but 3 months should be adequate in most cases.

Long-term anticoagulation has been used for secondary prevention following acute myocardial infarction. The WARIS trial (Jafri et al, 1992) found that long-term warfarin therapy following acute myocardial infarction reduced the number of deaths and strokes, although the AFTER study (Julian et al, 1996) did not find any difference between aspirin and warfarin. Routine anticoagulant treatment of all post-infarction patients is not practicable, in terms of numbers alone, but perhaps should be considered in 'high-risk' patients.

ANTIDYSRHYTHMIC THERAPY

Patients are at increased risk of potentially fatal dysrhythmias following acute myocardial infarction. The first 48 h constitute the highest risk period, although ventricular tachycardia and fibrillation accounts for almost three-quarters of sudden deaths in the first 12 months following discharge from hospital. Early trials on prophylactic suppression of these dysrhythmias using drugs such as lidocaine (MacMahon et al, 1988), encainide and flecainide (Echt et al, 1991) actually increased mortality, and routine use of these agents is not recommended. For sustained ventricular tachycardia or repeated short salvos of ventricular tachycardia, lidocaine remains widely used. Intravenous amiodarone is a useful alternative, particularly in those with heart failure and recurrent ventricular ectopic activity (Cairns et al, 1997; Julian et al, 1997). Automatic implantable cardiodefibrillators may offer improved survival over antidysrhythmic drugs in high-risk groups with malignant ventricular dysrhythmias following acute myocardial infarction (see Ch. 13).

IMPORTANT PHYSICAL FINDINGS IN THE POST-INFARCTION PATIENT

A low-grade fever is often seen in the first 3 days after myocardial infarction, and is more common with large myocardial infarctions. Other causes of fever, such as deep vein thrombosis and infection, should be excluded, especially if the pyrexia exceeds 38°C. Chest and urinary tract infections are common, and bacteraemia may be caused by intravenous cannulae, pacing wires or urinary catheters. Occasionally, drugs may be the cause of late or unusual fevers.

HYPERTENSION

Many patients with myocardial infarction are found to be hypertensive on admission to coronary care. This may represent pre-existing hypertension, or may be a response to the stress of myocardial infarction with sympathetic over-activity. Coronary mortality is higher in hypertensive patients, and a systolic blood pressure of more than 160 mmHg persisting for more than 3 h after admission predisposes to cardiac rupture. If the blood pressure does not settle after relief of pain and anxiety, drug treatment should be commenced, and should be considered as urgent when ischaemic pain continues, or there is heart failure. Intravenous beta-blockade is desirable.

RESPIRATORY SYSTEM
Pulmonary embolism

Thromboembolic phenomena have become less frequent since the introduction of thrombolysis, prophylactic low-dose heparin therapy and early mobilisation. The diagnosis of pulmonary embolism must be considered in any patient with recurrent chest pain, particularly if associated with dyspnoea, tachycardia and fever. Physical examination is often unhelpful, unless there is pulmonary infarction and a pleural rub. It is probably better to treat on clinical suspicion, rather than relying on lung scans.

Chest infections

Chest infections are common, especially in the elderly, the obese and smokers. Pulmonary congestion and left ventricular failure predispose to infection, and opiate therapy is associated with small areas of atelectasis and ventilation/perfusion abnormalities in the lungs. Aspiration pneumonia may follow cardiopulmonary resuscitation.

Pneumothorax

This complication may follow central venous catheterisation, temporary cardiac pacing or cardiopulmonary resuscitation. Aspiration should be carried out if required.

GASTROINTESTINAL TRACT

Gastric dilatation may sometimes result from nasal administration of oxygen, leading to discomfort nausea or vomiting. Constipation and occasional paralytic ileus may result from bedrest or opiate therapy. Straining at stool must be avoided to prevent excessive vagal stimulation by the Valsalva manoeuvre.

Gastro-oesophageal reflux is a common coexistent cause of chest pain, and even endoscopic evidence of oesophagitis does not exclude the diagnosis of concomitant myocardial ischaemia. Stress ulceration of the oesophagus, stomach or duodenum may occur, sometimes causing gastrointestinal haemorrhage. This latter complication may be occult, presenting with tachycardia, hypotension and shock in a previously stable patient. This may be misdiagnosed as cardiac failure or cardiogenic shock.

URINARY TRACT

Urinary problems may result from drug therapy or bladder catheterisation. Atropine and opiates may precipitate urinary retention, especially in the elderly male, which is often exaggerated by a sudden response to diuretics. Catheterisation may be necessary, although it is not without risk of introducing infection and vagal stimulation.

Acute renal failure may result from prolonged hypotension or renal arterial embolisation from left ventricular mural thrombi.

Urinary albumin excretion increases following acute myocardial infarction, high excretion levels being associated with an increased mortality (Berton et al, 2001). Increased albumin excretion may be assessed by estimating the urinary albumin:creatinine ratio during the first week. There is a strong relationship with heart failure, which may explain some of the increased mortality.

NERVOUS SYSTEM

Alterations in mental state are common on intensive care units, where there may be anxiety or even hostility arising as a response to psychological stress. Decreased cerebral perfusion may give rise to psychiatric symptoms and is predisposed to by pre-existing cerebrovascular disease. Hypoxaemia and deteriorating left ventricular function will exaggerate these effects. Narcotics and anxiolytic drugs may alter perception, and intravenous lidocaine can produce hallucinations and seizures. Mural thrombi may give rise to cerebral embolisation and stroke, and cerebral haemorrhage is a recognised complication of thrombolytic therapy, particularly in the elderly.

THE METABOLIC SYSTEM

Myocardial infarction, cardiogenic shock or cardiac arrest is associated with a metabolic acidosis, because hypoxia associates with accumulation of organic acids, particularly lactic acid (Box 7.3). The clinical picture of lactic acidosis is usually dominated by shock, with Kussmaul respiration, in the presence of high blood concentrations of hydrogen ions (a low pH), and should be treated with oxygen and inotropic support. Sodium bicarbonate may be used to correct the acidaemia, and is best given in small hypertonic concentrations (e.g. 50–100 ml of an 8.4% solution). Great care is needed in order to avoid sodium and fluid overload.

Myocardial infarction may precipitate or worsen hyperglycaemia. The blood glucose concentration should be checked routinely and

---

> **Box 7.3** Some causes of lactic acidosis
>
> **Due to impaired tissue oxygenation**
> Myocardial infarction
> Left ventricular failure
> Pulmonary embolism
> Shock
> Sepsis
> Pancreatitis
>
> **Other causes**
> Diabetes mellitus
> Renal failure
> Liver disease
> Drugs
>   Biguanides
>   Alcohol
>   Cyanide (sodium nitroprusside)
>   Aspirin

monitored if elevated. Hyperglycaemia of greater than 10 mmol/l on admission either represents pre-existing diabetes mellitus, or may be a marker of pre-infarction insulin resistance, which is known to associate with increased hypercoagulability, decreased fibrinolysis and endothelial dysfunction. Stress hyperglycaemia with or without diabetes is associated with an increased mortality both at 30 days and at 1 year following acute myocardial infarction (Capes et al, 2000). High admission blood sugars are frequent in those developing cardiogenic shock and those who will need temporary cardiac pacing (Jowett et al, 1989).

Potassium–insulin–glucose infusions in acute myocardial infarction

Metabolic modulation with potassium–insulin–glucose (PIG) to improve peri-infarction cardiac dysfunction is based on two principles. First, insulin stimulates the uptake of potassium, which helps stabilise the cell membrane and reduce the incidence of dysrhythmias. Second, insulin stimulates the myocardial uptake of glucose. High intracellular glucose concentrations protect myocytes from the toxic effects of high levels of intracellular calcium induced by ischaemia. Insulin also has an effect on the high

concentrations of free fatty acids that are generated by release of the stress hormones (especially catecholamines). High concentrations of free fatty acids depress the myocardium, predispose to dysrhythmias and endanger the recovery of ischaemic but viable tissue.

There is increasing evidence to support the beneficial effects of PIG infusions in acute myocardial infarction and cardiogenic shock. This was first described in the 1960s (Sodi-Pallares et al, 1969), but the beneficial effects were not confirmed, and the use of PIG was abandoned. In 1997, a meta-analysis showed a reduction in mortality of 28% in patients with acute myocardial infarction treated with PIG (Fath-Ordoubadi and Beatt, 1997). This is equivalent to 49 lives saved per 1000 patients treated. Two PIG regimens have been described (Diaz et al, 1998):

- High-dose (glucose 25%, soluble insulin 20 units, potassium chloride 80 mmol/l) infused at 1.5 ml/kg/h for 24 h.
- Low-dose (glucose 10%, soluble insulin 20 units, potassium chloride 50 mmol/l) infused at 1 ml/h for 24 h.

Both high-dose and low-dose infusions are beneficial, producing the same reduction in in-hospital mortality, but high-dose infusion produces a better outcome at 1 year. Even though the time from onset of symptoms to time of infusion was 10–11 h, the combined end-points of death, severe heart failure and non-fatal ventricular fibrillation were reduced by 40%.

Generally, PIG infusions should continue for 24 h with an insulin infusion rate of about 5–10 units/h. The rate may need adjusting to maintain the blood glucose concentration under 10 mmol/l and the serum potassium between 4 and 5 mmol/l. Frequent monitoring of the serum glucose and potassium concentrations is required, and should continue after the infusion stops in case of any rebound effect.

PIG infusions may also help in the period of myocardial ischaemia during reperfusion in patients following cardiac surgery and in those with chronic congestive cardiac failure (Broomhead and Colvin, 2001). This safe and cheap intervention may have major implications for future coronary care.

POST-INFARCT CARE

Most units have guidelines for a gradual return to physical activity (Table 7.8). The usual period on the unit is about 24–48 h, although longer admissions will be needed for those patients with extensive myocardial infarction, severe heart failure or recurrent serious dysrhythmias. About half of the coronary admissions will have an uncomplicated course and probably need little intensive care.

The patient and family will need support and advice on life-style and secondary prevention measures. Ideally, an assessment of prognosis should be made prior to discharge, preferably aided by exercise stress testing, echocardiography and Holter monitoring. Long-term therapy

Table 7.8   Typical physical activity plan following acute myocardial infarction

Time	Activity
Day 1	Bed–chair rest
Day 2	Sit out of bed or chair; discharge from coronary care unit
Day 3	Walk around ward and to toilet
Day 4	Try stairs
Days 5–7	Discharge home
Days 7–14	Exercise within home and garden
Days 14–28	Gradual increased walking outside home Enrol in rehabilitation programme
Days 28–35	Exercise stress test[a]
Weeks 4–6	Outpatient review Return to work Recommence driving (in line with DVLA regulations)

[a]Pre-discharge exercise stress testing may be preferable if resources allow.

with aspirin, statin, ACE inhibitor or beta-blocker improves survival.

REFERENCES

ACC/AHA (1999) Guidelines for the management of patients with acute myocardial infarction: executive summary and recommendations. *Circulation*, **100:** 1016–1030.

Adams J, Trent R, Rawles J (1993) Earliest electrocardiographic evidence of myocardial infarction: implications for thrombolytic treatment. The GREAT Group. *BMJ*, **307:** 409–413.

AIRE (Acute Infarction Ramipril Efficacy) Investigators (1993) Effect of ramipril on mortality and morbidity of survivors of acute myocardial infarction with clinical evidence of heart failure. *Lancet*, **342:** 821–828.

Antiplatelet Trialists' Collaboration (1994) Overview I: Prevention of death, myocardial infarction and stroke by prolonged antiplatelet therapy in various categories of patients. *BMJ*, **308:** 81–106.

Appleby MA, Angeja BG, Dauterman K et al (2001) Angiographic assessment of myocardial perfusion: TIMI myocardial perfusion (TMP) grading system. *Heart*, **86:** 485–486.

Arntz H, Bossaert L, Carli P et al (1998) The pre-hospital management of acute heart attacks. Recommendations of a Task Force of the European Society of Cardiology and the European Resuscitation Council. *European Heart Journal*, **19:** 1140–1164.

ASSENT-2 Investigators (1999) Single-bolus tenecteplase compared with front-loaded alteplase in acute myocardial infarction: the ASSENT-2 double-blind randomised trial. *Lancet*, **354:** 716–722.

ASSENT-3 Investigators (2001) Efficacy and safety of tenecteplase in combination with enoxaparin, abciximab, or unfractionated heparin: the ASSENT-3 randomised trial in acute myocardial infarction. *Lancet*, **358:** 605–613.

Baigent C, Collins R, Appleby MA on behalf of the ISIS-2 Collaborative Group (1998) ISIS-2: 10 year survival among patients with suspected myocardial infarction in randomised comparison of intravenous streptokinase, oral aspirin, both or neither. *BMJ*, **316:** 1337–1343.

Bergin-Blohm M, Hartford M, Karlson BW et al (1996) An evaluation of the results of media and educational campaigns designed to shorten the time taken by patients with acute myocardial infarction to decide to go to hospital. *Heart*, **76:** 430–434.

Berton G, Coriano R, Palmieri R et al (2001) Micro-albuminaemia during acute myocardial infarction. *European Heart Journal*, **22:** 1466–1475.

Blankenship JC, Almquist AK (1989) Cardiovascular complications of thrombolytic therapy in patients with a mistaken diagnosis of acute myocardial infarction. *Journal of the American College of Cardiology*, **14:** 1579–1582.

Blumgart HL, Gilligan R, Schlesinger MJ (1941) Experimental studies on the effect of temporary occlusion of coronary arteries. II. The production of myocardial infarction. *American Heart Journal*, **22:** 374–389.

Bode C, Smalling RW, Berg G et al (1996) Randomised comparison of coronary thrombolysis achieved with double bolus reteplase (recombinant plasminogen activator) and front-loaded accelerated alteplase (recombinant tissue plasminogen activator) in patients with acute myocardial infarction. The RAPID II investigators. *Circulation*, **94:** 891–898.

Boersma E, Maas ACP, Deckers JW et al (1996) Early thrombolytic treatment in acute myocardial infarction: reappraisal of the golden hour. *Lancet*, **348:** 771–775.

Boersma E, Maas ACP, Grijseels EWM et al (1998) Benefits and risks of possible pre-hospital thrombolysis strategies – the role of the electrocardiogram. *Cardiologie*, **5:** 562–568.

Braunwald E (1993) The open artery theory is alive and well – again. *New England Journal of Medicine*, **329:** 1650–1652.

Broomhead CJ, Colvin MP (2001) Glucose, insulin and the cardiovascular disease. *Heart*, **85:** 495–496.

Brugada R, Wenger NK, Jacobson TA et al (1996) Changes in plasma cholesterol levels after hospitalization for acute coronary events. *Cardiology*, **87:** 194–199.

Burnett RE, Blumenthal JA, Mark DB et al (1995) Distinguishing between early and late responders to symptoms of acute myocardial infarction. *American Journal of Cardiology*, **75:** 1019–1022.

Cairns JA, Connolly SJ, Roberts R et al for the Canadian Amiodarone Myocardial Infarction Arrhythmia Trial Investigators (1997) Randomised trial of outcome after myocardial infarction in patients with frequent or repetitive ventricular premature depolarisations CAMIAT. *Lancet*, **349:** 675–682.

Capes SE, Hunt D, Malmberg K et al (2000) Stress hyperglycaemia and increased risk of death after myocardial infarction in patients with and without diabetes: a systematic overview. *Lancet*, **355:** 773–778.

CAPRIE Steering Committee (1996) A randomised blinded trial of clopidogrel versus aspirin in patients at risk of ischaemic events – CAPRIE. *Lancet*, **348:** 1329–1339.

Chambless L, Keil U, Dobson A et al (1997) Population versus clinical view of case fatality from acute coronary disease. Results from the WHO MONICA Project 1985–1990. *Circulation*, **96:** 3849–3859.

Chapman GD, Ohman EM, Topol EJ et al (1993) Minimising the risk of inappropriately administering thrombolytic therapy (TAMI study group). *American Journal of Cardiology*, **71:** 783–787.

Chowdhury TA, Lasker SS, Dyer PH (1999) Comparison of secondary prevention measures after myocardial infarction in subjects with and without diabetes mellitus. *Journal of Internal Medicine*, **245:** 565–570.

Cobbe SM (1994) Thrombolysis in myocardial infarction. *BMJ*, **308:** 216–217.

Collins R, Peto R, Baigent C et al (1997) Aspirin, heparin and fibrinolytic therapy in suspected acute myocardial infarction. *New England Journal of Medicine*, **336:** 847–860.

Collinson PO (1998) Troponin T or troponin I or CK-MB (or none)? *European Heart Journal*, **19:** N16–N24.

Cross D (1993) Repeat thrombolysis. *Australian and New Zealand Journal of Medicine*, **23:** 740–752.

CURE (2001) Effects of clopidogrel in addition to aspirin in patients with acute coronary syndromes without ST elevation. *New England Journal of Medicine*, **345:** 494–502.

Davidson JAH, Hosie HE (1993) Limitations of pulse oximetry: respiratory insufficiency – a failure of detection. *BMJ*, **307:** 372–373.

Davies MJ, Thomas AC (1985) Plaque fissuring – the cause of acute myocardial infarction, sudden death and crescendo angina. *British Heart Journal*, **53:** 363–373.

de Belder MA (2001) Acute myocardial infarction: failed thrombolysis. *Heart*, **85:** 104–112.

de Bono DP (1987) Coronary thrombolysis. *British Heart Journal*, **57:** 301–305.

Department of Health (2000) *National Service Framework for Coronary Heart Disease*. London: The Stationery Office. Ch.3.

Dewar HA, Stephenson P, Horler AR et al (1963) Fibrinolytic therapy of coronary thrombosis. *British Medical Journal*, **1:** 915–920.

de Wood MA, Spores J, Notske R et al (1980) Prevalence of total coronary occlusion during the early hours of transmural myocardial infarction. *New England Journal of Medicine*, **303:** 897–902.

Diaz R, Paolasso EA, Piegas LS et al (1998) Metabolic modulation of acute myocardial infarction. *Circulation*, **98:** 2227–2234.

Drenth JP, Uppelschgoten A, Hooghoudt TE et al (1998) Rescue thrombolysis may work even though primary thrombolysis has failed (letter). *BMJ*, **317:** 147.

Echt DS, Liebson PR, Mitchell LB et al (1991) Mortality and morbidity in patients receiving encainide, flecainide or placebo: the Cardiac Arrhythmia Suppression Trial (CAST). *New England Journal of Medicine*, **324:** 781–788.

EMIP (1993) Pre-hospital thrombolytic therapy in patients with suspected acute myocardial infarction. *New England Journal of Medicine*, **329:** 383–389.

Fath-Ordoubadi F, Beatt K (1997) Glucose–insulin– potassium therapy for treatment of myocardial infarction: an overview of randomised-placebo controlled trials. *Circulation*, **96:** 1074–1077.

Fibrinolytic Therapy Trialists' Collaborative Group (1994) Indications for fibrinolytic therapy in suspected acute myocardial infarction: collaborative overview of early and major morbidity results from all randomised trials of more than 1000 patients. *Lancet*, **343:** 311–322.

Fitzpatrick B, Watt G, Tunstall-Pedoe H (1992) Potential impact of emergency intervention on sudden deaths from coronary heart disease in Glasgow. *British Heart Journal*, **67:** 250–254.

Fletcher AP, Alkjaersig N, Smyrniotis FE et al (1958) The treatment of patients suffering from early myocardial infarction with massive and prolonged streptokinase therapy. *Transcripts of the Association of American Physicians*, **71:** 287–295.

Francis GS (2001) Diabetic cardiomyopathy: fact or fiction? *Heart*, **85:** 247–248.

Freemantle N, Cleland J, Young P et al (1999) Beta-blockade after myocardial infarction: systematic review and meta-regression analysis. *BMJ*, **318:** 1730–1737.

French JK, Williams BF, Hart HH et al (1996) Prospective evaluation of eligibility for thrombolytic therapy in acute myocardial infarction. *BMJ*, **312:** 1637–1641.

Friemark D, Behar S, Matetsky S et al (1998) Time dependent effect of treatment with ASA during thrombolytic therapy in acute myocardial infarction. *Journal of the American College of Cardiology*, **31:** 231A.

Fromm R, Meyer D, Zimmerman J et al (2001) A double-blind, multicentered study comparing the accuracy of diagnostic markers to predict short- and long-term clinical events and their utility in patients presenting with chest pain. *Clinical Cardiology*, **24:** 516–520.

Furberg CD, Herrington DM, Psaty BM (1999) Are drugs within a class interchangeable? *Lancet*, **354:** 1202–1204.

Gallagher E, Lombardi G, Gennis P (1995) Effectiveness of bystander cardiopulmonary resuscitation and survival following out-of-hospital cardiac arrest. *JAMA*, **274:** 1922–1925.

Gandhi MM (1997) Clinical epidemiology of coronary heart disease in the UK. *British Journal of Hospital Medicine*, **58:** 23–27.

Gheorghiade M, Shivkumar K, Schultz L (1993) Prognostic significance of ECG persistent ST depression in patients with their first myocardial infarction in the placebo arm of the Beta-Blocker Heart Attack Trial. *American Heart Journal*, **126:** 271–278.

GISSI Study Group (1987) Long-term effects of intravenous thrombolysis in acute myocardial infarction: final report of the GISSI study. *Lancet*, **ii:** 871–874.

GISSI-3 (1994) Effect of lisinopril and transdermal glyceryl trinitrate singly and together on 6 week mortality and ventricular function after acute myocardial infarction. *Lancet*, **343:** 1115–1122.

Goldberg RJ, Gore JM, Alpert J et al (1988) Incidence and case fatality rates of acute myocardial infarction (1975–1984): the Worcester Heart Attack study. *American Heart Journal*, **115:** 761–767.

Goldman L, Cook EF (1984) The decline in ischaemic heart disease mortality rates. *Annals of Internal Medicine*, **101:** 825–836.

GREAT Study Group (1992) Feasibility, safety and efficacy of domiciliary thrombolysis by general practitioners: the Grampian Regional Early Anistreplase Trial. *BMJ*, **305:** 548–553.

Grijseels EW, Boutne MJ, Lenderink T et al (1995) Pre-hospital thrombolytic therapy with either alteplase or streptokinase. Practical applications, complications and long-term results in 529 patients. *European Heart Journal*, **16:** 1833–1838.

Gurble PA, Serebruany VL, Shustov AR for the GUSTO III Investigators (1998) Effects of reteplase and alteplase on platelet aggregation and major receptor expression during the first 24 hours of acute myocardial infarction treatment. The GUSTO III platelet study. *Journal of the American College of Cardiology*, **31:** 1466–1473.

GUSTO (1993) An international randomised trial comparing 4 strategies for acute myocardial infarction. *New England Journal of Medicine*, **329:** 673–682.

GUSTO Angiographic Investigators (1993) The effects of tPA, streptokinase or both on coronary artery patency, ventricular function and survival after acute myocardial infarction. *New England Journal of Medicine*, **329:** 1615–1622.

Hall AS, Murray GD, Ball SG (1997) Follow up study of patients randomly allocated ramipril or placebo for heart failure after acute MI: AIRE Extension (AIREX) Study. *Lancet*, **345:** 669–685.

Heart Outcomes Prevention Study (HOPE) Investigators (2000) Effects of an angiotensin converting enzyme inhibitor, ramipril, on cardiovascular events in high-risk patients. *New England Journal of Medicine*, **342:** 145–153.

ISIS-2 Collaborative Group (1988) Randomised trial of intravenous streptokinase, oral aspirin, both or neither amongst 17,187 cases of suspected acute myocardial infarction. *Lancet*, **ii:** 349–360.

ISIS-3 (Third International Study of Infarct Survival) Collaborative Group (1992) A randomised comparison of streptokinase vs tissue plasminogen activator vs anistreplase and of aspirin plus heparin vs aspirin alone among 41,299 cases of suspected myocardial infarction. *Lancet*, **339:** 753–770.

ISIS-4 Collaborative Group (1995) A randomised trial assessing early oral captopril, oral mononitrate and intravenous magnesium sulphate in 58,050 patients with suspected acute myocardial infarction. *Lancet*, **345:** 669–685.

Jafri SM, Gheorghiade M, Goldstein S (1992) Oral anti-coagulation for secondary prevention after myocardial infarction with special reference to the Warfarin Re-infarction Study (WARIS). *Progress in Cardiovascular Disease*, **34:** 317–324.

Jowett NI, Thompson DR, Bailey SW (1985) Electrocardiographic monitoring. I. Static monitoring. *Intensive Care Nursing*, **2:** 71–76.

Jowett NI, Stephens JM, Thompson DR et al (1986) Do indwelling cannulae on coronary care need a heparin flush? *Intensive Care Nursing*, **2:** 16–19.

Jowett NI, Thompson DR, Pohl JEF (1989) Temporary transvenous cardiac pacing: 6 years' experience in one coronary care unit. *Postgraduate Medical Journal*, **65:** 211–215.

Julian DG, Chamberlain DA, Pocock SJ for the AFTER study (1996) A comparison of aspirin and anticoagulation following thrombolysis for myocardial infarction: a multi-centre unblinded randomised clinical trial. *BMJ*, **313:** 1429–1431.

Julian DG, Camm AJ, Frangin G et al for the European Myocardial Infarction Amiodarone Trial Investigators (1997) Randomised trial of the effect of amiodarone on mortality in patients with left ventricular dysfunction after recent myocardial infarction: EMIAT. *Lancet*, **349:** 667–674.

Klein HO, Tordjman T, Ninio R et al (1983) The early recognition of right ventricular infarction: diagnostic accuracy of the V_{4R} lead. *Circulation*, **67:** 558–565.

Klootwijk P, Langer A, Meij S et al (1996) Non-invasive prediction of reperfusion and coronary artery patency by continuous ST monitoring in the GUSTO-1 trial. *European Heart Journal*, **17:** 689–698.

Kober L, Torp-Pedersen C, Carlsen JE et al (1995) A clinical trial of the angiotensin converting enzyme inhibitor trandolapril in patients with left ventricular dysfunction after myocardial infarction. Trandolapril Cardiac Evaluation (TRACE) Study Group. *New England Journal of Medicine*, **333:** 1670–1676.

Kostuk W, Barr JW, Simon AL et al (1973) Correlation between the chest film and haemodynamics in acute myocardial infarction. *Circulation*, **48:** 624–632.

Kovlack JD, Gershlick AH (2001) How should we detect and manage failed thrombolysis? *European Heart Journal*, **22:** 450–457.

Krone RJ, Greenberg H, Dwyer EM (1993) Long-term prognostic significance of ST segment depression during acute myocardial infarction. *Journal of the American College of Cardiology*, **22:** 361–367.

Lawson-Matthew PJ, Wilson AT, Woodmansey PA et al (1994) Unsatisfactory management of patients with acute myocardial infarction admitted to general medical wards. *Journal of the Royal College of Physicians of London*, **28:** 49–51.

Lynch M, Gammage MD, Lamb P et al (1993) Acute myocardial infarction in diabetic patients in the thrombolytic era. *Diabetic Medicine*; **11:** 162–165.

McGuire DK, Emanuelsson H, Granger CB et al (2000) Influence of diabetes mellitus on clinical outcomes across the spectrum of acute coronary syndromes: findings from the GUSTO-IIb study. *European Heart Journal*, **21**: 1750–1758.

MacMahon S, Collins R, Peto R et al (1988) Effects of prophylactic lidocaine in suspected myocardial infarction: an overview of results from the randomised controlled trials. *JAMA*, **260**: 1910–1916.

Mahaffey KW, Granger CB, Toth CA et al (1997) Diabetic retinopathy should not be a contraindication to thrombolytic therapy in acute myocardial infarction: review of ocular hemorrhage incidence and location in the GUSTO-1 trial. *Journal of the American College of Cardiology*, **30**: 1606–1610.

Mak KH, Moliterno DJ, Granger CB et al (1997) Influence of diabetes mellitus on clinical outcome in the thrombolytic era of acute myocardial infarction. *Journal of the American College of Cardiology*, **30**: 171–179.

Malmberg K for the DIGAMI Study Group (1997) Prospective randomised study of intensive insulin treatment on long-term survival after acute myocardial infarction in patients with diabetes mellitus. *BMJ*, **314**: 1512–1515.

Maroko PR, Radvany P, Braunwald E (1975) Reduction in infarct size by oxygen inhalation following acute coronary occlusion. *Circulation*, **52**: 360–368.

Maynard SJ, Menown IBA, Adgey AAJ (2000) Troponin T or troponin I as cardiac markers in ischaemic heart disease. *Heart*, **83**: 371–373.

Ng SM, Krishnaswamy P, Morissey R et al (2001) Ninety-minute accelerated critical pathway for chest pain evaluation. *American Journal of Cardiology*, **88**: 611–617.

Norris RM (1998) Fatality outside hospital from acute coronary events in three British health districts 1994–95. *BMJ*, **316**: 1065–1070.

Ohman EM, Califf RM, Topol EJ et al (1990) Consequences of re-occlusion after successful reperfusion therapy in acute myocardial infarction. *Circulation*, **82**: 781–791.

Oldroyd KG (2000) Identifying failure to achieve complete (TIMI-3) reperfusion following thrombolytic treatment: how to do it, when to do it, and why it's worth doing. *Heart*, **84**: 113–115.

Pantridge JF, Adgey AAJ (1969) Pre-hospital coronary care: the mobile coronary care unit. *American Journal of Cardiology*, **24**: 666–673.

Pell ACH, Miller HC, Robertson CE et al (1992) Effect of 'fast-track' admission for acute myocardial infarction on delay to thrombolysis. *BMJ*, **304**: 83–87.

Petersen S, Mockford C, Rayner M (2002) *Coronary Heart Disease Statistics*. London: British Heart Foundation Statistics Database. (www.dphpc.ox.ac.uk/bhfhprg).

Pfeffer MA, Braunwald E, Moyle LA et al (1992) Effect of captopril on mortality and morbidity in patients with left ventricular dysfunction after myocardial infarction: results of the survival and ventricular enlargement trial (SAVE). *New England Journal of Medicine*, **327**: 669–677.

Reffelmann T, Kloner RA (2002) The 'no-flow' phenomenon: basic science and clinical correlates. *Heart*, **87**: 162–168.

Rodrigues EA, Dewhurst NG, Smart LM et al (1986) Diagnosis and prognosis of right ventricular infarction. *British Heart Journal*, **56**: 19–26.

Ross AM, Lundergan CF, Rohrbeck SC et al (1998) Rescue angioplasty after failed thrombolysis: technical and clinical outcomes in a large thrombolysis trial (GUSTO-1). *Journal of the American College of Cardiology*, **31**: 1511–1517.

Ross AM, Molhoek P, Lundergan C et al (2001) Randomised comparison of enoxaparin, a low molecular weight heparin with unfractionated heparin adjunctive to recombinant tissue plasminogen activator thrombolysis and aspirin. Second Trial of Heparin and Aspirin Reperfusion Therapy (HART II). *Circulation*, **104**: 648–658.

Rutherford JD (2001) Diabetes and coronary artery disease – therapy and outcomes. *Coronary Artery Disease*, **12**: 149–152.

Ryan TJ, Anderson JL, Antman EM et al (1996) ACC/AHA guidelines for the management of patients with acute myocardial infarction: executive summary. A report of the American College of Cardiology/American Heart Association Task Force on Practice Guidelines (Committee on Management of Acute Myocardial Infarction). *Circulation*, **94**: 2341–2350.

Shotliff K, Kaushal R, Dove D et al (1998) Withholding thrombolysis in patients with diabetes mellitus and acute myocardial infarction. *Diabetic Medicine*, **15**: 1028–1030.

Sodi-Pallares D, Ponce de Leon J, Bisteni A et al (1969) Potassium, glucose and insulin in acute myocardial infarction. *Lancet*, **1**: 1315–1316.

St John Sutton M (1994) Should ACE inhibitors be used routinely after infarction? Perspectives from the SAVE trial. *British Heart Journal*, **71**: 115–118.

Sutton AG, Campbell PG, Price DJ et al (2000) Failure of thrombolysis by streptokinase: detection with a simple electrocardiographic method. *Heart*, **84**: 113–115.

Squire IB, Lawley W, Fletcher S et al (1999) Humoral and immune responses up to 7.5 years after administration of streptokinase for acute myocardial infarction. *European Heart Journal*, **20**: 1245–1252.

Swedberg K, Held P, Kjekshus J et al (1992) Effects of the early administration of enalapril on mortality in patients with acute MI: results of the Co-operative New Scandinavian Enalapril Survival Study II (Consensus II). *New England Journal of Medicine*, **327**: 678–684.

TEAHAT Study Group (1990) Very early thrombolysis in suspected myocardial infarction. *American Journal of Cardiology*, **65**: 401–407.

Tenerz A, Lonneberg I, Berne C et al (2001) Myocardial infarction and prevalence of diabetes mellitus: is increased casual blood glucose at admission a reliable criterion for the diagnosis of pre-existing diabetes? *European Heart Journal*, **22**: 1102–1110.

Thompson DR, Jowett NI, Folwell AM et al (1989) A trial of povidone–iodine antiseptic solution for the prevention of cannula-related thrombo-phlebitis. *Journal of Intravenous Nursing*, **12**: 99–102.

THRIFT II (Thrombo-embolic Risk Factors) Consensus Group (1998) Risk of and prophylaxis for venous thromboembolism in hospital patients. *Phlebology*, **13**: 87–97.

Topol EJ (2000) Acute myocardial infarction: thrombolysis. *Heart*, **83**: 122–126.

van Belle E, Leblanche JM, Bauters C et al (1998) Coronary angioscopic findings in the infarct-related vessel within 1 month of acute myocardial infarction: natural history and the effect of thrombolysis. *Circulation*, **97**: 26–33.

Vermeer F, Oude Ophuis AJ, van den Berg EJ et al (1999) Prospective randomised comparison between thrombolysis, rescue PTCA and primary PTCA in patients with extensive myocardial infarction admitted to a hospital without PTCA facilities: a safety and feasibility study. *Heart*, **82**: 426–431.

Volmink JA, Newton JN, Hicks NR et al (1998) Coronary events and case fatality rates in an English population: results of the Oxford Myocardial Infarction Incidence study. *Heart*, **80**: 40–44.

Waine C, Hannaford P, Kay C (1993) Early thrombolysis therapy: some issues facing general practitioners. *British Heart Journal*, **70**: 218.

Weaver WD (1995) Time to thrombolytic treatment: factors affecting delay and their influence on outcome. *Journal of the American College of Cardiology*, **25**: 35–95.

Weaver WD, Litwin PE, Martin JS et al (1991) Effect of age on use of thrombolytic therapy and mortality in acute myocardial infarction. The MITI Project Group. *Journal of the American College of Cardiology*, **18**: 657–662.

Weaver WD, Simes J, Betriu A et al (1997) Comparison of primary coronary angioplasty and intravenous thrombolytic therapy for acute myocardial infarction. A quantitative review. *JAMA*, **278**: 2093–2098.

Wilcox RG, Olsson CG, Skene AM et al (1988) Trial of tPA for mortality reduction in acute myocardial infarction (ASSET). *Lancet*, **ii**: 525–530.

Woods KL, Fletcher S, Roffe C et al (1992) Intravenous magnesium sulphate in suspected acute myocardial infarction: results of the second Leicester Intravenous Magnesium Trial (LIMIT-2). *Lancet*, **339**: 1553–1558.

Wu KC, Zerhouni EA, Judd RM et al (1998) Prognostic significance of micro-vascular obstruction by magnetic resonance imaging in patients with acute myocardial infarction. *Circulation*, **97**: 765–772.

8

Management of unstable angina and non-ST elevation myocardial infarction

The majority of patients presenting with an acute coronary syndrome will have either unstable angina (UA) or non-ST elevation myocardial infarction (NSTEMI), conditions that currently account for more than 130 000 admissions to UK hospitals every year. These two conditions can be considered together since their pathogenesis and presentation are similar, although they differ in the severity of the ischaemic insult. In patients with NSTEMI, this has been sufficient to produce detectable myocardial injury. Previously covered by terms such as crescendo angina, pre-infarction angina or acute coronary insufficiency, the term 'unstable coronary syndromes' may be more useful to describe UA/NSTEMI.

The unstable coronary syndromes are high-risk conditions, and admission coronary care is required for urgent intervention to prevent progression to transmural myocardial infarction or any complication associated with severe myocardial ischaemia, such as dysrhythmias, heart failure or death. Without early treatment around 5–10% of these cases progress to myocardial infarction or death within 30 days, and 12.2% of patients within 6 months (Collinson et al, 2000). Even with optimal medical treatment, up to half the patients will experience recurrent ischaemia, and require revascularisation.

The management of patients with unstable angina and NSTEMI remains controversial because of the heterogeneous nature of these

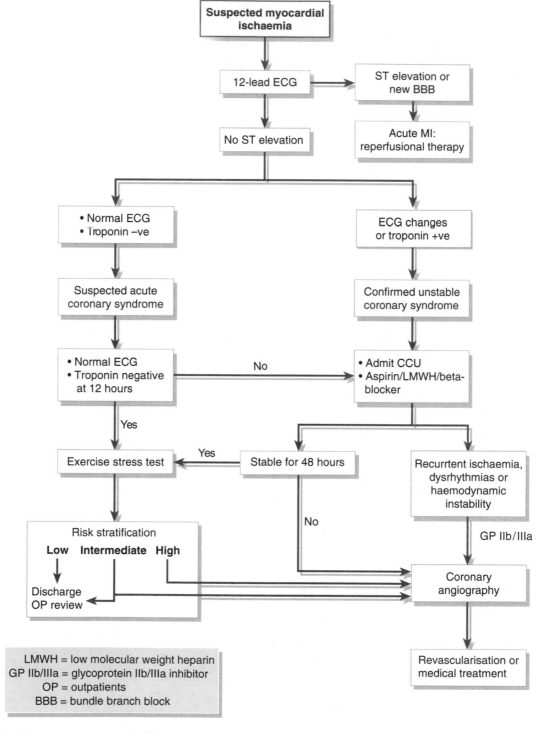

Figure 8.1 Management of patients with suspected acute coronary syndrome without ST segment elevation on the presenting ECG. MI, myocardial infarction; CCU, coronary care unit.

syndromes, and evolving modalities of therapy. An overview of management is shown in Fig. 8.1.

PATHOLOGY

Unstable coronary syndromes are caused by acute or subacute coronary arterial occlusion, precipitated by erosion or fissuring of an atherosclerotic plaque (Davies and Thomas, 1985). There is associated thrombosis, vasoconstriction and micro-embolisation of differing proportion and severity. In the majority of cases, the degree of arterial stenosis would have been unlikely to produce symptoms when the plaque was stable, and not even a target for angioplasty or bypass surgery if previously demonstrated at angiography. The risk of plaque rupture does not depend on the total number or size of the atheromatous plaques in the coronary tree, but on the number of vulnerable plaques (Falk et al, 1995). These have a thin fibrous cap and a large lipid pool, and often do not appear significant at angiography.

The unstable plaque is packed with activated macrophages, suggesting a major role for inflammation as a precipitating event. These macrophages express tissue factor that is strongly prothrombotic, although the associated thrombus does not usually occlude the whole vessel. Angioscopic studies show that the thrombus is white, reflecting a platelet-rich composition, unlike the thrombin-rich red cell mass seen in acute myocardial infarction (Mizuno et al, 1992). This different composition of the thrombus in unstable angina may explain why thrombolysis does not appear to be beneficial.

In cases of stable angina, a fixed stenosis in one or more coronary arteries causes an imbalance between myocardial oxygen supply during exercise. In contrast, myocardial ischaemia in patients with unstable angina is caused by a reduction in coronary flow rather than increased myocardial demand. Erratic coronary perfusion is caused by:

- Intermittent coronary occlusion due to waxing and waning of the thrombus
- Intense vasoconstriction
- Platelet embolisation.

Coronary arterial spasm and platelet embolisation usually occur in association with eccentric type I atheromatous lesions where the plaque is simply eroded, but, in most cases, the vessels show type II plaques undergoing deep fissuring. Following plaque disruption, there is platelet aggregation and activation. Release of vasoactive substances produces coronary arterial spasm with distal micro-embolisation of thrombus, platelets and debris into small myocardial vessels. The consequences of plaque disruption will depend upon many factors, including:

- The size of the artery
- The proximity of the occlusion
- The degree of pre-existing stenosis
- The extent of thrombus formation
- The presence or absence of collateral vessels.

Although the degree of myocardial damage is usually smaller following NSTEMI than in cases of acute transmural infarction, the long-term mortality is higher (Herlitz et al, 2001). This probably relates to persistence of the underlying unstable plaque, which unless modified may lead to another acute coronary syndrome, and possibly re-infarction. Prognosis is particularly bad in those who suffer myocardial infarction with ST depression on the presenting ECG. These patients often have multivessel coronary disease or pre-existing myocardial damage.

DIAGNOSIS

Unstable coronary syndromes may present in many different ways. About half the patients have warning symptoms, the commonest of which is worsening angina, although the significance is sometimes not realised. Indeed, the condition may be missed in patients with no previous history of cardiac disease as both they and their doctors (if consulted) may not consider the diagnosis.

The severity of anginal symptoms has been graded by the Canadian Cardiovascular Society (Table 8.1). Most patients with NSTEMI present following an episode of prolonged anginal pain at rest (over 20 min). In about a fifth of patients,

Table 8.1 Canadian Cardiovascular Society (CCS) grading of angina (Campeau, 1976)

Class	
I	Angina occurring with strenuous, but not with ordinary, activities
II	Slight limitation of ordinary activities, e.g. angina after two flights of stairs
III	Marked limitation of ordinary activities, e.g. angina after one flight of stairs
IV	Angina precipitated by any activity, or at rest

the presentation is with new-onset and severe angina (CCS III or IV). In other cases, there has been recent destabilisation of angina to at least CCS III, or a change in character of the anginal symptoms.

Sometimes the presentation is atypical, particularly in women, young men and those with diabetes. Symptoms may then be described as stabbing chest pain, recent-onset indigestion, epigastric pain, pleuritic chest pain or increasing dyspnoea. In a multicentre chest pain study (Lee et al, 1985), evidence of acute myocardial ischaemia was found in 22% of patients presenting with stabbing or sharp pains, in 13% with pleuritic type pain, and in 7% with tenderness of the chest wall on palpation. Elderly patients may present with unexplained dyspnoea, fatigue, nausea, vomiting or sweating. Such 'angina equivalents' may be difficult to diagnose, particularly if there is no exertional precipitation.

Physical examination may be normal, but may help exclude non-cardiac causes of the chest pain such as aortic dissection, pneumonia or pneumothorax. Anxiety, sweating and a tachycardia are usual. Signs of haemodynamic instability or left ventricular failure indicate poor left ventricular function, and indicate high risk. Cardiogenic shock may develop in up to 5% of patients with NSTEMI, and carries a mortality of over 60%.

ECG CHANGES

An early 12-lead ECG is vital to make the diagnosis, and provide prognostic information. Further recordings may be made during pain or other symptoms, and then compared with tracings taken when symptom-free. This is particu-

larly useful when the patient had a previously abnormal ECG. Between episodes of ischaemic pain, the ECG may be normal, although nonspecific changes are often present. During pain the ECG may show ST elevation, indicating transmural ischaemia, but more usually there is planar or down-sloping ST depression. T waves may be flattened, peaked or inverted. These ECG changes may be transitory, and serial ECGs may show both ST elevation and depression. The appearance of Q waves usually implies infarction, although this may be a transient manifestation of ischaemia (Goldberger, 1979). The changes in the ECG during pain do not always predict subsequent angiographic findings, but widespread ST depression and anterior T wave inversion usually associate with severe coronary disease, and a poorer outcome. Deep symmetrical T waves in the anterior leads often relate to a proximal stenosis in the left anterior descending coronary artery. A normal ECG in pain does not exclude an unstable coronary syndrome.

Each ECG provides a brief view of a dynamic process, and continuous 12-lead ECG monitoring may identify abnormalities not captured on the standard ECG. Two-thirds of all ischaemic episodes in unstable angina are brief and painless, and are thus unlikely to be recorded unless there is continuous multilead electrocardiographic monitoring. Using this technique, 15–30% of patients with unstable angina may be shown to have fleeting ST depression, which associates with high risk (Andersen and Eriksson, 1996).

TROPONIN

Positivity of troponin associates with increased risk for infarction or death, and the higher the value the greater the risk (Ohman et al, 1996). This is independent of other risk factors. Troponin testing therefore realises both diagnosis and prognosis at the same time. In addition, positivity of troponin identifies those who will benefit from treatment with low molecular weight heparin and glycoprotein inhibitors. An initial rise of troponin may be detectable in the blood as early as 3–4 h after the onset of chest pain, and persists for up to 2 weeks because of proteolysis of the contractile apparatus.

RISK ASSESSMENT

Patients who present with an acute coronary syndrome are a heterogeneous group of individuals with varying degrees of severity and extent of coronary atheroma, and differing degrees of acute 'thrombotic' risk. It is important to determine those who are most at risk of myocardial infarction or death. Such evaluation needs to be made early and repeated in the light of clinical, ECG and biochemical evaluation. Patients are already at risk if there is a prior history of coronary heart disease, heart failure, hypertension, or if they are already taking aspirin. Elderly patients, particularly men, are more likely to have established and extensive coronary disease.

The two most important high-risk features are ST segment depression on the presenting ECG and troponin positivity. Additional risk factors include advanced age, pain at rest, haemodynamic instability and serious dysrhythmias. Patients at intermediate risk include those with post-myocardial infarction angina (i.e. within 2 months), patients with recurrent pain after admission, those with diabetes, or patients with established coronary disease, especially if they have had previous bypass surgery. Patients are at intermediate levels of risk if they have one but not all the high-risk features.

Low-risk patients are usually younger, have no rest pain, a normal presentation ECG and a negative troponin. They may declare themselves at higher risk if they become unstable during observation, or have a positive exercise stress test.

TREATMENT

Since the unstable coronary syndromes are essentially caused by non-occlusive thrombus formation on a ruptured and inflamed atherosclerotic plaque, treatment requires deactivation of the platelets, and dissolution of the thrombus with measures to 'calm' the plaque. Additional therapy is needed to relieve the symptoms and effects of myocardial ischaemia. Oxygen therapy is usual, although not all patients will need it. Patients with obvious cyanosis or dyspnoea should be treated with oxygen during initial assessment, and others if arterial saturation falls below 90%.

ANALGESIA

Intravenous diamorphine should be used for those whose pain does not respond to initial sublingual nitrates. Diamorphine has potent analgesic and anxiolytic effects, as well as haemodynamic effects that may be valuable in the unstable coronary syndromes. It produces venodilation, reduces the blood pressure and slows the heart rate by increasing vagal tone. The fall in blood pressure reduces myocardial oxygen demand, although care is required as blood pressure reduction may be profound if there is volume depletion or in the presence of other vasodilators. Doses of 2.5–5 mg may be given every 5–30 min until pain is relieved, and to maintain comfort. Significant respiratory depression is unusual, but may be reversed with naloxone 0.4–2.0 mg intravenously. Diamorphine is not a substitute for anti-ischaemic agents.

ANTI-ISCHAEMIC AGENTS

These are utilised to reduce myocardial oxygen consumption by decreasing the heart rate, depressing contractility or lowering the blood pressure. Some vasodilate the coronary arteries to promote oxygen delivery.

Beta-blockers

Beta-blockers are the mainstay of therapy for unstable angina; they will control pain in about three-quarters of patients, and produce a 13% reduction in the risk of myocardial infarction (Yusuf et al, 1988). Beta-blockers act predominantly at beta-1 receptors and reduce the heart rate, blood pressure, myocardial contractility and hence myocardial oxygen consumption. There is a small theoretical disadvantage of unopposed alpha-adrenergic vasoconstriction precipitating coronary arterial spasm and leading to worsening myocardial ischaemia, but most patients will be treated concurrently with nitrates and calcium antagonists. In the absence of contraindications, beta-blockers should be given as early as possible, preferably by the intravenous route, and then changed to oral therapy. No particular beta-blocker has been shown to be of value in unstable angina, but those without intrinsic sympathomimetic activity should be avoided (e.g. labetalol, acebutolol). Metoprolol, atenolol or propranolol are the usual agents, and the ultra-short-acting beta-blocker esmolol may be used initially if there are concerns over adverse reactions. For metoprolol, the dose is 5 mg intravenously over 2 min, with frequent checks on blood pressure and heart rate. If necessary, the initial dose is followed by further doses after 5 min at 1 mg/min to a total dose of 15 mg, to bring the pulse rate to a target of 50–60 beats/min. Oral metoprolol may be started at the same time at an initial dose of 25 mg qds for 24 h, 50 mg qds for 24 h, and then continued at a dose of 100 mg twice daily. Contraindications to beta-blockers include severe left ventricular failure, asthma or significantly impaired atrioventricular conduction.

Nitrates

Nitrates work predominantly by venodilation, with arteriolar dilatation at higher doses. They thus relieve cardiac preload and afterload, and thereby reduce myocardial oxygen consumption. Subendocardial blood flow is also improved by dilatation of normal, collateral and atherosclerotic coronary arteries. Some of these effects may be offset by an increase in heart rate, so that nitrates should be co-prescribed with a beta-blocker or diltiazem. The intravenous route may be used initially to allow rapid titration. The starting dose of intravenous nitrate should be low (around 2–5 µg/min), and may be increased in increments of 5–10 µg/min every 3–5 min until symptoms are relieved or until the blood pressure is affected. Once a partial blood pressure response is observed, the rate of increase should be slowed. If anginal symptoms continue, it may be neces-

sary to increase to as much as 200 µg/min, although this may be limited by headache and hypotension. The systolic blood pressure should not be allowed to fall below 100 mmHg or by more than 25% of the initial blood pressure, or coronary perfusion pressures will fall which may worsen myocardial ischaemia. If hypotension develops at low doses of nitrate therapy, it may be advisable to insert a Swan–Ganz catheter so that unsuspected hypovolaemia is not missed, and to ensure that the patient has an adequate left ventricular filling pressure. Abrupt cessation of intravenous nitrates may produce rebound ischaemia, and the dose should be weaned rather than stopped abruptly. Tolerance to the effects of nitrates is duration-dependent, and patients who require more than 24 h of intravenous therapy may require periodic increases in the infusion rate to maintain efficacy. Long-acting oral nitrates may be commenced before stopping intravenous nitrates. There is some evidence to suggest that nitrates have an anti-aggregatory action on platelets (Chirkov et al, 1993).

Nicorandil is a potassium channel activator with nitrate-like action, and may be used as an alternative. Tolerance does not occur, and, when given with beta-blockers or calcium channel blockers, nicorandil reduces the frequency of angina, ischaemia and dysrhythmias in patients with unstable angina (Patel et al, 1999).

Calcium channel blockers

The calcium channel blockers work by producing vasodilatation, and some will affect heart rate and atrioventricular conduction. They are used for symptom relief in patients already on beta-blockers and nitrates. They may also be of benefit in those who cannot tolerate beta-blockade, and both verapamil and diltiazem have been shown to be useful agents in reducing ischaemic episodes in patients with unstable angina. Calcium channel blockers have not been shown to reduce infarction or death rates, but diltiazem may be beneficial in non-ST elevation myocardial infarction (Boden et al, 2000). The main groups of calcium blockers are the dihydropyridines (e.g. nifedipine), the phenylalkylamines (e.g. verapamil) and the benzothiazepines (e.g. diltiazem). Short-acting dihydropyridines, such as nifedipine, nicardipine and nisoldipine, should not be used unless the patient is already on a beta-blocker, because they induce a tachycardia. Amlodipine and felodipine appear to be well tolerated if there is left ventricular dysfunction, but verapamil is not.

ANTITHROMBIN THERAPY

Intracoronary thrombus consists of fibrin and platelets, and formation and dissolution may be promoted by inhibition of thrombin, fibrinolytic drugs and antiplatelet agents.

Heparin

Both intravenous unfractionated heparin and subcutaneous low molecular weight heparin (LMWH) are effective in reducing risk when given in combination with aspirin. Subcutaneous LMWH has the advantages of being easier to administer, having a more constant antithrombin effect and not needing routine anticoagulant monitoring. LMWH is of greatest benefit in those with positive troponins, and should be given for at least 2 days and longer in cases of recurrent ischaemia. In high-risk patients, LMWH should be continued until angiography is undertaken, and, if revascularisation is judged not to be feasible, LMWH should be continued for a period of at least 2 weeks (Wallentin et al, 2000).

Aspirin

Unstable angina is associated with enhanced platelet reactivity and increased production of the powerful vasoconstrictor thromboxane A_2, which may aggravate the degree of coronary obstruction. Aspirin is an irreversible inhibitor of platelet cyclo-oxygenase-1 that prevents the formation of thromboxane A_2, and thus reduces platelet aggregation. In the presence of strong thrombogenic stimuli, the antiplatelet effect of aspirin may be overcome.

Aspirin reduces death and progression to myocardial infarction in patients with unstable angina by 36% (Anti-platelet Trialists' Collaboration, 1994). This effect is maintained for up to 2 years. Low-dose treatment (75 mg) is probably sufficient, provided a loading dose of at least 300 mg has been given, although no trial on different doses has been carried out in patients with unstable angina. Aspirin should be given as soon as the diagnosis of an acute coronary syndrome is considered, either dissolved in water or chewed to enhance absorption.

Clopidogrel

Clopidogrel is a platelet adenosine diphosphate inhibitor that helps prevent platelet aggregation, and is often used as an alternative to aspirin (CAPRIE Steering Committee, 1996). The CURE trial (CURE Investigators, 2001) showed that co-prescribing clopidogrel with aspirin in unstable angina significantly reduced the risk of myocardial infarction and recurrent ischaemia. The benefits start early, so all patients presenting with an unstable coronary syndrome should be given aspirin 300 mg and clopidogrel 300 mg immediately. Both drugs should be continued at 75 mg/day for at least 9 months.

Glycoprotein IIb/IIIa receptor blockers

The glycoprotein IIb/IIIa receptor is found in abundance on platelet membrane surfaces. When activated, the receptor attracts fibrinogen, cross-linking platelets and binding them together. Blocking these sites with glycoprotein IIb/IIIa inhibitors will inhibit platelet aggregation by antagonising the formation of these fibrinogen bridges between activated platelets. Glycoprotein IIb/IIIa receptor blockers may result in a reduction of non-fatal myocardial infarction and death in acute coronary syndrome patients by up to 25% compared with conventional treatment of aspirin and heparin alone (Verheugt, 1999; Boersma et al, 2002).

Abciximab is a monoclonal antibody that is used at the time of percutaneous coronary intervention (PCI). *Tirofiban* and *eptifibatide* are small molecules suitable for repeated intravenous administration, but their value in those who are already destined to receive abciximab is unclear. Currently, benefits of the glycoprotein IIa/IIIb receptor blockers are mostly in those undergoing early percutaneous coronary intervention, where using these agents intravenously, in addition to heparin and aspirin, reduces complications in high-risk patients (Knight, 2001). Although we do not yet have evidence of major benefit in those who do not go on to intervention (Simoons, 2001), a recent meta-analysis suggests widening their use to all high-risk patients until a decision is made regarding revascularisation (Boersma et al, 2002). Oral IIb/IIIa inhibitors have not been found to be beneficial.

Thrombolysis

Fibrinolytic therapy is not recommended for acute coronary syndromes without ST segment elevation. The Fibrinolytic Therapy Trialists' overview (Fibrinolytic Therapy Trialists' Collaborative Group, 1994) showed that mortality following thrombolysis in patients with suspected myocardial infarction and ST depression was 15.2%. Mortality in those not treated with thrombolysis was 13.8%.

Oxygen

Supplementary oxygen may be helpful. Oxygen should be given at 2–4 litres/min via nasal prongs until stability, particularly if there is hypotension or heart failure, and should aim to ensure an SaO_2 of over 90%.

LIPID-LOWERING THERAPY

Reduction in plasma lipids has profound effects on plaque morphology. Apart from reducing the size of the lipid pool, macrophage numbers are reduced, and smooth muscle cell numbers and collagen content rise. These plaque-stabilising effects can take up to 18 months, and may explain why the secondary prevention trials do not show separation of survival curves until 1–2 years after starting statin therapy. However, observational studies have suggested improvements in outcome in statin-treated patients compared with untreated patients after acute coronary syndromes (Waters and Hsue, 2001). Improved outcome may then not be related to atherosclerosis regression, but may be due to passivation of the inflamed plaque, reversal of endothelial dysfunction or a decrease in prothrombotic factors (Rossouw, 1995). The Myocardial Ischemia Reduction with Aggressive Cholesterol Lowering (MIRACL) trial demonstrated that intensive cholesterol lowering with atorvastatin administered immediately after hospitalisation for unstable angina or NSTEMI reduced the incidence of recurrent ischaemic events over the next 4 months (Schwartz et al, 2001).

STABILISATION

A *refractory acute coronary syndrome* describes patients with recurrent symptoms or ECG changes despite medical therapy. These are patients with the worst prognosis, particularly if this occurs soon after myocardial infarction, or where there is already a history of coronary heart disease (van Miltenberg-van Zijl et al, 1995). A *stabilised acute coronary syndrome* describes patients with unstable angina or non-ST elevation infarction whose condition has become stable with initial therapy. If, at least 12 h after the onset of symptoms of a suspected acute coronary syndrome the ECG remains unchanged, the symptoms have not recurred and the cardiac enzymes and troponin are negative, the patient can be mobilised. Stress testing is vital to detect patients who have otherwise not declared increased risk. This should take place at least 48 h after stabilisation, but always prior to discharge. Its main value is high negative predictive value. A submaximal test is usual, stopping with the development of ECG changes, chest pain or attainment of 85% of predicted maximal heart rate. Those with positive tests at low work rate (less than 5 METS) should be referred for angiography. If ischaemia appears at high workloads, or the test is terminated at low workloads, but there are no ECG changes, the results are intermediate, and angiography may or may not be needed. Those who cannot exercise may be at high risk, declared by inability to undergo the test. For tests that are interpretable or in those who cannot use the treadmill, perfusion scanning with dipyridamole or adenosine, or stress echocardiography may be used. Stress echocardiography may be the best way of assessing risk in patients with unstable angina (Lin et al, 1998). Left ventricular dysfunction signals high risk. This may be defined clinically, but stress echocardiography may show localised wall motion abnormalities that are not otherwise detectable.

Intra-aortic balloon counter-pulsation

Counter-pulse balloon pumping is occasionally utilised where other medical therapies have failed, particularly if there is haemodynamic instability. These pumps can stabilise most patients with unstable angina in the short term, but they cannot usually be weaned off without sudden deterioration, often associated with cardiogenic shock. As a consequence, once the balloon has been inserted, there is little choice but to proceed to cardiac catheterisation and surgery (either coronary artery bypass grafting or angioplasty).

Coronary angiography

Routine early angiography and revascularisation have not been shown to alter outcome in all cases of unstable coronary syndrome, and limiting this approach in those deemed to be at high risk is appropriate (Braunwald et al, 2000). Angiography with a view to PCI or surgical revascularisation should be performed during initial hospitalisation in those with:

- Recurrent ischaemia (symptomatic or ECG evidence)
- Haemodynamic instability
- Early post-infarction unstable angina
- Major dysrhythmias
- Previous coronary artery bypass graft or recent PCI (less than 6 months)
- Diabetics.

Culprit lesions are usually identified by their appearance, which is typically eccentric with irregular borders. Occasionally, occlusive thrombus is seen. Angiographically significant disease is usually defined as a visually assessed stenosis greater than 70% of the diameter, or over 50% in the left main stem. Between 20% and 25% of patients will be shown to have significant triple-artery or left main stem disease and need bypass surgery. About a quarter of all patients presenting with unstable angina have diabetes, and at angiography will be shown to have more severe coronary disease, with more ulcerated plaques and intracoronary thrombus. As a group, patients with diabetes obtain a better outcome with bypass surgery than with PCI.

Up to a fifth of patients who present with an unstable coronary syndrome will have angiographically normal coronary arteries, or only minor irregularities within the major epicardial vessels. Although the absence of major stenoses does not exclude an acute coronary syndrome, the diagnosis needs to be reviewed. In selected patients, an ergonovine provocation test may detect or exclude important coronary spasm. Variant angina normally presents with chest pain at rest and reversible ST elevation on the ECG. The majority of these have significant coronary disease, but sometimes spasm alone is seen, often at the site of an insignificant coronary arterial plaque.

Revascularisation

If major coronary stenoses are demonstrated at angiography, the choice of revascularisation procedure is not very different from patients without unstable angina. Those found to have left main stem disease, severe proximal left anterior descending coronary artery disease, triple coronary artery disease or ventricular aneurysms are usually considered for early bypass surgery (ACC/AHA, 1999). If possible, bypass surgery should be delayed until medical stabilisation, since instability is associated with a greater risk of peri-operative complications. Those previously referred for and awaiting bypass surgery should be given waiting list priority over patients with stable angina, because they are at increased risk of dying.

In single-vessel disease, PCI of the culprit lesion is the preferred option. If there is important other disease, then a staged procedure may be considered, with angioplasty and stenting of the culprit lesion and subsequent delayed PCI or coronary surgery. This approach may also be used in patients with co-morbidities that preclude surgery.

Management of patients who have had previous bypass surgery

About a fifth of patients presenting with unstable coronary syndromes will have had previous bypass surgery, often only with saphenous vein grafts. These are a high-risk group, because of more extensive native coronary disease and impaired left ventricular function, and outcomes are not as good as for patients who have not had previous surgery. Atherosclerosis may have developed in native vessels, or in the vein grafts. Lesions in these grafts are complex, and more likely to result in occlusion. Re-operation or PCI is usually needed.

LONG-TERM MANAGEMENT

Although the majority of patients settle with conservative management in the first 24 h, this does not mean the plaque has stabilised. The period of plaque healing is not known, and there is potential for rapid progression of the culprit lesion despite medical intervention. Most recurrent cardiac events occur soon after the initial presentation (Theroux and Fuster, 1998), so at-risk patients will need to be identified before discharge from hospital. Many of these will undergo immediate angiography and revascularisation, but the remainder should be reviewed within 1–2 weeks of going home. If angina remains a problem, either during day-to-day activity, or provoked at low workloads on formal exercise stress testing, then early angiography is indicated.

The acute phase of the unstable coronary syndromes is usually about 2 months, during which there is an increased risk of progression to myocardial infarction or death. After this time, risks decline to those of patients with stable angina. A *recurrent acute coronary syndrome* is defined as a return of symptoms, or ischaemic changes on the ECG despite drug therapy within 2 months of a confirmed acute coronary syndrome. Patients who were initially managed medically should undergo coronary angiography.

Active rehabilitation may prepare the patient for returning to normality and gives an opportunity for evaluating long-term care, with aggressive and long-term risk factor modification. Smoking must stop completely, and suitable advice on nicotine replacement therapy is needed. Pravastatin or simvastatin should be continued to reduce the admission total cholesterol by 30% or to under 5 mmol/l, whichever is greater. The blood pressure must be maintained below 140/85 mmHg. The benefit of ACE inhibitors probably goes beyond blood pressure control, and may relate to plaque stabilisation. This is supported clinically by the Heart Outcome Prevention Evaluation (HOPE) trial (HOPE Investigators, 2000) where ramipril reduced cardiovascular deaths and myocardial infarction in at-risk patients. Aspirin should continue indefinitely, and clopidogrel for at least 9 months. Given the evidence of beta-blockade improving prognosis following myocardial infarction, these drugs should be continued indefinitely.

General measures such as counselling and rehabilitation should be undertaken as for those who have had a myocardial infarction. Daily walking is important, and patients will require specific advice on driving and return to work. They should also be instructed on what to do if there are recurrent symptoms on return home; there is a significant risk of recurrent unstable angina, myocardial infarction and death in this group of patients, although full risk stratification should lead to fewer at-risk patients going home.

REFERENCES

ACC/AHA (1999) Guidelines for coronary artery bypass graft surgery: executive summary and recommendations. *Circulation,* **100:** 1464–1480.

Andersen K, Eriksson PMD (1996) Ischaemia detected by continuous on-line vector-cardiographic monitoring predicts unfavorable outcome in patients admitted with probable unstable coronary artery disease. *Coronary Artery Disease,* **7:** 753–760.

Anti-platelet Trialists' Collaboration (1994) Overview I: prevention of death, myocardial infarction and stroke by prolonged anti-platelet therapy in various categories of patients. *BMJ,* **308:** 81–106.

Boden WE, Van Gilst WH, Scheldewaert RG et al (2000) Diltiazem in acute infarction treated with thrombolytic drugs: a randomised placebo-controlled trial. INTERCEPT. *Lancet.* **355:** 1751–1756.

Boersma E, Harrington RA, Moliterno DJ et al (2002) Platelet glycoprotein IIb/IIIa inhibitors in acute coronary syndromes: a meta-analysis of all major randomised clinical trials. *Lancet,* **359:** 189–198.

Braunwald E for the ACC/AHA committee on management of patients with unstable angina (2000) ACC/AHA guidelines for unstable angina and non-ST elevation myocardial infarction. *Journal of the American College of Cardiology,* **36:** 970–1062.

Campeau L (1976) Grading of angina. *Circulation,* **54:** 522–523.

CAPRIE Steering Committee (1996) A randomised double blind trial of clopidogrel versus aspirin in patients at risk of ischaemic events. *Lancet,* **348:** 1329–1339.

Chirkov YY, Naujalis JI, Sage RE et al (1993) Antiplatelet effects of nitroglycerine in healthy subjects and in patients with stable angina pectoris. *Journal of Cardiovascular Pharmacology,* **21:** 384–389.

Collinson J, Flather M, Fox KA et al (2000) Clinical outcomes, risk stratification and practice patterns of unstable angina and myocardial infarction without ST elevation: Prospective Registry of Acute Ischaemic Syndromes in the UK (PRAIS-UK). *European Heart Journal,* **21:** 1450–1457.

CURE Investigators (2001) Effects of clopidogrel in addition to aspirin in patients with acute coronary syndromes without ST-segment elevation. *New England Journal of Medicine,* **345:** 494–502.

Davies MJ, Thomas AC (1985) Plaque fissuring – the cause of acute myocardial infarction, sudden ischaemic death and crescendo angina. *British Heart Journal,* **53:** 363–373.

Falk E, Shah PK, Fuster V (1995) Coronary plaque disruption. *Circulation,* **92:** 657–671.

Fibrinolytic Therapy Trialists' (FTT) Collaborative Group (1994) Indications for fibrinolytic therapy in suspected acute myocardial infarction: collaborative overview of early mortality and major morbidity results from all randomised trials of over 1000 patients. *Lancet,* **343:** 311–322.

Goldberger AL (1979) *Myocardial Infarction: Electrocardiographic Differential Diagnosis.* St Louis: CV Mosby.

Herlitz K, Karlson BW, Sjolin M et al (2001) Ten year mortality in sub-sets of patients with an acute coronary syndrome. *Heart,* **86:** 391–396.

HOPE Investigators (2000) Effects of an angiotensin-converting-enzyme inhibitor, ramipril, on cardiovascular events in high-risk patients: the Heart Outcome Prevention study investigations. *New England Journal of Medicine,* **342:** 145–153.

Knight CJ (2001) National Institute for Clinical Excellence guidance: too NICE to glycoprotein IIb/IIIa inhibitors? *Heart,* **85:** 481–483.

Lee T, Cook F, Erb R (1985) Acute chest pain in the emergency room. *Archives of Internal Medicine,* **145:** 65–69.

Lin SS, Lauer MS, Marwick TH (1998) Risk stratification of patients with medically treated unstable angina using exercise echocardiography. *American Journal of Cardiology,* **82:** 720–724.

Mizuno K, Satomura K, Miyamoto A et al (1992) Angioscopic evaluation of coronary artery thrombi in acute coronary syndromes. *New England Journal of Medicine,* **326:** 287–291.

Ohman EM, Armstrong PW, Christenson RH et al (1996) Cardiac troponin T levels and risk stratification in acute myocardial ischemia. *New England Journal of Medicine,* **335:** 1333–1341.

Patel DJ, Purcell HJ, Fox KM (1999) Cardio-protection by opening of the kATP channel in unstable angina. Is this a clinical manifestation of myocardial preconditioning? Results of a randomised study with nicorandil. *European Heart Journal* **20:** 51–57.

Rossouw JE (1995) Lipid-lowering interventions in angiographic trials. *American Journal of Cardiology* **76:** 86c–92c.

Schwartz GG, Olsson AG, Ezekowitz MD et al for the Myocardial Ischemia Reduction with Aggressive Cholesterol Lowering (MIRACL) Study Investigators (2001) Effects of atorvastatin on early recurrent ischemic events in acute coronary syndromes: the MIRACL study: a randomised controlled trial. *JAMA,* **285:** 1711–1718.

Simoons ML (2001) Effect of glycoprotein IIb/IIIa receptor blocker abciximab on outcome in patients with acute coronary syndromes without coronary revascularisation: the GUSTO IV-ACS randomised trial. *Lancet,* **357:** 1915–1924.

Theroux P, Fuster V (1998) Acute coronary syndromes: unstable angina and non-ST elevation myocardial infarction. *Circulation,* **97:** 1195–1206.

van Miltenberg-van Zijl AJ, Simoons ML, Veerhoek RJ et al (1995) Incidence and follow up of Braunwald subgroups in unstable angina pectoris. *Journal of the American College of Cardiology,* **25:** 1286–1292.

Verheugt FWA (1999) Acute coronary syndromes: drug treatments. *Lancet,* **353** (suppl II): 20–23.

Wallentin L, Lagerqvist B, Husted S et al (2000) Outcome at one year after an invasive compared with a non-invasive strategy in unstable coronary artery disease: the FRISC II invasive randomized trial. *Lancet,* **356:** 9–16.

Waters DD, Hsue PY (2001) What is the role of intensive cholesterol lowering in the treatment of acute coronary syndromes? *American Journal of Cardiology,* **88** (suppl): 7J–16J.

Yusuf S, Wittes J, Friedman L (1988) Overview of results of randomised clinical trials in heart disease, II: unstable angina and heart failure. Primary prevention with aspirin and risk factor modification. *JAMA,* **260:** 2259–2263.

9

Nursing patients with acute coronary syndromes

Nursing management is designed to help the patient overcome various physical and psychological reactions to the myocardial infarction. Therapeutic goals are broadly designed to promote healing of the damaged myocardium, prevent complications (e.g. dysrhythmias, heart failure and shock) and facilitate the patient's rapid return to normal health and life-style (Webster and Thompson, 1992).

Meeting the basic needs of the patient, such as comfort, rest, sleep and elimination, forms an essential component of nursing intervention. Some of these needs will require immediate attention, whereas others will be dealt with in later days. The nurse should be aware of what will be required and should be able to anticipate problems, rather than waiting for them to occur.

Patients are bound to be under a great deal of stress and anxiety, both during their hospital stay and often after discharge. There will be uncertainty about their surroundings, fear of what has happened to them and worry about lack of control over what may occur in the following days. The situation may be exacerbated by lack of information, pain, discomfort or inability to obtain adequate rest. Patients' perceptions of the cardiac care unit have been linked to recovery (Proctor et al, 1996). Nurses need to demonstrate a calm, confident approach and, while needing the knowledge and skills to interpret and act on a wide variety of variables, they should also be sensitive to patient signals such as facial expression and body posture.

The acute illness brings changes for the patient and family in terms of usual patterns of living, which, although hopefully only short-term, may persist after discharge from hospital. Acute myocardial infarction, in particular, poses major threats to the patient, usually because of the suddenness of the illness, and because of the connotations that heart disease carries. Fear of sudden death is the immediate worry, usually followed by a realisation that the patient will have to cope with a chronic disease for many years to come. Apart from these changes in self-image, there are also feelings of loss in terms of status within the family unit, working environment and social circle. The secure knowledge of a regular financial income, the ability to care for the family and continuing full physical fitness are no longer present.

The responses that individual patients make to these threats include emotional crisis, defence mechanisms and coping behaviours. The patient's personal beliefs, attitudes, responsibilities, values and experiences will all influence how he perceives and responds to the acute illness. In the unfamiliar and frightening environment of the coronary care unit, the nurse needs to establish a close rapport with the patient and family in order to be effective in reducing anxiety and fear, promoting the resolution of losses, encouraging adjustment to change and planning together for complete recovery and successful rehabilitation. This will include detailed explanations about the significance of the illness, the nature of coronary heart disease and the goals of treatment, including the part that the coronary care unit plays. The personnel involved in the provision of care will need introducing, and the roles of these people and the surrounding equipment should be fully explained. The encouragement of independence and the fostering of a realistic, but optimistic, outlook are of great importance. Such interventions should involve the nurse in providing care in an individualised and flexible fashion, rather than the traditional rigid task-orientated system. The coronary care unit is an ideal setting for the nurse, patient and family to meet and discuss progress and future management. Care plans should be based upon an assessment completed within the initial hours of admission, so that priorities of care can be established early and modified as the patient improves.

It can thus be seen that nursing intervention involves many challenges in the management of acute myocardial infarction. A considerate and sensitive approach to the patient and family is required to permit full evaluation of present and potential problems, and to establish an overall plan of care, which may overcome them.

Care planning for patients on the cardiac care unit should consider the following:

1. The reduction or control of stressful physical (e.g. temperature and pain) and sensory (e.g. noise and lighting) stimuli is desirable. Specific sources should be identified in the assessment plan.

2. The preservation, where possible, of patients' routines. In coronary care units, patients' eating, toileting and resting habits will be very different, sometimes resulting in disorientation or physical complications.

3. The adherence to life-style changes and drug regimens. The nurse needs to ensure that the patient listens to, understands and retains information, and adheres to advice.

4. Encouragement of the patient and family to participate in care planning with the aim of taking responsibility for their own health.

There are many types of format for recording data, defining problems and outlining goals and intervention strategies. Although different units or wards may have their own care plans, it is desirable to have some degree of standardisation to facilitate the transfer of patients between wards, units and hospitals, if required. The care plan is the major tool for communicating instructions and providing a permanent and legal record. Entries should be written concisely, legibly and systematically, avoiding jargon and abbreviations to minimise ambiguity about care. The care plan should be kept up to date and made flexible to meet the patient's changing needs.

COMMUNICATION

If nursing intervention is to be effective, communication between the nurse, the patient, the family and other personnel involved in care has to be effective. Communication can take many forms – structured or informal, verbal or non-verbal – and tends to be a continuous process in situations where individuals are working within the same environment. Thus, much of nursing management will be directly or indirectly concerned with communication at some level.

There are various reasons why nurse–patient communication is often inadequate in coronary care. These include the short duration of the patient's stay on the unit, the severity of the patient's condition and, often, the nurse's preoccupation with handling technical rather than personal requirements. Staff need to judge the timing and content of their communication with patients (Svedlund et al, 1999). In a review of staff–patient communication in coronary care, Ashworth (1984) sees the aims of communication as being:

- For the patient to perceive the nurse as friendly, helpful, competent and reliable
- For the nurse to recognise the patient's individuality, perceived needs and other needs.

Coronary care patients are often brought suddenly into the unfamiliar environment of hospital. They change from a position of being in control of their lives to one of having to accept the submissive role of a patient. Effective communication can really only be achieved if patients are allowed to retain their individuality. The nurse should work with the patient to effect positive adaptation and coping mechanisms by education and counselling. Liaison with the patient and family is required to ensure that they are aware of the objective of the cardiac unit and understand the various procedures and treatments. A realistic outlook for the future, based on knowledge and understanding, may then be achieved. It is important for communication to be clear and comprehensible, using language familiar to the patient (at whatever level) and avoiding the use of jargon. Simple explanations need to be reiterated, since retention of verbal information is seldom for long. Reassuring patients that survival and recovery are fully anticipated should encourage an atmosphere of optimism.

Cardiac nurses themselves need to be able to demonstrate credibility in their role as communicators. Communication is a two-way process, and there is a need to interact with the patient, adapting the approach to meet changing needs.

Some patients may not possess the necessary skills to be able to communicate successfully. They may be too ill or anxious, they may be physically disabled or have learning difficulties, or they may lack the knowledge and understanding to be able to make realistic decisions regarding their future. This may equally apply to the relatives, who can find the hospital environment imposing. Nurses have an important role to play as advocates of the patient and relatives, basing advice on experience, knowledge of the illness and the individual patient. As well as structured planned communication to convey specific points, there is also day-to-day conversation, interaction and non-verbal communication. Human contact is important in a technical environment such as coronary care. Patients are likely to appreciate knowing that a nurse is near at hand, especially if they are bedridden, when communication is perhaps the only way in which some patients can influence their environment and routine.

In the highly technical and invasive atmosphere of coronary care, there is sometimes a need to stand back and think carefully about what is the best treatment or strategy for the patient. Allowing a critically ill patient to die with peace and dignity is not a failure and may be a better course of action than prolonging life with multiple therapies, which mislead the relatives into thinking there is hope (Thompson, 1995). Discussing such subjects openly in a constructive fashion with medical colleagues, in a detached and unemotional manner, involves a sensitive and professional approach, which is necessary but seldom easy.

Smooth and effective communication between nurses and other personnel is likely to result in better nurse–patient communication. There is a need in cardiac care units to ensure that the medicotechnical aspects do not detract from the physical and emotional requirements of patients.

INFORMATION

In most studies of the self-perceived needs and concerns of post-infarct patients and their families, information needs rank as the highest priority (Moser et al, 1993). Many patients understand little of what has happened to them or how to manage their lives in the aftermath (Calkins et al, 1997). Many require more information than they usually receive in the course of their care (Jaarsma et al 1995; Thompson et al, 1995; Turton, 1998). They need different kinds of information at different times and for different purposes. Some items might be readily understood, whereas others might need to be reiterated, especially when a patient's receptivity is limited by physical debility and emotional distress.

Determining the most important information for patients to know and communicating it effectively are crucial elements to improving the quality of healthcare. Healthcare staff should communicate accurate, relevant and timely information to patients at their own level of understanding. Now that patient turnover is becoming more rapid and hospital stay shorter, nurses have less time for verbal information giving. They are having to become more reliant on written information as a supplement. However, it is vital that such materials are of the highest quality, taking into account issues such as format and presentation as well as content (Walsh and Shaw, 2000).

HEALTH BELIEFS

An important issue in information giving is that of beliefs and misconceptions that patients and relatives may have. Indeed, nurses often have as many, or even more, misconceptions than their patients (Newens et al, 1997). Early, in-hospital counselling, commencing in the cardiac care unit and aimed at correcting misconceptions, dispelling myths and allaying fears has been shown to be effective in improving knowledge and satisfaction and reducing psychological distress in patients and partners (Thompson, 1990). Delivering routine health information by audiotape is a useful adjunct to personally tailored advice. This would allow the information to be delivered early, in a standardised fashion, and repeated whenever necessary at the patient's convenience. Such an approach is appreciated by patients and reduces the number of misconceptions they may have (Lewin et al, 2002).

ASSESSMENT OF PAIN

Pain is a complex and personal experience, and it is usually the nurse who is near at hand when the patient experiences pain and who is responsible for its evaluation and for providing relief. However, pain assessment and management by nurses is often suboptimal (Meurier et al, 1998), but may lend itself to numerical or graphic measurement by using a visual analogue scale or 'pain ruler' (Huskisson, 1974).

The assessment of pain should include the patient's own description of it and observation of his reaction to it. It is not always possible to make this evaluation on admission to coronary care if the patient is critically ill, but later on it will be important to determine whether the pain the patient is still suffering is ischaemic or pericarditic pain, or is just due to anxiety. Each of these will have different specific antidotes, such as aspirin for pericarditis, or diazepam for anxiety, although the disinterested may simply choose to obliterate all possibilities with a large dose of diamorphine.

In addition to the traditional provision of analgesia with drug therapy, there is a wide range of pain-relieving strategies that can be instituted by the nurse:

- Ensuring peace and comfort
- Careful positioning of the patient
- Reassurance
- Protection from stressful situations

- Limitation of unnecessary activity
- Promotion of sleep.

If the patient fully understands the pain and its cause, it may then become less distressing. Coping strategies such as therapeutic touch, relaxation techniques and distraction are useful, as are guided imagery, hypnosis and transcutaneous electric nerve stimulation, which may be used alone or in conjunction with drugs.

COMFORT

The promotion of relaxation and comfort is an essential and fundamental component of nursing. Unfortunately, such skills tend to be overlooked on coronary care units. Careful positioning of the patient, reassurance and the presence of a caring nurse assume a high priority to ensure complete comfort. Careful bed-making, regulation of light, temperature and noise, and the provision of hot milky drinks in the evening may seem mundane and obvious but are often delegated to the most junior nurse as a low priority in the 'high-tech' environment of coronary care. Other comforting strategies such as massage have been shown to be effective in promoting sleep and recovery in critically ill patients (Richards, 1998). The effects of massage and associated therapeutic touch have been shown to reduce anxiety and promote comfort and rest in intensive care units (Cox and Hayes, 1998).

Attached monitoring equipment, or frequent disturbances that occur when routine observations are made, may compound a patient's discomfort. Invasive monitoring devices and intravenous lines often result in the general enforced immobilisation of the patient, which carries with it the attendant risk of pressure sores. Thus, frequent changing of the patient's position in bed and the use of pressure-relieving devices are important in reducing discomfort. Consideration should be given to the siting of intravenous cannulae and the use of nasal cannulae rather than oxygen masks.

Rest has to be both physical and mental and can be achieved by a variety of factors, including:

- Adequate pain relief
- Promotion of relaxation, comfort and sleep
- Ensuring that noise is kept at a low level
- Control of temperature, light and humidity
- Planned rest periods during the day.

A warm, stimulating environment should be encouraged, where patients feel they can relax and chat with fellow patients, staff and relatives. Nursing interventions such as music and relaxation can be comforting and reduce anxiety in patients with myocardial infarction (White, 1999; Biley, 2000).

BEDREST AND ACTIVITY

Bedrest is usual, but recent trends are towards early mobilisation, with slower schedules being reserved for those with complications. Hospitalisation and enforced bedrest can produce their own problems, such as constipation, bone resorption, thromboembolism, pulmonary atelectasis, pressure sores and urinary retention. It is important, therefore, that patients mobilise as soon as possible, particularly the elderly, who fare worse from complications due to enforced rest than they would otherwise do as a result of myocardial infarction alone. Active and passive leg movements should be encouraged, and early chest physiotherapy is advisable, especially in smokers. Rotation of the shoulders is also advisable to prevent 'frozen' shoulders and the shoulder–hand syndrome.

Although the coronary care unit should theoretically be the ideal environment for resting, in practice it rarely is because of the non-stop activity in and around the patients. Amongst its many other benefits, the purpose of rest following myocardial infarction is to decrease the myocardial demand for oxygen and limit myocardial work. Inactivity is a major problem, in that it serves as a source of frustration and boredom. It is therefore important to stress to patients the need for temporary limitation, but to reassure them that bedrest is only temporary and is in their own best interest. Enforced bedrest will only have adverse effects on people who are normally active, by making them perceive themselves as more seriously ill. Relaxation, deep breathing and active and passive leg exercises are useful in reducing boredom and mood changes, as well as the risk of physical complications of bedrest. Such activities will boost patients' morale by making them feel that they are playing an active part in the recovery process.

It is preferable that the patient sits upright in bed rather than lying flat, because the latter requires more myocardial work to pump blood through the excess pool of tissue fluid in the lungs. Thus, patients with uncomplicated infarcts should sit out as early as possible. Some patients may feel reluctant or hesitant to resume activity, whereas others are overzealous.

There is no reason why most patients cannot wash, eat and shave. In fact, it is likely that there is danger of more stress resulting from not being allowed to do such activities than the actual performance of them. Patients may require some assistance from the nurse if they are severely restricted by equipment, such as short monitor cables, intravenous infusions, pacemaker units, etc, or if they are feeling weak or are generally too ill. The nurse should, in any case, offer to assist, as some patients may feel unable to ask. If the patient is bed-bound, the nurse needs to ensure that he has everything needed within easy reach.

EARLY AMBULATION

Only 40 years ago, patients with acute myocardial infarction were kept on strict bedrest for 2 months, all activities being performed by attending nursing staff, with limited mobilisation over the following year. The concern was that early mobilisation would lead to dysrhythmia, heart failure, rupture of the heart or formation of a left ventricular aneurysm. The period of strict rest was based upon pathological studies, which indicated that 6 weeks were required for a firm scar to form from the necrotic myocardium. However, it soon became apparent that this form of therapy led to an increased incidence of thromboembolic disorders, chest infections and musculoskeletal disorders. Alteration in vasomo-

tor reflexes and hypovolaemia also occur with prolonged bedrest, leading to tachycardia, hypotension and unsteadiness on standing. The highly controversial approach to early mobilisation in the early 1960s (Cain et al, 1961) was regarded as reckless and dangerous: uncomplicated infarct patients were allowed out of bed after only 15 days.

The emphasis today is on early mobilisation and discharge, especially for those who have an uncomplicated hospital course. This type of approach minimises physical and psychological disability, and reduces the risk of thromboembolism.

Peri-infarction mortality is higher in patients who have had complications such as prolonged or recurrent chest pain, left ventricular failure, significant dysrhythmia (e.g. ventricular tachycardia or fibrillation), or those with complicating disease, particularly diabetes. Early mobilisation should be delayed in these patients, even when the underlying complication has been corrected. However, most of these potential high-risk cases may be identified in the first 24 h following admission, and provisional selection for early discharge may be made within 48 h.

Nursing should reflect the current pattern of care for coronary patients, which has been characterised by an increase in physical activity soon after infarction and has led to a decrease in imposed invalidism and an earlier discharge from hospital. Patients with an uncomplicated infarct are kept in bed for a maximum of 24–48 h only. Indeed, in some units, patients are encouraged to sit out on the day of admission, providing they are free of pain and significant dysrhythmia. Gradual but early mobilisation should certainly encourage patients to walk around the ward by the end of a few days, and it is important that an individualised approach takes preference over a strict regime.

When the patient resumes activity, it is helpful if the nurse knows the normal activity levels and habits of the patient. This should have been ascertained during the nursing assessment. A plan can then be developed by the nurse and patient to provide a framework as to what level of activity he can realistically be expected to achieve by a specific time. This will need to be a tentative plan, and it is important to stress that only guidelines and not strict regimes can be formulated, because each patient will be different in his abilities.

The stress that various activities have on the body can be assessed by observing heart rate and rhythm, respiratory rate and blood pressure. However, these should be monitored in an informal manner to avoid unduly worrying the patient. Symptoms such as chest pain, shortness of breath, palpitations or faintness are indications to cease activity. The patient should be made aware of this and encouraged to inform the nurse if such symptoms occur.

In uncomplicated cases, patients should be encouraged to climb one or two flights of stairs before they are discharged home. They will need to be advised about what they will be able to do at home, including information on eating, drinking and driving. A realistic appraisal of the prospect of a full recovery and early return to work is essential.

SLEEP

The function of sleep is unknown and there is debate about whether it is concerned with bodily and brain restitution, energy conservation or as an occupier of time (Horne, 1988). Sleep may be roughly divided into two broad stages:

- *Non-REM* (rapid eye movement) or orthodox sleep
- *REM* or paradoxical sleep.

Non-REM sleep is characterised by lowering of the blood pressure, heart and respiratory rates, whereas REM sleep is characterised by the opposite and is strongly correlated with dreaming. Many people experience onset or worsening of an illness during the night. Cardiovascular events often occur with a high frequency during sleep, especially REM sleep. Patients with nocturnal angina are more likely to suffer their attacks during periods of REM sleep, and there is also an increase in the frequency of ventricular ectopic activity. The onset of symptoms of acute myocardial infarction is more frequent in bed, especially just after falling asleep and on waking (Thompson et al, 1991).

It is clear that coronary patients experience marked sleep disturbances in hospital, particularly in specialised units (Broughton and Baron, 1978). Additionally, much of this sleep is desynchronised and, therefore, less effective. The reasons for this poor sleep are many. Sleep may be affected by several factors, including age, noise, temperature, comfort, pain and anxiety (Webster and Thompson, 1986). Patients will be able to sleep better if they are comfortable, free from pain and in a quiet and peaceful environment. The promotion of comfort and relaxation are important, as discussed in the previous section, with control of environmental factors (e.g. reduced noise, regulated room temperature and dimmed lights) needed. Pain relief is, of course, essential. Unnecessary nursing or medical observations or interventions disrupt the continuity and efficiency of patients' sleep, and essential procedures should be organised in a fashion that ensures that patients are only minimally disturbed. With current advanced technology, multichannel monitoring facilities make many routine observations easy to perform without waking the patient.

Nursing assessment should incorporate information about the patient's usual sleeping habits and patterns, such as quality and quantity of normal sleep and the identification of any routines that the patient feels will enhance his ability to sleep. Hot, milky drinks often form part of the night-time ritual and have been shown to improve sleep significantly. The use of a sleep questionnaire, such as the St Mary's Hospital Sleep Questionnaire (Ellis et al, 1981), is a useful adjunct in the assessment of sleeping habits.

DIET

Although diet is not usually considered in the early stages following myocardial infarction, there are many reasons why adjustments may need to be made. In the early hours following admission, nausea and vomiting are common, and there is a higher risk of cardiorespiratory arrest, which may lead to bronchial aspiration of gastric contents. A liquid diet is, therefore, probably best given initially until a normal diet can be instituted. Caffeine should be avoided because of its possible dysrhythmic effect, and salt should be avoided because of its deleterious effect on cardiac failure. In order to assist the healing process, adequate and appropriate nutrition is essential. The nurse should possess some of the knowledge and skills necessary to assess and advise on the nutritional requirements of the patient. Nurses, by the very nature of their close involvement with the patient and family, are ideally placed, yet all too often they seem to ignore their responsibility in this area, prematurely enlisting the help of a dietitian. A careful assessment of the patient's usual eating habits and lifestyle is essential. Many patients will have preconceived ideas obtained from their relatives and the media about good dietary habits. Nurses play a major role in nutrition education and often have to perform the notoriously difficult task of persuading the patient to consider a change in dietary habits. The major difficulty is not in giving the advice to patients and their relatives, but in achieving the appropriate behavioural responses that should be in their own interests.

Many misconceptions regarding diet litter the popular press and even the fringe scientific literature. The problem is compounded by conflicting and unsubstantiated information and advice given by friends, relatives or health professionals, particularly with regard to coronary heart disease.

Other considerations in relation to diet include the following:

1. Patients on coronary care units feel nauseated or not hungry. Nourishing drinks and small snacks at times other than established meal times may be more appreciated.

2. Patients from ethnic groups will require special consideration, and relatives need to be consulted, as they can offer valuable advice and assistance by bringing in meals.

3. Although some patients may require parenteral or nasogastric feeding, these methods should not be undertaken lightly. Not only are they likely to be stressful to the patient, they may also be associated with metabolic disturbance and infection.

4. Fluid restriction may be warranted if the patient is in heart failure. Such patients will require thoughtful mouth care, including mouthwashes and sips of cold or iced water. Confiscating the water jug is not sufficient; the patient should be informed of what is being done and why.

ELIMINATION

Prolonged bedrest or general physical inactivity should be avoided, as this inhibits gastrointestinal motility and leads to constipation. The faeces may, additionally, become hardened because of increased water resorption or use of diuretics. The constipated patient will strain at stool, with excessive isometric work, which leads to vagal stimulation. This is likely to produce bradycardia or heart block and may severely compromise venous return, with dramatic falls in cardiac output. A 'bedpan' vasovagal collapse may result, but staff should be aware that patients with acute pulmonary emboli often call for a bedpan as a terminal event. Similar vasovagal effects may result with the use of a bedpan, upon which most patients seem to strain, whether constipated or not. They are most uncomfortable and stressful contraptions, which probably need banning. Using a bedside commode is easier and more comfortable and places the patient in a more familiar position for defecation (Winslow et al, 1984). In fact, there appears to be little scientific evidence to support the use of a bedpan in preference to the commode. Laxatives may be warranted to prevent excessive straining at stool and may be helped by careful attention to the fluid and fibre content of the diet. The patient needs to be reassured that many patients have altered bowel habit following admission to hospital. This may simply be due to different dietary habits or enforced bedrest, but certain drugs can alter normal elimination habits. For instance, opiates cause constipation and broad-spectrum antibiotics may cause diarrhoea. Additionally, many patients feel extremely embarrassed about using a commode or urinal in the vicinity of others. This in itself may give rise to constipation or retention. They are more likely to feel at ease in a private room or cubicle than in the middle of an open-plan area, even if they do have the benefit of partially closed curtains through which different faces keep appearing. Perhaps more patients should be permitted to use a toilet at an earlier stage.

Careful recording of fluid balance is essential for patients on diuretic therapy. Daily weighing of the patient may be more accurate than a fluid balance chart for assessment in congestive cardiac failure. The patient should be warned of the resulting increase in quantity and frequency of urine. Consideration regarding the timing of diuretic administration should be given so that the patient is minimally disturbed during the night. Bumetanide (Burinex) is probably a shorter-acting loop diuretic than frusemide (Lasix) and will limit the duration of diuresis.

HYGIENE

BATHING AND HYGIENE

Many patients admitted to coronary care have been unprepared for admission because of the sudden onset of symptoms and may feel acutely embarrassed and uncomfortable, particularly if they are sweating, have vomited or are partly naked. Patients are likely to be feeling too unwell in the immediate stages to look after themselves, but, although the nurse will need to assist acutely, she should avoid encouraging the patient to become dependent on her help. The psychological aspects of bathing and hygiene are important. For example, patients feel better after a shower or bath and appreciate simple things such as being offered handwashing facilities after using the commode, without having to ask.

ORAL HYGIENE

Mouth toilet should be offered to all patients, especially those who wear dentures, or are on fluid restriction or have been vomiting. Patients with dentures are often very embarrassed about cleaning them in the presence of others and should be afforded the necessary privacy and facilities.

USE OF THE BATH AND SHOWER

It appears that coronary patients move more slowly and deliberately than normal when bathing in order to conserve energy (Winslow et al, 1985). Patients may prefer to shower if this has been their normal domestic routine, particularly during the later stages of their stay in hospital. However, oxygen consumption of coronary patients is higher in patients who shower than in those who use a bath, and this should be taken into consideration. The isometric activity required by some patients to get out of a bath may result in a steep rise in arterial blood pressure, which increases myocardial work. Hence, before a patient is first bathed, the nurse needs to evaluate any potential difficulties. If the patient is weak, obese or generally likely to have difficulties, bathing is probably contraindicated.

EMOTIONAL DISTURBANCES

Emotional disturbances after myocardial infarction may adversely influence subsequent recovery and health outcome (Thompson and Lewin, 2000). They are extremely common in patients admitted to coronary care. Anxiety is, not surprisingly, very common, especially in women (Kim et al, 2000), and many patients are depressed, agitated or even openly hostile. Many complain of difficulty in concentrating, and nearly half the patients will have difficulty with sleep. If anxiety is unrelieved, depression usually supervenes, and both may persist for long periods of time in many patients (Lane et al, 2002).

The nurse needs to be able to recognise verbal and non-verbal cues to emotional distress and understand the basic mechanisms that the patient is using to cope. Three of the most common acute responses following acute myocardial infarction are fear, dependency and disorientation. These may later be replaced by anxiety and depression.

FEAR

The patient's immediate reaction is usually fear, not only of death, but also of the threat the illness poses to his life-style (Thompson, 1995). This fear can be reduced by an explanation of the purpose of coronary care, the monitoring equipment and the high nurse:patient ratio. Patients need to be warned of and informed about routine observations, investigations and drug administration. Knowing the names of staff and the ease of summoning them increases their security. In general, the unit environment should become more reassuring than frightening to the patient, and later also to his family.

DEPENDENCY

This can be reduced by encouraging the resumption of usual activities as soon as possible in an attempt to minimise the sense of damage and helplessness. Involving the patient in planning his own care helps to increase feelings of self-worth and independence. Involving the partner or other family members is a useful adjunct.

DISORIENTATION

Disorientation, together with social isolation, can be reduced by the provision of a suitable environment, which includes calendars, clocks, radios, televisions, newspapers and windows with a view of the outside world. The additional comforts and provision of items such as personal photographs indicate extra thoughtfulness.

ANXIETY

Anxiety is a normal but complex human phenomenon, which is difficult to define exactly. Mild anxiety is part of normal everyday life, but, in excess, it impairs physical and mental performance. Empirically, anxiety is used to describe an unpleasant emotional state, although it is also used to describe differences in anxiety-proneness as a personal characteristic.

Anxiety is certainly the most common initial response to acute myocardial infarction. Its main source is the prospect of sudden death, and the signs of anxiety are more likely to be noticed during the initial phase of the illness, when recurrent symptoms such as chest pain or shortness of breath develop, or when special procedures such as the insertion of a temporary pacemaker or cardioversion are required. A less obvious symptom that evokes anxiety is the feeling of weakness and complete exhaustion. Patients who have normally been fit and strong, but are now feeling weak as a consequence of an infarct, may experience extreme anxiety and frustration. Anxiety about transfer to the ward and discharge home is likely to be particularly high if the patient is discharged abruptly with little or no warning.

Anxiety can be identified subjectively and objectively. Subjectively, patients will appear tense, apprehensive and restless. They may have a sustained tachycardia, sweat freely and constantly seek reassurance. Care must be taken not to mistake these symptoms for heart failure. Objectively, anxiety can be measured in a variety of ways, including physiological and biochemical indices, such as blood pressure, heart rate and plasma or urinary catecholamine levels. However, in cardiac patients, such methods are more likely to reflect the physical than the psychological state. Questionnaires such as the Hospital Anxiety and Depression Scale (Zigmond and Snaith, 1983) or visual analogue scales may prove more practical and quicker to use.

Once anxiety has been assessed, intervention can be more specifically tailored to the patient's needs. The patient with a mild level of anxiety is usually alert and able to absorb information and solve problems, even though he may be restless and irritable. In contrast, the patient with a very high level of anxiety is often terrified and much too distressed to perceive and communicate normally.

A reduction of anxiety can usually be achieved in the majority of patients by considerate, attentive and competent nurses, who can be a major source of reassurance. Close and consistent nurse–patient contact increases the patient's feelings of security (Thompson, 1990). Relaxation techniques involving progressive muscle relaxation may be effective in minimising undue stress.

DEPRESSION

Depression is common in coronary patients and will often follow anxiety, especially if the latter is untreated. It is reactive rather than endogenous depression and seldom assumes psychotic status. It is an understandable response to myocardial infarction because of the implied loss of health, loss of earning capacity, impairment of physical activity and diminution of general status within family and society. It is important that depression is recognised and dealt with promptly, because it may interfere with the recovery process. Patients who are depressed make the poorest long-term recovery, as measured by their ability to return to work and resume sexual activity. They may experience sadness, disinterest, sleep disturbances and loss of appetite. In the acute phase, depression usually appears on the third to fifth day, when the patient is at an emotional low ebb. Denial is the most common coping mechanism and can often be recognised by statements the patient makes. There may be refusal to acknowledge that he has suffered a heart attack and is becoming depressed as a consequence. Denial is usually a temporary phenomenon and may serve to protect the patient from further psychological deterioration. Gradual acceptance of the illness and active participation in recovery usually follow. However, denial is dangerous to the patient when its presence allows him to engage in some form of behaviour that threatens his welfare, such as trying to take too much exercise too soon. The nurse needs to examine to what extent denial is interfering with the treatment and endangering the patient.

Depression is often accompanied by anxiety. Some patients may be irritable, oversensitive or prone to bouts of tearfulness. Others may experience feelings of hopelessness and helplessness, which results in them forming a generally pessimistic outlook. A full assessment of the patient's situation is required to ascertain whether the depression is part of the normal process of adapting to illness or whether it is related to other events. It may be helpful for the nurse to sit quietly with the patient and attempt to determine the major worries. Many of his fears may be quite realistic, and are likely to prove difficult to resolve or alleviate. Some concerns may be unfounded, and, once these are identified, the nurse can help correct any misconceptions that the patient may hold. Having someone to talk with, or to hold or cry with, may enable the patient to organise his thinking and help him to reassess his future positively. An optimistic but realistic outlook, which conveys hope and gives him energy and enthusiasm, is usually what is required. Probably the best antidote is early mobilisation, to counter the physical and psychological problems associated with immobility. The sooner the patient is back on his feet, the sooner will feelings of self-worth and self-esteem return. The nurse will need to avoid overprotection or the encouragement of dependency.

ANGER AND HOSTILITY

Once patients are aware of the fact that they have had a heart attack (and what this may imply), it is possible that their reaction may be one of anger, hostility or both. There is much emphasis and media coverage today on healthy living, and patients who consider that they have taken special care of their health may feel cheated that this has happened to them. Anger occurs in response to frustration, threat or injury. It may be expressed actively or passively or may be self-directed. Active expressions of anger include sarcasm, criticism, irritability and argument. Passively, it may be expressed through non-compliance, boredom, withdrawal or forgetfulness. Self-directed anger is manifested as depression, self-depreciation, accident proneness and somatic symptoms such as headaches and dizziness.

It is often difficult to remain objective, especially when the patient is critical of the care he is receiving or of the personnel who provide it. The attending medical staff and others may feel powerless or may experience anger themselves. They need to try to help the patient clarify his ideas and feelings, and explain constructive ways of dealing with such feelings. A consistent approach should be adopted towards the patient, and staff should not allow themselves to be played off against each other.

THE REACTION OF THE FAMILY

Hospital is a frightening place for the majority of the general public, especially cardiac intensive care and high-dependency units – their very titles are suggestive of danger and bodily assault. The family will have more time to sit and think about the implications of these titles and may actually fear the coronary care unit more than the patient, who is usually too busy being ill. Relatives often feel that their loved one has been taken away and isolated from them. They frequently feel helpless, frightened and unnecessarily excluded from close involvement with their loved one. All members of the family (especially the partner) may fear that the patient may die, and there may be many recriminations and feeling of guilt if there have been recent family arguments or upsets.

Professional support from nurses and doctors is sadly lacking where the family is concerned and that which they do get is often inadequate or inappropriate (Thompson et al, 1995). Nursing intervention is aimed at assessing and supporting the family's coping mechanisms by providing information and reassurance and involving other appropriate professional help and opinion. Family members may view the patient's illness as a loss; they may feel they have lost the security of having certain needs, especially economic and emotional security, consistently and reliably met. They are, therefore, likely to need information, reassurance and support, but often feel reluctant to seek out staff and indicate their concerns. Many feel that by doing so they may be in the way, stopping important work, or that they may cause friction with the staff, resulting in a deterioration of their relative's care. It is, important, therefore, for the coronary care staff to take the initiative in making and maintaining contact with the family, especially the partner, who is most likely to benefit from involvement in the care of the patient. The partner can also provide a unique service by giving insight into the patient's preferences, dislikes and frame of mind and by generally supporting recovery. Unnecessary distress may be prevented by including the partner in discharge planning and preparing the family for the patient's homecoming (Thompson, 2002). Anticipation of any difficulties will facilitate a smooth and continuous transition from hospital to home.

The reaction of the partner to the illness is likely to be influenced by a number of factors, not least of which will be the general state of the marriage. Partners will need to be warned that they are likely to experience emotional and physical responses to their loved one's illness, such as fatigue, anxiety, depression, difficulty in sleeping, weight loss and sexual difficulties. These are expected stress reactions to the patient's return home. Partners will often feel that, if they show concern, they may be accused of being overprotective, and, if they do not, they may be regarded as callous and unsympathetic.

Once the patient returns home, family members are often afraid to express their true feelings to the patient in case they induce another heart attack. Such cautious suppression of feelings inhibits frank and easy communication within the family and often results in a general atmosphere of tension. Both partners and their families should be invited to follow-up visits to continue education and to provide an opportunity to discuss their problems and receive advice about possible resolution (Thompson, 1990; Johnston et al, 1999). Groups for the partners of post-infarction patients may be beneficial in offering support, providing information and encouraging changes in life-style.

TRANSFER FROM THE CORONARY CARE UNIT

Although transfer to the ward may be interpreted by the patient as evidence of improvement, it may sometimes be viewed as an indication of lack of care or rejection. There is a perception amongst some patients and family members that units such as coronary care are secure, safe and familiar (Coyle, 2001). Anxiety and even fear about transfer are not uncommon, and likely to be compounded if the patient is transferred abruptly or during the night. Such negative reactions can be alleviated by careful preparation and explanation at the time of transfer.

It is important to warn the patient and family that, after transfer, there is usually a marked change in daily routine, with fewer nurses and doctors on hand and possible changes in medication, diet and activity. Most patients assume that they must have virtually recovered, since they no longer have monitoring equipment, cannulae or high nurse:patient ratios. Ward staff may assume

likewise and there is a real danger that the patients will be left alone to 'self-care', in the belief that they require minimal nursing contact. It is vital that, during handover from the unit to the ward, a full explanation of what has happened to the patient, and what is required in terms of care and treatment, is given. A fully documented up-to-date care plan, with a suggested plan of further management and expected outcome, is highly desirable. Ideally, such a handover should involve the patient, who can clarify any points and make a valid contribution.

Preparing patients for transfer from coronary care forms an important part of nursing management and requires more attention than is frequently afforded. There is certainly a need for a systematic evaluation of this process.

REFERENCES

Ashworth PM (1984) Staff–patient communication in coronary care units. *Journal of Advanced Nursing*, **9**: 35–42

Biley FC (2000) The effects on patient well-being of music listening as a nursing intervention: a review of the literature. *Journal of Clinical Nursing*, **9**: 668–677.

Broughton R, Baron R (1978) Sleep patterns in the ICU and on the ward after acute myocardial infarction. *Electroencephalography and Clinical Neurophysiology*, **45**: 348–360.

Cain HD, Frasher WG, Stivelman R (1961) Graded activity program for safe return to self-care after myocardial infarction. *JAMA*, **171**: 111.

Calkins DR, Davis RB, Reiley P et al (1997) Patient–physician communication at hospital discharge and patients' understanding of the postdischarge treatment plan. *Archives of Internal Medicine*, **157**: 1026–1030.

Cox C, Hayes J (1998) Experiences of administering and receiving therapeutic touch in intensive care. *Complementary Therapies in Nursing and Midwifery*, **4**: 128–133.

Coyle MA (2001) Transfer anxiety: preparing to leave intensive care. *Intensive and Critical Care Nursing*, **17**: 138–143.

Ellis BW, Johns MW, Lancaster R et al (1981) The St Mary's Hospital Sleep Questionnaire: a study of reliability. *Sleep*, **4**: 93–97.

Horne JA (1988) *Why We Sleep*. Oxford: Oxford University Press.

Huskisson EC (1974) Measurement of pain. *Lancet*, **ii**: 1127–1131.

Jaarsma T, Kastermans M, Dassen T et al (1995) Problems of cardiac patients in early recovery. *Journal of Advanced Nursing*, **21**: 21–27.

Johnston M, Foulkes J, Johnston DW et al (1999) Impact on patients and partners of inpatient and extended cardiac counseling and rehabilitation: a controlled trial. *Psychosomatic Medicine*, **61**: 225–233.

Kim KA, Moser DK, Garvin BJ et al (2000) Differences between men and women in anxiety early after acute myocardial infarction. *American Journal of Critical Care*, **9**: 245–253.

Lane D, Carroll D, Ring C et al (2002) The prevalence and persistence of depression and anxiety following myocardial infarction. *British Journal of Health Psychology*, **7**: 11–21.

Lewin RJP, Thompson DR, Elton RA (2002) Trial of the effects of an advice and relaxation tape given within the first 24 h of admission to hospital with acute myocardial infarction. *International Journal of Cardiology*, **82**: 107–114.

Meurier CE, Vincent CA, Parmar DG (1998) Perceptions of causes of omissions in the assessment of patients with chest pain. *Journal of Advanced Nursing*, **28**: 1012–1019.

Moser DK, Dracup KA, Marsden C (1993) Needs of recovering cardiac patients and their spouses: compared views. *International Journal of Nursing Studies*, **30**: 105–114.

Newens AJ, McColl E, Lewin R et al (1997) Cardiac misconceptions and knowledge in nurses caring for myocardial infarction patients. *Coronary Health Care*, **1**: 83–89.

Proctor T, Yarcheski A, Oriscello RG (1996) The relationship of hospital process variables to patient outcome post-myocardial infarction. *International Journal of Nursing Studies*, **33:** 121–130

Richards K (1998) Effect of a back massage and relaxation intervention on sleep in critically ill patients. *American Journal of Critical Care*, **7:** 288–299.

Svedlund M, Danileson E, Norberg A (1999) Nurses' narrations about caring for inpatients with acute myocardial infarction. *Intensive and Critical Care Nursing*, **15:** 34–43.

Thompson DR (1990) *Counselling the Coronary Patient and Partner*. London: Scutari Press.

Thompson DR (1995) Fear of death. In: O'Connor S (ed.). *The Cardiac Patient: Nursing Interventions*. London: Mosby. pp. 117–126.

Thompson DR (2002) Involvement of the partner in rehabilitation. In: Jobin J, Maltaais F, Poirier P et al (eds). *Advancing the Frontiers of Cardiopulmonary Rehabilitation*. Champaign, IL: Human Kinetics.

Thompson DR, Lewin RJP (2000) Management of the post- myocardial infarction patient: rehabilitation and cardiac neurosis. *Heart*, **84:** 101–105.

Thompson DR, Sutton TW, Jowett NI et al (1991) Circadian variation in the frequency of onset of chest pain in acute myocardial infarction. *British Heart Journal*, **65:** 177–178.

Thompson DR, Ersser SJ, Webster RA (1995) The experiences of patients and their partners 1 month after a heart attack. *Journal of Advanced Nursing*, **14:** 686–693.

Turton J (1998) Importance of information following myocardial infarction: a study of the self-perceived needs of patients and their spouse/partner compared with the perception of nursing staff. *Journal of Advanced Nursing*, **27:** 770–778.

Walsh D, Shaw DG (2000) The design of written information for cardiac patients: a review of the literature. *Journal of Clinical Nursing*, **9:** 658–667.

Webster RA, Thompson DR (1986) Sleep in hospital. *Journal of Advanced Nursing*, **11:** 447–459.

Webster RA, Thompson DR (1992) *Caring for the Coronary Patient*. Oxford: Butterworth Heinemann.

White JM (1999) Effects of relaxing music on cardiac autonomic balance and anxiety after acute myocardial infarction. *American Journal of Critical Care*, **8:** 220–230.

Winslow EH, Lane LD, Gaffney FA (1984) Oxygen consumption and cardiovascular response in patients and normal adults during in-bed and out-of-bed toileting. *Journal of Cardiac Rehabilitation*, **4:** 348–354.

Winslow EH, Lane LD, Gaffney FA (1985) Oxygen uptake and cardiovascular responses in control adults and acute myocardial infarction patients during bathing. *Nursing Research*, **34:** 164–169.

Zigmond AS, Snaith RP (1983) The Hospital Anxiety Depression Scale. *Acta Psychiatrica Scandinavica*, **67:** 361–370.

10

Complications of acute myocardial infarction and their management

There are numerous complications that may arise as a consequence of acute myocardial infarction. The risk of complications is mostly dependent upon:

- The size of the myocardial infarction
- The cumulative loss of functional myocardium following previous ischaemic damage
- The extent and severity of coronary arterial disease.

Abnormal electrical activity within ischaemic or necrotic cardiac tissue can precipitate disturbances in cardiac rate, rhythm and conduction (the 'dysrhythmias'); the loss of left ventricular myocardium associates with pump malfunction ('heart failure').

Dysrhythmias are the most common complication of myocardial infarction. A classification is shown in Box 10.1. These will need treating if there is deterioration in circulatory function with hypotension, heart failure or syncope, or if the rate is increasing myocardial work such that ischaemia is worsened. Many dysrhythmias can be prevented or abolished by relief of pain and anxiety, correction of hypoxaemia and treatment of heart failure.

Cardiac arrest complicates about 3% of cases that reach hospital and may be recurrent. Circulatory standstill is usually associated with ventricular fibrillation, asystole or pulseless electrical activity, although many other dysrhythmias

---

Box 10.1 A classification of cardiac dysrhythmias

Abnormal impulse formation and ectopic beats

At the sinus node

Sinus arrhythmia
Sinus bradycardia
Sinus tachycardia
Sinus arrest

In the atria

Atrial ectopic beats
Atrial tachycardia
Atrial flutter
Atrial fibrillation
Wandering atrial pacemaker

In the AV node

Nodal ectopic beats
Junctional rhythm
Junctional tachycardia

In the ventricles

Ventricular ectopic beats
Idioventricular rhythm
Ventricular tachycardia
Ventricular fibrillation

Conduction disturbances

In the sinus node

SA block

In the AV node

First-, second- and third-degree AV block

In the bundle of His

Left bundle branch block
Right bundle branch block
Left anterior and posterior hemiblocks

Others

Intra-atrial block
Ventricular pre-excitation
AV dissociation

---

can have serious haemodynamic consequences during the acute phase of myocardial infarction.

Heart failure complicates about one-quarter to one-half of cases of acute myocardial infarction, and is caused by loss of contractility of damaged myocardium. As a result, the ejection fraction falls and there is a concomitant rise in the left ventricular end diastolic pressure. A fall in the arterial blood pressure reduces coronary artery perfusion, and this, with arterial hypoxaemia and acidosis, leads to a further reduction in myocardial performance. The development of heart failure is primarily determined by the extent of myocardial necrosis, although hypoperfusion of the adjacent surviving myocardium may compromise its contractility (myocardial hibernation or stunning).

THE DYSRHYTHMIAS

Disturbances of cardiac rhythm are particularly common in the first 24 h following myocardial infarction. Detection and prompt treatment of these was the primary reason for the creation of coronary care units. Early-phase dysrhythmias are largely a result of micro re-entry, and it is probable that both the size and the location of the infarction play a part in their occurrence. Important contributory factors include electrolyte imbalance, hypoxia, acidosis and free radicals released following reperfusion of ischaemic myocardium. Most patients have enhanced activity of the autonomic nervous system. Parasympathetic (vagal) overactivity is particularly common following inferior and posterior myocardial infarction, marked by sinus bradycardia, heart block or hypotension. Sympathetic overactivity is evident by tachycardia, and transient hypertension may be present in nearly half of all patients, particularly those with anterior infarction, and lowers the threshold for ventricular fibrillation. Most patients will have frequent ectopic beats, 15% will have atrial fibrillation and 20% will have potentially life-threatening dysrhythmias. Slow rhythms affect about a third of patients, particularly those with inferior myocardial infarction, and about 5–10% will have an episode of heart block.

CONSEQUENCES OF CARDIAC DYSRHYTHMIAS

Clinical consequences of cardiac dysrhythmias are extremely variable, but are always more pronounced in patients with chronic heart disease. Although the healthy heart can withstand many abnormal rhythms, the diseased heart cannot, and sustained tachycardias may lead to ischaemic pain, heart failure or circulatory collapse. Any circulatory embarrassment is serious following acute myocardial infarction, since it may compromise perfusion in areas of marginally ischaemic myocardium. If these then become infarcted, the cycle may be repeated.

Tachycardias are particularly serious, since increases in heart rate lead to a reduction in diastolic timing. Ventricular filling is therefore reduced, with a fall in cardiac output. Coronary arterial blood flow also takes place during diastole, and a shortened perfusion time reduces oxygen supply to the myocardium at a time when demand is high.

MANAGEMENT OF ACUTE DYSRHYTHMIAS

The treatment of acute rhythm disturbances usually aims to restore normal sinus rhythm and prevent recurrence of the dysrhythmia. Establishment of sinus rhythm is sometimes not possible (e.g. in atrial fibrillation), and treatment is then designed to slow the ventricular rate and improve cardiac output. Treatment is either electrical or pharmacological. If drugs are used, they are usually given intravenously, since absorption by other routes may be slowed because of a low cardiac output, which impairs tissue perfusion in muscle and the gut. Wherever possible, attention should be directed towards the precipitating cause. Pain, fear, hypoxia, acidosis and electrolyte imbalance should be considered. Restoring and maintaining normal cardiac rhythm will be difficult if these factors remain uncorrected.

THE BRADYCARDIAS

Slow heart rates (bradycardias) occur as a result of sino-atrial (SA) dysfunction, when generation of the impulse at the sinus node is inhibited, or when conduction through the heart is slowed or blocked (heart block). Bradycardia predisposes to cardiac standstill.

SINUS BRADYCARDIA

Sinus bradycardia is defined arbitrarily as a sinus rhythm slower than 60 beats/min. Bradycardia occurs in about 30–40% of patients following acute myocardial infarction and normally indicates parasympathetic overactivity, with release of acetylcholine from autonomic fibres in the atria and atrioventricular (AV) node. Because afferent vagal fibres are more common on the inferior surface of the heart, vagal overactivity and consequent bradycardia often accompany inferior myocardial infarction, particularly in the first hour. Although slowing of the heart is useful in protecting the injured heart, by limiting myocardial work, it may result in hypotension secondary to a reduced cardiac output. Escape rhythms are also more likely to occur, which can predispose to ventricular tachycardia and fibrillation. Sinus bradycardia may sometimes occur following reperfusion of the right coronary artery (Bezold–Jarish reflex).

Sinus bradycardia is usually asymptomatic, but sudden onset of any bradycardia may result in hypotension or syncope. No treatment is required unless there are signs of low cardiac output, when a small dose of atropine (0.3–0.6 mg) is usually sufficient to raise the pulse and restore the blood pressure to normal. Further doses may be given at 2–3-min intervals, up to a total dose of 2.4 mg. Adrenaline (epinephrine) may be used to maintain heart rate, but increases myocardial work, and may precipitate ventricular dysrhythmias. Cardiac pacing should be considered if the sinus rate is poorly tolerated, or there is evidence of ectopic (escape) ventricular activity. This will often control the ectopic rhythm without resort to antidysrhythmic agents. If sinus bradycardia complicates anterior myocardial infarction, external pacing pads should be applied, since sudden complete heart block may follow. Endocardial pacing should be considered (Jowett et al, 1989).

SINO-ATRIAL BLOCK

If the sinus node fails to initiate one or more stimuli, or if there is block of transmission of the impulse into the atria, SA block is said to occur (Fig. 10.1). The atria and ventricles will not be depolarised, and long pauses in the pulse may result.

Block at the sinus node is classified in the same way as block at the AV node, although first-degree SA block cannot be recognised electrically.

Second-degree SA block may occur in one of two forms:

1. The PP interval becomes progressively shorter until a long pause occurs between two beats (sino-atrial Wenckebach). This is very similar in appearance to sinus arrest.
2. Long pauses occur regularly following multiple normal PP cycles. Although this most frequently happens every 3–4 beats and has little effect on the pulse rate, the pulse rate will be halved if it occurs with alternate beats.

Third-degree SA block (sinus arrest) is characterised by cardiac standstill for varying periods of time. Escape beats from the atria, AV node or ventricles then take over pacemaker function. Since the right coronary artery usually supplies the sinus node, SA block is particularly common following inferior myocardial infarction. Drugs may sometimes be implicated.

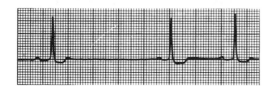

Figure 10.1 ECG: sinoatrial (SA) block.

No treatment is required if the pauses are short and asymptomatic. If drugs are responsible, they should be stopped or the dose reduced. Atropine, adrenaline (epinephrine) and pacing may be required, as for sinus bradycardia.

JUNCTIONAL BRADYCARDIA
(Fig. 10.2)

The AV node is the second major site of impulse formation. If the sinus node fails to initiate an impulse, and no other focus arises in the atria, the AV junction takes over pacemaker function. This most commonly arises following acute myocardial infarction, particularly if the patient is acidotic or hypoxic. AV junctional rhythms are relatively slow (40–60 beats/min), but may speed up by enhanced automaticity to produce either a relative junctional tachycardia (60–100 beats/min), or junctional tachycardia (over 100 beats/min).

If junctional rhythm is present, the nodal pacemaker may stimulate the atria and ventricles at the same time. The stimulus passes normally into the ventricles, producing a normal QRS complex, but there is also retrograde activation of the atria by the same impulse, such that a P wave may appear slightly before, after or buried in the QRS complex, depending upon the velocity of forward (antegrade) and backward (retrograde) conduction. The retrograde spread of the atrial impulse may also be recognised by the shape of the P wave, which is abnormal and usually inverted.

Because the atria and ventricles beat simultaneously, atrial contraction takes place against closed mitral and tricuspid valves. Blood is then pumped backwards into the superior vena cava,

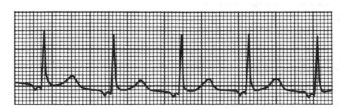

Figure 10.2 ECG: junctional bradycardia. The junctional focus has also activated the atria, as shown by the fact that each ventricular complex is preceded by an inverted P wave.

resulting in giant venous 'v' waves in the venous pulse. Junctional rhythm is usually short-lived, and no treatment is required apart from stopping any medication that may be depressing the sinus node. Atropine may restore sinus rhythm, if necessary.

HEART BLOCK

Heart block exists when conduction from the atria to the ventricles is either slowed down or completely blocked. The conduction disturbance may arise within or just below the AV node (high block), or below the divisions of the bundle of His and involving the bundle branches (low block). Inferior infarction is usually associated with high block, and anterior infarction is associated with low block. Inter-His and multisite block may occur. Heart block usually results in bradycardia, with or without hypotension and reduced cardiac output. Alternatively, ventricular standstill and sudden death may follow.

Heart block develops in approximately 10% of patients with acute myocardial infarction and is associated with an increased risk of in-hospital death that relates more to the extent of myocardial damage than to the conduction problem. This probably explains why temporary cardiac pacing has not been shown to reduce mortality.

ATRIOVENTRICULAR BLOCK

AV heart block may be transient, intermittent or permanent, and the dysfunction has been classified as first-, second- or third-degree AV block.

First-degree heart block (Fig. 10.3)

During first-degree heart block, the impulse passing from the atria to the ventricles is delayed at the AV node (or rarely in the atria or bundle of His), resulting in prolongation of the PR interval on the ECG. The PR interval varies with age, but does not usually exceed 0.2 s. First-degree heart block is asymptomatic, since it produces no change in heart rate, and the abnormality may only be appreciated electrocardiographically. It complicates up to 14% of acute myocardial infarcts and is more common with inferior myocardial infarction. Approximately 40% will progress to higher degrees of AV block.

Any cause of increased vagal tone can delay AV conduction and prolong the PR interval. Drugs, such as digoxin, diltiazem and beta-blockers, which affect the AV node, may also produce first-degree heart block.

Second-degree heart block

This is a partial AV block, which results in some atrial impulses failing to reach the ventricles. It is usually asymptomatic, unless it is associated with a slow ventricular rate. There are two electrocardiographically recognised types of second-degree heart block, although histological and electrophysiological distinction is not quite so clear-cut.

Möbitz type I (Wenkebach) AV block (Fig. 10.4)

About 90% of cases of second-degree heart block are Möbitz type I, where each successive stimulus from the atria finds it more difficult to pass through the AV junction, reflected as a progressive

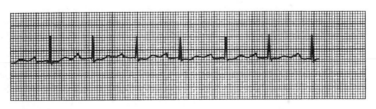

Figure 10.3   ECG: first-degree AV block.

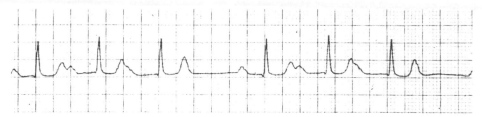

Figure 10.4   ECG: second-degree AV block (Möbitz type I).

prolongation of the PR interval on the ECG. Eventually, the stimulus is completely blocked, and a QRS complex does not follow the atrial P wave. When the next atrial impulse reaches the AV junction, it is able to pass through normally, since conductivity is restored, and the cycle then repeats. The frequency of dropped beats varies, and may be numerous or very few.

This dysrhythmia often complicates inferior myocardial infarction, and may precede complete heart block. It is usually responsive to atropine, but, if complicating anterior myocardial infarction, temporary pacing pads should be applied, with consideration for prophylactic endocardial pacing. Other causes of Möbitz I block include electrolyte imbalance or drugs that suppress AV conduction, such as digoxin and diltiazem. It may also be benign, particularly if observed during sleep, when it is due to high vagal tone.

Möbitz type II AV block (Fig. 10.5)

Here, the AV junction does not respond to every atrial stimulus because of infranodal blockade in the bundle of His or bundle branches, rather than in the AV node. The observed rhythm may be called 2:1 or 4:1 heart block, to denote the ratio of atrial to ventricular beats. The pulse is regular but slow. The QRS complex is often widened, denoting that blockade is at the level of the bundle branches. This is why this form of block is more serious, as bundle branch disease associates with slow ventricular rates, Stokes–Adams attacks and sudden death. Temporary pacemaker prophylaxis is advisable.

Third-degree (complete) heart block (Fig. 10.6)

In complete heart block, atrial impulses are totally blocked, either at or below the AV junction

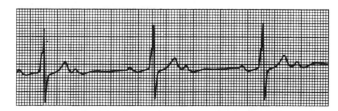

Figure 10.5   ECG: second-degree AV block (Möbitz type II), with 2:1 AV conduction.

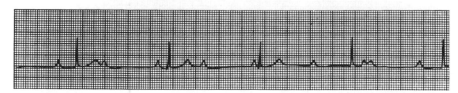

Figure 10.6   ECG: third-degree AV block.

(nodal or infranodal block). An escape rhythm takes over from within the distal AV node, the His–Purkinje system or the ventricles. P waves occur regularly but have no relationship to the slower ventricular QRS complexes. Complete heart block can also occur with atrial fibrillation, in which case there are no P waves, and it can then only be recognised by appreciation of the ectopic ventricular pacemaker, which will be slow and with abnormal QRS morphology. The heart rate and QRS morphology vary in complete heart block, depending upon the origin of the secondary pacemaker. If the block is within the AV node, the QRS complex is usually normal, unless there is co-existent bundle branch block. However, if the block is infranodal, the ectopic pacemaker usually arises in either the left or right bundle, producing widened QRS complexes at a slower rate. In general, the lower down the conducting system that the secondary pacemaker arises, the slower the rate, the wider the complex and the higher the associated mortality. Lower pacemakers are often irregular, with a propensity to interposed ventricular ectopic beats and ventricular standstill.

Following acute inferior infarction, complete heart block usually develops slowly following first- and second-degree heart block. The pacemaker is usually high nodal rate producing a regular and haemodynamically stable rhythm at 40–60 beats/min. However, complete heart block following acute anterior myocardial infarction usually results from massive septal necrosis and infarction of the bundle branches. The onset often occurs without warning, with escape rhythms originating low down in the ventricles. As such, they are slow (fewer than 45 beats/min), irregular, and often precede ventricular standstill. Following inferior myocardial infarction, recovery of AV node function usually occurs within a few hours or days, although it may take up to 3 weeks. However, most patients who develop complete heart block following anterior myocardial infarction usually die within 3 weeks. Insertion of a prophylactic permanent pacemaker does not seem to alter prognosis, and the associated extensive myocardial damage usually causes heart failure and ventricular fib-

rillation. If sinus rhythm does return, bifascicular block often persists, and complete heart block may recur weeks or months later.

Complete heart block may be asymptomatic if there is an efficient ventricular escape rhythm, and not all cases of AV block complicating acute myocardial infarction require pacing (Jowett et al, 1989). Drugs affecting AV conduction, such as digoxin, diltiazem and beta-adrenergic blocking agents, should be stopped.

In patients without myocardial infarction, fibrosis of the AV junction is the most common cause of complete heart block. It is probably a degenerative process and predominantly affects men. Patients often present to coronary care.

TRIFASCICULAR DISEASE

Patients with conduction problems in all three fascicles are said to have *trifascicular disease*. At any one time, one of the three fascicles is capable of intermittent conduction, and this is recognised on the ECG as sinus rhythm with bifascicular block. As a result, trifascicular disease is usually suggested by:

- Left bundle branch block with a prolonged PR interval
- New right bundle branch block and left posterior hemiblock
- New right bundle branch block with left anterior hemiblock and a prolonged PR interval
- Alternating right and left bundle branch block.

Following acute myocardial infarction, patients with evidence of trifascicular disease should be paced temporarily, because progress to complete heart block is very common. Prognosis depends upon the extent of coronary disease and left ventricular function.

Indications for temporary and permanent cardiac pacing are discussed in detail in Ch. 13.

ATRIOVENTRICULAR DISSOCIATION
(Fig. 10.7)

Atrioventricular dissociation (AVD) is a non-specific term used when the atria and ventricles

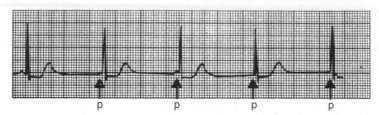

Figure 10.7 ECG: AV dissociation, with atrial and ventricular rates of 49/min and 51/min, respectively. The last two P waves are covered by superimposed QRS waves.

are activated by independent pacemakers, the ventricular rate being the same or slightly faster than the atrial rate. The rhythm is mostly regular and manifests as normal P waves that bear no relation to the QRS complexes. As the atrial rate is slower than the ventricular rate, the PP interval is longer than the RR interval, and the P waves gradually overtake, or 'march through', the QRS complexes. The PR interval diminishes, until the P wave becomes superimposed upon the QRS complex and eventually appears on the other side. When the P wave is far enough beyond the QRS complex, the sinus beat will 'capture' the next QRS complex, resulting in an early PQRST complex. Hence, AVD should always be expected when the PR interval progressively shortens. Occasionally, synchronous discharge of the atria and ventricles will result in the two impulses meeting and interfering with each other's progress, resulting in a wide, abnormal QRS complex (fusion beat). Demonstrating AVD is very important in the diagnosis of ventricular tachycardia.

AVD is usually benign, but is often confused with complete heart block, as both show independent atrial and ventricular activity. However, in AVD, the ventricular rate is usually faster than the atrial rate, and there is no block at the AV junction, unless both the ventricular and atrial impulse stimulate the AV node at the same time, when it will become refractory.

No treatment is required, unless drugs are a contributing cause, in which case they should be withdrawn.

VENTRICULAR STANDSTILL AND ASYSTOLE (Fig. 10.8)

If supraventricular impulses fail to reach the ventricles, or impulse formation ceases, *ventricular standstill* results. If the problem is primarily in the conduction system, atrial P waves may continue to occur, but there will be no ventricular activity unless a ventricular pacemaker takes over. There is no cardiac output, and cardiac arrest results. More often, there is no evidence of either atrial or ventricular electrical activity, and the term *asystole* is used. This form of cardiac arrest has a poor prognosis and has many causes, such as metabolic acidosis, electrolyte imbalance, hypoxia and drugs, and/or acute myocardial infarction. About 25% of in-hospital and 10% of out-of-hospital cardiac arrests are due to asystole. Management is for cardiac arrest, as described in Ch. 11.

Following cardiac arrest, an apparent rhythm called *dying heart rhythm* is sometimes seen. True

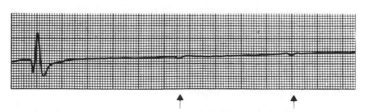

Figure 10.8 ECG: ventricular asystole. The arrows indicate residual atrial complexes.

stimulation of the heart does not occur, and irregular, bizarre complexes continue for several minutes, even though the patient is dead. For this reason, it may be better to turn the monitor off, particularly if relatives are present.

THE TACHYCARDIAS

An increase in pulse rate (tachycardia) is the normal response of the heart to increased physical work, so that cardiac output may be increased. However, abnormal tachycardias are often associated with a diminished cardiac output. At different heart rates, systolic timing remains remarkably constant, so that increases in heart rate occur at the expense of diastolic timing. Since ventricular filling takes place in diastole, ventricular filling time falls as the heart rate increases, and hence cardiac output is diminished. Furthermore, since coronary blood flow takes place during diastole, coronary insufficiency may result, causing ischaemic chest pain. Symptoms provoked by tachycardia may thus include angina, dyspnoea, palpitation or syncope.

MECHANISMS OF TACHYCARDIAS

Most abnormal tachycardias are produced by one of two pathophysiological mechanisms: re-entry and enhanced automaticity.

Re-entry

Re-entry may occur within the atria or the ventricles, or may involve the AV junction. A circuit exists by the presence of two or more conduction pathways with different electrical characteristics. This is best understood by explaining the mechanism in relation to junctional tachycardias.

Junctional tachycardias are caused by the circulation of an impulse between the atria and the ventricles. This may occur if there are two separate connections between the atria and the ventricles, one allowing forward (antegrade) conduction and the other allowing return (retrograde) conduction. In the minority of cases, this is due to an anatomically separate conduction

pathway, such as occurs in the Wolff–Parkinson–White or Lown–Ganong–Levine syndrome (AV re-entry tachycardias). However, most are caused by the establishment of a circuit within or around the AV node itself (AV nodal re-entry tachycardias). These are probably caused by part of the node becoming refractory, allowing a bypass circuit to be established (Fig. 10.9).

The rapid passage of the circulating impulse between the atria and ventricles results in what is sometimes called a *reciprocating tachycardia*.

Enhanced automaticity

Automaticity describes the inherent ability of specialised cardiac tissue to initiate electrical impulses. The cells responsible are known as pacemaker or automatic cells. In the sinus node,

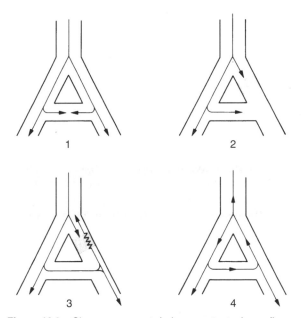

Figure 10.9 Circus movement during re-entry tachycardia. (1) Normal electrical conduction through a common proximal piece of tissue, which splits into two pathways. (2) A unidirectional block develops in one limb of tissue (possibly because of a slowing in the refractory period) and this fails to conduct the impulse. The other pathway conducts normally. (3) The normal conduction wave is carried round to the proximal side of the block, which, if it has recovered functionally, will transmit the impulse in a retrograde direction. (4) If the normal limb of tissue has recovered, it can be stimulated by the returning impulse and a circus movement about the area of conducting tissue is set up, which is self-propagating. This gives rise to a re-entrant dysrhythmia.

these will discharge spontaneously at about 80/min, but elsewhere automatic cells have a slower discharge rate. For example, in the AV node, this may be at about 60/min, and within the ventricles, 30/min. This back-up system of escape rhythms exists to prevent rhythm failure should the sinus node fail to discharge. In this instance, an alternative pacemaker usually takes over, and, although the rate will initially be slow, there is a tendency for the rate of this abnormal pacemaker to speed up because of enhanced automaticity. When an ectopic site takes over pacemaker function, it is denoted by the prefix 'idio' (e.g. idionodal tachycardia and idioventricular tachycardia). Attempting to terminate these dysrhythmias using drugs that suppress re-entry circuits will be ineffective, although the ventricular response may be slowed.

NARROW-COMPLEX TACHYCARDIAS

The main narrow-complex tachycardias are junctional tachycardias, atrial flutter and atrial fibrillation. Other atrial causes of fast or irregular pulses include sinus tachycardia and multiple ectopic beats. With the exception of atrial fibrillation, most narrow-complex tachycardias are regular, and the P wave may or may not be visible. If seen, it is usually different from the sinus rhythm P wave. AV block may occur during the tachycardia. Sometimes it is not possible to determine the exact atrial rhythm during tachycardias unless specialised ECG leads are used.

The term supraventricular tachycardia is still often used, but it is anatomically incorrect because most narrow-complex tachycardias incorporate both ventricular and atrial myocardium within the circuit. The term narrow-complex tachycardia may be useful to describe the ECG appearances, but it should be remembered that some supraventricular tachycardias might appear as broad-complex tachycardias.

Narrow-complex tachycardias may present acutely as a sustained or paroxysmal tachycardia. Treatment is usually directed towards the restoration of sinus rhythm, although, in chronic or unstable rhythms, treatment aims to control the ventricular rate.

Junctional tachycardias

Junctional tachycardia is characterised by the sudden onset of a tachycardia greater than 150 beats/min (Fig. 10.10). In some patients there may be no symptoms, but in the context of acute myocardial infarction there is often ischaemic pain, dyspnoea or syncope.

There are three forms of junctional tachycardia:

- AV nodal re-entry tachycardia (AVNRT)
- AV re-entry tachycardia (AVRT)
- Paroxysmal atrial tachycardia (PAT).

AV nodal re-entry tachycardia

Most junctional tachycardias are due to AV nodal re-entry. AVNRTs originate from a focus within, or immediately adjacent to, the AV node. The re-entry circuit usually comprises a slow antegrade limb and a fast retrograde limb, resulting in almost simultaneous atrial and ventricular activation. The ECG shows rapid normal QRS complexes at a rate of 160–220 beats/min, with the P wave buried in the QRS complex. The onset is usually associated with a premature atrial beat, which, if recorded, is seen to conduct to the ventricles with a prolonged PR interval. Sometimes, the antegrade limb is fast and the retrograde limb is slow (long RP tachycardia). Atrial depolarisation is late, and there are inverted P waves in the inferior leads half way between the QRS complexes. The PR interval is less than the RP interval.

AV re-entry tachycardia

AVRTs are associated with the presence of an accessory AV connection or pathway, such as the bundle of Kent in the Wolff–Parkinson–White syndrome. This diagnosis is often made from the sinus rhythm ECG that characteristically shows a

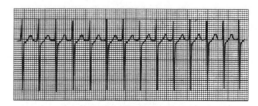

Figure 10.10 ECG: junctional tachycardia.

short PR interval and a delta wave. During the tachycardia, slow antegrade conduction occurs through the AV node, and the fast retrograde pathway is through the extranodal accessory pathway. Atrial and ventricular activation are thus separated in time, which results in the P wave occurring between the QRS complexes. The rate is typically 150–250 beats/min, with a 1:1 AV conduction relationship. The P waves may be difficult to see, but brief interruptions of the tachycardia using carotid sinus massage or adenosine may be very helpful. Because the antegrade conduction is normal, there is no delta wave during the tachycardia.

Accessory pathways are not infrequent. About 2 in 1000 people have the Wolff–Parkinson–White syndrome, although less than 25% have sustained tachycardias, in part because the ability to conduct via the accessory pathway declines with age.

Paroxysmal atrial tachycardia (Fig. 10.11)

The term paroxysmal atrial tachycardia (PAT) was often incorrectly applied to AVNRTs in the past. True PAT is much less common and is caused by the rapid discharge of an atrial pacemaker arising from one or more foci in the atria (usually the interatrial septum) at a rate of 150–250/min. It is thus a true supraventricular tachycardia. An intra-atrial re-entry circuit is usually present, although a few cases of atrial tachycardia may be caused by enhanced automaticity of an atrial focus that speeds up. Second- or third-degree AV block is often present, so the ventricular response is usually not rapid and causes little systemic upset. Although 'PAT with block' is described classically in relation to digitalis toxicity, this is only the case in about 10% of episodes.

The treatment of junctional tachycardias

The urgency of treatment depends upon symptoms. Cardiac output falls as the heart rate rises, due to loss of atrial transport. Ischaemic pain may be produced, and, in the peri-infarction period, ventricular work must be limited to prevent infarct extension. Electrical cardioversion is then the treatment of choice, regardless of prior digitalisation.

Carotid sinus massage may terminate re-entry tachycardias or increase AV block to allow differentiation from atrial flutter (Fig. 10.12). The carotid sinus is located anterior to the sternomastoid muscle, at the upper level of, or just above, the thyroid cartilage. The carotid artery is massaged against the transverse process of the 6th vertebra for 10–20 s by direct pressure. The patient should be lying flat, and only one side should be massaged at a time. Other methods of vagal stimulation are the Valsalva manoeuvre,

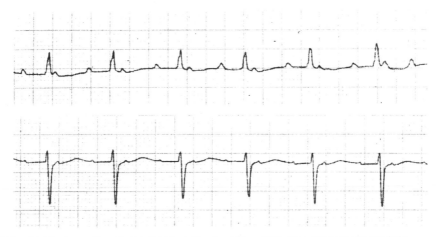

Figure 10.11 ECG: atrial tachycardia with 2:1 AV block (leads aVF and VI). The atrial rate is 175/min.

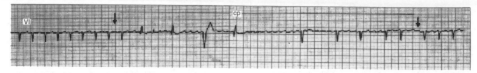

Figure 10.12 ECG: supraventricular tachycardia slowed by pressure on the carotid sinus (cp, carotid pressure). This has increased the block at the AV node, showing that the underlying rhythm is atrial flutter.

splashing cold water on the face, or stimulation of the soft palate, which causes the gag reflex.

Drug treatment is usually very effective, and long-term treatment should be considered for repeated and poorly tolerated attacks. The drug of choice for terminating acute narrow-complex tachycardias is adenosine, particularly if there is left ventricular dysfunction or hypotension. Adenosine is sometimes used in broad-complex tachycardias, if they are thought to be due to an aberrantly conducted supraventricular tachycardia. Intravenous adenosine may induce atrial fibrillation or even asystole, but this is usually short-lived. Flushing or transient chest pain may occur. When given to patients in sinus rhythm, adenosine may be utilised to reveal otherwise latent pre-excitation (e.g. Wolff–Parkinson–White syndrome).

A bolus injection of verapamil (5–10 mg) may be preferable in patients with asthma, as adenosine can cause bronchospasm. Verapamil usually restores sinus rhythm within 2 min. It should never be given for broad-complex tachycardias.

Beta-blockers are often successful, but should be avoided if there is uncontrolled cardiac failure or in patients who have been pre-treated with verapamil. Refractory tachycardias usually respond to amiodarone. Overdrive or underdrive cardiac pacing may be effective in selected cases.

Almost all recurrent regular supraventricular tachycardias can be treated simply with catheter ablation, and this form of treatment should be considered for all recurrent attacks, or where drug control is suboptimal or producing side-effects (Schilling, 2002).

Atrial flutter (Fig. 10.13)

During atrial flutter, there is a re-entry circuit in the right atrium that spreads to the left atrium to cause contraction at a rate of 220–350 beats/min, in response to a macro re-entry circuit within the atrium. The ECG shows flutter (F) waves, which have a saw-tooth appearance in the inferior leads. Leads V1 and V2 often appear to show large, discrete biphasic P waves. The QRST complex may obscure flutter waves if the rate is very fast, and, because atrial activity is concealed, sinus tachycardia of 150 beats/min may be diagnosed. In such cases, F waves may be revealed by carotid sinus massage, which will transiently increase AV blockade and slow the ventricular response. If this is not effective, alternate F waves should be sought; these are often found hidden in the preceding T wave, and this can be confirmed by measuring the interval between the P wave and the following T wave peak. It should be precisely the same as the interval between the T wave peak and the following P wave.

Although the AV node can respond to atrial rates of about 300 beats/min, there is some degree of AV blockade. In the healthy AV node

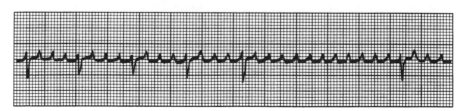

Figure 10.13 ECG: atrial flutter, with varying degrees of AV block.

unaffected by drugs, this results in a ventricular rate of about 150 beats/min (i.e. there is 2:1 block). Higher degrees of AV blockade usually occur in the presence of drugs or when there is damage to the conducting system, although 3:1 conduction is unusual. Although the pulse is usually regular, AV conduction ratios may vary, giving rise to varying RR intervals on the ECG and an irregular pulse. Exercise decreases AV blockade and may lead to a doubling of the pulse rate. As a result, the apparently normal patient with a pulse rate of 75 beats/min may feel faint on exercise when switching from 4:1 block to 2:1 conduction. During 2:1 conduction, ventricular conduction may become aberrant, and the widened QRS complexes may give the appearance of ventricular tachycardia.

Atrial flutter is unstable, and should always be converted to sinus rhythm, unless it has been present for many months or years. Carotid sinus massage will not usually restore sinus rhythm but may reveal the true nature of the atrial dysrhythmia by increasing AV block, allowing F waves to be seen more easily. Verapamil can also be used to increase AV block temporarily, and it produces sinus rhythm in 20% of cases. Otherwise, the treatment of atrial flutter is the same as for atrial fibrillation. Low-energy DC cardioversion is especially useful. Rapid atrial pacing is also effective.

Atrial fibrillation (Fig. 10.14)

Paroxysmal or sustained atrial fibrillation is one of the most common cardiac dysrhythmias. Its incidence increases with age, occurring in about 4% of patients under the age of 59 years and in 16% of patients over the age of 70 years. Atrial fibrillation associated with acute myocardial infarction most often occurs within the first 24 h and is usually transient, but may recur. The incidence of AF complicating acute myocardial infarction ranges from 5% to 18%, but the higher estimates probably include those with pre-existing atrial fibrillation. The dysrhythmia occurs for many different reasons, including left ventricular dysfunction, atrial ischaemia, right ventricular infarction or hypoxia. It thus occurs more often in patients with larger infarcts, those anterior in location, and in patients whose hospital course is complicated by heart failure, complex ventricular arrhythmias, advanced AV block, atrial infarction, or pericarditis. Atrial fibrillation may also occur in patients with inferior myocardial infarction due to involvement of the SA node artery, which provides the major blood supply to the atria. The incidence of atrial fibrillation after acute myocardial infarction has decreased since routine thrombolysis, but it is still indicative of a poor prognosis (Pizzetti et al, 2001).

During atrial fibrillation, a disorganised and continuous series of irregular fibrillation waves (350–600/min), caused by multiple and changing micro re-entry circuits, replaces normal atrial contraction. Myocardial contraction is ineffective for atrial emptying, and the atria remain functionally in diastole. Because the ventricles are incompletely filled by atrial systole prior to ventricular contraction, the presence of atrial fibrillation reduces cardiac output by about 10–20%. Although atrial fibrillation makes the heart less efficient, the most important consequence is that of thromboembolism, especially stroke. The incidence of peripheral embolisation is particularly high in patients with paroxysmal atrial fibrillation, atrial infarction or previous rheumatic heart valve disease.

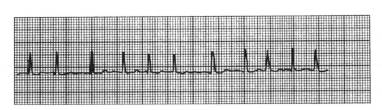

Figure 10.14   ECG: atrial fibrillation.

The ECG in atrial fibrillation shows the replacement of P waves by small irregular undulations of the baseline ('f' waves), which represent the only evidence of atrial activity. These are not usually visible in all leads, and, at fast heart rates, the ventricular response becomes more regular and 'f' waves are not visible. Differentiation from a nodal tachycardia may then be difficult, and often it is only a slight irregularity in the ventricular rate that allows the correct diagnosis to be made. Sometimes, the 'f' waves are very coarse and may be mistaken for normal P waves or flutter (F) waves. If the atrial 'f' waves have a rate of more than 350/min, atrial fibrillation is more likely, particularly if the ventricular response is totally irregular. The ventricular response in the untreated patient is usually at a rate of about 100–180 beats/min, and the QRS is normal, except when the rate is so fast that aberrant conduction occurs.

Because atrial fibrillation complicating myocardial infarction is often transient, it may be enough to control the ventricular rate with a small dose of beta-blocker, if required. Digoxin should be avoided, because it is poor at controlling the ventricular rate following myocardial infarction, does not encourage a return to sinus rhythm and may worsen acute ischaemia due to its positive inotropic action, which in turn may lead to ventricular dysrhythmias. Intravenous amiodarone rapidly slows the ventricular rate, and will convert 75% of patients back to sinus rhythm within 4 h.

In patients with atrial fibrillation of more than 1–2 days' duration, the risks of embolisation following cardioversion (either electrically or pharmacologically) are 3–5%. Prior anticoagulation is therefore advisable.

If atrial fibrillation is producing haemodynamic deterioration, intravenous amiodarone or DC cardioversion should be considered. The energy required to cardiovert atrial fibrillation is very variable, and most would start at 360 J.

SINUS TACHYCARDIA

Sinus tachycardia is arbitrarily defined as a sinus rhythm greater than 100 beats/min and commonly ranges between 100 and 150 beats/min. The P waves are normal and have a 1:1 relationship with the QRS complexes. The PR and QT intervals decrease as the heart rate increases, such that, during tachycardia, the P wave tends to merge with the preceding T wave. It may then be difficult to ascertain whether the rhythm is arising from the sinus node or elsewhere, but there may be clues. During sinus tachycardia, the heart rate is usually less than 140 beats/min at rest and varies with respiration (sinus arrhythmia). The tachycardia does not start or finish abruptly. 'Sinus' rates of 150 beats/min are, on closer inspection, usually due to atrial flutter with 2:1 block.

A sinus tachycardia is found in one-third of patients with acute myocardial infarction and represents an attempt to maintain cardiac output in the face of reduced stroke volume. The tachycardia may be worsened by fear, anxiety or pain. A sinus tachycardia may be a sign of impending left ventricular failure. Incipient heart failure is more likely in the presence of tachypnoea, a wide pulse pressure and a loud first heart sound.

Adequate analgesia will often settle a sinus tachycardia following myocardial infarction, and also helps with associated anxiety. The use of intravenous beta-blockade has been shown to improve prognosis in patients with acute myocardial infarction by limiting heart rate, myocardial work and limiting infarct size (Freemantle et al, 2001). The mortality of patients with sinus tachycardia is higher than for those with sinus bradycardia, and death is usually due to left ventricular failure. Beta-blocking agents should, therefore be given in small and frequent doses to reduce the pulse rate to about 60 beats/min. Both atenolol and metoprolol have been utilised following acute myocardial infarction. The ultra-short-acting beta-blocker esmolol is safe and effective if there is any doubt about cardiac decompensation.

ATRIAL ECTOPIC BEATS (Fig. 10.15)

Atrial extrasystoles are very common in both health and disease, and occur when an atrial focus discharges before the sinus pacemaker.

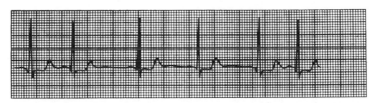

Figure 10.15   ECG: atrial ectopic beats. Note that the ectopic P waves are slightly different from those of SA origin.

Atrial ectopic beats are seen on the ECG as premature, often abnormally shaped, P waves, usually followed by normal QRS complexes. The further the ectopic focus is from the sinus node, the greater the abnormality in shape of the P wave and the shorter the PR interval. An incomplete compensatory pause follows the ectopic beat, because the premature impulse depolarises the SA node, which must recover before it is able to initiate another sinus beat. The PP interval between three consecutive P waves (i.e. two complete PQRST complexes) is, therefore, only slightly longer than the interval between two normal PQRST complexes. Complete compensatory pauses are a feature of ventricular ectopic beats.

Conduction of atrial impulses to the ventricles depends upon the recovery status of the AV node. If the atrial ectopic beat arises near the AV node (seen as an abnormal P wave and short PR interval), the AV node may be refractory. The impulse is therefore blocked, and no QRS follows. If the AV node is partially refractory, a prolonged PR interval is seen, because conduction of the ectopic beat is delayed. Other parts of the conducting system below the AV node may also be refractory, even when the AV node is able to convey the supraventricular impulse, and an aberrantly conducted impulse is then seen on the ECG.

Atrial ectopics are very commonly seen following acute myocardial infarction, often indicating sympathetic overactivity, hypoxia or anxiety. They are usually asymptomatic and cause no haemodynamic upset. With relief of pain, sedation and beta-blockade, they usually disappear, but, if they reflect progressive atrial dilatation, treatment of heart failure is necessary.

Atrial ectopics often precede reciprocating tachycardias by initiation of a re-entry circuit.

Aberrant conduction is the term applied when a widened and abnormal QRS complex is seen following a supraventricular impulse. It is the result of the unequal recovery periods of the right and left bundle branches. If a supraventricular stimulus is conducted to the bundles before both have recovered, bundle branch block will occur. This is usually of the right bundle branch block pattern, since the right bundle has a longer refractory period than the left bundle. Differentiating ventricular ectopic beats from aberrantly conducted supraventricular beats may be difficult. With aberrantly conducted beats, P waves may be seen, and the QRS is usually of the right bundle branch block pattern. In the chest lead V1, the R' wave is larger than the secondary R wave (i.e. the right 'rabbit's ear' is longer). In contrast, ventricular ectopics usually show monophasic or biphasic QRS patterns in chest lead V1, and the left 'rabbit's ear' is larger. P waves are not seen, and the ectopic beat is followed by a full, rather than an incomplete, compensatory pause.

IDIONODAL TACHYCARDIA
(Fig. 10.16)

The normal discharge rate from the AV node is about 50–60 beats/min. If there is suppression of sinus or atrial pacemaker function, the AV node may take over as the pacemaker. Because of enhanced automaticity, the rate may increase gradually to 70–100 beats/min. The sinus node often continues to discharge at a slower rate, and there is a propensity to AV dissociation. Idionodal rhythm arises as a consequence of

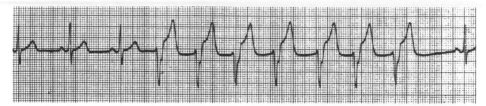

Figure 10.16 ECG: accelerated idioventricular rhythm.

sinus node depression following myocardial infarction, or secondary to drugs.

VENTRICULAR DYSRHYTHMIAS

Ventricular dysrhythmias include ventricular ectopics, ventricular tachycardia, ventricular flutter and ventricular fibrillation. The detection and prompt treatment of serious ventricular dysrhythmias was the primary reason for the creation of coronary care units.

COMMON FACTORS PREDISPOSING TO VENTRICULAR DYSRHYTHMIAS

Myocardial ischaemia

Myocardial ischaemia may result from occlusive or non-occlusive changes in the coronary vasculature that impair the blood supply to the myocardium. Ischaemia predisposes to cardiac dysrhythmias, regardless of whether or not myocardial necrosis takes place. Normal electrical conduction pathways may alter with ischaemia, providing a focus for dysrhythmias. Myocardial irritability following acute myocardial infarction is, of course, the major cause of ventricular dysrhythmia. Necrotic myocardial tissue provides a focus for this ectopic activity, and myocardial hypoxia associated with exaggerated catecholamine release compounds the situation.

Electrolyte and acid–base imbalance

Hypokalaemia is probably the most common electrolyte disturbance seen on the coronary care unit. It is often associated with prior diuretic therapy, although the infarction itself may produce a transient fall in serum potassium. Hypokalaemia may be a marker for the severity of the infarct, reflecting a catecholamine-induced shift of potassium into cells.

Hypokalaemia can lead to complex ventricular ectopic beats, ventricular tachycardia and ventricular fibrillation. The risk of ventricular fibrillation is approximately 10-fold in patients with a serum potassium of less than 3 mmol/l following acute myocardial infarction, compared to those whose potassium level is greater than 4 mmol/l (Campbell et al, 1987). Potassium replacement depends upon the initial serum level and the urgency of the situation. The maximum safe intravenous infusion rate of potassium chloride is about 30 mmol/h. Potassium canrenoate can be given faster than other potassium salts (400 mg intravenously over 5 min) in urgent situations.

Hyperkalaemia may be found in those on angiotensin-converting enzyme (ACE) inhibitors, in renal failure or because of acidaemia following cardiac arrest. The QRS widens, indicating an intraventricular conduction block. If untreated, the QRS duration continues to increase, and ventricular fibrillation ensues. Intravenous calcium gluconate (10 ml of a 10% solution given over 3 min) will protect the heart from asystolic arrest, and glucose and insulin may then be used to control the serum potassium level.

The effect of drugs

Many drugs, both cardiovascular and non-cardiovascular, may predispose the patient to cardiac dysrhythmias. Furthermore, many drugs prescribed as antidysrhythmic agents may sometimes produce serious dysrhythmias (proarrhythmic effect). Torsade de pointes may be precipitated by drugs that affect the QT interval such as disopyramide and flecainide. It is likely that severe left ventricular dysfunction predisposes to this dysrhythmia, which is often selfterminating but may progress to ventricular fibrillation.

VENTRICULAR ECTOPICS
(Fig. 10.17)

Ventricular extrasystoles occur when an ectopic ventricular focus discharges prematurely anywhere within the His–Purkinje system or the ventricles. They can occur at any time in diastole. The QRS complex is premature, widened to over 0.12 s, slurred and usually notched. There is no preceding P wave, and the following T wave usually points in the opposite direction.

Although infrequent ventricular ectopics do not adversely affect cardiac output, attention has previously been focused on them as 'warning dysrhythmias' (Lown et al, 1967). Ventricular ectopic beats that are frequent, multifocal, occurring in salvoes or showing the R-on-T phenomenon (ventricular ectopics occurring on the apex of the preceding T wave) are termed 'complex', and considered to be precursors of cardiac arrest. However, these warning dysrhythmias only occur in about half of patients who develop ventricular fibrillation.

Treatment of ventricular ectopic beats

Although no antidysrhythmic drug has yet been shown to decrease mortality when used to suppress ventricular ectopics (apart from betablockers), drug therapy should be considered for ventricular ectopics that produce haemodynamic disturbances or repetitive short episodes of ventricular tachycardia and perhaps R-on-T ectopics. Lidocaine (lignocaine) is probably the most frequently, and most controversially, used prophylactic agent. Lidocaine (lignocaine) may be of value in preventing recurrent ventricular fibrillation, following cardiac arrest, although the trend these days is to give smaller doses for shorter times (<12 h). Side-effects are then reduced, without an apparent increase in further episodes of ventricular fibrillation. Care is needed in the elderly and in those with hypotension or conduction defects.

Serious ventricular dysrhythmias can occur after patients leave hospital. Early exercise stress tests, 24-h ECG monitoring or electrophysiological testing may be helpful in identifying patients at risk (see Ch. 15). Patients with ventricular aneurysms may benefit from surgery, as may those with chronic recurrent ventricular tachycardia. Scarred or ischaemic areas of the myocardium may act as a focus for dysrhythmias, and coronary artery bypass grafting, with or without removal of an irritable focus, may be of benefit. Resistant, life-threatening dysrhythmias may be an indication for implantation of a cardioverter defibrillator.

PARASYSTOLE (Fig. 10.18)

Parasystole is a relatively uncommon dysrhythmia, but is often seen following myocardial infarction, particularly in patients taking digoxin.

It is a dual rhythm, in which two pacemakers concurrently and independently govern the

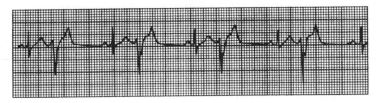

Figure 10.17   ECG: ventricular ectopic beats (ventricular bigeminy).

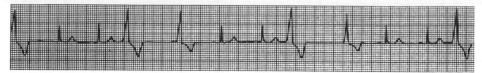

Figure 10.18 ECG: parasystole.

rhythm of the heart. During parasystole, an ectopic ventricular focus discharges regularly and competes with another focus, which may be in either the atria or the ventricles. The competition is usually with normal sinus rhythm, the ventricular rhythm mostly being at a slightly faster rate. The interval between successive ventricular ectopic beats is the same or a multiple of that interval, and, since this parasystolic focus is independent of the regular heart rhythm, there is no fixed relationship between the two rhythms, and the coupling interval (i.e. the interval between the ectopic beat and the sinus beat) varies.

It might be expected that the dominant pacemaker would take over cardiac rhythm and suppress the ectopic focus. However, during parasystole, the ectopic focus is protected by 'entrance block', a unidirectional block in the vicinity of the ectopic focus. Outward conduction from the ectopic focus is normal and forms the secondary pacemaker. Two pacemakers therefore exist, each discharging at its own independent rate and depolarising the myocardium if it is in a responsive state. If the two pacemakers discharge simultaneously, each activates the adjacent myocardium, and a 'fusion beat' will arise as the two discharge waterfronts collide. A QRS complex intermediate in appearance between a normal sinus beat and a ventricular ectopic results. No treatment is required, and parasystole normally resolves spontaneously.

VENTRICULAR TACHYCARDIA

Ventricular tachycardia (VT) is a life-threatening re-entry dysrhythmia, and is usually defined as a succession of four or more beats arising from one or more foci in the ventricles at a rate of over 100 beats/min. Several definitions have been used

for VT in the setting of acute myocardial infarction, but it is commonly referred to as non-sustained VT (lasting less than 30 s), or sustained VT (lasting more than 30 s, and/or causes earlier haemodynamic compromise requiring immediate intervention). The majority of post-infarction VT occurs within the first 48 h following the infarct, and seldom recurs. Short bursts of up to 5 beats of non-sustained VT are particularly common within the first 24 h, but this does not require specific therapy. It does not reflect infarct size or prognosis, and long-term prophylaxis is not indicated.

In contrast, late sustained or monomorphic VT at rates of less than 170 beats/min deserves careful evaluation, including consideration of electrophysiological studies. Recurrence is likely in the post-infarction period, days, weeks or even months later. Late VT is usually related to re-entry associated with scar tissue at the interface between infarcted and normal myocardium, and associates with larger infarcts.

During VT, the ECG will show widened QRS complexes to over 0.16 s, which are regular, at a rate of 100–250 beats/min. The atria continue to beat independently from the ventricles, and dissociated P waves may be seen (AV dissociation). The atrial rate is usually slower than the ventricular rate, as it originates at the sinus node. However, there may be co-existent atrial tachycardia, junctional rhythm or atrial fibrillation. Occasionally, ventricular beats may pass back through the AV node to stimulate the atria, and inverted P waves then appear after the QRS complex, or concealed in the terminal part of the QRS complex. Fusion and capture beats may be present, which helps in distinguishing VT from other broad-complex tachycardias:

- *Fusion beats* occur when a normal supraventricular stimulus meets a ventricular stimulus being conducted retrogradely. The resulting QRS complex looks partly like a normal QRS complex and partly like a ventricular ectopic beat.

- *Capture beats* occur when an atrial stimulus arrives at a non-refractory AV node and is conducted normally to the ventricles. This results in a normal P wave followed by a normal (narrow) QRS complex.

There are four types of ventricular tachycardia:

- Monomorphic ventricular tachycardia
- Polymorphic ventricular tachycardia
- Accelerated idioventricular tachycardia
- Ventricular flutter.

Monomorphic ventricular tachycardia
(Fig. 10.19)

This is the most common form of VT. The ventricular complexes are of uniform appearance (monomorphic), and each episode of VT continues for a variable time, usually terminating in a long pause before sinus rhythm returns. Each paroxysm of tachycardia starts with a ventricular ectopic beat, which occurs at the same fixed interval from the previous QRS complex.

Polymorphic ventricular tachycardia
(Fig. 10.20)

Whereas monomorphic VT consists of QRS complexes of the same configuration, the QRS complexes in a polymorphic VT undulate around the isoelectric line, with a marked change of amplitude occurring every 5–30 beats. Treatment following acute myocardial infarction is similar to that for monomorphic VT.

Torsade de pointes ('turning of the points') is a dangerous form of polymorphic VT characterised by paroxysms of VT when the QT interval is prolonged during sinus rhythm. Prolongation of the QT interval implies prolongation of repolarisation. Although this may affect the whole myocardium, polymorphic VT is more likely to occur when different regions of the myocardium repolarise at different rates. Although QT prolongation is uncommon in the setting of acute myocardial infarction, episodes of torsade de pointes may be precipitated following administration of drugs that prolong the QT interval (e.g. class 1 antidysrhythmic agents), or by electrolyte imbalance.

Torsade de pointes usually terminates spontaneously but may precede ventricular fibrillation. Antidysrhythmic drugs should be stopped, and

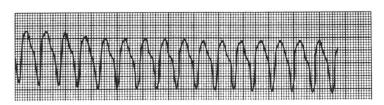

Figure 10.19 ECG: monomorphic ventricular tachycardia.

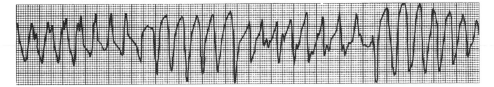

Figure 10.20 ECG: torsade de pointes.

increasing the heart rate to over 100 beats/min by pacing or isoprenaline will often prevent the tachycardia until the precipitating drugs are metabolised.

Accelerated idioventricular tachycardia (Fig. 10.21)

When escape rhythms arise in the ventricles or His–Purkinje system, they are called idioventricular rhythms. Idioventricular rhythm often occurs in association with successful thrombolysis, is benign and requires no treatment. The rate is usually slow, at about 60 beats/min, sometimes referred to as 'slow VT'. After about 30 beats, sinus rhythm usually takes over. Occasionally, the rhythm accelerates, although the rate does not usually exceed 120 beats/min. Rarely, sustained VT or ventricular fibrillation may replace accelerated idioventricular tachycardia.

Ventricular flutter (Fig. 10.22)

This is characterised by a rapid ventricular rate of 180–250 beats/min, in which it is not possible to differentiate the QRS complexes from the ST segments or T waves. The pattern of oscillating waves of large amplitude has been likened to

rows of hairpins. It often precedes ventricular fibrillation, and for practical purposes does not differ from ventricular fibrillation.

THE DIAGNOSIS OF BROAD-COMPLEX TACHYCARDIAS (Fig. 10.23)

Differentiating VT from other broad-complex tachycardias is important, both in the management of the acute dysrhythmia and for long-term therapy to prevent recurrence.

Regular broad-complex tachycardias may be due to:

- Ventricular tachycardia
- Supraventricular tachycardia with pre-existent bundle branch block
- Supraventricular tachycardia with rate-related bundle branch block.

Irregular broad-complex tachycardias may be due to:

- Atrial fibrillation with pre-existing bundle branch block
- Atrial fibrillation with rate-related bundle branch block
- Torsade de pointes.

VT is often misdiagnosed as having a supraventricular origin (Dancy et al, 1985),

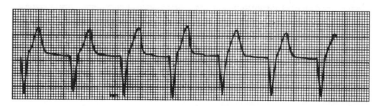

Figure 10.21 ECG: idioventricular tachycardia.

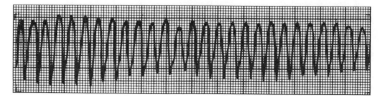

Figure 10.22 ECG: ventricular flutter.

which is of major concern since treatment and prognosis are markedly different. Generally speaking, if the patient is known to have cardiac disease, the broad-complex tachycardia is due to VT. If the patient is thought to have a normal heart, the tachycardia is likely to be supraventricular in origin. Differentiation relies heavily on the demonstration of independent atrial and ventricular activity (AV dissociation), although VA conduction may sometimes occur in VT. A full 12-lead ECG should always be recorded, providing the patient is well enough during the tachycardia. If the QRS in sinus rhythm is of normal duration, QRS duration greater than 160 ms usually indicates a ventricular origin of the tachycardia. However, VT arising close to the interventricular conducting tissue may have a QRS duration of under 140 ms. Ventricular concordance (uniformly positive or negative QRS complexes) in the chest leads almost always indicates VT. The RR interval is regular unless there are capture beats and, in contrast to supraventricular tachycardias that are affected by respiration, does not vary by more than 0.04 s.

It is important to realise that the clinical condition of the patient is not helpful. Some patients tolerate VT extremely well, whereas others may be severely haemodynamically compromised by a rapid supraventricular tachycardia. *If in doubt, broad-complex tachycardias should be treated as VT.*

Guidelines for diagnosis are shown in Box 10.2.

TREATMENT OF VENTRICULAR TACHYCARDIA

Treatment of VT depends on the haemodynamic status of the patient. Short salvoes of non-sustained VT do not usually require treatment, but most sustained ventricular dysrhythmias are accompanied by moderate to severe haemodynamic decompensation and require immediate termination. The treatment of choice in such circumstances is cardioversion. An initial shock of no less than 100 J should be used, as lesser charges may induce ventricular fibrillation. Where a defibrillator is not immediately available, a precordial blow is sometimes effective (Caldwell et al, 1985), as may lying flat with the

---

> **Box 10.2**   Features of ventricular tachycardia
>
> **Clinically**
> - The venous pulse rate is slower than the arterial pulse rate
> - There are irregular cannon waves seen in the venous pulse
> - There is varying intensity of the first heart sound
>
> **In the 12-lead ECG**
> - There is usually left axis deviation (QRS < −30°)
> - The QRS duration is >0.14 s (140 ms)
> - There are multiple QRS morphologies
> - There is concordance of the QRS vector in the chest leads (i.e. they are all in the same direction)
> - In chest lead V1, the R wave is taller than the R′ wave (the left 'rabbit's ear' is longer)
> - Dissociated P waves may be seen (AV dissociation)
> - Blocked, fusion and capture beats may be present
> - There is a Q wave in V6, or a notch on the downstroke of the S wave in V1/V2

legs raised. Coughing (cough CPR – see Ch. 11) may maintain a cardiac output until cardioversion.

Stable ventricular tachydysrhythmias in the presence of good cardiac output and stable blood pressure can be treated either electrically or pharmacologically. An approach to the management of regular, acute, broad-complex tachycardias is shown in Fig. 10.23.

Many antidysrhythmic drugs have been used for acute treatment and control of recurrent VT, but lidocaine (lignocaine) remains the first choice in most coronary care units. Although it only has a 20% response rate, it is usually safe and has a short half-life of about 6 min. Unlike other class 1 drugs, it has a vasoconstrictor action, and is less likely to produce hypotension. A 50-mg bolus may be given at 5-min intervals to a maximum of 200 mg, followed by a continuous infusion of 1–4 mg/min if necessary. Side-effects are rare and include dizziness, tremor and agitation. Amiodarone is highly effective and is a suitable second choice. Third choice drugs include flecainide, disopyramide and mexiletine. Bretylium is a final choice, but may take 20–30 min for effect.

VENTRICULAR FIBRILLATION
(Fig. 10.24)

Electrically and mechanically, the heart is completely disorganised when in ventricular

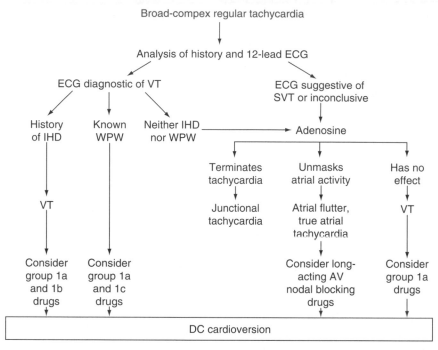

Figure 10.23 An approach to the management of acute broad-complex regular tachycardia. SVT, supraventricular tachycardia; IHD, ischaemic heart disease; WPW, Wolff-Parkinson-White syndrome.

fibrillation (VF), and cardiac arrest results. The ECG shows fine or coarse waves of irregular size, shape and rhythm. Fine VF may mimic asystole and produce an apparently flat line on the ECG. About 90% of deaths following acute myocardial infarction are due to VF, most occurring immediately (primary VF).

Primary VF is the term used if the heart was functioning normally when in sinus rhythm. Primary VF usually occurs within the first 12 h of acute myocardial infarction. It is usually associated with a good prognosis, as the heart is often still functioning well and those who survive to hospi-

tal discharge have the same long-term prognosis as patients who do not experience primary VF.

Reperfusional VF may occur following thrombolysis, but this probably reflects a good prognosis as it implies that the infarct-related artery has been opened.

Secondary or late VF describes fibrillation in hearts whose function has been severely compromised by the infarct. These patients usually have been hypotensive and in heart failure. The prognosis is poor.

The management of cardiac arrest from VF is discussed in Ch. 11.

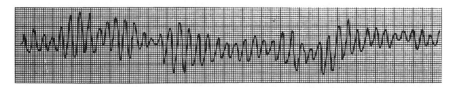

Figure 10.24 ECG: ventricular fibrillation.

PROPHYLAXIS AGAINST VENTRICULAR FIBRILLATION FOLLOWING ACUTE MYOCARDIAL INFARCTION

Randomised trials of prophylaxis with lidocaine (lignocaine) suggested a reduction in the incidence of primary VF, but this was offset by a trend toward increased mortality from fatal episodes of bradycardia and asystole. With the high doses required to obtain this result, side-effects due to toxicity are frequent. Routine administration of lidocaine (lignocaine) to all patients with known or suspected myocardial infarction has been abandoned in most contemporary coronary care unit protocols because of this unfavourable risk:benefit ratio and because it has not been shown to improve survival. Routine administration of intravenous beta-blockers in the acute phase of myocardial infarction seems to reduce the incidence of serious dysrhythmias and is attributable, in part, to the inherent antidysrhythmic properties of these drugs, as well as limiting infarct size. Sotalol may be of particular advantage where recurrent VT or VF has complicated myocardial infarction.

Many other drugs (e.g. flecainide, encainide, mexiletine and moricizine) have been tried as prophylaxis against ventricular dysrhythmias following myocardial infarction, but short-term mortality does not seem to differ with or without treatment (Reiffel et al, 1994). Amiodarone may be the exception to this (CASCADE Investigators, 1993).

HEART FAILURE

Acute left ventricular failure and congestive heart failure are often the presenting problems of patients admitted directly to the coronary care unit. This may or may not be a consequence of acute myocardial infarction. Chronic heart failure punctuated by acute exacerbations is the most common form of heart failure seen in-hospital (Remme and Swedberg, 2001); this is discussed in Ch. 12.

Heart failure following acute myocardial infarction is caused by a combination of loss of myocardial tissue and decreased myocardial contractility. This may be compounded by dysrhythmias, or from drugs that either depress myocardial contractility or produce salt and water retention. Heart failure following acute myocardial infarction is a poor prognostic feature, and there is a close relationship between the degree of left ventricular dysfunction and subsequent mortality. The Killip classification (Killip and Kimball, 1967) shows this relationship (Table 10.1).

Acute left ventricular failure may present suddenly, with marked breathlessness, anxiety and tachycardia. When accompanied by hypotension and oliguria, the syndrome constitutes cardiogenic shock.

Mild heart failure should not be based upon a few crackles at the lung bases alone, as this may simply reflect prior lung disease. A prominent third heart sound, especially with a tachycardia (gallop rhythm), is usually diagnostic, particularly when it occurs with crackles at the lung bases that do not clear with coughing. The chest X-ray appearance may be supportive.

Left ventricular failure may lead to frank pulmonary oedema as a result of transudation of fluid into the pulmonary alveoli. There is decreased airflow to and from the alveoli, because oedema of the pulmonary membranes causes airway narrowing. The lung compliance ('stiffness') increases, making breathing more difficult, and alveolar flooding reduces gaseous exchange within the alveoli. This leads to dyspnoea with arterial hypoxaemia. Increased mucus production may precipitate cough and wheeze

Table 10.1 The Killip classification of heart failure following acute myocardial infarction

Killip class	Clinical status	Mortality (%)
1	No failure	6
2	Mild/moderate heart failure	17
3	Severe heart failure	38
4	Cardiogenic shock	81

(cardiac asthma), and the sputum may be tinged with blood from small haemorrhages in the congested bronchial mucosa.

TREATING HEART FAILURE

The aims of treatment are to relieve symptoms by:

- Reducing intracardiac pressures and volume overload
- Increasing salt and water excretion.

Although assisting impaired left ventricular contraction with positive inotropes would seem logical, myocardial stimulation increases oxygen consumption in the areas of borderline perfusion, and also increases the potential for dysrhythmias. Treatment is therefore aimed at reducing volume overload with diuretics and increasing capacitance with vasodilators.

The patient should be sat upright, and given high concentrations of oxygen to breathe. This is particularly important following acute myocardial infarction, since hypoxaemia will worsen already impaired left ventricular function by increasing areas of critical myocardial ischaemia. Ventilatory function will already be compromised by the combined action of reduced pulmonary compliance, pulmonary vascular congestion and respiratory depression from injected opiates.

Loop diuretics work by decreasing cardiac preload, partly by venodilatation and partly by volume depletion. Intravenous bumetanide and furosemide (frusemide) reduce pulmonary venous pressure within 15 min. Relief of symptoms occurs before the onset of diuresis, probably due to a direct vasodilatory effect on the capillary beds.

Diamorphine may be an important adjunct in certain cases by relieving anxiety and pain and reducing myocardial oxygen demand. Opiates produce transient venodilation; this may be helpful, but may aggravate bradycardia and suppress ventilation, and should be used sparingly.

Nitrates are venodilators, and reduce cardiac filling pressures. Since most episodes of cardiac failure are due to fluid redistribution rather than fluid overload, high-dose nitrates, preferably given as repeated intravenous boluses, may be very beneficial in early treatment (Northridge, 1996; Sharon et al, 2000).

Sodium nitroprusside is a potent dilator of arteries and veins that acts by direct action on vascular smooth muscle, with a rapid onset and rapid cessation of action when infusions are turned on and off. Administration requires close supervision. The major side-effect is cyanide toxicity, but limiting infusions to less than 1 per 48 h can reduce cyanide levels. Hydroxocobalamin (vitamin B_{12}) infusions reduce cyanide concentrations and may be given concurrently.

Assisted ventilation

Assisted ventilation should be considered in severe cardiogenic pulmonary oedema. Formal intubation and ventilation may have detrimental cardiovascular effects due to sedation, hypotension and reduced cardiac output secondary to high intrathoracic pressures. On the other hand, non-invasive positive pressure ventilation improves oxygenation, corrects acidosis and improves left ventricular function (Cooper and Jacob, 2002). As yet, few coronary care units use non-invasive biphasic positive pressure ventilation in acute left ventricular failure, but it is likely to become more frequent.

Further management

Bedrest is valuable until signs and symptoms of cardiac failure improve. Recumbency reduces metabolic demand and increases renal perfusion, and thus decreases myocardial work and improves diuresis. Passive leg exercises and enoxaparin are recommended to prevent deep vein thrombosis. Anticoagulation with warfarin should be considered for patients with enlarged hearts, atrial fibrillation, anterior myocardial infarction or generally poor left ventricular function. This last group is prone to deep vein thrombosis, pulmonary emboli, left ventricular thrombus and peripheral embolisation.

All patients with left ventricular dysfunction should be started on an ACE inhibitor to reduce mortality and future serious cardiovascular events (Packer, 1992). There is no urgency for this, and it is better to await haemodynamic stability before instituting therapy.

POST-INFARCT ANGINA

If flow in the infarct-related artery is not fully restored, there is a risk of re-occlusion. Cases of re-infarction are more likely to develop cardiogenic shock; they have a poor prognosis and a 2.5 times greater risk of death or further myocardial infarction within 1 year. Symptomatic coronary re-occlusion usually occurs within 24 h, although asymptomatic re-occlusion may occur later (Ohman et al, 1990).

Of course, post-infarction chest pain may be due to many causes, such as pericarditis, pulmonary embolism or dyspepsia, so a definite diagnosis is needed. Transient ECG changes and response to glyceryl trinitrate are the main confirmatory features. Post-infarction angina may affect up to one-third of patients, and the risk of re-infarction in these patients is considerable. This is particularly so in those who suffer a non-Q wave infarction. They should be treated for unstable angina, and glycoprotein IIb/IIIa antagonists are particularly useful. Coronary angiography followed by reperfusional therapy is needed in most cases.

CARDIOGENIC SHOCK

Shock is a complex syndrome associated with inadequate perfusion of vital organs, most significantly the brain, the kidneys and the heart. Cardiogenic shock is essentially a disease of inadequate pump function associated with massive cardiac damage (more than 40% of the left ventricular myocardium), but can occur with major pulmonary emboli, cardiac tamponade or following cardiac surgery. The presence of diabetes, established cardiovascular disease and the female sex all place the patient at increased risk. Some patients are admitted to coronary care already in shock, and most cases develop the syndrome

within 24 h. About 15% may develop shock more than 7 days later. Pre-shock is a cardiological emergency and requires aggressive management aimed at preventing deterioration into established cardiogenic shock, which is difficult to reverse (Box 10.3). Despite advances in the treatment of acute myocardial infarction with thrombolysis and other reperfusion therapies, there has been no significant change in the incidence of cardiogenic shock, which has remained at between 7% and 10% for the last 20 years. Hospital mortality was over 90% in the 1970s and is still in the region of 45–80% (Goldberg et al, 1999). It is thus a major contributor to overall cardiovascular morbidity and mortality.

There are typically five types of conditions that predispose to cardiogenic shock:

1. *Recent massive myocardial infarction.* The affected vessel is usually the main stem of the left coronary artery, which will generally result in 40–50% of the left ventricular myocardium being damaged.
2. *Acute-on-chronic infarction.* This occurs when there is a smaller myocardial infarction, which takes the cumulative damage to more than 40% of the ventricular myocardium. These patients are more likely to have pre-existing hypertension and multiple coronary artery disease.
3. *Myocardial infarction with mechanical complication.* Here, acute myocardial infarction is complicated by a mechanical defect, such as a ruptured mitral valve, ruptured septum or acute left ventricular aneurysm.
4. *Myocardial infarction with recurrent dysrhythmias.* Dysrhythmias, especially

---

Box 10.3 Key management of cardiogenic shock

- Rapid admission to a coronary care unit
- Control dysrhythmias
- Echocardiography
- Invasive haemodynamic assessment
- Haemodynamic stabilisation (fluids/inotropic support/vasodilators)
- Reperfusion (primary angioplasty or thrombolysis)
- Cardiac catheterisation, to define coronary anatomy and mechanical defects
- Cardiac surgery or coronary angioplasty

ventricular dysrhythmias, reduce cardiac output and increase myocardial work and oxygen consumption, so may extend the size of the area originally infarcted. Extension of the infarction is common in patients who die from cardiogenic shock.

5. *Extensive right ventricular infarction.*

The syndrome presents with:

- Systemic hypotension (systolic blood pressure less than 90 mmHg)
- Oliguria (urine less than 20 ml/h)
- Arterial vasoconstriction, leading to hypoperfusion of the vital organs and peripheries.

The patient is cold, sweaty and cyanosed, with rapid shallow respiration, hypotension and tachycardia. Mental changes reflecting poor cerebral perfusion are usually present, including irritability, restlessness and, later, coma. Shunting of blood occurs, particularly in the lungs, and the resulting decreased tissue flow causes hypoxia, anaerobic metabolism and a propensity for lactic acidosis that further embarrasses left ventricular function. The fall in blood pressure compromises coronary flow, which worsens the ischaemia to the rest of the myocardium, and worsens function. A vicious cycle is set up, whereby arterial hypotension leads to coronary hypoperfusion and poor myocardial perfusion that produces left ventricular dysfunction. This in turn results in worsening heart failure, hypoxia, acidosis and hypotension, and so on. Additional factors such as the severity of disease in the other coronary arteries, dysrhythmias, and infarct expansion all come into play. The frequent finding of infarct extension in these patients is relevant. Salvage of the border zone of infarction by revascularisation, even late after coronary occlusion, may prevent infarct expansion and aneurysm formation, and may salvage enough myocardium to provide an adequate contractile mass.

MANAGEMENT OF CARDIOGENIC SHOCK

Since the mortality from established cardiogenic shock is so high, the best approach is prevention.

This relies on early intervention to bring about reperfusion of the ischaemic or infarcting myocardium to arrest the inevitable progress to loss of left ventricular myocardium. Thrombolysis has been proven to reduce development of cardiogenic shock, but is unlikely to benefit those who present with cardiogenic shock (Fibrinolytic Therapy Trialists' Collaborative Group, 1994). Special attention is needed in the relief of ischaemia, control and prevention of dysrhythmias, optimisation of haemodynamic variables by inotropic support, and the use of glucose–insulin–potassium infusions to support viable myocardial function (Fath-Ordoubadi and Beatt 1997; Diaz at al, 1998). Unfortunately, patients are seldom seen early enough, and once cardiogenic shock is established the prognosis is dire, even with aggressive intervention.

High concentration oxygen should be given, and some patients will benefit from non-invasive ventilation. Immediate echocardiography is vital to assess the major haemodynamics and may later be confirmed by insertion of a Swan–Ganz catheter (Table 10.2). The abrupt loss of myocardial contractility usually results in a significant rise in intracardiac pressures and a critical fall in arterial blood pressure and cardiac output. However, left ventricular filling pressures and the cardiac index can vary widely, and it is not wise to assume that cardiac output is low or the filling pressures high. Hypovolaemia and low filling pressures may be found in patients with unsuspected right ventricular infarction and patients taking diuretics or antihypertensive agents. Echocardiography will also exclude pericardial tamponade and provides information about left ventricular function and size. Mechanical defects may also be defined. A chest X-ray can give information about heart size, lung

Table 10.2 Assessment of cardiogenic shock

Determinant	Method
Preload	Swan–Ganz catheter
Afterload	Arterial catheter
Heart rate	ECG monitoring
Contractility	Echocardiography
Infarct size	ECG, cardiac enzymes and ventriculography

fields and aortic root size. An increase in the latter may suggest aortic dissection as a cause of the shock.

All drugs commonly prescribed during acute myocardial infarction need reviewing. Opiates, ACE inhibitors, beta-blockers, nitrates and calcium antagonists need to be used very cautiously in these patients because they can worsen hypotension and cardiogenic shock (Williams et al, 2000).

Inotropic support with drugs such as dopamine and dobutamine may provide temporary stabilisation until other measures can be instituted. If the blood pressure on maximal inotropic stimulation fails to exceed 100/70 mmHg and the patient is still clinically hypoperfused (i.e. oliguric, peripherally shut down), the patient is unlikely to survive on medical treatment alone. However, revascularisation will not benefit all patients with cardiogenic shock. The SHOCK and SMASH trials randomly allocated patients with cardiogenic shock to early revascularisation or medical treatment, and the results showed no major difference in outcome with any intervention (Hochman 1995; Urban et al, 1999). This is probably because those with little or no myocardial contractile reserve are unlikely to have enough salvageable myocardium for revascularisation to have a major impact on survival.

Patients who are responsive to inotropic stimulation and show adequate cardiac reserve may be suitable for early revascularisation to salvage the still viable myocardium, provided they have presented early enough. Those seen within 6 h of the onset of infarction, and with features suggestive of ongoing ischaemia, should be seriously considered for revascularisation, but usually require chemical and mechanical inotropic support (intra-aortic balloon pumping).

Intra-aortic balloon pumping

Since its introduction in the 1960s (Kantrowitz et al, 1968), intra-aortic balloon counter-pulsation has been recognised as an effective treatment for patients with unstable ischaemic syndromes and cardiogenic shock. Modern intra-aortic balloons are inserted percutaneously without arterial cutdown. Fluoroscopy is generally used, but blind insertion is possible. The narrow balloon catheter is inserted via the femoral artery and advanced retrogradely to lie in the descending aorta, just below the aortic arch (Fig. 10.25). The two basic phases of counter-pulsation are inflation during diastole and deflation during systole. During systole, sudden deflation allows blood to be ejected from the left ventricle around the deflated balloon. Before deflation, the balloon protects

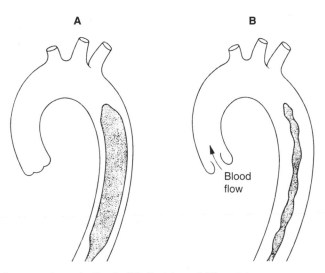

A   B

Blood flow

Figure 10.25   Intra-aortic balloon counter-pulsation in (A) diastole and (B) systole.

the aortic outflow, so afterload is low, which promotes left ventricular emptying. At the onset of diastole, an ECG-activated trigger causes the balloon to inflate with helium, just after the dicrotic notch of aortic valve closure, and occludes the aorta. Approximately 50 ml of blood are pushed up towards the closed aortic valve; this actively propels blood into the coronary arteries to promote myocardial perfusion, and, additionally, improve cerebral blood supply. When the balloon deflates again, the intra-aortic pressure is low, and blood is ejected with minimal extra cardiac work and oxygen consumption. Pulmonary congestion is relieved, and global myocardial perfusion, often including collateral circulation to the infarcted area, is improved. Cardiac output may increase by up to 50%, allowing improved blood flow to the vital organs. The mean arterial blood pressure increases as myocardial function improves by up to 15 mmHg, and shock quickly stabilises.

Counter-pulsation was first used as a stand-alone modality to treat patients with post-infarct cardiogenic shock, but it is currently used as a stabilising device or bridge to facilitate diagnostic angiography and revascularisation or repair (Kumar and Roberts, 2001). Recommendations for intra-aortic balloon counter-pulsation now include:

- Cardiogenic shock not quickly reversed with pharmacological therapy as a stabilising measure before angiography and revascularisation
- Acute mitral regurgitation or septal rupture complicating myocardial infarction, as a stabilising therapy for angiography and repair/revascularisation
- Recurrent intractable ventricular arrhythmias with haemodynamic instability
- Refractory post-infarct angina as a bridge to angiography and revascularisation.

Unfortunately, although balloon pumping may improve the initial mortality for patients in cardiogenic shock, 'balloon dependence' is common, so, when this support is withdrawn, shock returns. Insertion should only be considered

where myocardial stunning is thought to play a major part, or where surgical intervention is possible. Left ventricular assist devices have also been used as holding measures until surgery can be performed (see Ch. 16). No study has yet shown that balloon pumping alone reduces mortality.

CARDIAC RUPTURE

After dysrhythmias and cardiogenic shock, the most common cause of death following acute myocardial infarction is cardiac rupture, which complicates up to one-quarter of cases. It usually occurs in the healing stages following infarction (3–5 days), although maximum risk seems to have moved towards the first 24 h since the introduction of thrombolytic therapy (ISIS-2 Collaborative Group, 1988). The risk of cardiac rupture may be decreased by early treatment with beta-blockers. Rupture is predisposed to by extensive infarction, prior hypertension, diffuse coronary heart disease and anticoagulant therapy. It is four times more common in women.

The most common site for rupture is through the free left ventricular wall, producing chest pain, hypotension, dyspnoea and distended neck veins. Death is rapid and caused by an acute haemopericardium, leading to cardiac tamponade. Recurrent chest pain without ECG changes may warn of imminent rupture, and cardiac collapse in the presence of normal complexes on the ECG is typical (pulseless electrical activity).

Rupture of the interventricular septum produces an intracardiac shunt, with blood being forced from the powerful left ventricle into the lower pressure right ventricle, resulting in a marked fall in cardiac output, with pulmonary circuit overload and severe pulmonary oedema. A loud pansystolic murmur is audible at the left sternal edge, with a systolic thrill.

The papillary muscles may become ischaemic and infarcted, like any other part of the ventricular myocardium, and rupture in the healing stages. Acute mitral regurgitation results, with a fall in cardiac output and acute pulmonary oedema. An apical pansystolic murmur develops, which radiates to the axilla or sometimes the left sternal edge (the regurgitant jet is often eccentric). The degree of mitral dysfunction depends upon whether the rupture is partial or complete. The prognosis is better than for septal rupture and depends upon the degree of left ventricular dysfunction.

MANAGEMENT OF CARDIAC RUPTURE

The management of mechanical defects following acute myocardial infarction is surgical (see Ch. 16); without operation, most patients with cardiac rupture will die.

RIGHT VENTRICULAR INFARCTION

Although myocardial infarction usually results in left ventricular dysfunction, the right ventricle may also be involved, either alone or with the left ventricle. Clinical consequences vary from none to cardiogenic shock. Estimates from post-mortem studies suggest that right ventricle infarction has an incidence of between 8% and 14% (Wartman and Hellerstein, 1948), but involvement via extension from acute inferior myocardial infarction is very common (Zehender et al, 1993). Some degree of right ventricular ischaemia may be demonstrated in half of all inferior infarcts, but only 10–15% will develop clinically important abnormalities. In most cases, the right ventricle becomes stunned, with normal function returning over a period of weeks to months. However, where there is right ventricular necrosis in association with inferior infarction, there is increased mortality.

The right coronary artery usually supplies most of the right ventricular myocardium, and right coronary occlusion proximal to the right ventricular branches will lead to right ventricular ischaemia. However, there is usually little haemodynamic consequence, as the right ventricle is relatively protected against the effects of acute ischaemia through extensive collateral flow from left to right, with coronary perfusion that

occurs in both systole and diastole. Oxygen demand is also not so high as for the left ventricle because the right ventricle has a much smaller muscle mass, with lower vascular resistance from the pulmonary circuit. These factors explain why right ventricular ischaemia usually passes unnoticed in most patients with proximal right coronary artery occlusion.

The clinical triad of hypotension, clear lung fields and elevated jugular venous pressure in the setting of an inferior myocardial infarction is characteristic of right ventricular infarction. Distended neck veins alone or the presence of Kussmaul's sign (distended neck veins which fail to empty on inspiration) are both sensitive and specific clinical clues for right ventricular involvement in these patients.

The ECG is usually unhelpful unless right-sided chest leads are used. Demonstration of 1-mm ST segment elevation in the right precordial lead V_{4R} is the single most predictive ECG finding in patients with right ventricular infarction, but it may be transient (Andersen et al, 1989).

Echocardiography is necessary to exclude cardiac tamponade, and may show right ventricular dilatation with abnormal interventricular and interatrial septal motion. The acutely ischaemic right ventricle dilates, but it is restrained by the pericardium. The increased intrapericardial pressure reduces the right ventricular systolic pressure and output, which in turn decreases left ventricular preload and stroke volume. There is paradoxical movement of the interventricular septum into the right ventricle during systole, providing a piston-like movement that helps right ventricular emptying (Goldstein et al, 1992). This compensatory mechanism will be lost if there is concomitant septal infarction, which may result in a major diminution of right ventricular output.

Treatment of right ventricular infarction aims to maintain the right ventricular filling pressure while reducing the right ventricular afterload. Drugs used routinely in the management of myocardial infarction, such as nitrates and diuretics that reduce preload, may diminish cardiac output and produce severe hypotension. Volume loading with normal saline alone often resolves accompanying hypotension and improves cardiac output. However, in some patients, volume loading further elevates the right-sided filling pressure and right dilatation, resulting in decreased left ventricular output. Thus, although volume loading (0.5–1 litre of normal saline) is a critical first step in the management of hypotension, inotropic support with dobutamine should be initiated promptly if cardiac output fails to improve after fluids have been given. Sodium nitroprusside or an intra-aortic balloon pump is often necessary to unload the heart, and measurement of intracardiac pressures with a Swan–Ganz catheter is of major value in balancing therapy to optimise cardiac output.

Atrial fibrillation occurs in up to one-third of patients with right ventricular infarction and may have profound haemodynamic effects. Prompt cardioversion should be considered. Similar haemodynamic deterioration may develop if there is complete heart block, which is a common complication of right coronary occlusion. Sequential AV pacing is preferable to ventricular pacing to maintain cardiac output. Prompt opening of the right coronary artery by thrombolysis or angioplasty reduces the incidence of heart block, and also improves right ventricular function.

Clinical and haemodynamic right ventricular dysfunction may persist for weeks or months following acute myocardial infarction. Recovery is helped by a gradual stretching of the pericardium with amelioration of its restraining effect on the heart. Improvement of concomitant left ventricular dysfunction helps reduce right ventricular afterload.

LEFT VENTRICULAR ANEURYSM

Left ventricular aneurysms more commonly develop following acute myocardial infarction in the presence of diffuse coronary heart disease, in hypertensive patients or where there has been extensive myocardial damage. The site is usually anterolateral (60%), and 20% occur in the inferior wall. The apex and septum may also be affected. Patients are often identified because of refractory left ventricular failure or because of persistent ST elevation on the ECG. In addition, the aneurysm may act as a focus for recurrent ventricular tachycardia, and also as a site for thrombus formation. Systemic embolisation complicates about 50% of cases of left ventricular aneurysm. Diagnosis may be confirmed by echocardiography, a MUGA scan or angiography. Where possible, surgical excision is usually combined with revascularisation procedures (see Ch. 16).

LEFT VENTRICULAR MURAL THROMBI AND SYSTEMIC EMBOLISATION

Left ventricular mural thrombus may develop over areas of acutely inflamed endocardium in the first 3 weeks following myocardial infarction, particularly in association with a left ventricular aneurysm. Most episodes of peripheral embolisation result in stroke. Overall, cerebral embolism affects 1–3% of patients with myocardial infarction, and usually occurs within the first 10 days. Large mesenteric emboli are generally fatal. Limb emboli may be removed surgically. Coronary emboli causing re-infarction are fortunately uncommon.

DEEP VEIN THROMBOSIS AND PULMONARY EMBOLISM

There are many reasons why deep vein thrombosis (DVT) is more likely following myocardial infarction, including immobility, increasing age, obesity and heart failure (THRIFT II Consensus Group, 1998). DVT is thought to complicate as many as one-third of cases of myocardial infarction, most of which are asymptomatic. Postmortem examinations have found pulmonary emboli in 8% of deaths associated with acute myocardial infarction (Griffin, 1996). Prophylaxis is therefore of major importance.

PROPHYLAXIS

Patients on the coronary care unit are at least at moderate risk of venous thromboembolism. Prophylaxis with subcutaneous low-dose unfractionated heparin (5000 U 8-hourly), or low molecular weight heparin (enoxaparin, 40 mg daily), should be used routinely in all patients, and full anticoagulation considered for those with prolonged immobilisation and heart failure. Graduated pressure stockings may also be useful. Early mobilisation is desirable for all patients, especially the elderly, provided there are no contraindications.

DIAGNOSIS OF ESTABLISHED DEEP VEIN THROMBOSIS

Clinical signs of DVT are not always reliable, but may include swelling, tenderness and redness of the affected limb. These signs are not specific, and clinical diagnosis is less than 50% accurate. The diagnosis must be supported by sensitive diagnostic tests. The role of D-dimer measurement following recent coronary thrombosis is limited, but a negative result may rule out active thrombosis, especially if clinical suspicion is low. *Compression ultrasound* of the legs is sensitive for detecting proximal DVT when carried out by an experienced practitioner. *Venography* may be used to demonstrate thrombosis in the deep veins, and, with modern image enhancement, excellent quality films may be obtained up to the inferior vena cava. The investigation is invasive and has the risk of producing thrombophlebitis in some patients. Spiral CT angiography can also be used.

MANAGEMENT

For initial treatment of DVT, low molecular weight heparin is effective and easier to administer than unfractionated heparin. Tinzaparin (175 IU/kg daily), dalteparin (200 IU/kg daily) and enoxaparin (100 IU/kg/12-h) are all suitable, and do not need monitoring. If unfractionated heparin is used, a bolus of 5000 U should be followed by an infusion of about 40 000 U/day,

adjusted to keep the activated partial thromboplastin time twice that of the control. Heparin should be continued for 4–5 days, and oral anticoagulants given at the same time. The INR (international normalised ratio) should be 2–3 for at least 2 days before heparin is discontinued. The optimum duration of anticoagulation is not clear, and depends upon clinical status of the patient and reversible risk factors. Typically, warfarin is continued for 6 weeks to 6 months (Jowett, 1999).

Physical measures are very important, but often forgotten. Bedrest is unnecessary, and indeed may be harmful in promoting venous stasis. Adequate analgesia is required, and the patient encouraged to walk in class II graduated compression stockings. In patients with severe oedema, high elevation of the affected leg will help reduce the swelling until a stocking can be worn. When not walking, the patient should return to bed with the leg elevated at a level higher than the heart. Sitting for long periods should be avoided as it encourages venous stasis and increases calf compartment pressures predisposing to limb ischaemia.

Thrombolysis is an attractive alternative to anticoagulation for DVT, as it will clear veins more quickly and preserve valve function (Jowett et al, 1998), but there have been concerns about precipitating pulmonary embolism when the clot breaks up (Armon and Hopkinson, 1996).

PERICARDITIS AND DRESSLER'S SYNDROME

Post-infarction pericarditis affects patients in the first week following acute transmural myocardial infarction, and is more common in those with larger infarcts and left ventricular failure. The erythrocyte sedimentation rate and white cell count may be elevated, and a small pericardial effusion seen on echocardiography. Sometimes, pericarditis and pleurisy recur 2 weeks to 3 months after myocardial infarction, a condition called *Dressler's syndrome*. Pericardial pain is accompanied by systemic symptoms, such as fever and malaise. Large pleural and pericardial effusions may develop. The mechanism is thought to be autoimmune, triggered by blood in the pericardial cavity or from antibodies to necrotic myocardium.

Treatment is with non-steroidal anti-inflammatory agents and bedrest. Echocardiography should be repeated to check for increasing pericardial effusion, particularly if the ECG shows progressive low-voltage reduction. The condition is self-limiting but may recur. It is best to discontinue anticoagulants, because of the risk of a haemorrhagic pericardial effusion. More resistant cases may need corticosteroid therapy.

SHOULDER–HAND SYNDROME

The shoulder–hand syndrome presents with stiffness and pain in the shoulder (usually the left side) 2–8 weeks after acute myocardial infarction, sometimes accompanied by pain and swelling of the hand. Physiotherapy and analgesia are all that is required. With early mobilisation of the post-coronary patient, this has become a rare complication.

DEPRESSION

Up to a third of patients develop depressive symptoms following acute myocardial infarction; this may result from denial or being too frightened to admit to problems. Early mobilisation, and information and education about their status can prevent depression. Early involvement of the rehabilitation team is vital.

SUDDEN CARDIAC DEATH

Sudden cardiac death (SCD) can occur at any stage following the onset of an acute coronary syndrome. Most of these deaths associate with malignant ventricular dysrhythmias, although they may be due to pulmonary embolism, or acute cardiac rupture. Primary ventricular fibril-

lation often occurs before admission to hospital, typically within the first 2 h following onset of symptoms. Reperfusional therapy has a clear role in reducing in-hospital mortality from reduction of cardiogenic shock and dysrhythmic death. Furthermore, early perfusion limits infarct size, ventricular enlargement and preserves left ventricular function, all of which help reduce late ventricular dysrhythmias.

Late ventricular dysrhythmias occur 10 days or more after myocardial infarction, a time when most patients have been discharged from hospital. The patient has often made normal post-infarction progress, and then suddenly collapses at home. Trying to identify this group of patients is difficult. Some of these patients are predisposed to ventricular dysrhythmias because of electrolyte imbalance, particularly hypokalaemia, which must be avoided in the peri-infarction period. Early exercise testing or Holter monitoring before discharge in selected high-risk cases (large infarcts, heart failure, diabetes) may help identify those prone to SCD.

Due to the complex mechanisms leading to SCD, a variety of therapeutic targets may be considered. The terms primary and secondary prophylaxis are used in the context of ventricular dysrhythmias. 'Primary' intervention is applied to patients at high risk who have not yet had a ventricular dysrhythmia. Secondary prophylaxis is applied to those who have already had a VF arrest, or ventricular tachycardia associated with hypotension and pre-syncope.

PRIMARY PROPHYLAXIS

ACE inhibition following acute myocardial infarction decreases progression to overt or worsening heart failure, and may reduce mortality from SCD by as much 30–54% (Kober et al, 1995).

Antidysrhythmic drugs have a limited role in prophylaxis against SCD post-infarction. The suppression of spontaneous non-sustained ventricular tachycardia does not affect outcome, and certain agents may be harmful (e.g. sodium channel blockers). Treatment with beta-blockers reduces all-cause mortality, some of which is related to reductions in SCD. The greatest benefits of beta-blockade have been shown in those with poor left ventricular function and heart failure, a subgroup who traditionally have been denied this therapy. Amiodarone may be safely administered for symptomatic non-sustained VT where beta-blockers are contraindicated.

Primary intervention trials of automatic implantable cardiodefibrillators (AICDs) show a reduction in all-cause mortality when compared with medical therapy, but identification of the ideal recipients is not yet decided.

SECONDARY PROPHYLAXIS

Patients who have a cardiac arrest or demonstrate sustained VT following acute myocardial infarction are most usefully treated by amiodarone or sotalol, but the recent trials with AICDs, may suggest that this approach is not necessarily the best. A meta-analysis of the major trials of secondary prevention showed a clear benefit of AICDs over amiodarone over a 6-year follow-up (Connolly et al, 2000). The role of AICDs is discussed in Ch. 13.

REFERENCES

Andersen HR, Falk E, Nielsen D (1989) Right ventricular infarction: diagnostic accuracy of electrocardiographic right chest leads V_{3R} to V_{7R} investigated prospectively in 43 consecutive fatal cases from a coronary care unit. *British Heart Journal*, **61:** 514–520.

Armon MP, Hopkinson BR (1996) Thrombolysis for acute deep vein thrombosis. *British Journal of Surgery*, **83:** 580–581.

Caldwell G, Millar G, Quinn E et al (1985) Simple mechanical methods for cardioversion: defense of the precordial thump and cough version. *BMJ*, **291:** 627–630.

Campbell RWF, Higham D, Adams P et al (1987) Potassium: its relevance for arrhythmias complicating acute myocardial infarction. *Journal of Cardiovascular Physiology*, **10:** S25–S27.

CASCADE Investigators (1993) Randomised anti-arrhythmic drug therapy in survivors of cardiac arrest: the CASCADE study. *American Journal of Cardiology*, **72:** 280–287.

Connolly SJ, Hallstrom AP, Cappato R et al (2000) Meta-analysis of the implantable cardioverter defibrillator secondary prevention trials. *European Heart Journal*, **21:** 2071–2078.

Cooper N, Jacob B (2002) Biphasic positive pressure ventilation in acute cardiogenic pulmonary oedema. *British Journal of Cardiology*, **9:** 38–41.

Dancy M, Camm AJ, Ward D (1985) Misdiagnosis of chronic recurrent ventricular tachycardia. *Lancet*, **ii:** 320–323.

Diaz R, Paolasso EA, Piegas LS et al (1998) Metabolic modulation of acute myocardial infarction. The ECLA (Estudios Cardiologicos Latino-America) Collaborative Group. *Circulation*, **98:** 2227–2234.

Fath-Ordoubadi F, Beatt KJ (1997) Glucose–insulin–potassium therapy for treatment of acute myocardial infarction: an overview of randomized placebo-controlled trials. *Circulation*, **96:** 1152–1156.

Fibrinolytic Therapy Trialists' Collaborative Group (1994) Indications for fibrinolytic therapy in suspected acute myocardial infarction: collaborative overview of early and major mortality from all randomised trials of more than 1000 patients. *Lancet*, **343:** 311–322.

Freemantle N, Cleland JG, Young P et al (2001) Beta-blockade after myocardial infarction: systematic review and meta-regression analysis. *BMJ*, **318:** 1349–1355.

Goldberg RJ, Samad NA, Yarzebski J et al (1999) Temporal trends in cardiogenic shock complicating acute myocardial infarction. *New England Journal of Medicine*, **340:** 1162–1168.

Goldstein JA, Tweddell JS, Barzilai B et al (1992) Importance of left ventricular function and systolic ventricular interaction to right ventricular performance during acute right heart ischemia. *Journal of the American College of Cardiology*, **19:** 704–711.

Griffin J (1996) *Deep Vein Thrombosis and Pulmonary Embolism*. London: Office of Health Economics.

Hochman JS, Boland J, Sleeper LA and the SHOCK Registry Investigators (1995) Current spectrum of cardiogenic shock and effect of early revascularisation on mortality: results of an international registry. *Circulation*, **91:** 873–881.

ISIS–2 Collaborative Group (1988) Randomised trial of intravenous streptokinase, oral aspirin, both or neither amongst 17,187 cases of suspected acute myocardial infarction. *Lancet*, **ii:** 349–360.

Jowett NI (1999) Use of anti-coagulants in the treatment of deep vein thrombosis. *Prescriber*, **6:** 57–74.

Jowett NI, Thompson DR, Pohl JEF (1989) Temporary transvenous endocardial pacing: six years experience in one coronary care unit. *Postgraduate Medical Journal*, **65:** 211–215.

Jowett NI, Robinson CGF, Clow WM (1998) Invasive management of deep vein thrombosis. *Postgraduate Medical Journal*, **74:** 311–312.

Kantrowitz A, Tjonneland S, Freed PS et al (1968) Initial clinical experience with intra-aortic balloon pumping in cardiogenic shock. *JAMA*, **203:** 113–118.

Killip T, Kimball JT (1967) Treatment of myocardial infarction in a coronary care unit: two years experience with 250 patients. *American Journal of Cardiology*, **20:** 457–464.

Kober L, Torp-Pedersen C, Carlsen JE et al (1995) A clinical trial of the angiotensin-converting-enzyme inhibitor trandolapril in patients with left ventricular dysfunction after myocardial infarction with clinical evidence of heart failure. Trandolapril Cardiac Evaluation (TRACE) study. *New England Journal of Medicine*, **333:** 1670–1676.

Kumar S, Roberts DH (2001) Intra-aortic balloon pulsation: an overview. *British Journal of Cardiology*, **8:** 658–663.

Lown B, Fakhro AM, Hood WB et al (1967) The coronary care unit: new perspectives and developments. *JAMA*, **199:** 188–198.

Northridge D (1996) Furosemide or nitrates for acute heart failure? Lancet, **347:** 667–668.

Ohman EM, Califf RM, Topol EJ et al (1990) Consequences of re-occlusion after successful reperfusion therapy in acute myocardial infarction. *Circulation*, **82:** 781–791.

Packer M (1992) Patho-physiology of chronic heart failure and treatment of heart failure. *Lancet*, **340:** 88–95.

Pizzetti F, Tarazza FM, Franzosi MG et al and behalf of the GISSI–3 Investigators (2001) Incidence and prognostic significance of atrial fibrillation in acute myocardial infarction: the GISSI–3 data. *Heart*, **86:** 527–532.

Reiffel JA, Estes NA, Waldo AL et al (1994) A consensus report on anti-arrhythmic drug use. *Clinical Cardiology*, **17:** 103–116.

Remme WJ, Swedberg K (2001) Guidelines for the diagnosis and treatment of chronic heart failure. *European Heart Journal*, **22:** 1527–1560.

Schilling RJ (2002) Which patients should be referred to an electrophysiologist: supraventricular tachycardia. *Heart*, **87:** 299–304.

Sharon A, Shpirer I, Kaluski E et al (2000) High dose intravenous isosorbide dinitrate is safer and better than Bi-PAP ventilation combined with conventional treatment for severe pulmonary oedema. *Journal of the American College of Cardiology*, **36:** 832–837.

THRIFT II (Thrombo-embolic Risk Factors) Consensus Group (1998) Risk of and prophylaxis for venous thromboembolism in hospital patients. *Phlebology*, **13:** 87–97.

Urban P, Stauffer JC, Bleed D et al (1999) A randomized evaluation of early revascularisation to treat shock complicating acute myocardial infarction. The (Swiss) Multicenter Trial of Angioplasty for Shock(S)MASH. *European Heart Journal*, **20:** 1030–1038.

Wartman WB, Hellerstein HK (1948) The incidence of heart disease in 2000 consecutive autopsies. *Annals of Internal Medicine*, **28:** 41–65.

Williams G, Wright DJ, Tan LB (2000) Management of cardiogenic shock complicating acute myocardial infarction: towards evidence-based medical practice. *Heart*, **83:** 621–626.

Zehender M, Kasper W, Kauder E et al (1993) Right ventricular infarction as an independent predictor of prognosis after acute inferior myocardial infarction. *New England Journal of Medicine*, **328:** 981–988.

11

Cardiopulmonary resuscitation

Cardiorespiratory arrest occurs when there is sudden cessation of spontaneous respiration and circulation. The most common reason is a cardiac dysrhythmia secondary to coronary heart disease, although only a minority will have had a recent myocardial infarction. Other frequent causes include pulmonary emboli, massive haemorrhage and trauma. Coronary care units were developed primarily to treat ventricular fibrillation and other serious dysrhythmias in the first few hours following myocardial infarction. Unfortunately, many episodes occur before admission to hospital, and three-quarters of all deaths from myocardial infarction occur after cardiac arrest in the community. This proportion is even higher in people under 55 years of age, in whom 91% of cardiac arrest deaths occur outside hospital. Bystander-initiated resuscitation more than doubles pre-hospital survival, but most patients do not receive this treatment (Ballew, 1997). Survival after cardiac arrest outside hospital remains low. People who suffer cardiac arrest outside hospital initially develop ventricular tachycardia before they progress to ventricular fibrillation. This will deteriorate to asystole within a few minutes if untreated. The most important predictors of survival are whether the arrest was witnessed, the time from collapse to defibrillation and the initial rhythm encountered by the emergency staff. Those who are already in asystole rarely survive.

The ambulance service in the UK has a statutory obligation to arrive at the scene of 50% of emergency calls within 7 min, and a target of 90% within 8 min is being contemplated. First-responders (fire-service, police and community volunteers) could be provided with automatic defibrillators to reduce the time to defibrillation.

Patients who suffer cardiac arrest outside hospital are relatively healthy, whereas those in hospital usually have an overt underlying illness. On the other hand, many more cardiac arrests in hospital are witnessed, and the speed to defibrillation is obviously faster. This is particularly so on coronary care units, intensive therapy units and high-dependency units. A proportion of cardiac arrests occur on the hospital wards, where it is the nursing staff that have the responsibility for carrying out basic life support before the arrival of the 'arrest team'. Undoubtedly, open-plan wards permit the rapid recognition of circulatory arrest and, from the point of view of resuscitation, it is a shame that so many four-bed or single-bed wards now exist. Simulated cardiac arrests may help in identifying any deficiencies or difficulties in resuscitation within such areas (Sullivan and Guyatt, 1986). The chances of initial survival after in-hospital arrest are about 1 in 8. Of these only 1 in 3 will survive to discharge (Ebell et al, 1998).

Since resuscitation by nurses is usual on high-dependency units, and early steps are commonplace on general medical wards (especially at night), it is essential that the nursing staff can cope with this task competently. Audit at our hospital shows that 71% of cardiac arrest calls are made during 'on-call' hours, when medical staff are not immediately available (17.00–09.00 h, and at weekends). Although chances of resuscitation should be optimal within hospital, there are often deficiencies in the knowledge of basic resuscitation skills (Hershey and Fisher, 1982). Studies have highlighted this inadequacy in both the nursing and the medical staff (Skinner, 1985; Kaye and Mancini, 1986; Wynne et al, 1987; David and Prior-Willeard, 1993). One of the principal functions of the coronary care unit and its specialist staff must be to train personnel in the basic resuscitation procedures (Jowett and Thompson, 1988a). All hospital staff, whatever their work, need to learn the rudiments of car-

diopulmonary resuscitation (CPR); it is one of the main life-saving procedures that can be carried out by everybody. In addition, junior medical staff and those in specialist areas (e.g. coronary care unit, intensive therapy unit or accident and emergency) need to be checked on their proficiency at these basic skills, the use of simple equipment (oxygen, suction and airways) and defibrillation procedures (Royal College of Physicians, 1987). As the staff become more senior and more experienced at attending arrests, increased confidence is not necessarily matched by an increase in skills (Marteau et al 1990; Berden et al, 1993), so that periods of retraining and retesting are required. The appointment of a resuscitation officer to address these problems is associated with improved survival to discharge following in-hospital cardiac arrest (McGowan et al, 1999). The deficiencies in resuscitation skills in junior doctors has been addressed by integrating resuscitation training into the undergraduate medical curriculum of most universities (Graham et al, 1994a,b). The amount of time required for dedicated teaching of medical undergraduates and house-officers alone justifies appointment of a resuscitation officer in most district general hospitals (Leah et al, 1998).

THE ETHICS OF RESUSCITATION

The Resuscitation Council (UK) together with the British Medical Association and the Royal College of Nursing updated their statement 'Decisions relating to cardiopulmonary resuscitation' in 2000, as a framework on which hospital and other trusts may build their own more detailed guidelines. The new guidance now avoids the term 'DNR' (do not resuscitate) in favour of 'DNAR' (do not attempt resuscitation). They have outlined three situations where a DNAR order is appropriate:

- If cardiopulmonary resuscitation (CPR) is unlikely to be effective
- If it is known that the patient does not wish to receive CPR

• If successful CPR would not result in a length, or more importantly a quality, of life that would be in the patient's best interest.

It must be fully understood by all (patients, doctors, nurses and relatives) that DNAR orders apply only to the decision whether or not to initiate CPR in the event of respiratory or cardiac arrest (Shepardson et al, 1999). The DNAR decision should not in any way limit other medical or nursing care that the patient receives. Hospitals should have written policies of when to start resuscitation, which need to be understood by all concerned. One study showed that one-quarter of nurses did not know or did not understand such orders written in the patients' notes (Jones et al, 1993).

WHEN IS RESUSCITATION INAPPROPRIATE?

All life ends with cardiopulmonary arrest, and CPR is not a treatment for death or for the dying. Resuscitation is best not attempted if a patient is found dead or if he is known to have a distressing or inevitably fatal illness. The age of the patient is immaterial. CPR is at best traumatic and often invasive, and failed attempts do little to enhance the dignity of death and may subject the patient and his relatives to added pain and misery (Candy, 1991). Those who have come to the end of their natural lives should be allowed to die as peacefully as possible.

There is a growing assumption that failure to initiate resuscitation may have legal repercussions and it is wiser for all patients who suffer a cardiopulmonary arrest to be resuscitated unless a DNAR order has been made. It must be remembered that nearly 90% of patients who arrest on general wards do not survive, and patients do not have a right to useless interventions, or doctors a duty to provide them on demand, if there is no reasonable prospect of success (Saunders, 2001). Currently, nursing staff are under professional and managerial obligations to initiate the process unless specifically instructed otherwise,

and should be supported in such circumstances. A DNAR order must therefore be clearly recorded and should be made whenever death can be anticipated and resuscitation judged pointless. We use a specific proforma (Fig. 11.1).

The responsibility for making a DNAR order is that of the doctor in charge of the case. Other medical and nursing staff may be involved, and the views of the patient, the relatives or close friends should be considered (Ebrahim, 2000). Such discussion with relatives helps to improve communication and keeps those who care for the patient fully informed, although it must be understood that no relative has a legal right to determine an adult patient's treatment. The responsibility for a DNAR decision may have to be delegated to the next most senior doctor on duty, but the ultimate responsibility remains with the consultant and should be confirmed as early as possible. The attending doctor must make the initial decision in the best interests of the patient where relatives are not present, and refrain from making a DNAR order because full discussion has not taken place. It should be remembered that most patients with cardiac arrest die despite intervention, and dramatic efforts might be inappropriate. The BRESUS study (Tunstall-Pedoe et al, 1992) showed that for every eight attempted resuscitations, there were only three immediate survivors. One of these would die within 24 h and another over the course of the following year. In the Netherlands, of 827 resuscitated patients, only 12% survived to 3 months (de Vos et al, 1999); 17% of these had cognitive impairment, and 16% depressive symptoms. Fewer than one in ten of the original group were capable of independent daily life.

DNAR orders should be clearly understood by the patient's carers and recorded formally in both the medical and nursing notes – a procedure that is not well adhered to (Aarons and Beeching, 1991). The rationale for the order, and any patient consultation, should also be noted. Such orders should be reviewed frequently and changed if there is any relevant change in the patient's condition or circumstances.

Do Not Attempt Resuscitation Order (DNAR)

Ymddiriedolaeth GIG
SIR BENFRO a DERWEN
PEMBROKESHIRE & DERWEN
NHS Trust

(Health Records Label may be attached)	In the event of a Cardio-Pulmonary Arrest, <u>no</u> active resuscitation should occur and 222 should <u>not</u> be dialled.
Name _____	
Address _____	
_____	Hospital _____
DOB _____ Number _____	Ward/deparment _____

| 1. This decision was discussed with the patient.

On _____ at _____ am / pm

No this was not discussed with the patient because:

_____
_____
_____
_____
_____
_____
_____ | 2 The decision has been discussed with the patient's Next of Kin

Mr/Ms/Miss _____

Relationship _____

On _____ at _____ am/pm

In person / by telephone / other
This was not discussed with the patient's relative because:

_____
_____
_____
_____ |

3. Date of commencement _____

   Time of commencement _____ am / pm

4. Signed _____ Name (Please print) _____

   Grade: SHO / SpReg / StaffGrade / GP / Consultant   (Please circle)

   NB: SHOs can only make a DNAR decision if prior delegation has been given by consultant.

5. **Planned review dates** 1 _____ Signature _____
   To be agreed and
   signed by Patient's   2 _____ Signature _____
   Consultant/GP at
   the earlist opportunity 3 _____ Signature _____

6. **THE ABOVE ORDER IS NOW CANCELLED**   Date _____ at _____ am/pm

   Signature _____ Print Name _____ Grade _____

This form is to be usedin accordance with the Trust Resuscitation Policy. For further information please contact the Resuscitation and Clinical Skills Training Officer via switchborad at Withybush General Hospital.

Figure 11.1 A DNAR ('do not attempt resuscitation') proforma. Reproduced with kind permission of Pembrokeshire and Derwen NHS Trust.

STANDARDS FOR CARDIOPULMONARY RESUSCITATION

The American Heart Association first published *'Standards for Cardiopulmonary Resuscitation and Emergency Cardiac Care'* in 1973. There was little evidence base for their recommendations, but they were generally followed around the world. In 1986, the Resuscitation Council of the United Kingdom was joined by a group representing five Nordic countries to produce guidelines more suited to European practice. The European Resuscitation Council (ERC) was officially established in 1989 as a multidisciplinary group representing many countries, and produced four sets of European guidelines between 1992 and 1998. Against this background, the International Liaison Committee On Resuscitation (ILCOR) was founded in 1992 with representatives from around the world, resulting in the first truly international guidelines in August 2000 (American Heart Association/ILCOR, 2000). These guidelines, which resulted from international consensus, have a stronger evidence base, but retain simplicity, and have at last achieved true international uniformity. The interpretation of these guidelines may differ in different countries due to local custom and availability of resources, but such differences are likely to be small, so standards will now be uniform throughout the world. Current guidelines issued by the Resuscitation Council (UK) may be viewed at http://www.resus.org.uk. Given that there is now international agreement, the contents of cardiac arrest boxes can be rationalised, and perhaps standardised with regard to content and appearance (Jowett et al, 2001).

PRINCIPLES OF RESUSCITATION

The basic principles of cardiopulmonary resuscitation (CPR) have arisen from research work over the last 40 years. The sequence of airway management, artificial respiration and external chest compression is now well established. Early manual methods of ventilation (e.g. Holger–Neilson) have been surpassed by expired air resuscitation methods ('mouth-to-mouth'), which have been shown to improve arterial oxygenation (Safar et al, 1958; Elam and Greene, 1961). Support of the arrested circulation has changed little since early descriptions by Kouwenhoven et al (1960) and Jude et al (1961), when it was believed that the heart was 'emptied' by being squeezed between the sternum and the thoracic spine. However, this 'cardiac pump' hypothesis assumes that the heart valves remain competent during external compression, which is not the case. Two-dimensional echocardiography has shown that the heart valves remain open, and there are no changes in left ventricular size, as might be expected were the heart acting as a pump (Rich et al, 1981). Although there is no difference in pressure within intrathoracic organs during compression, there is between intrathoracic and extrathoracic vessels. As a result, chest compression squeezes the heart and great vessels like a pump during external compression, propelling blood forwards by the production of an intermittent pressure gradient between the inside of the chest and the rest of the body (the 'thoracic pump' mechanism). The mitral and aortic valves remain open, and partial closure of the pulmonary valve, with collapse of the great veins, helps to prevent retrograde blood flow (Rudikoff et al, 1980). The heart fills passively on recoil. Active decompression has been studied with the hope of increasing negative intrathoracic pressure, and thus improving cardiac filling. However, active compression–decompression does not seem to be an improvement over conventional CPR (Stiell et al, 1996).

External chest compression only produces a cardiac output of about 25% of normal, which provides poor perfusion of the carotid and coronary arteries (Niemann, 1984), and hence methods to augment this have been sought. The term 'new CPR' has arisen following research into new techniques for improving blood flow during resuscitation (Varon and Fromm, 1993). These have included simultaneous chest compression and ventilation, abdominal compression with synchronised ventilation, interposed abdominal compression, continuous abdominal binding and unsynchronised CPR for intubated patients with continuous chest compressions at 100/min and 10–12 ventilations/min.

Abdominal binding or abdominal compression may help by raising intra-abdominal diastolic pressure within the aorta and promoting coronary and cerebral perfusion (Chandra et al, 1981). However, the central venous pressure is also elevated, and this may compromise coronary perfusion. Abdominal compression requires a third resuscitator, which might delay implementation of normal resuscitative measures, and may cause intra-abdominal trauma, including laceration of the liver. However, one small study did suggest that interposed abdominal compression may improve survival, and further trials need to be carried out (Sack et al, 1992).

Open chest cardiac massage has been practised since the 19th century and became the routine procedure until 1960, when closed chest compression was introduced. Access to the heart is via a left thoracotomy, which can be easily taught to and performed by those without formal surgical training. Despite open massage being probably more efficient, it is probably best reserved for cases with a recent sternotomy (following cardiac surgery), suspected cardiac tamponade or rigid chest walls, when external chest compression may be ineffective (Robertson and Holmberg, 1992).

DEFINITIONS AND AETIOLOGY OF CARDIAC ARREST

Cardiac arrest is the cessation of effective cardiac contraction, with a consequent and lethal fall in cardiac output. In clinical practice, this implies either ventricular standstill (asystole) or ventricular fibrillation, although there may be virtual circulatory arrest with profound bradycardias or ventricular tachycardia. Electromechanical dissociation describes a state in which normal electrical complexes continue to show on the ECG but there is no effective pulse or blood pressure. This is now referred to as pulseless electrical activity,

and may complicate many primary disorders, including cardiac rupture or tamponade, severe haemorrhage, pulmonary embolism and electrolyte imbalance.

The majority of cardiac arrests occur outside hospital, and 'sudden deaths' are usually due to ventricular dysrhythmias. Cardiac arrest may be due to problems arising within the heart (e.g. myocardial infarction) or elsewhere in the body (e.g. hypovolaemia, hypoxia or hyperkalaemia). Common precipitating causes are acute myocardial ischaemia, valvular heart disease (especially aortic stenosis), cardiomyopathy, chronic obstructive airways disease and drugs. In hospital, conditions commonly associated with cardiac arrest include myocardial infarction, pulmonary embolism, valvular heart disease, post-operative hypoxia and some investigative procedures.

Occasionally, there are warning signs preceding cardiac arrest, which experienced personnel can often recognise. In the monitored patient, certain rhythm disturbances, especially R-on-T ectopic beats, left ventricular ectopic beats and multifocal ectopic beats, have long been associated with the onset of ventricular fibrillation. Unfortunately, many cases of ventricular fibrillation occur with no warning.

There are two main phases of CPR:

- Basic life support (BLS)
- Advanced life support (ALS).

These form links on the chain of survival, which starts with early access, then BLS, early defibrillation and ALS.

BASIC LIFE SUPPORT

The main objective of CPR is to provide oxygen to the vital organs (brain, heart and kidneys) until spontaneous oxygenation returns or until definitive medical treatment (ALS) can be initiated. The lungs can withstand long periods of anoxia, although the heart and kidneys can only survive for 30 min before irreversible ischaemic changes result. Unfortunately, and perhaps crucially, the cerebral cortex can only withstand anoxia for about 5 min. The critical factor in BLS, therefore, is speed. This applies not only within hospital, but also in the community, where bystander resuscitation may be used to good effect (Myerburg et al, 1982).

BLS comprises an initial assessment, then airway maintenance, expired air ventilation (rescue breathing) and finally chest compression. The term 'basic life support' implies that there is no use of supportive equipment. If simple airways or face masks are used, the term 'BLS with airway adjunct' is used. BLS will occasionally reverse the cause of collapse, but more often it is a holding intervention until ALS can be instituted. The speed of application is vital, since irreversible anoxic brain damage may occur in as little as 3–4 min.

THE FIRST ABC OF BASIC LIFE SUPPORT

BLS has traditionally been taught by an ABC sequence of Airway, Breathing and Circulation. We teach our staff to precede this with another ABC as follows:

A: Ascertain arrest

An assessment phase is critical. This must start with ensuring the safety of rescuer and patient. The next stage is the recognition and confirmation of cardiopulmonary arrest. The alternative term 'assess responsiveness' is sometimes used.

Recognition

During cardiac arrest, there is ineffective mechanical activity of the heart, a reduced cardiac output and cerebral hypoperfusion. Loss of consciousness, apnoea (or gasping respiration) and loss of pulses occur within seconds. Other signs, such as cyanosis and dilatation of the pupils, take much longer and should not be awaited. Speed in initiating CPR is essential, and any delay may be fatal; a false alarm is better than a dead patient. Cardiac arrest does not necessarily reflect serious myocardial damage, but the neurones of the cerebral cortex undergo irreversible changes after 3–5 min. If prompt and efficient CPR is not started within

this time, permanent cerebral damage will occur. Hence, cardiac arrest must be assumed to have occurred with:

- Any sudden loss of consciousness
- Sudden onset of a seizure in a non-epileptic patient
- Sudden onset of cyanosis or respiratory distress.

Other underlying causes (e.g. syncope, cerebrovascular accidents, haemorrhage or epilepsy) may be responsible, but, if there is any doubt, CPR should be instituted immediately.

Confirmation

Immediate clinical assessment of a patient who has suffered a cardiac arrest will show:

- A rapidly deteriorating level of consciousness
- A change in skin colour: pallor or cyanosis
- Absence of a pulse (put an ear to the chest; time should not be wasted in trying to feel peripheral pulses)
- Absence of respiration (note that a spontaneous 'gasping' ineffective respiration may occur for a few minutes following circulatory arrest).

The international committee have de-emphasised the need for checking the carotid pulse to ascertain arrest. In normal volunteers following prolonged palpation, 45% of carotid pulses were pronounced absent (Priori et al, 2001). The term 'look for signs of circulation' is now preferred. If in doubt, resuscitation should be started.

B: Bang on chest

The precordial thump is not included in the current recommendations for BLS but should be considered by professional healthcare providers. Since this manoeuvre takes only a few seconds, and is only of value very early on (within 30 s of arrest), it is probably more relevant for mention here so that it may be employed by more experienced rescuers, particularly on coronary care units, where it may be used while the defibrillator is charging.

Schott, who terminated a Stokes–Adams attack with a precordial blow, reported using a precordial thump for restoring sinus rhythm in 1920. This method of restoring sinus rhythm was widely practised until it was suggested that such a manoeuvre might convert ventricular tachycardia to ventricular fibrillation. However, the potential benefit of the precordial thump to mechanically cardiovert ventricular fibrillation to sinus rhythm greatly outweighs its risks (Caldwell et al, 1985). About 40% of patients with ventricular tachycardia and 2% of patients with ventricular fibrillation will cardiovert into sinus rhythm. A similar mechanical stimulus may be given by raising the legs to promote venous return and may terminate ventricular tachycardia. Conscious patients with ventricular tachycardia may restore sinus rhythm by forceful coughing, and some patients can maintain cerebral circulation by repeated coughing (cough CPR). By using the pressure changes in the chest, coughing can produce arterial pressures of 100 mmHg, and gives scientific support to the thoracic-pump theory of chest compression in CPR (Criley et al, 1976).

C: Call for help

Once cardiac arrest is confirmed, help will be required for basic and advanced resuscitation: shout for immediate help and make sure that an 'arrest call' is put out. If there is no-one immediately available to fetch help, it is better to leave the victim to ensure help is coming, because it is a defibrillator that will save the life ('call first, call fast'). BLS is just a holding measure until it arrives.

THE SECOND ABC OF BASIC LIFE SUPPORT

The second ABC refers to the basic resuscitation skills of Airway clearance, initiating artificial Breathing and Circulation.

A: Airway

Effective CPR requires the patient to be supine and on a flat, firm surface. The head must not be raised above the level of the thorax, or the brain will not be perfused. Pillows and the backrest need to be removed, cot sides lowered and bed brakes engaged.

The most important initial action is to open the airway. In 90% of unconscious patients, the upper airway will be obstructed, usually by the tongue, which falls back into the pharynx when muscle tone is lost, allowing its supporting structure to relax. Since the tongue is attached to the lower jaw, moving the jaw forward will lift the tongue away from the back of the throat and open the airway. There are two main ways of opening the airway (Fig. 11.2):

1. *Head-tilt/chin-lift manoeuvre*. The head is tilted back by firm backward pressure on the patient's forehead with the palm of the hand. The fingers of the other hand are used to lift the chin forward so that the teeth almost close together. This supports the jaw and helps to hold the head back.

2. *Head-tilt/jaw-thrust*. The mandible is pulled forward by grasping the angle of the jaw on both

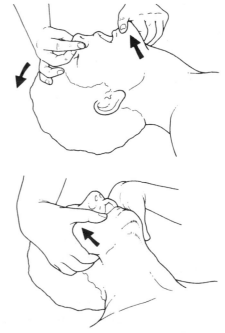

Figure 11.2 Opening the airway: the head-tilt/chin-lift and head-tilt/jaw-thrust methods.

sides and tilting the head back. This may be made easier if the rescuer's elbows are allowed to rest on the floor close to the patient's head.

The simplest method is the head-tilt/chin-lift method, although medically trained staff may find the head-tilt/jaw-thrust method more useful. The latter is technically more difficult and tiring, but is highly effective and especially useful if neck injury is suspected, since it may be used without hyperextending the neck.

B: Breathing

The absence of respiration is deduced by the lack of chest movement and by listening and feeling for expired air from the mouth and nose ('look–listen–feel'). The presence of vomit or foreign bodies (e.g. dentures) should be suspected if the airway is not cleared after proper positioning of the head and neck. The mouth should be checked for obvious obstruction, but, if none is found, the possibility of inhalation exists. The application of chest or abdominal thrusts is more efficient than traditional blows to the back for dislodging foreign bodies in the airway. BLS often needs to be instituted when equipment is not always to hand, and the use of mouth-to-mouth and mouth-to-nose respiration is of great emergency benefit. However, not only does the sight of vomit and blood usually deter the most hardened resuscitator, the theoretical transmission risks of serum hepatitis, herpes simplex and AIDS (the acquired immune deficiency syndrome) have now also to be contended with. Nevertheless, delay should not be allowed to occur, since there is still very little evidence of disease transmission during mouth-to-mouth ventilation. Most cases of cardiac arrest occur at home, and the previous health of the victim is often known. Within hospital, the number of occasions upon which any individual is called to administer mouth-to-mouth ventilation is few, and again the health of the patient is usually known.

Mouth-to-mouth ventilation should be started immediately and may be made easier with an oropharyngeal airway. While maintaining the airway using the head-tilt/chin-lift technique, the nose is pinched, and one or two slow breaths are delivered in succession (2 s each), with the lips sealed over the patient's mouth. It is almost impossible to inflate the lungs in under a second, and attempts at faster inflation simply force air down the oesophagus, leading to gastric dilatation, which promotes vomiting and limits full expansion of the lungs. The chest should be observed for equal and satisfactory movements, and expiration of air should be heard when the chest falls. If these do not occur, the airway is obstructed and should be cleared. Subsequent inflation of the patient's lungs should be slow, to minimise pressure on the pharynx and hence reduce the risk of gastric dilatation. The expired volume should be approximately 700–1000 ml in an adult, which is enough just to raise the chest visibly (Wenzel et al, 2001). The normal adult tidal volume is 400 ml, and the forced vital capacity is 4500 ml (3200 ml in women), so that it can be seen that a full, forced expiration is not required, but rather a slow exhalation, following a quick intake of breath. Each sequence of 10 breaths should take between 40 and 60 s; however, timing is not important, and it is best to wait for the chest to fall.

Mouth-to-nose respiration may be more effective than mouth-to-mouth ventilation and is associated with a lower incidence of regurgitation of gastric contents. It is, additionally, of great value in cases of oral trauma or trismus. The mouth is sealed around the patient's nose, and ventilation is carried out as previously described.

C: Circulation

Circulatory arrest may be assessed by palpation of the carotid artery, which lies in the groove between the trachea and the sternomastoid (strap) muscles in the neck. However, the assessment of the carotid pulse at times of high drama is time-consuming and leads to an incorrect conclusion (present or absent) in half of all cases. Peripheral pulses should not be used, as low-output states may masquerade as cardiac arrest. If there are no signs of circulation, or if there is uncertainty, and the precordial thump is unsuccessful, external chest compression should be started.

External chest compression

The application of compressions over the lower half of the sternum has been used to effect artificial circulation for over 40 years (Kouwenhoven et al, 1960). The heel of the hand nearest the patient's head is placed over the lower half of the sternum, and the other hand is placed over the top, with the fingers either extended or interlocked (but not in contact with the chest). Pressure of the fingers on the ribs or lateral pressure increases the possibility of rib fractures or costochondral separation. The arms should be kept straight, with the elbows locked, so that pumping action is delivered in a straight line from the shoulders by pivoting at the hips to depress the sternum 4–5 cm in adults.

Compressions should be smooth, regular and uninterrupted, at a rate 100/min. Although some studies have suggested using 'high-impulse CPR', with compression rates of over 120/min, this is very difficult to achieve or maintain in practice (Maier et al, 1986).

At the end of each compression, relaxation must be complete, to allow adequate refilling of the thoracic pump, although the hands should not lose contact with the patient in case the correct position is lost. Applying cardiac massage at the wrong site may lead to laceration of the liver, fractured ribs, pneumothorax or lung contusion.

The ratio of 15 compressions to 2 breaths is used. As the chances of restoring cardiac rhythm without defibrillation are remote, time should not be wasted in trying to assess the pulse. Resuscitation must be continuous, rhythmic and uninterrupted. If, however, the patient tries to breathe spontaneously, or moves, the pulse should be assessed; this should not take more than 10 s. An algorithm for BLS is shown in Fig. 11.3.

THE NEXT STEPS

The design of BLS does not require the use of equipment, although the highest priority must be given to early defibrillation. The use of other adjuncts is useful, although not so critical, and basic resuscitation should never be neglected because of the absence of medical aids. Once instituted, therapy should be continued until admission to a specialist unit or until a decision is made for life support to be terminated.

The arrival of help should, ideally, lead to advanced resuscitative measures. These include:

- Securing an airway (preferably with an endotracheal tube)
- Augmentation of oxygenation with portable oxygen
- Recognition of cardiac rhythms with an ECG
- Treatment of dysrhythmias with drugs and electrical defibrillation
- Cardiovascular stabilisation to allow transport of the patient to a high-dependency unit.

ADVANCED LIFE SUPPORT

Advanced life support (ALS) combines basic life support (BLS) with the use of specialist techniques and equipment for maintaining circulation and respiration. The key components are:

- Early defibrillation
- Ensuring an adequate airway
- Establishing intravenous access
- ECG monitoring
- Pharmacological therapy.

AIRWAY MANAGEMENT

The airway can be cleared in most patients by correct positioning of the head and neck, and suction. However, securing the airway and improving oxygenation are vital. Expired air has a fractional inspired oxygen (FiO_2) of only about 0.16, so that enrichment with portable oxygen is highly desirable. All airways should use 100% oxygen wherever possible (FiO_2 of 1.0). Oropharyngeal airways should be used only in unconscious patients, as they may otherwise induce vomiting. Care and practice is required for correct insertion, or the tongue may be dis-

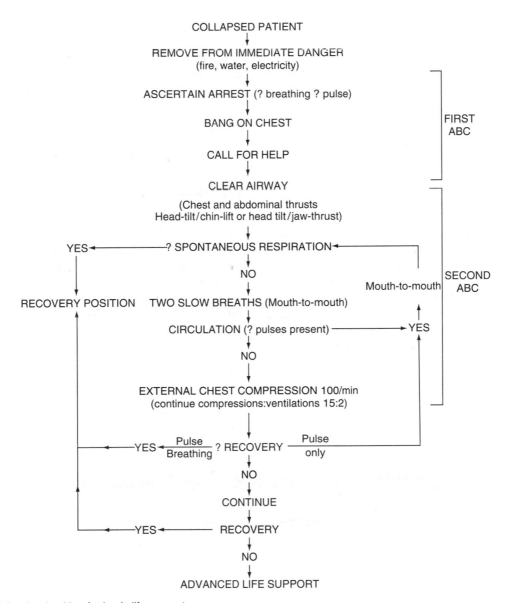

Figure 11.3 An algorithm for basic life support.

placed backwards into the pharynx and obstruct the airway.

Self-inflating bag–valve–mask units can deliver higher oxygen concentrations providing an oxygen reservoir is used ($FiO_2 > 0.6$), but most people accept that successful application needs two people to be effective. One rescuer maintains the jaw-thrust position and ensures a tight seal between the mask and the patient's face, while the other inflates the lungs by squeezing the bag with a tidal volume of 700–1000 ml delivered over 2 s. Once supplementary oxygen is attached, the tidal volume can be reduced to 400–600 ml.

Laerdal pocket masks are extremely effective for mouth-to-mask ventilation and should be carried by all would-be resuscitators. In hospital, where oxygen is readily available, an oxygen inlet nipple enables increased oxygen concentrations to be dispensed. For a single rescuer, the pocket mask is superior to the bag–valve–mask unit in all but the most experienced hands.

The main disadvantage of mask ventilation is gastric distension, leading to diaphragmatic splinting and oesophageal regurgitation.

Alternatives to tracheal intubation

Because of the difficulties associated with laryngoscopy and intubation, simpler methods of securing an airway have been investigated. The introduction of the oesophageal obturator and oesophageal gastric tube airways (Jowett and Thompson, 1988b) have led to more promising devices, such as the oesophageal tracheal double-lumen airway (Combitube) and laryngeal mask airway (LMA). These devices have specific problems regarding placement and use, and require more training. The LMA device consists of a plain flexible tube with a distal inflatable silicone ring diagonally attached (Fig. 11.4). The ring is designed to obliterate the hypopharynx and oesophageal isthmus, achieving a low-pressure seal between the tube and trachea and reducing the risk of gastric regurgitation and

aspiration. The use of any ventilatory devices that imperfectly protect the patient's airway should be avoided wherever possible, and any preliminary steps should be converted to endotracheal intubation as soon as possible. The LMA may have an important role in those unskilled in endotracheal intubation, and even as an alternative in cases of difficult intubation because of anatomical problems (Baskett, 2001).

Endotracheal intubation

The best means of securing and maintaining an airway is endotracheal intubation. This ensures delivery of high concentrations of oxygen and provides an alternative route for drug administration. The procedure requires skill, which can only be gained by practice. Repeated attempts to intubate should not be made by unskilled operators, and the maximum interruption in ventilation should be 30 s. Endotracheal tubes are labelled with the internal diameter in millimetres and should be cut to appropriate lengths. Female patients will require the 7.0–8.0 mm size, and male patients the 8.0–9.0 mm size. Passage of the tube may sometimes be aided by external

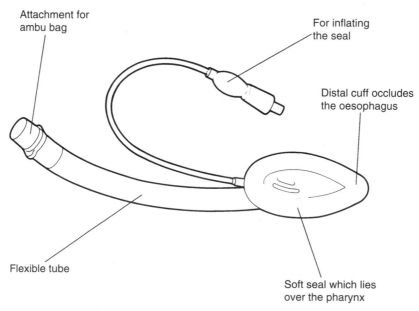

Figure 11.4 The laryngeal mask airway.

pressure on the cricoid cartilage (the Sellick manoeuvre), which occludes the upper part of the oesophagus and prevents aspiration of gastric contents (Sellick, 1961).

After intubation, the position of the tube should be verified by watching for equal expansion of both sides of the chest and listening over the lungs with a stethoscope. Ventilation should be about 12–15 inflations/min and can be performed independently of chest compression.

INTRAVENOUS ACCESS

Intravenous access is essential for the administration of fluids and drugs. Peripheral lines are the simplest, since the veins are easily seen, despite their tendency to collapse following cardiac arrest. The site of choice is the antecubital fossa, since cannulation of the subclavian and neck veins needs practice and may require a temporary halt of CPR. Peripheral administration of drugs may cause significant delay (1–2 min) in arrival at the heart, even with optimal external cardiac massage. Drugs administered peripherally should be followed by a flush with at least 20 ml of 0.9% saline. A central line provides the optimal route for delivering drugs into the central circulation, but placement may be difficult and could cause complications. If skills and equipment are available, an additional central line is often very useful, since the larger veins will allow faster infusion of fluids and drugs into the central circulation, and may additionally be used for transvenous pacing, if required.

Regardless of the aetiology of the arrest, increased vascular permeability allows plasma proteins and water to pass into the extravascular spaces, leading to intravascular hypovolaemia. However, caution is advised in routinely administering large volumes, since cerebral and myocardial blood flow may be diminished. Expansion of circulating blood volume is, of course, critical in patients with severe acute blood loss, and cardiac arrest in these patients is often marked by pulseless electrical activity (see below).

CARDIAC MONITORING

Most sudden deaths are due to malignant ventricular dysrhythmias, especially in the early period following myocardial infarction, when rhythm disturbances are usually abrupt and without warning. ECG monitoring should be established as soon as possible in all patients following myocardial infarction or sudden collapse (Jowett et al, 1985).

Heart rhythms associated with cardiac arrest may be broadly divided into two groups:

- Ventricular fibrillation/pulseless ventricular tachycardia
- Pulseless electrical activity and asystole.

However, there are other serious dysrhythmias that may be precursors of cardiac arrest or associated with a critical fall in cardiac output (e.g. profound bradycardia or paroxysmal ventricular tachycardia).

Arrest rhythms

Ventricular fibrillation/pulseless ventricular tachycardia

Ventricular fibrillation (VF) is the most common arrest dysrhythmia in adults. A period of ventricular tachycardia (VT), or other dysrhythmias may precede it. There is a total breakdown of ordered electrical activity within the heart, and contraction of individual myocardial fibres is random and independent. The generated work is counter-productive, and cardiac output falls dramatically. The ECG shows random waves, which will usually diminish into asystole if left untreated. Consciousness is lost within 20 s. Although there is co-ordinated muscle activity during pulseless VT, the ventricles are beating too fast to sustain a cardiac output. In the context of cardiac arrest, the rhythm does not differ effectively from VF.

Asystole

Asystole is characterised by ventricular standstill due to suppression of the cardiac pacemakers by myocardial disease, anoxia, electrolyte imbalance or drugs. Strong cholinergic activity may depress the sinus and atrioventricular (AV) nodes following myocardial infarction or episodes of myocardial ischaemia.

Asystole may occur without warning, or may be preceded by various types of heart block, and is found in about 25% of hospital cardiac arrest (10% outside hospital). It often represents massive cardiac damage and sometimes appears as the last dying rhythm of the heart following prolonged VF. Survival is less than 4%. The ECG shows a flat trace, which must be differentiated from fine VF or, sometimes, from faulty connection of the leads and monitor. Asystole must be confirmed by checking the leads, checking the gain and viewing the rhythm through two separate leads. If there is any doubt over whether the rhythm may be fine VF, VF should be assumed and treated by defibrillation. Shocking a heart in asystole will not worsen the situation.

Pulseless electrical activity

Previously known as electromechanical dissociation, pulseless electrical activity (PEA) is characterised by regular complexes on the ECG in the presence of circulatory failure. It may complicate anoxia, hypovolaemia, tension pneumothorax, severe acidosis or pulmonary embolism, and the patient's best chances of survival depend upon identification and treatment of the underlying problem. The occurrence of PEA following myocardial infarction usually signifies a terminal event, such as rupture of the heart or cardiac tamponade.

PEA is rare outside hospital practice, but occurs in about 5% of hospital cardiac arrests. The prognosis is very poor.

TREATMENT OF CARDIAC ARREST

The treatment of cardiac arrest requires identification of any potential or aggravating factors, and re-establishing cardiorespiratory function. The UK Resuscitation Council suggests four 'H's and four 'T's to help resuscitators consider potentially reversible causes:

- Hypoxia
- Hypovolaemia
- Hyperkalaemia (hypocalcaemia, acidaemia)
- Hypothermia.

- Tension pneumothorax
- Tamponade
- Toxins
- Thrombo-embolism

The outcome from non-VF/VT rhythms is poor unless underlying precipitants are detected and treated. For VF/VT arrests, the chances of successful resuscitation depend on the speed of defibrillation. Effective myocardial function depends on the co-ordinated contraction of myocardial fibres. VF is the extreme example of disorganisation, which will result in death due to total abolition of cardiac output. Prompt therapy is mandatory. There are essentially two methods of restoring normal cardiac rhythm: electrical and pharmacological. Defibrillation is the cornerstone of advanced resuscitation (Zoll et al, 1956), and the earlier this is performed, the more likely sinus rhythm is to result. Any delay allows further myocardial ischaemia, anoxia and acidaemia, which will inhibit the restoration of normal rhythm. Defibrillation should, therefore, be carried out with or without ECG confirmation of VF.

Defibrillation

The defibrillator basically consists of a large capacitor for storing electrical energy and two conductive paddles for delivering this energy to the heart. The energy delivered is usually measured in joules (volts × amps × time) and is displayed on a meter. The pulse width is usually fixed at 3 ms and is not variable. The shock is delivered by the two hand-held paddles, which are well insulated. Two buttons are usually built into the handles of the paddles for delivery of the defibrillating shock; both must be pressed to prevent inadvertent defibrillation. In most machines, these paddles can act simultaneously as electrodes for ECG monitoring and, when not transmitting electricity to the patient, can convey the electrical activity within the heart back to a conventional oscilloscope to show the cardiac rhythm ('quick-look paddles').

Solid conducting gel pads should be placed directly onto the skin to improve contact. Paddle position is important, in order to maximise the energy delivered to the heart. Standard placement is shown in Fig. 11.5a, with one paddle placed to the right of the upper sternum inferior

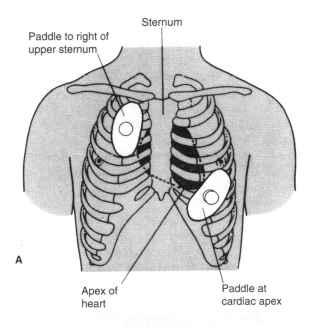

A

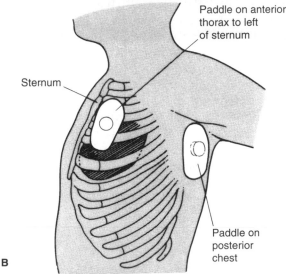

B

Figure 11.5 Positioning of defibrillation paddles.

to the clavicle over the 2nd–3rd intercostal space, with the other to the left of the nipple, with the centre of the paddle in the mid-axillary line. Successful defibrillation requires depolarisation of a critical mass of myocardium, which is more likely to be achieved if the paddles are placed correctly. Incorrect positioning means that a greater proportion of the charge will not pass through the heart, and will associate with failed defibrillation. Observational studies suggest that paddles are not positioned correctly during defibrillation in many cases (Heames et al, 2001).

The paddles should be placed firmly against the skin with at least 25 lb (about 10 kg) of pressure, to prevent loss of current. Obese patients have increased transthoracic resistance, and the *apicoposterior* position may be more useful, particularly for elective cardioversion (Fig. 11.5b). Here, one paddle is placed at the cardiac apex, and the other to the right of the spine (which would otherwise prevent good skin contact), below the scapula (Ewy, 1994). Transthoracic resistance can also be overcome by using higher energies or multiple discharges, or by shortening the intervals between shocks (Kerber et al, 1981).

The amount of energy required to restore sinus rhythm without producing myocardial damage is very difficult to calculate and depends upon such variables as paddle size and position, blood pH and drugs. The sequence of energies is now conventional (200 J, 200 J, 360 J), unless using defibrillators with alternative waveforms. Repeated biphasic shocks at less than 200 J have an equivalent or higher success for defibrillation than monophasic waveforms of increasing energy.

The rationale for starting at lower energies was originally based upon the slow charging speed of older equipment. This is no longer a problem with modern equipment, and all units must have defibrillators that can recharge rapidly and must be capable of delivering the first three shocks within 30–45 s. Starting the sequence at a lower energy level is retained in current guidelines, since a balance between successful defibrillation and myocardial damage may be important. A defibrillation algorithm is shown in Fig. 11.6. The operator should stand well clear of the patient and bed and ensure that colleagues do too. This

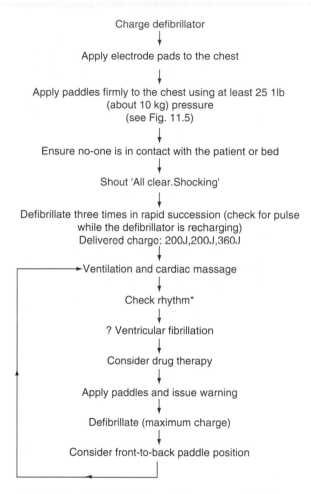

Charge defibrillator
↓
Apply electrode pads to the chest
↓
Apply paddles firmly to the chest using at least 25 1lb
(about 10 kg) pressure
(see Fig. 11.5)
↓
Ensure no-one is in contact with the patient or bed
↓
Shout 'All clear.Shocking'
↓
Defibrillate three times in rapid succession (check for pulse
while the defibrillator is recharging)
Delivered charge: 200J,200J,360J
↓
Ventilation and cardiac massage
↓
Check rhythm*
↓
? Ventricular fibrillation
↓
Consider drug therapy
↓
Apply paddles and issue warning
↓
Defibrillate (maximum charge)
↓
Consider front-to-back paddle position

* Note that a brief period of asytole is common following
defibrillation. No therapy other than basic life support is
required or further ventricular fibrillation may be induced.

Figure 11.6   Procedure for defibrillation.

applies especially to the anaesthetist, who may be hand-ventilating the patient.

Automatic and semi-automatic defibrillators

Because two of the best predictors of survival of cardiac arrest are time to defibrillation and initial rhythm, decreasing the time to defibrillation will increase survival rates. The chances of successful defibrillation decline by about 7–10% with each minute. Although BLS helps to sustain a shockable rhythm, it is the time to the first defibrillatory shock that is critical, and logistic problems limit this. Automatic external defibrillators (AEDs)

were designed and developed for paramedical staff, but have been shown to be useful in other circumstances (Cummins et al, 1986). For example, using a defibrillator in semi-automatic mode may be more rapid than a fully manual machine. Rather than using traditional 'paddles', large adhesive chest pads are applied; these can both monitor heart rhythm and, additionally, conduct a defibrillatory shock to the patient. A computer decides whether or not a shock should be delivered, based upon the recorded cardiac rhythm. This is delivered either automatically or semi-automatically, when it is up to the operator whether to discharge the defibrillator. Energy levels are usually preset, and warning buzzers sound to make sure that no one is in contact with the patient at the time of defibrillation. A manual override facility is required in case the machine misinterprets dysrhythmias such as ventricular flutter, allowing operator-instituted defibrillation.

Following the introduction of AEDs in Scottish front-line ambulances, it has become clear that this system can be easily and effectively introduced for out-of-hospital cardiac arrest since ambulance technicians can defibrillate without the need for full paramedic training. Of 1476 patients admitted to a hospital ward following cardiac arrest treated by AEDs, about 40% were discharged without major neurological disability (Cobbe et al, 1996). AEDs also have an educational role for 'showing' the decision-making process, to help the confidence of new resuscitators. There has been an expanding role of AEDs to first responders not trained in ALS, including the general public. The operator simply has to check that there is no pulse, place the device on the patient, and turn it on. It senses cardiac rhythm, and if identified as VT or VF delivers a shock. Operators therefore need little training. A meta-analysis of seven prospective studies of AEDs found an 8.5% reduction in relative risk with early defibrillation by emergency medical technicians compared with BLS alone (Auble et al, 1995).

Drug therapy

The value of drug therapy for treatment of cardiac arrest is probably minimal, and the importance of BLS with early defibrillation cannot be stressed enough. In recent years, numerous controversies have arisen about whether pharmacological intervention is required at all and, if it is, about the optimal route for delivery (Gonzales, 1993; Jaffe, 1993).

Pharmacological intervention may be used during cardiac arrests to:

- Correct hypoxia and acidosis
- Accelerate or reduce the heart rate
- Suppress ectopic activity
- Stimulate the strength of myocardial contraction.

Because of the haemodynamic changes during CPR, the administration of drugs into the central circulation is preferable, although gaining access is often difficult and should not be allowed to hinder BLS or defibrillation.

Adrenaline (epinephrine)

Adrenaline (epinephrine) has strong alpha- and beta-adrenergic agonist activity, with a powerful vasoconstrictor action. When used with effective chest compressions, adrenaline (epinephrine) produces peripheral vasoconstriction, which helps divert blood to the brain and coronary vessels. The beta-agonist properties (positive chronotropic and inotropic effects) help myocardial function following attainment of sinus rhythm. Experimentally, vasopressin (40 U) leads to higher coronary perfusion pressures, and has been suggested as an alternative to adrenaline (epinephrine).

Adrenaline (epinephrine) is the first drug given for all types of cardiac arrest. The recommended dose in adults is 1 mg (10 ml of a 1:10 000 solution), which may be repeated every 2–3 min.

Sodium bicarbonate

With effective BLS, deterioration in blood gases and pH is slow in previously well patients. With prolonged resuscitation, particularly in those who may have been unwell prior to cardiac arrest, efforts to combat the metabolic acidosis that accompanies poor tissue perfusion is needed. Acidosis result from the build-up of lactic acid, and with increased levels of carbon dioxide depresses myocardial contractility, produces vasodilatation and capillary leakage, inhibits catecholamine activity and increases the likelihood of dysrhythmias.

Intravenous sodium bicarbonate has been widely used in the past for correcting the metabolic acidosis during cardiac arrest, but there is little evidence that this therapy improves outcome. Hence, routine administration of sodium bicarbonate is no longer recommended because of the frequent occurrence of deleterious side-effects, including increasing carbon dioxide levels, hypernatraemia, inactivation of concurrently administered catecholamines, and tissue necrosis if accidentally given extravascularly.

Critically ill patients in hospital may warrant early therapy with sodium bicarbonate if there is developing hyperkalaemia or acidosis that might precede a cardiac arrest, but these occasions are now the exception rather than the rule.

When given, small aliquots should used (50 mmol) to patients in one of the following groups:

- Severe acidosis (pH < 7.1)
- Cardiac arrest associated with hyperkalaemia
- Cardiac arrest associated with tricyclic antidepressant overdose
- Blind administration after prolonged resuscitation (10–20 min).

The principal method of correcting acidosis is by establishing adequate alveolar ventilation. Hyperventilation corrects respiratory acidosis by removing carbon dioxide, which freely diffuses across cell membranes. Optimal oxygenation, ventilation and airway control are, therefore, vital.

Antidysrhythmic agents

When considering these drugs, there are certain basic principles:

- Immediate treatment will depend upon whether the patient is stable or unstable
- Cardioversion is preferable in most cases, and especially if the patient is unstable

- All drugs used for treating dysrhythmias are potentially pro-arrhythmic
- Most drugs impair myocardial function
- Cocktails of different agents are dangerous; if one drug fails, cardioversion is the next best option.

Amiodarone

Amiodarone (300 mg) may be considered in VF and pulseless VT refractory to the initial three defibrillatory shocks (Kudenchuk et al, 1999). The initial dose should be diluted to a volume of 20 ml with 5% dextrose, and may be given by a peripheral vein. Pre-filled syringes are available. This initial dose may be followed by a further 150 mg followed by an infusion of 1 mg/min for 6 h and then 0.5 mg/min to a maximum of 2 g in 24 h.

Magnesium

Magnesium (8 mmol) should be given for refractory VF if there is any suspicion of hypomagnesaemia. This may be assumed if patients have been taking potassium-losing diuretics.

Lidocaine (lignocaine)

Lidocaine (lignocaine) has been used for many years for the control of ventricular dysrhythmias complicating cardiac arrest and myocardial infarction. Its major action during cardiac arrest is to inhibit the initiation of re-entry dysrhythmias in the ischaemic myocardium, but its use makes defibrillation more difficult. Its routine use is now discouraged, unless amiodarone is not available. Lidocaine (lignocaine) should not be given in addition to amiodarone. When used, bolus therapy at a dose of 0.5 mg/kg every 10 min is usual. Reduced hepatic circulation may make lidocaine (lignocaine) toxicity more likely, and no more than 3 mg/kg should be administered.

Procainamide

This is an alternative to amiodarone, but is seldom used in Europe.

Bretylium

Bretylium is no longer recommended.

Atropine

Atropine lowers vagal tone, although its value after the first few minutes following cardiac arrest is unclear, since significant vagotonia is unlikely to be present. However, a single dose of 3 mg is still recommended in asystolic and bradycardiac arrest, to ensure that vagal tone is fully blocked. Repeat doses should be avoided, since they may reduce the electrical stability of the heart, making VF more likely (Cooper and Abinader, 1979). For symptomatic bradycardia, aliquots of 500 µg may be given to a total dose of 3 mg. Otherwise, transcutaneous pacing should be employed, or an infusion of adrenaline (epinephrine) 1–10 µg/min intravenously while transvenous pacing is being arranged. This has replaced isoprenaline because supplies of this drug are limited.

Transbronchial administration of drugs

Adrenaline (epinephrine) can also be given transbronchially via the endotracheal tube in two to three times the intravenous dose, diluted with 5–10 ml of water. Lidocaine (lignocaine) can also be given in this way; its onset of action is as rapid as an intravenous bolus, and its effect is twice as long. Other agents that can be given transbronchially are atropine and naloxone. Bicarbonate, calcium carbonate, amiodarone and noradrenaline (norepinephrine) must not be given via the endotracheal tube, as they are very irritant to the tissues. Drug absorption from the bronchial tree is erratic and impaired by pulmonary oedema, atelectasis and, perhaps, the drugs themselves; for example, adrenaline (epinephrine) causes local vasoconstriction. After instillation, five inflations should be given to aid distribution and absorption. Intracardiac adrenaline (epinephrine) is no longer recommended, since major complications may occur, including coronary laceration, pericardial effusion and tamponade.

THE RESUSCITATION ALGORITHM

The ALS resuscitation algorithm assumes that the preceding step has been unsuccessful. The precordial thump may be considered in witnessed arrests, or in monitored VF, and should be used rather than BLS. BLS should be instituted if the defibrillator arrival is delayed or if the defibrillator is not charging fast enough (Jowett and Thompson, 1988a). The next important step is to assess the rhythm by attachment to a monitor. The treatment pathways essentially follow one of two directions: VF/VT arrest, or non-VT/VF arrest (Fig. 11.7).

The treatment of VF/VT arrests

Spontaneous reversion from VF is rare, and immediate defibrillation gives the best chance of restoring normal rhythm in VF/VT arrests. The speed with which this is done is critical, and it should be given highest priority. Although successful defibrillation can take place for several minutes following cardiac arrest, the chances of success and favourable outcome are considerably reduced if the first shock is delayed by as little as 90 s, with the chances diminishing by 7–10% for every minute.

The three initial shocks (200 J, 200 J, 360 J) are now conventional and should be given in rapid succession, since this will lower transthoracic resistance and hence maximise energy delivery to the heart. If VT/VF persists, further shocks are given at 360 J or the biphasic equivalent. It should be possible, with modern equipment, to deliver the first three shocks within 30–45 s, and BLS between shocks is not necessary. These shocks may therefore be given without removing the paddles from the chest. The ECG rhythm should be checked between shocks, although there may be a brief delay for the ECG tracing to return. There is often a period of electromechanical stunning, resulting in an isoelectric line on the ECG trace. This does not mean that the rhythm has converted to asystole, or coordinated rhythm. If it persists for more than one sweep of the monitor screen, further chest compressions should be given.

At this point, a brief attempt to intubate the patient and obtain intravenous access should be made. Neither procedure should interfere with BLS or further defibrillation shocks; 15–20 s is perhaps the maximum time allowable.

If normal rhythm has not returned after the initial three shocks, the chances of recovery are less than 20%. If appropriate, continuing resuscitation must change priorities to preserving cerebral and myocardial perfusion. This is best done by administration of adrenaline (epinephrine), combined with BLS. The VF algorithm, therefore, enters a loop, which includes administration of 1 mg of adrenaline (epinephrine) every 3 min, further ventilation and further shocks (all now at 360 J). The time interval between the third and fourth shocks should not exceed 2 min. Palpation of the pulse is restricted to the start of each loop (i.e. after every third defibrillation). During this time, it is important that potential causes or aggravating factors, such as toxins or electrolyte imbalance, are considered. Antidysrhythmic agents may be considered after the first two sets of three shocks.

Torsade de pointes is a polymorphic VT associated with a prolonged QT interval and is characterised by gradual alteration in the amplitude and direction of the electrical activity. Antidysrhythmic drugs, many of which prolong the QT interval, often cause it. Treatment is as for VF if the patient is compromised; intravenous magnesium sulphate may be useful. Atrial pacing or isoprenaline infusion may also be used.

The treatment of non-VT/VF rhythms

If VF/VT has been excluded, defibrillation is not indicated as a primary intervention. Fine VF may often appear as asystole, so that a defibrillatory shock should always be considered. If an additional monitor lead is connected, the rhythm can be checked in two leads, and if 'quick-look' paddles are being used, they should be rotated through 90° to confirm the rhythm. The detection and treatment of underlying causes of non-VT/VF arrests is much more important, because, without this intervention, outlook is very poor (10–15% survival). While these are being

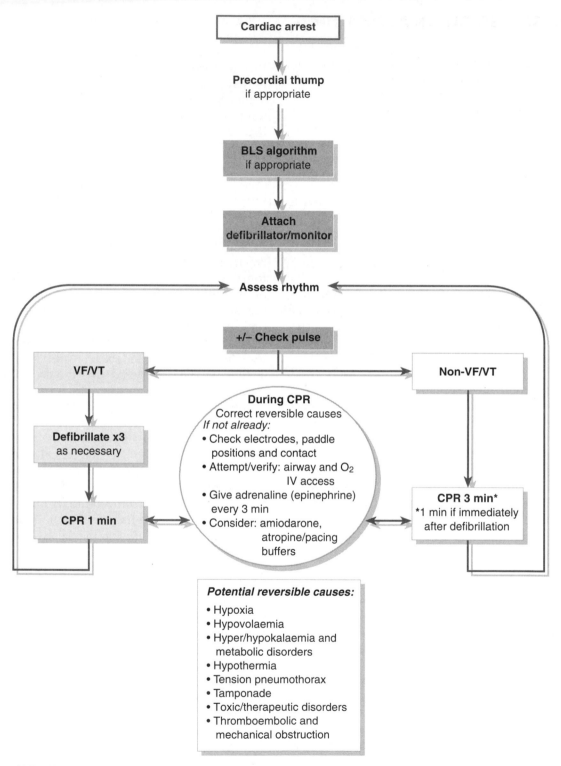

Figure 11.7 Algorithm for management of cardiac arrest.

considered, BLS with adrenaline (epinephrine) 1 mg intravenously every 3 min is recommended. Atropine 3 mg is recommended as a single intravenous dose at the end of the first CPR cycle.

Pacing is perhaps a more logical approach to treating asystole if there is evidence of atrial activity, which may indicate trifascicular block. The occasional QRS complex may also give some hope of the successful use of pacing, which may be carried out transoesophageally, transvenously or transthoracically. Pacing is usually ineffective if the arrest is due to extensive myocardial damage. External cardiac percussion ('fist' or 'thump' pacing) may generate QRS complexes with cardiac output if cardiac contractility is not severely compromised (Dowdle, 1996). This involves softer blows over the heart (not the sternum) at 100/min. Conventional CPR should be instituted if QRS complexes and an output are obtained.

If there is no sign of activity after initial resuscitation, further loops may be considered, but recovery is very rare.

The prognosis of PEA (pulseless electrical activity) is equally grave, and an aggressive search for possible underlying causes should be made. These include severe acidosis, hypoxia, hypovolaemia, tension pneumothorax, cardiac tamponade and pulmonary embolus. Calcium may help, especially if the QRS complex is widened to greater than 0.12 s (Camm, 1986). Sodium bicarbonate may be needed if there is severe acidosis.

Peri-arrest dysrhythmias

Dysrhythmias in the peri-arrest period may need treatment to prevent recurrent cardiac arrest or to obtain haemodynamic stability after resuscitation. The choice of treatment depends on the nature of the dysrhythmia and the overall status of the patient. The presence or absence of adverse signs or symptoms will dictate the appropriate treatment for most rhythm disturbances.

Treatment is usually advised if there is excess tachycardia or bradycardia, and particularly if there is evidence of low cardiac output or heart failure. Oxygen is always needed in the peri-arrest period, and close attention should be paid to the correction of electrolyte abnormalities.

The major peri-arrest dysrhythmias are:

- Atrial fibrillation
- Other narrow-complex tachycardias
- Broad-complex tachycardias
- Excess bradycardia.

Atrial fibrillation/atrial flutter

The two main consequences of atrial fibrillation or atrial flutter are an adverse haemodynamic effect and the increased risk of thromboembolism. Patients who have been in atrial fibrillation for more than 24 h may have an atrial thrombus, which could embolise as sinus rhythm is restored. It is therefore preferable to control the ventricular rate, and not attempt to restore sinus rhythm. The heart rate may be slowed with beta-blockers, verapamil, diltiazem or digoxin, and elective cardioversion should not be attempted until the patient has been anticoagulated for a period of 3–4 weeks.

If the onset of the atrial fibrillation is known to be within the last 24 h, the patient may be heparinised and an attempt made to restore sinus rhythm using amiodarone 300 mg over 1 h, repeated once if necessary. Synchronised DC cardioversion is an alternative.

If the patient is haemodynamically compromised, the approach depends upon the ventricular rate, and the degree of haemodynamic upset. In those with mild symptoms, and a ventricular rate under 150 beats/min, rate control may be enough. However, if the ventricular response is over 150 beats/min, particularly if there is chest pain, there should be immediate heparinisation and attempted cardioversion with a synchronised DC shock. If attempted cardioversion fails or the atrial fibrillation recurs, amiodarone 300 mg can be given intravenously over 1 h before a further attempt at cardioversion. A second dose of 300 mg amiodarone can be given if necessary.

Narrow-complex tachycardias

Narrow-complex tachycardias, which associate with haemodynamic collapse, should undergo immediate synchronised cardioversion.

If the tachycardia is being tolerated, vagal manoeuvres may terminate the tachycardia in up to 25% of cases. Carotid sinus massage should not be attempted by the unskilled. Strong vagal manoeuvres may cause a sudden and profound bradycardia. This may in turn trigger VF in the context of acute ischaemia. A case report in 1985 speculated that carotid sinus massage might cause disruption of atheromatous carotid plaques (Bastulli and Orlowski, 1985). As a result, the UK Resuscitation Council advises caution in patients with carotid bruits. However, significant carotid stenoses may occur in the absence of a bruit, so perhaps caution is required, particularly in the elderly, but there is no proof that carotid massage causes stroke. Interestingly, the patient described in the case report had no evidence of carotid disease at angiography!

Probably a safer vagal stimulant is the Valsalva manoeuvre (forced expiration against a closed glottis). This manoeuvre is sometimes hard to explain, and even harder to get patients to perform. It thus has a low success rate in clinical practice. Asking patients to blow up a balloon is probably helpful, and perhaps balloons should be kept on the resuscitation trolley.

If vagal stimulation is unsuccessful, the drug of first choice is adenosine (Camm et al, 1992). It should be given as a rapid bolus into a fast running intravenous infusion, or followed by a saline flush. An initial 6-mg dose may be followed by up to three doses each of 12 mg every 1–2 min. Patients should be warned of transient unpleasant side-effects, in particular nausea, flushing and chest discomfort. It should not be given to patients with asthma, patients on dipyridamole or carbamazepine. Esmolol, verapamil, amiodarone or digoxin are second-line choices.

Broad-complex tachycardia

Broad-complex tachycardias in the peri-arrest period should be assumed to be ventricular in origin. If there is no pulse, defibrillation should be carried out immediately, followed by the usual protocol for VF/VT cardiac arrest.

In the presence of a pulse, cardioversion is often the best option, which can be carried out semi-electively. It is the best option if there is chest pain, breathlessness, hypotension and cardiac failure.

Following appropriate sedation, synchronised cardioversion should be attempted with increasing monophasic energies of 100 J, 200 J and 360 J, or the biphasic equivalent. Further cardioversion can be undertaken if necessary. In refractory cases, amiodarone 150 mg may be given intravenously, or overdrive pacing can be considered.

If the patient is stable, drug therapy may be considered as first-line. Amiodarone 150 mg intravenously over 10 min is the best option. Amiodarone should be administered preferably through a central line, but in more urgent cases it should be given through a peripheral line because the significant risk of causing a pneumothorax outweighs the risk of thrombophlebitis from peripheral intravenous amiodarone.

Lidocaine 50 mg intravenously over 2 min, repeated every 5 min to a maximum dose of 200 mg is an alternative to amiodarone.

Bradycardia

Bradycardia is defined strictly as a heart rate of < 60 beats/min, but clinically the degree of slowing of the heart rate may be of importance when the heart rate is inappropriately slow for the haemodynamic state of the patient. A slow pulse is therefore important if there is:

- Systolic blood pressure < 90 mmHg
- Heart rate < 40 beats/min
- Ventricular arrhythmias requiring suppression
- Heart failure.

Atropine 500 µg intravenously is usually effective.

Patients with bradycardia following acute myocardial infarction should be assessed to determine the risk of asystole. This is signalled by:

- Recent asystole
- Möbitz type II AV block
- Complete (third-degree) heart block with broad-complex QRS
- Ventricular pause > 3 s.

If atropine is ineffective, or the risk of asystole is judged to be high, a transvenous pacing wire should be inserted. If there is haemodynamic deterioration in the intervening period, repeated doses of intravenous atropine 500 µg may be given to a total dose of 3 mg.

Adrenaline (epinephrine) infusions are now recommended rather than isoprenaline to help maintain cardiac rhythm if the above interventions are not effective until a transvenous wire can be placed. It is infused at a rate of 2–10 µg/min, depending upon response. Transcutaneous pacing is another option.

Complete heart block with a narrow QRS complex is not, in itself, an indication for pacing, particularly following inferior myocardial infarction (Jowett et al, 1989). AV junctional ectopic pacemakers with a narrow QRS usually provide a reasonable and stable heart rate.

CHANCES OF SUCCESS WITH CPR

The likelihood of survival following cardiac arrest is dependent on many variables, the most important of which are:

- Where the arrest takes place
- The patient's overall physical fitness
- The underlying pathology
- The patient's condition after arrest.

The development of out-of-hospital resuscitation has been shown to be of benefit in reports from the USA, the UK and Sweden (Geddes, 1986), with immediate bystander CPR doubling the percentage of survivors. The improved prognosis noted in these speedily resuscitated patients might be because early CPR limits the extent of myocardial damage by establishing early reperfusion.

Most patients who arrest in hospital have recently sustained a myocardial infarction, hence the importance of coronary care units and special observation of these patients, especially those with hypotension and heart failure. Warning dysrhythmias will not always precede ventricular fibrillation. 'Step-down' coronary units, between the coronary care unit and the ward, are

now recommended (Department of Health, 2000).

The prognosis of patients resuscitated within hospital is often governed by where the arrest takes place. The time between collapse and initiation of resuscitation is critical. Long-term survival in ward patients is only 2–3% (Hershey and Fisher, 1982), probably reflecting the increased time spent in confirmation of diagnosis and initiation of definitive therapy. Initial success rates in all cases of adult resuscitation may be as low as 30%, falling to 10% in the long term (Peatfield et al, 1977). Nevertheless, these poor results should not discourage attempts at resuscitation, since there are many full cardiac arrests that can be averted in the early stages when warning dysrhythmias or pure respiratory arrest have occurred. The best results may be obtained if resuscitation equipment is readily available and the nursing staff are able to defibrillate on their own initiative. The resuscitation rate then approaches 75%, 50% of all arrest cases being discharged from hospital (Mackintosh et al, 1979).

POST-ARREST MANAGEMENT

The treatment of a patient following resuscitation depends on the initial outcome of CPR. Full recovery from cardiac arrest is rarely immediate and can only be said to have occurred when the patient is fully conscious, with full cardiac, cerebral and renal function. This will be more likely if prompt CPR and defibrillation are carried out and if the underlying dysrhythmia was ventricular fibrillation. Around a third of patients who have return of spontaneous circulation die a neurological death. A third more long-term survivors have recognisable motor or cognitive deficits. After stabilisation, all standard care should be given (preferably in an intensive care environment), although the amount of care patients require following a cardiac arrest varies enormously (Box 11.1).

Following successful resuscitation, the patient's condition may be broadly classified into four groups:

Box 11.1 First steps after resuscitation

1. Check ventilation is adequate:
   - Endotracheal tube is correctly placed
   - 100% oxygen
   - Breath sounds heard in all areas of the chest
2. Obtain blood gases and potassium
3. Insert urinary catheter
   - Measure hourly output
4. Insert nasogastric tube
   - Aspirate gas and fluid
5. Obtain ECG and chest X-ray
6. Consider need for:
   - Low-dose dopamine infusion
   - Lidocaine (lignocaine) infusion

- Immediate recovery with no sequelae.
- Unconscious for a few hours. These patients may well be amnesic but some suffer anxiety, confusion, delusions and difficulty in concentrating for several months.
- Unconscious for more than 24 h. These patients often exhibit signs of spasticity, stroke or incoordination. The prognosis is variable.
- Decerebrate. Death is usual within a few days.

The patient should be examined to assess haemodynamic status and to look for complications of the resuscitation procedure, such as bleeding in thrombolysed patients, aspiration of gastric contents or pneumothorax (secondary to rib fracture or central venous catheterisation). An underlying cause for the arrest, such as anoxia or drug toxicity, should be considered. Elective ventilation and prophylactic drug therapy may be required. The routine use of lidocaine (lignocaine) remains controversial; the property of negative inotropy should be weighed against the presence or intended suppression of ventricular dysrhythmias. It must be remembered, however, that there will be impaired renal and hepatic flow, and drug pharmacokinetics will alter.

Special attention should be given to the following.

CARDIOVASCULAR SYSTEM

A full ECG and chest X-ray should be obtained. Blood should be sent for analysis of blood gases and electrolytes. An adequate blood pressure and cardiac output must be obtained to allow renal, coronary and cerebral perfusion. Formal haemodynamic monitoring with a Swan–Ganz catheter and arterial lines may be needed (Stokes and Jowett, 1985). Low-dose dopamine is often of value in promoting renal perfusion to avert acute renal failure. It is important to maintain an adequate and stable blood pressure at a level as close to the patient's norm as possible. Cerebral autoregulation will be impaired, and both cerebral hypoperfusion and oedema need to be avoided.

RESPIRATORY SYSTEM

Ventilation/perfusion defects are common in both lungs following resuscitation, and oxygen therapy should always be given. Pulse oximetry is very helpful, but arterial blood gases should be measured at least once to check gases and the acid–base status. Artificial ventilation may be required if saturations are not maintained over 93%. Hyperventilation to lower the PCO_2 may be useful in reducing cerebral oedema acutely. A chest X-ray is needed to exclude pneumothorax.

RENAL SYSTEM

Adequate renal perfusion must be obtained as a priority and an adequate blood pressure should produce a urine output of 40–50 ml/h. Catheterisation of the bladder will usually be required, with urine output measured at hourly intervals to detect early signs of renal failure. Some authorities advocate the use of furosemide (frusemide) or mannitol to prevent renal shutdown or cerebral oedema. Low-dose dopamine may also be considered. Renal failure should be treated along conventional lines. Careful consideration must be given to the use of drugs excreted by the kidneys and those with potential nephrotoxic side-effects.

CENTRAL NERVOUS SYSTEM

Primary cerebral damage may be caused by hypoxia during the arrest. Secondary damage may also occur after circulation is restored if the injured brain becomes oedematous. A flat trace on the EEG is seen within 10 s of loss of cerebral circulation, and cerebral glucose is depleted within 1 min. Micro-thrombi may form in the small cerebral vessels when blood flow ceases, which compromises cerebral perfusion when circulation is restored. Micro-emboli may also be ejected from the heart and great vessels during cardiac massage. Adequate arterial oxygenation is of great importance, if necessary using mechanical ventilation. Cerebral oedema may be reduced by the use of intravenous mannitol (200 ml of 20% solution) and dexamethasone (10 mg intravenously, followed by 4 mg orally every 6 h). Limitation of intravenous fluids and elevation of the head to 30° to increase venous drainage may also help. An EEG may be of prognostic importance.

Convulsions increase cerebral metabolic requirements and intracranial pressures, contributing to brain damage. They should be controlled in the usual way.

ACID–BASE STATUS

The acid–base balance must be assessed urgently, and plasma potassium must be measured immediately and frequently after the arrest. Both should be corrected as required. The serum potassium should be maintained above 4 mmol/l. Hyperkalaemia over 6 mmol/l should be treated with a glucose–insulin infusion. Giving 10 ml of 10% calcium chloride intravenously over 5 min will offer some cardioprotection. Any significant metabolic acidosis should be treated by alveolar hyperventilation. Care is required in administration of sodium bicarbonate, since it can lead to a rapid fall in plasma potassium levels and a rise in PCO_2 (thereby worsening cerebral oedema).

WHEN TO STOP

The decision to terminate resuscitation is a medical one and should be made by the most senior physician present, in consultation with other members of the resuscitation team. This decision should follow an assessment of the patient's cerebral and cardiovascular status, as well as prognosis (Baskett, 1986). Patients with non-VF arrests seldom recover after 15–20 min, unless the arrest was associated with drugs or hypothermia. For those with persistent VF, the situation is potentially reversible, but outcome remains poor. Prolonged resuscitation is seldom justified; the mortality following an arrest of over 15 min is 90% (Bedell et al, 1983). Patients with hypothermia are a special group, and may still recover after prolonged resuscitation, and attempts should continue until the core temperature is over 36°C and the arterial pH and serum potassium are normal.

All patients who die suddenly should be considered as potential organ donors, and visceral perfusion and oxygenation should be maintained until a decision is made.

It is appropriate for all team members to be thanked for their efforts by the team leader. All tubes, lines and leads should be removed prior to the patient being 'laid out'. A senior doctor should discuss the death with relatives as soon as possible, and the presence of an experienced nurse is of great value.

AUDIT

Open discussion by all members of an arrest team (preferably immediately after an arrest) is of value, to identify weaknesses and allay anxieties. Misplaced confidence may be unmasked, since, although regular attendance at cardiac arrests increases confidence, it is not necessarily matched by increased competence (Wynne et al, 1987; Marteau et al, 1990). There is no substitute for training, retraining and feedback via the audit process (Berden et al, 1993).

OUT-OF-HOSPITAL RESUSCITATION

Survival after cardiac arrest varies from 5% to 60% and is influenced both by the conditions that preceded the arrest and by the efficiency of CPR. The time to defibrillation is accepted as the single most important determinant. Before the introduction of automatic external defibrillators, only 15% of patients with out-of-hospital cardiac arrest had restoration of spontaneous circulation, and reached hospital alive, and only half of these survived to discharge.

The typical out-of-hospital arrest happens at home, during the daytime in men over 50 years of age with a previous history of cardiovascular disease. This is important for teaching citizen CPR, as the key people to teach are thus housewives and other close family of patients with cardiac disease.

The concept of the 'chain of survival' describes interventions for optimal survival rates. Weakness in any link will compromise a satisfactory outcome. These links are:

1. Early recognition of the collapse and calling for emergency help
2. Early bystander BLS
3. Early defibrillation
4. Early ALS.

DEFIBRILLATION AND CARDIOVERSION

The use of an electric current to terminate ventricular fibrillation in man was first reported in 1947 by Beck et al, who applied 120 V directly to the ventricles. Later an alternating current (AC) defibrillator was developed for terminating ventricular fibrillation by passing a current across the chest at 720 V (Zoll et al, 1956). The modern direct current (DC) defibrillator was developed by Lown in 1962, and had the advantages of being smaller, chargeable with batteries and (because smaller currents were being employed) less likely to cause myocardial damage or precipitate dysrhythmias. This type of defibrillator is still the most common, and employs a monophasic waveform shock. Smaller *biphasic* defibrillators were developed during the design of implantable defibrillators and were found to have equal efficacy at reduced strength. Unlike traditional defibrillators, which send a high-energy electrical charge in a single direction,

biphasic external defibrillators use a lower-energy self-reversing (biphasic) waveform. Biphasic waveforms deliver current that first flows in a positive direction for a specified duration. In the second phase the device reverses the direction of current so that it flows in a negative direction. Biphasic shocks appear to achieve the same defibrillation success rates as monophasic waveforms but at significantly lower energy levels. Lower-energy devices are smaller, lighter, less expensive and less demanding of batteries, with fewer maintenance requirements. On average, two-thirds less current is required for the equivalent effect, and biphasic shocks of 200 J or less are as safe and as effective as monophasic shocks of 360 J (Mittal, 1999; Tang et al, 2001). The combination of increased efficacy, with decreased current requirements make biphasic defibrillators more efficient than monophasic defibrillators, and this type of defibrillator is recommended by the International Resuscitation Committees (ILCOR).

Electrical defibrillation depolarises myocardial tissue ahead of the intrinsic depolarisation wave, making it refractory to conduction. The whole myocardium is thus suddenly depolarised and awaits intrinsic pacemaker function to return, hopefully from the SA node. It follows that, if an insufficient current is applied, not all the myocardium will be depolarised, and defibrillation will not result. Successful defibrillation occurs when the current delivered exceeds the defibrillation threshold. Transthoracic impedance resists this, and varies considerably between patients (e.g. poor skin contact, large patient, large bone mass, etc). Biphasic defibrillation has been found to be particularly advantageous in those with high transthoracic impedance. The device can adjust the amount and duration of current delivered, based on impedance measurements performed twice during every shock. This unique combination of biphasic waveform shocks and impedance adjustment or compensation provides equivalent defibrillation success at lower energy levels than those of monophasic shocks and eliminates the need to increase the energy for persistent VF.

ELECTIVE CARDIOVERSION

Following its application to cardiac arrest, the defibrillator was applied to other dysrhythmias with marked success. Electrical treatment of cardiac dysrhythmias has marked advantages over drugs, in that it is free from pharmacological side-effects (especially depression of myocardial contractility), and it is useful for the treatment of both supraventricular and ventricular tachydysrhythmias. Typical indications include atrial flutter, ventricular tachycardia and supraventricular tachycardia unresponsive to drug therapy. Atrial fibrillation is usually initially treated with drugs to slow the ventricular rate, but electrical or chemical cardioversion may be employed for recent-onset atrial fibrillation (especially peri-infarction), after therapy for heart failure has reduced cardiac size or after cardiac surgery. Anticoagulants should not be necessary for recent-onset atrial fibrillation, but other cases should be given warfarin for 3–4 weeks before cardioversion and a month after.

METABOLIC AND DRUG CONSIDERATIONS

Patients with hypoxaemia and acidaemia are difficult to defibrillate. For successful defibrillation, attention needs to be directed to these metabolic upsets. Careful attention should also be paid to electrolyte levels, particularly those of potassium. Drugs may also influence the success of cardioversion. Digoxin reduces the energy threshold required for defibrillation, and much smaller currents should be delivered. In contrast, quinidine, lidocaine (lignocaine) and phenytoin all increase the threshold and higher energies will be needed to restore sinus rhythm.

TECHNIQUE

The procedure should be explained to the patient and consent obtained. The patient should be fasted for 6–8 h. A standard 12-lead ECG should be recorded before and after cardioversion, and a rhythm strip should be recorded during the procedure. An anaesthetist should be in attendance to administer a short-acting anaesthetic, and resuscitation equipment must be on hand. It is usual to pre-oxygenate the patient, and oxygen should be delivered throughout the procedure and during recovery.

There are two main methods of paddle placement, although there appears to be no superiority in either method:

- *Anteroanterior*: one paddle is applied close to the sternum over the right 2nd–3rd intercostal space and the other just below the apex of the heart in the mid-axillary line
- *Apicoposterior*: one paddle is placed at the apex, and the other to the right of the spine (which would otherwise prevent good skin contact), below the scapula (Ewy, 1994).

The technique is the same as used for defibrillation, as in the first part of Fig. 11.6, but the defibrillator will need to be set in 'synchronised' mode. Unsynchronised shocks could potentially precipitate ventricular fibrillation, if delivered to the heart at a time coincident with the vulnerable 30 ms preceding the apex of the T wave of the cardiac cycle (R-on-T). This can be avoided by synchronising the defibrillators to trigger the shock just after the R wave. It is therefore best to ensure that the ECG is set so that the QRS complex displays the most upright R wave, to ensure safe triggering. A practical point is that the discharge will not necessarily occur as soon as the button is pressed, and the operator must not be tempted to release pressure on the paddles until after the shock has been delivered.

Because myocardial damage increases with the amount of energy applied, the shock should be 'titrated' against the type of dysrhythmia; typical monophasic energy levels required are:

- Atrial fibrillation: at least 200 J; consider starting at 360 J (Joglar et al, 2000)
- Atrial flutter, supraventricular tachycardias: start at 100 J
- Ventricular tachycardia: at least 100 J
- Ventricular fibrillation: normal rapid sequence (200 J, 200 J, 360 J).

If the shock causes a stable rhythm to deteriorate into ventricular fibrillation, an immediate unsynchronised shock of at least 200 J should be delivered.

Antidysrhythmic drugs are occasionally needed between shocks, to help to restore sinus rhythm, and these are always worth trying if the first two or three attempts fail. Administration of a suitable antidysrhythmic agent such as lidocaine (lignocaine) is particularly recommended if multiple ventricular ectopic beats develop after an unsuccessful shock.

After restoration of sinus rhythm, a further 12-lead ECG should be obtained, vital signs recorded and arrangements made for monitoring for a few hours.

COMPLICATIONS

Dysrhythmias may occur after cardioversion, either because the underlying problem that precipitated the original dysrhythmia is still present or as a direct consequence of cardioversion.

Bradydysrhythmias frequently occur immediately following cardioversion and are self-limiting. Sinus bradycardias, wandering pacemakers and junctional rhythms are not serious and can be treated with atropine if they persist. A few ventricular ectopic beats may also be seen and, again, are usually self-limiting. However, runs of ectopics, ventricular tachycardia and fibrillation need treating along usual lines. Because these complications may develop up to 8 h after cardioversion, prolonged monitoring is indicated. This is particularly the case if antidysrhythmic drugs have also been used or if hypokalaemia is present. The risk of ventricular fibrillation and ventricular tachycardia is increased if the patient has been taking digoxin, and, although many discontinue the drug prior to cardioversion, this is not required, and the procedure is well tolerated, providing there are

no signs of digoxin toxicity (Dalzell et al, 1990). Injury to the myocardium may occur, especially with multiple shocks (Dahl et al, 1974), and makes subsequent dysrhythmias more likely. It is therefore advisable to start defibrillation at lower energies and allow 2–3 min to elapse before the next shock is given. Clinical signs of myocardial injury are not usually evident, even after multiple shocks, and microscopic evidence has not been demonstrated. Transient ST–T wave changes may be seen on the ECG but CK-MB and troponin levels are only rarely elevated.

Thromboembolic complications may occur in those restored to sinus rhythm, and may occur at any time in the first 10 days following the procedure (Berger and Schweitzer, 1998). Patients at risk are those with atrial flutter and atrial fibrillation, particularly if the left atrium is enlarged, or the left ventricle is dilated or dyskinetic. The risk may be minimised by prior anticoagulation for 3 weeks before and 4 weeks after cardioversion (ACC/AHA/ESC, 2001). Paddle burns are uncommon if careful attention is paid to application of the electrodes, and gel pads. Any inflammation will quickly respond to topical steroid cream such as 1% hydrocortisone.

CARDIOVERSION IN A PATIENT WITH A PACEMAKER

Modern pacemakers and implanted defibrillators have circuitry to protect against external defibrillation, although reports of pacemaker damage have been reported. It is, therefore, a good idea routinely to assess pacemaker function prior to discharge from hospital. External defibrillation pads should be placed away from the pulse generator, and it may be necessary to use the anteroposterior paddle positions if the generator is in the right infraclavicular area.

REFERENCES

Aarons EJ, Beeching NJ (1991) Survey of 'do not resuscitate' orders in a district general hospital. *BMJ*, **303:** 1504–1506.

ACC/AHA/ESC (2001) Joint guidelines for the management of patients with atrial fibrillation. *European Heart Journal*, **22:** 1852–1923.

American Heart Association in collaboration with the International Liaison Committee on Resuscitation (2000) Guidelines 2000 for cardiopulmonary resuscitation and emergency cardiovascular care. An international consensus on science. *Resuscitation*, **46:** 1–448.

Auble TE, Menegazzi JJ, Paris PM (1995) Effect of out of hospital defibrillation by basic life support providers on cardiac arrest mortality: a meta-analysis. *Annals of Emergency Medicine*, **25:** 642–648.

Ballew KA (1997) Cardiopulmonary resuscitation. *BMJ*, **314:** 1462–1465.

Baskett PJF (1986) The ethics of resuscitation. *BMJ*, **293:** 189–190.

Baskett PJF (2001) The respiratory system during resuscitation: a review of the history, risk of infection during assisted ventilation, respiratory mechanics, and ventilation strategies for patients with an unprotected airway. *Resuscitation*, **49:** 123–134.

Bastuli JA, Orlowski JP (1985) Stroke as a complication of carotid sinus massage. *Critical Care Medicine*, **13:** 869.

Beck CS, Prilchard WH, Feil HS (1947) Ventricular fibrillation of long duration abolished by electric shock. *JAMA*, **135:** 985–986.

Bedell SE, Delbanco TL, Cook EF et al (1983) Survival after cardiopulmonary resuscitation in hospital. *New England Journal of Medicine*, **10:** 569–576.

Berden HJJM, Willems FF, Hendrick JMA et al (1993) How frequently should basic CPR training be repeated to maintain adequate skills? *BMJ*, **306:** 1576–1577.

Berger M, Schweitzer P (1998) Timing of thrombo-embolic events after elective cardioversion of atrial fibrillation or flutter: a retrospective analysis. *American Journal of Cardiology*, **82:** 1545–1547.

Caldwell G, Millar G, Quinn E et al (1985) Simple mechanical methods for cardioversion: defense of the precordial thump and cough version. *BMJ*, **291:** 627–630.

Camm AJ (1986) ABC of resuscitation: asystole and electromechanical dissociation. *BMJ*, **292:** 1123–1124.

Camm AJ, Malcolm AD, Garratt CJ (1992) Adenosine and cardiac arrhythmias. The preferred treatment for supraventricular tachycardia. *BMJ*, **305:** 3–4.

Candy CE (1991) 'Not for resuscitation': a student nurse's viewpoint. *Journal of Advanced Nursing*, **16:** 138–146.

Chandra N, Snyder L, Weisfeldt ML (1981) Abdominal binding during CPR in man. *JAMA*, **246:** 351–353.

Cobbe SM, Dalziel K, Ford I et al (1996) Survival of 1476 patients initially resuscitated from out of hospital cardiac arrest. *BMJ*, **312:** 1633–1637.

Cooper MJ, Abinader EG (1979) Atropine-induced ventricular fibrillation: case report and review of the literature. *American Heart Journal*, **99:** 225–228.

Criley JM, Blaufuss AH, Kissel GL (1976) Cough-induced cardiac compression. *JAMA*, **236:** 1246–1250.

Cummins RO, Eisenberg MS, Shultz KR (1986) Automatic external defibrillators: clinical issues in cardiology. *Circulation*, **73:** 381–385.

Dahl CF, Ewy GA, Warner ED (1974) Myocardial necrosis from direct current countershock: effect of paddle electrode size and time interval between discharge. *Circulation*, **50:** 956–961.

Dalzell GW, Anderson J, Adgey AA (1990) Factors determining success and energy requirements for cardioversion in atrial fibrillation. *Quarterly Journal of Medicine*, **76:** 903–913.

David J, Prior-Willeard PFS (1993) Resuscitation skills of MRCP candidates. *BMJ*, **306:** 1578–1579.

Department of Health (2000) *National Service Framework for Coronary Heart Disease*. London: The Stationery Office.

de Vos R, Koster RW, de Haan RJ et al (1999) In-hospital cardiopulmonary resuscitation: pre-arrest morbidity and outcome. *Archives of Internal Medicine*, **159:** 845–850.

Dowdle JR (1996) Ventricular standstill and cardiac percussion. *Resuscitation*, **32:** 31–32.

Ebell MH, Becker LA, Barry HC et al (1998) Survival after in-hospital cardiopulmonary resuscitation. A meta-analysis. *Journal of General Internal Medicine*, **13:** 805–816.

Ebrahim S (2000) Do not resuscitate decisions: flogging dead horses or a dignified death? *BMJ*, **320:** 1155–1156.

Elam JO, Greene DG (1961) Mission accomplished. Successful mouth-to-mouth resuscitation. *Anesthesia and Analgesia (Current Research)*, **40:** 440–442, 578–580, 672–676.

Ewy GA (1994) The optimal technique for electrical cardioversion of atrial fibrillation. *Clinical Cardiology*, **17:** 79–84.

Geddes JS (1986) Twenty years of pre-hospital coronary care. *British Heart Journal*, **56:** 491–495.

Gonzales ER (1993) Pharmacological controversies in CPR. *Annals of Internal Medicine*, **22:** 317–323.

Graham CA, Guest KA, Scollon D (1994a) Cardiopulmonary resuscitation. Paper 1: A survey of undergraduate training in UK medical schools. *Emergency Medicine Journal*, **11:** 162–164.

Graham CA, Guest KA, Scollon D (1994b) Cardiopulmonary resuscitation. Paper 2: A survey of basic life support training for medical students. *Emergency Medicine Journal*, **11:** 165–167.

Heames RM, Sado D, Deakin CD (2001) Do doctors position defibrillation paddles correctly? Observational study. *BMJ*, **322:** 1393–1394.

Hershey CO, Fisher L (1982) Why outcome of CPR in general wards is poor. *Lancet*, **i:** 31–34.

Jaffe AS (1993) The use of anti-arrhythmics in advanced cardiopulmonary resuscitation. *Annals of Emergency Medicine*, **22:** 307–316.

Joglar JA, Hamdan MH, Ramaswamy K et al (2000) Initial energy for elective external cardioversion of persistent atrial fibrillation. *American Journal of Cardiology*, **86:** 348–350.

Jones A, Peckett W, Clark E et al (1993) Nurses' knowledge of the resuscitation status of patients and action in the event of cardiorespiratory arrest. *BMJ*, **306:** 1577–1578.

Jowett NI, Thompson DR (1988a) Basic life support. The forgotten skills? *Intensive Care Nursing*, **4:** 9–17.

Jowett NI, Thompson DR (1988b) Advanced cardiac life support: current perspectives. *Intensive Care Nursing*, **4:** 71–81.

Jowett NI, Thompson DR, Bailey SW (1985) Electrocardiographic monitoring. I. Static monitoring. *Intensive Care Nursing*, **2:** 71–76.

Jowett NI, Thompson DR, Pohl JEF (1989) Temporary transvenous endocardial pacing: six years experience in one coronary care unit. *Postgraduate Medical Journal*, **65:** 211–215.

Jowett NI, Turner AM, Hawkins D et al (2001) Emergency drug availability for the cardiac arrest team: a national audit. *Resuscitation*, **49:** 179–181.

Jude JR, Kouwenhoven WB, Knickerbocker GG (1961) Cardiac arrest. Report of application of external cardiac massage in 118 patients. *JAMA*, **178:** 1063–1070.

Kaye W, Mancini ME (1986) Retention of cardiopulmonary resuscitation skills by physicians, registered nurses and the general public. *Critical Care Medicine*, **14:** 621–623.

Kerber RE, Grayzel J, Hoyt R (1981) Transthoracic resistance of human defibrillation: influence of body weight, chest size, serial shocks, paddle size and paddle contact pressure. *Circulation*, **63:** 676–682.

Kouwenhoven WB, Jude JR, Knickerbocker GG (1960) Closed chest cardiac massage. *JAMA*, **173:** 1064–1067.

Kudenchuk PJ, Cobb LA, Copass MK et al (1999) Amiodarone for resuscitation after out-of-hospital cardiac arrest due to ventricular fibrillation. *New England Journal of Medicine*, **341:** 871–878.

Leah V, Whitbread M, Coats TJ (1998) Resuscitation training for medical students. *Resuscitation*, **39:** 87–90.

Mackintosh AF, Crabb ME, Brennan H et al (1979) Hospital resuscitation from ventricular fibrillation in Brighton. *BMJ*, **1:** 511–513.

Maier GW, Newton JR, Wolfe JA et al (1986) The influence of manual chest compression rate on hemodynamic support during cardiac arrest: high impulse cardiopulmonary resuscitation. *Circulation*, **74**(suppl IV): 51–59.

Marteau TM, Wynne G, Kaye W et al (1990) Resuscitation: experience without feedback increases confidence but not skills. *BMJ*, **300:** 849–850.

McGowan J, Graham CA, Gordon MW (1999) Appointment of a resuscitation training officer is associated with improved survival from in-hospital ventricular fibrillation/ventricular tachycardia cardiac arrest. *Resuscitation*, **41:** 169–173.

Mittal S, Ayati S, Stein KM et al (1999) Comparison of a novel rectilinear biphasic waveform with a damped sine wave monophasic waveform for transthoracic defibrillation. *Journal of the American College of Cardiology*, **35:** 1595–1601.

Myerburg RJ, Kessler KM, Zarman L et al (1982) Survivors of pre-hospital cardiac arrest. *JAMA*, **247:** 1485–1490.

Niemann JT (1984) Differences in cerebral and myocardial perfusion in closed chest resuscitation. *Annals of Emergency Medicine*, **13:** 849–853.

Peatfield RC, Sillett RW, Taylor D et al (1977) Survival after cardiac arrest in hospital. *Lancet*, **i:** 1223–1225.

Priori SG, Aliot E, Blomstrom-Lundqvist C et al (2001) Task force on sudden cardiac death of the European Society of Cardiology. *European Heart Journal*, **22:** 1374–1450.

Rich S, Wix HL, Shapiro EP (1981) Clinical assessment of heart chamber size and valve motion during cardiopulmonary resuscitation by two-dimensional echocardiography. *American Heart Journal*, **102:** 367–373.

Robertson C, Holmberg S (1992) Compression techniques and blood flow during cardiopulmonary resuscitation. *Resuscitation*, **24:** 123–132.

Royal College of Physicians (1987) Resuscitation from cardiopulmonary arrest. Training and organisation. *Journal of the Royal College of Physicians*, **21:** 175–182.

Rudikoff MT, Maughan WL, Effron M et al (1980) Mechanisms of blood flow during cardiopulmonary resuscitation. *Circulation*, **61:** 345–352.

Sack JB, Kesselbrenner MB, Bregman D (1992) Survival from in-hospital cardiac arrest with interposed abdominal counter-pulsation during CPR. *JAMA*, **267:** 379–385.

Safar P, Escarra L, Elam J (1958) A comparison of the mouth to mouth and mouth to airway methods of artificial respiration with the chest pressure arm-lift method. *New England Journal of Medicine*, **258:** 671–677.

Saunders J (2001) Perspectives on CPR: resuscitation or resurrection? *Clinical Medicine*, **1:** 457–460.

Sellick BA (1961) Cricoid pressure to control regurgitation of stomach contents during induction of anaesthesia. *Lancet*, **ii:** 404–406.

Shepardson LB, Youngner SJ, Speroff T et al (1999) Increased risk of death in patients with do-not-resuscitate orders. *Medical Care*, **37:** 722–726.

Skinner DV (1985) Cardiopulmonary skills of pre-registration house officers. *BMJ*, **290:** 1549–1550.

Stiell IG, Herbert PC, Wells GA et al (1996) The Ontario trial of active compression-decompression cardiopulmonary resuscitation in hospital and pre-hospital arrests. *JAMA*, **275:** 1417–1423.

Stokes PH, Jowett NI (1985) Haemodynamic monitoring using the Swan–Ganz catheter. *Intensive Care Nursing*, **1:** 9–17.

Sullivan MJJ, Guyatt GH (1986) Simulated cardiac arrests for monitoring quality of in-hospital resuscitation. *Lancet*, **ii:** 618–620.

Tang W, Weil MH, Sun S et al (2001) A comparison of biphasic and monophasic waveform defibrillation after prolonged ventricular fibrillation. *Chest*, **120:** 948–954.

Tunstall-Pedoe H, Bailey L, Chamberlain DA et al (1992) Survey of 3765 cardiopulmonary resuscitations in British Hospitals (the BRESUS study): methods and overall results. *BMJ*, **304:** 1347–1351.

Varon J, Fromm RE (1993) Cardiopulmonary resuscitation. New and controversial techniques. *Postgraduate Medical Journal*, **93:** 235–239.

Wenzel V, Idris AH, Dörges V et al (2001) The respiratory system during resuscitation: a review of the history, risk of infection during assisted ventilation, respiratory mechanics and ventilation strategies for patients with an unprotected airway. *Resuscitation*, **49:** 123–134.

Wynne G, Marteau TM, Johnston M et al (1987) Inability of trained nurses to perform basic life support. *BMJ*, **294:** 1198–1199.

Zoll PM, Linenthal AJ, Gibson W et al (1956) Termination of ventricular fibrillation in man by externally applied counter shock. *New England Journal of Medicine*, **254:** 727–732.

12

Management of other conditions presenting to the coronary care unit

Patients are usually admitted to the coronary care unit because of chest pain, breathlessness, a rhythm disturbance or sometimes all three.

HEART FAILURE

Heart failure is now recognised as a major and rapidly increasing problem in industrialised countries. Improved treatment for coronary heart disease has reduced mortality, but increased survival means that many more patients are living on with complications, and the number of patients with chronic heart failure is increasing. In addition, the elderly population is increasing, and this group has the highest incidence of cardiovascular diseases, including the most common precursors of heart failure: coronary artery disease and hypertension. An important consequence is that the mean age of patients with heart failure in the community is now 76 years, an age group not studied in most heart failure trials (Cowie et al, 1999).

Chronic heart failure punctuated by acute exacerbations is the most common form of heart failure seen in hospital (Remme and Swedberg, 2001), and most patients are admitted directly to the coronary care unit. An average district general hospital can be expected to manage over 1000 deaths and discharges related to heart failure every year (Cleland et al, 2000). The condition is serious. Many patients die within 3 months of diagnosis, rising to approximately 60% within 5 years (McMurray and Stewart, 2000). In contrast, the overall 5-year mortality related to cancer is under 50%.

AETIOLOGY

Heart failure is a clinical syndrome that results from an inability of the heart to provide an adequate cardiac output for metabolic needs. The majority of cases are of *systolic heart failure*, which occurs when the ventricular pump is weakened and cannot eject enough blood. This is usually caused by loss of normal myocardial tissue secondary to myocardial infarction, or is due to decreased myocardial contractility as a result of ischaemia or cardiomyopathy. A reduced cardiac output may also result from drugs that depress myocardial contractility.

Common precursors of chronic heart failure are:

- Coronary artery disease (especially following acute myocardial infarction)
- Hypertension
- Cardiomyopathy
- Valve disease
- Cardiac arrhythmias/conduction disturbance (e.g. heart block and atrial fibrillation)
- Pericardial disease (e.g. pericardial effusion, constrictive pericarditis)
- Infection (e.g. rheumatic fever, viral myocarditis, HIV)
- Alcohol and drugs (e.g. cancer chemotherapy).

Over 80% of cases of heart failure are due to coronary artery disease, and associate with poor ventricular contraction. However, the Framingham Investigators found that half their cohort with heart failure had an ejection fraction of over 50% (Vasan, 1999). The assumption was that heart failure in these cases must be due to diastolic dysfunction (Gaasch, 1994). *Diastolic heart failure* occurs when the left ventricle cannot relax sufficiently in diastole, which compromises filling. Increased stiffness of the ventricular wall is sometimes found in the elderly, patients with hypertension or other fibrotic heart diseases, and is apparent on echocardiography or nuclear scanning. However, it is not widely accepted that

most patients presenting with pulmonary congestion and normal systolic function have isolated diastolic dysfunction as a cause for heart failure (Caruana et al, 2000), and optimal therapy is not known even if it is diagnosed.

High-output heart failure is uncommon, but may occur in sepsis, anaemia, thyrotoxicosis and Paget's disease. There is a high cardiac output, but signs of heart failure because the high metabolic needs are not being fulfilled. The underlying cause needs treatment.

THE RESPONSE TO HEART FAILURE

The symptoms of heart failure are usually not due to a low ejection fraction, but rather to the compensatory mechanisms that the body employs to maintain an adequate cardiac output. The fall in blood pressure caused by a diminished cardiac output stimulates the baroreceptors, producing increased catecholamine secretion, with tachycardia, increased myocardial contractility and a rise in systemic vascular resistance. Selective arterial vasoconstriction redistributes the cardiac output, so that flow to the gut and liver is reduced, with preferential perfusion of the brain and heart. The heart dilates, increasing myofibril stretch, which increases the force of myocardial contraction (Starling's Law), and augments cardiac output. A further adaptation is seen in the arterioles, particularly those supplying skeletal muscle and kidneys, where the vessel walls become oedematous and less responsive to circulating vasodilators. Reduced renal blood flow stimulates the renin–angiotensin–aldosterone system to release high levels of angiotensin II and aldosterone, causing widespread vasoconstriction, with sodium and water retention. *Endothelins* are secreted by the vascular endothelium and also cause vasoconstriction and fluid retention. Endothelin-1 levels in the blood are increased in proportion to the severity of heart failure, and are of prognostic significance.

These effects are antagonised by *natriuretic peptides*, which produce many effects, including diuresis, vasodilatation and increased sodium excretion. There are three natriuretic hormones:

- *Atrial natriuretic peptide* (ANP), which is released from the atria in response to stretch
- *Brain natriuretic peptide* (BNP), which is released both by the brain and the left ventricle
- *C-type natriuretic peptide*, which is found in the vascular endothelium and central nervous system, but only has weak actions.

Measuring BNP in the blood may become useful in the diagnosis of asymptomatic heart failure, or in predicting outcome in those with established heart failure (Latini et al, 2001). A normal BNP concentration virtually excludes heart failure, but high concentrations exist in many other cardiac problems (Cowie, 2000). High plasma BNP concentrations measured within 7 days of myocardial infarction indicate adverse left ventricular remodelling, and predict 1-year mortality (Crilley and Farrar, 2001). Measuring BNP concentrations following myocardial infarction may help target patients who will benefit from angiotensin-converting enzyme (ACE) inhibition. NT-proBNP (N-terminal pro-B-type natriuretic peptide) is more cardiospecific and easier to measure, and may replace standard BNP assays.

INVESTIGATIONS

The ECG is usually abnormal, so normality suggests an alternative diagnosis. A chest X-ray is useful to detect cardiac enlargement and pulmonary congestion. Echocardiography gives objective evidence of cardiac dysfunction, and excludes valvular disease. Nuclear scanning can also be used to assess cardiac function, and myocardial perfusion. Baseline renal function tests should be taken before long-term treatment with diuretics and ACE inhibitors. Exercise stress testing provides an objective measure of functional impairment in heart failure.

CLINICAL FEATURES OF HEART FAILURE

There is a poor relationship between symptoms and the severity of heart dysfunction.

The usual presentation of left ventricular failure is dyspnoea caused by increased pulmonary vascular engorgement, with decreased compliance of the lungs. Blood gases remain normal or near normal during exercise, but ventilatory reflexes are exaggerated. Paroxysmal nocturnal dyspnoea results when nocturnal absorption of oedema fluid increases the intravascular volume, waking the patient with gasping respiration, cough and wheeze. Fatigue and lethargy are marked, caused by low blood flow to exercising muscles and structural and metabolic changes within the muscles. Muscle wasting is associated with poor prognosis. Swelling of the ankles is common, but non-specific.

The Criteria Committee of the New York Heart Association has used symptoms and exercise capacity to classify the severity of heart failure (see Table 14.1; page 294).

Acute left ventricular failure is a medical emergency; its management is discussed in Ch. 10.

Right ventricular failure usually occurs secondary to left heart failure, but can occur alone following right ventricular infarction, pulmonary embolism, pulmonary valve disease or chronic lung disease (cor pulmonale). Symptoms are due to high systemic venous pressure. Oedema, with elevation of the jugular venous pressure, is usual. The liver becomes engorged, enlarged and may be tender. Functional tricuspid incompetence occurs, and the dilated right ventricle often produces a right parasternal heave. Pleural effusions and ascites are common.

TREATING HEART FAILURE

The aims of treatment are to relieve symptoms by:

- Increasing salt and water excretion
- Reducing intracardiac pressures and volume overload
- Increasing myocardial contractility.

Bedrest reduces metabolic demand, increases renal perfusion, and is valuable until signs and symptoms improve. However, passive leg exercises are recommended to prevent deep vein thrombosis, and subcutaneous heparin should be considered for inpatients. Anticoagulation with warfarin is needed for patients with enlarged hearts, atrial fibrillation and very poor left ventricular function.

Diuretics

Diuretics provide the mainstay of treatment for heart failure, giving symptomatic relief and improving exercise capacity. They do not effect long-term outcome. Diuretics inhibit sodium resorption by the kidney, and reduce intravascular volume and hence cardiac preload. There is loss of sodium from arteriolar walls, allowing vasodilatation and a reduction in afterload. Potassium intake needs to be increased to prevent hypokalaemia.

Potassium-sparing diuretics such as amiloride are usually not needed if ACE inhibitors are co-prescribed. However, low-dose spironolactone (25 mg/day) should be used in addition to standard heart failure therapy to reduce morbidity and mortality in patients with moderate to severe heart failure (Pitt et al, 1999). Hyperkalaemia is more frequent because of the combination of spironolactone with ACE inhibitors, and electrolytes need to be checked frequently.

In severe heart failure, the gut wall becomes oedematous, limiting absorption of orally administered drugs. Intravenous diuretics will get round this problem, switching to oral therapy once the diuresis has started. Over-diuresis should be avoided, since a depleted plasma volume will reactivate the renin–angiotensin–aldosterone system, and stimulate fluid retention and vasoconstriction. The dose of diuretic must be reduced to just sufficient to prevent salt and water retention.

Vasodilators

It has become apparent that many episodes of pulmonary oedema that punctuate chronic heart failure are not caused by fluid overload, but rather fluid redistribution that is directed to the lungs. Acute on chronic heart failure is characterised by a sudden reduction in stroke volume that triggers increased sympathetic activity, resulting in tachycardia and an abrupt increase in systemic vascular resistance (Kramer et al, 2000). The combination of tachycardia and increased peripheral resistance shifts fluid centrally. Because of impaired left ventricular function, the heart cannot cope with this sudden fluid overload and pulmonary oedema results, even though there is no excess fluid retention (Northridge, 1996). This is why treatment with vasodilators is probably more effective than diuretics in acute heart failure.

There are many vasodilators that can be used in the management of heart failure, and their haemodynamic effects depend on their ability to affect arterioles or venules (Table 12.1). The most important vasodilator group are the ACE inhibitors.

ACE inhibitors

The benefits of ACE inhibitors for patients with heart failure in terms of mortality, morbidity and quality of life are unequivocal (Packer, 1992), and these agents should be introduced at an early stage. The ACE inhibitors inhibit production of the potent vasoconstrictor angiotensin II, and increase bradykinin concentrations by inhibiting its breakdown. Although bradykinin is probably responsible for the common dry cough commonly seen with ACE inhibitors, it has been shown to have beneficial effects on endothelial function. Venous and arterial blood pressure falls, allowing an increase in cardiac output and renal blood flow. Aldosterone levels also fall, reducing fluid retention and allowing a reduction in the dose of diuretics.

The use of ACE inhibitors is often limited by side-effects, including cough, renal impairment and symptomatic hypotension, but they should be prescribed for all patients with heart failure if there are no contraindications. The dose should be titrated up to the doses shown to be effective in the controlled trials, and not to the level that relieves symptoms. The evidence-based ACE inhibitors are captopril 50 mg tds, lisinopril 30–40 mg daily, enalapril 20 mg bd, ramipril 5 mg bd and trandolapril 4 mg daily.

Table 12.1 Commonly used vasodilators

Drug	Mechanism	Dosage	Onset of action	Precautions
Nitroprusside	Direct action	IV only 0.5–1 µg/kg/min Titrate for effect	Immediate	Sudden hypotension – requires close monitoring Cyanide and thiocyanate toxicity
Nitrates	Direct action	IV, SL, B, O, TD Wide range of doses	Minutes	Headache, flushing, hypotension
Hydralazine	Direct action	IV, 10–20 mg IM, 10–20 mg	Minutes	Tachycardia may produce angina Lupus-like syndrome Blood dyscrasias
Prazosin	Alpha-adrenergic blocker	O, 25–100 mg three times a day O, 0.5–5.0 mg three times a day	0.5–2 h	First-dose hypotension Tachyphylaxis in heart failure
Captopril	ACE inhibitor	O, 6.25–50.00 mg three times a day	0.5–1.5 h	First-dose hypotension Altered taste Rashes Proteinuria
Enalapril	ACE inhibitor	2.5–40.0 mg daily	1–2 h	Hypotension if patient is sodium-depleted
Nifedipine	Calcium channel blocker	O, 5–160 mg three times a day SL, 5 mg	15–30 min 2–5 min	Hypotension and tachycardia Headache Ankle oedema Negative inotropic effect in high doses
Nicardipine	Calcium channel blocker	O, 20–30 mg three times a day	30–60 min	As nifedipine, but little inotropic effect

IV, intravenous; IM, intramuscular; B, buccal; O, oral; SL, sublingual; TD, transdermal.

Other vasodilators

Angiotensin II receptor blockers are a new class of drug, with clinical effects similar to those of the ACE inhibitors, but with fewer side-effects. It is unknown whether the benefits of the ACE inhibitors in heart failure can be extended to this group of agents, particularly with regard to improved prognosis (Miller and Srivastava, 2001).

Hydralazine improves cardiac output by arteriolar vasodilatation, but may produce reflex tachycardia. This would be unhelpful in increasing myocardial work and oxygen consumption.

Nitrates predominantly affect venous capacitance vessels. Intravenous nitrates are particularly helpful in acute left ventricular failure to reduce cardiac preload.

Calcium channel blocking agents do not have a specific role in heart failure. Although there may be a favourable acute response, long-term results have been disappointing, possibly because of negative inotropic activity. Nifedipine and verapamil are poorly tolerated in patients with heart failure, but the second-generation calcium antagonists, such as felodipine and amlodipine, have little cardiodepressant activity.

Positive inotropic agents

Logically, the use of positive inotropic agents should be of value in the treatment of heart failure to promote cardiac output. However, most of the drugs that have been tried so far have been associated with decreased survival in the long term (Felker and O'Connor, 2001). Inotropic support may be of value in the short term in patients following acute myocardial infarction or cardiac surgery, or for those awaiting operation (including transplantation).

Digoxin

The role of digoxin in heart failure remains controversial, particularly following acute myocardial infarction (Spargias et al, 1999). The Digitalis Investigation Group (1997) showed that digoxin does not reduce mortality in patients with heart failure, but did reduce hospitalisation for worsening heart failure. The main role of digoxin is in patients with permanent atrial fibrillation and heart failure.

Beta-adrenergic agonists

Although short-term haemodynamic improvements may be seen in patients with heart failure, long-term use of beta-adrenergic agonists is limited by peripheral vasoconstriction. Dopamine and dobutamine are relatively cardioselective beta-1 stimulants and are especially useful in patients with heart failure and cardiogenic shock following myocardial infarction. Preferential arterial vasodilatation with low-dose dopamine may help renal, coronary and cerebral hypoperfusion. Significant vasoconstriction is, fortunately, only present with higher doses of dopamine, allowing the benefits of positive inotropism to improve renal perfusion and cardiovascular haemodynamics. Dobutamine is similar, and does not seem to affect the pulse rate so much.

Phosphodiesterase inhibitors

Phosphodiesterase inhibitors, such as enoximone, are employed for short-term intravenous use in patients with heart failure on intensive care units. These agents strengthen cardiac contraction and dilate peripheral vessels, reducing ventricular preload and afterload with little effect on blood pressure. Although they may be useful in the short term, there is no evidence that they improve survival. On the contrary, milrinone may produce a significant increase in mortality (Nony et al, 1994).

Beta-adrenergic blockers

Increased cardiac stimulation by catecholamines has adverse effects in patients with heart failure. Activation of adrenergic receptors can lead to myocyte toxicity. Beta-blockade has always appeared desirable, but until recently was contraindicated in the treatment of heart failure. However, beta-blockers are now established evidence-based and recommended treatment, because of beneficial effects on total and cardio-vascular mortality (Tendera and Ochala, 2001). All patients with chronic, stable heart failure (NYHA II/III) and depressed left ventricular function on ACE inhibitors and diuretics should be offered treatment with beta-blockers. Long-term treatment improves left ventricular function, reduces hospital admissions and associates with a reduction in all-cause mortality of about 12%. Contraindications include chronic obstructive pulmonary disease, hypotension (systolic blood pressure under 90 mmHg), bradycardia less than 50 beats/min or heart block. Therapy should be started with a very small dose and titrated up very slowly to maximal dosage, and continued indefinitely.

Initiation and uptitration of beta-blockers

Beta-blockade is underutilised in heart failure because it is generally assumed that initiation and uptitrating is difficult, or that there are too many contraindications. Patients should be on standard heart failure treatment with ACE inhibitors and diuretics before therapy is started. Initial doses must be small, then doubled every 2–4 weeks to target (Table 12.2).

During titration there may be transient worsening of heart failure symptoms, fluid retention, bradycardia or hypotension. Hence:

- If *heart failure symptoms* worsen, the dose of diuretics should be increased, with a temporary reduction in the dose of beta-blocker if needed
- If there is *symptomatic hypotension*, the dose of vasodilators should be reduced, and the dose of beta-blocker reduced if required
- If *symptomatic bradycardia* occurs, the dose of beta-blocker should be reduced.

Table 12.2 Starting and target doses of beta-blockers approved for the treatment of heart failure

Drug	Starting dose	Target dose
Metoprolol CR/XL	12.5–25 mg once daily	200 mg once daily
Bisoprolol	1.25 mg once daily	10 mg once daily
Carvedilol	3.125–6.25 mg twice daily	50 mg once daily

When the patient is stable, uptitration can be attempted again. Increasing availability of the relevant beta-blockers in appropriate formulations has helped this.

Antidysrhythmic agents

Atrial fibrillation is present in about a third of patients with heart failure, and many have complex ventricular dysrhythmias, which are not always symptomatic. Sudden death is the most common cause of death in patients with heart failure (up to 70%), presumably secondary to sustained ventricular tachycardia or fibrillation. The role of antidysrhythmic agents is not clear since most agents are negatively inotropic, and in some cases are pro-arrhythmic. Class 1 agents have been shown to increase mortality, but amiodarone might improve prognosis, and make patients less likely to go into atrial fibrillation. The increasing and routine use of beta blockers to improve survival and symptoms may exert some of their effect by their antidysrhythmic actions, although sotalol was found to increase mortality when used in heart failure trials.

Patients with heart failure who have been resuscitated from sudden cardiac death should be considered for an automatic implantable cardiodefibrillator.

New drug therapies

Endothelin antagonists, natriuretic peptides and calcium promoters are three new classes of drug under investigation. Endothelin is the strongest vasoconstrictor known, and antagonists have been found to reduce systemic and pulmonary vascular resistance and increase cardiac output. *Neiseritide* is a natriuretic peptide with vasodilatory effect; *lovosimendan* is a calcium promoter that enhances myocardial troponin binding and improves contractility.

Non-drug therapy in heart failure

The use of non-invasive positive airway pressure ventilation in acute pulmonary oedema helps improve oxygen saturation without adversely affecting cardiac output. Salt and water restriction may be beneficial, reducing fluid intake to 1–1.5 litres/24 h, and avoiding high-salt foods such as cheese, sausages, tinned soup and vegetables, chocolate, crisps and peanuts. Fresh produce such as fruit, vegetables, eggs and fish have relatively low salt content. Prostaglandin inhibitors, such as the non-steroidal anti-inflammatory agents, inhibit production of renal vasodilators, and antagonise the effect of loop diuretics.

Effective education and counselling of patients is important and enhances long-term adherence to complex drug regimens, and there is an important role here for specialist heart-failure nurses. Chronic heart failure predisposes to and can be exacerbated by pulmonary infection. Influenza and pneumococcal vaccination is advisable. Exercise training and rehabilitation may improve symptoms and quality of life, but no effect has been shown on survival.

Surgical approaches

Surgical treatment should be directed towards the underlying cause and mechanisms. If coronary heart disease is the underlying cause of heart failure, patients may benefit from revascularisation. This may be especially important where there is hibernating myocardium, or in patients presenting with heart failure secondary to silent ischaemia. Valve surgery or repair may be of value in selected cases. Cardiomyoplasty and the Batista operation are currently not recommended. Cardiac transplantation, sometimes with prior ventricular support, is an established therapy for severe heart failure. The role of surgery is discussed in Ch. 16.

Pacemaker therapy

About a third of patients with heart failure have intraventricular conduction defects resulting in discoordinated ventricular contraction. This may be partially overcome with biventricular pacing to resynchronise ventricular contraction. Several small trials indicate acute improvement in symptoms and exercise tolerance, but long-term results, especially effects on mortality, are not yet available.

HYPERTENSION

In adults, the considered upper limit of normal systemic blood pressure is 130–139/85–89 mmHg, and pressures consistently above these levels are defined as hypertension. Hypertension is more common in urban populations than in rural populations, and in those with diabetes, obesity or positive family histories. In over 90% of hypertensive patients there is no identifiable cause; these patients are said to have essential hypertension.

Occasionally, patients may be admitted to hospital with marked elevation of the blood pressure. When associated with certain symptoms, including headache, vomiting, retinal haemorrhages and disturbances of consciousness, the term *malignant hypertension* is used.

There are two groups of hypertensive emergencies seen on coronary care:

1. *Those with hypertensive heart failure.* Pulmonary oedema and hypertension often co-exist, and the blood pressure usually falls with effective treatment of left ventricular failure. Parenteral vasodilator therapy with nitrates is first-line treatment, particularly if there is co-existent myocardial ischaemia. Sodium nitroprusside is an alternative.

2. *Those with hypertension complicating acute coronary syndromes.* Many patients with acute myocardial infarction will be hypertensive on admission to hospital. Hypertension will often respond to pain relief and sedation, but those whose systolic blood pressure remains over 160 mmHg should be treated to reduce the risk of several cardiac complications, including cardiac rupture. Hypertension in the early stages of acute myocardial infarction increases the risk of stroke following thrombolysis, and uncontrolled severe hypertension therefore provides a relative contraindication to thrombolytic therapy. Beta-blockers are first-line therapy because of their prognostic benefits. Intravenous nitrates can also be used acutely.

Emergency treatment of hypertension aims to lower the blood pressure as safely as possible, rather than as quickly as possible. In patients with chronic hypertension, sudden reduction of the blood pressure may cause cerebral infarction. This is because cerebral autoregulation is set to higher levels (Fig. 12.1) and 'normal' blood pressures will be insufficient to perfuse the brain. Controlled reduction over the course of several hours is desirable.

CHEST PAIN

Acute chest pain is a very common reason for emergency hospital admission, and most patients are admitted directly to the coronary care unit. The prevalence of central chest pain in the community in the 40–60-year-old age group is about 8%. Half of these patients have 'typical' anginal pain, but only one-quarter will have coronary heart disease. The association between typical anginal symptoms and coronary artery disease is stronger in men than in women. In many people, the chest pain initially believed to be due to coronary heart disease is later shown to have other causes. The negative coronary angiography rate in the UK is 10%, but in the USA it is over 30%!

Formulating the initial diagnosis is sometimes very difficult given the number of possible sources of pain, including the heart, the pericardium, the lungs and pleura, the oesophagus, the spine and the chest wall. Many patients who arrive on the coronary care unit prove subsequently not to have had a heart attack, and many do not even have a cardiac cause of pain (see Table 4.1; page 66). Patients with chest pain of unknown cause are a particular management challenge.

STABLE ANGINA

Heberden introduced the term 'angina pectoris' in 1772 to characterise a syndrome in which there was 'a sense of strangling and anxiety' in the chest, especially in association with exercise (Heberden, 1772). We now know that the cause of the syndrome is myocardial ischaemia, although similar symptoms may be caused by disorders of the oesophagus, lungs or chest wall.

Angina may be defined as symptomatic coronary ischaemia of less than 5 min duration that is consistently precipitated by exercise or stress (over 90% of episodes), or infrequently at rest

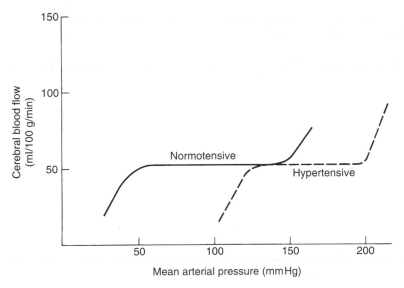

Figure 12.1   Cerebral autoregulation.

(under 10% of episodes). Angina is regarded as stable if it has been occurring over several weeks without major deterioration, although symptoms may vary depending upon many factors, including ambient temperature and emotion. The severity of stable angina has been classified by the Canadian Cardiovascular Society (see Table 8.1; page 166).

Angina is a common and disabling manifestation of coronary artery disease, with an estimated prevalence in the UK of 30 000–40 000 cases per million population. It is more common in men and with increasing age. Patients are often admitted to coronary care with new angina, or a severe attack of otherwise stable angina.

CAUSES OF ANGINA

Angina results from an imbalance of oxygen supply and demand to the myocardium. In most cases, this is due to fixed atheromatous deposits in the major epicardial arteries. Myocardial ischaemia leads to left ventricular dysfunction, which further impairs coronary blood flow and sets up a vicious cycle. Recurrent episodes of ischaemia lead to adaptive changes in myocardial metabolism termed 'hibernation', a chronic, but potentially reversible, state of myocardial dysfunction. On the other hand, periods of sublethal ischaemia may make the myocardium resistant to infarction, a situation termed *ischaemic pre-conditioning* (Yellon, 1995).

It is usually considered that a coronary artery must be narrowed by at least 50–70% in luminal diameter before coronary blood flow is inadequate to meet the metabolic needs of the heart during exertion, but this may depend upon on the number and length of the stenoses. Additionally, eccentric stenoses are not fixed and may alter with changes in coronary tone. Coronary arterial spasm most often occurs in association with an atheromatous plaque.

Prinzmetal (variant) angina describes a syndrome characterised by episodes of acute myocardial ischaemia associated with transient ST segment elevation on the ECG. These episodes may last several minutes, and resolve spontaneously, or may be aborted by glyceryl

trinitrate (GTN). About 0.5–1% of patients admitted to hospital with ischaemic chest pain have variant angina. Typically, Prinzmetal attacks occur at night, often waking the patient in the early morning. Ischaemic pain usually lasts longer than other types of angina, but almost always responds to GTN. Although the underlying problem is coronary artery spasm, the precipitants are not fully understood. No single mechanism has been demonstrated, but a history of migraine or Raynaud's disease is common, suggesting it may be part of a generalised vasospastic disorder. Symptoms wax and wane, with several attacks in a short space of time and then long periods of remission. Coronary spasm can also occur on exertion, and probably reflects a degree of underlying coronary atherosclerosis at the site of spasm. In patients with known coronary disease, the same picture can be produced by transient non-occlusive thrombosis. Some patients describe dyspnoea during attacks, presumably caused by transient rises in left ventricular filling pressures.

ECG during an episode of chest pain usually shows ST elevation, indicating transmural ischaemia, although ST depression may also occur in the same patient at different times. Spasm subsides spontaneously in most cases, but sometimes it may be so severe as to result in myocardial infarction (1.2% per year) and sudden death (0.5% per year).

Microvascular angina (syndrome X) is a condition, usually of women, where there is anginal pain in association with normal epicardial arteries.

INVESTIGATION OF PATIENTS WITH ANGINA

The history is the most important part of assessment. The ECG at rest may be normal, even in the presence of severe coronary artery disease. An abnormal ECG both supports the diagnosis and identifies those with a poorer prognosis. Exercise stress testing is appropriate in most cases, but is of limited usefulness in those with a low pre-test probability of coronary heart disease (e.g. young women). Radionuclide myocardial perfusion scintigraphy or stress echocardiography are alternatives. In many patents these may precede coronary angiography, although this investigation may be needed without prior functional testing for those with more severe symptoms. Angiography is justifiable in all cases where it would alter patient management. It carries a mortality of 0.1%.

MANAGEMENT

General management includes risk factor intervention, with particular regard to cholesterol, smoking and hypertension. Aspirin should be administered in all cases unless contraindicated (de Bono, 1999). Nitrates and calcium channel blockers are effective in controlling symptoms, but there is no evidence of superiority of any of these agents. Beta-blockade may reduce the incidence of cardiac events and improve survival (Nidorf et al, 1990), and should perhaps be used as first-line therapy along with sub lingual GTN as required. A resting heart rate below 60 beats/min is not an indication for dose reduction or failure to titrate to maximal doses. Diltiazem should be considered where beta-blockers are contraindicated. When combined with other anti-anginal therapy, nicorandil reduces symptoms and may reduce coronary deaths and non-fatal myocardial infarcts.

Both angioplasty and bypass surgery relieve symptoms, although those undergoing percutaneous coronary intervention (PCI) are more likely to need repeated intervention. In certain groups, coronary bypass surgery improves survival (ACC/AHA, 1999), but evidence is lacking in women or those aged over 65 years. Operative mortality from coronary artery bypass graft is around 1%. In patients with moderate or poorly controlled angina, PCI is appropriate and is more effective than medical therapy (Bucher et al, 2000).

PCI is unlikely to improve prognosis. The biological features of the lesion and not the degree of stenosis determine the probability of plaque rupture and coronary occlusion. Treatment of a single stenosis is unlikely to affect prognosis unless it is in the proximal left coronary artery.

NON-CARDIAC CHEST PAIN

Many patients admitted to coronary care do not have an acute cardiac problem, but may have other serious conditions requiring diagnosis and treatment. The most important of these are:

- Pulmonary embolism
- Dissecting aortic aneurysm
- Pericarditis
- Oesophageal pain
- Pneumothorax
- Abdominal pain.

PULMONARY EMBOLISM

Pulmonary emboli are common, and up to one-third are fatal, contributing to approximately 15–20% of all hospital deaths. In the UK, there are an estimated 20 000 deaths per year from pulmonary embolism, as well as a further 40 000 non-fatal cases. Most patients have clinical risk factors, including immobility, recent surgery or recent myocardial infarction. The most common source of emboli is the deep veins of the legs, although clinical evidence is lacking in over half the patients presenting with pulmonary embolism. Emboli may originate from the right ventricle in some patients following myocardial infarction.

Signs and symptoms

Pulmonary emboli may cause varying degrees of symptoms and signs, depending upon their size; many may not be detected clinically. *Acute minor pulmonary emboli* present with pleuritic chest pain and some breathlessness, but little haemodynamic disturbance. There may be tachycardia, gallop rhythm and a raised jugular venous pressure. *Acute major pulmonary emboli* will obstruct the major pulmonary vessels and produce sudden circulatory arrest, syncope, cyanosis and cardiac arrest (often marked by pulseless electrical activity on the ECG).

Investigations

The diagnosis of pulmonary emboli is not easy. Most diagnostic tests are non-specific and are prone to misinterpretation, and many patients correctly diagnosed have negative investigations.

Electrocardiography

The ECG is vital to exclude myocardial infarction, but there are no diagnostic changes of pulmonary embolism. The ECG is usually normal in acute minor pulmonary embolism. Non-specific findings include sinus tachycardia, widespread T wave inversion (especially in leads V1–V4), right axis deviation, right bundle branch block and the classical $S_1Q_3T_3$ pattern of acute cor pulmonale. Atrial fibrillation is precipitated in about 5% of cases.

Arterial blood gases

Since pulmonary emboli can give rise to both vascular and airway changes, blood gas alterations are variable, and often within normal limits. The classical abnormalities are hypoxaemia and hypocapnia. Patients with heart failure or chronic lung disease may also have pre-existing abnormalities.

Radiology

The chest X-ray is often normal, but may reveal an alternative diagnosis, such as pneumothorax or pneumonia. Loss of lung volume (e.g. an elevated hemidiaphragm) is the most common radiological sign of significant pulmonary embolism, and there may be pulmonary opacities (not necessarily wedge-shaped) or linear atelectasis with a small pleural effusion. Larger emboli will produce an area of oligaemia with a 'plump' hilum.

A ventilation/perfusion (V/Q) lung scan is usually the next investigation. The patient is injected with technetium-labelled macro-aggregates of albumin, which lodge in the pulmonary capillaries and show the distribution of pulmonary blood flow. The distribution of the trapped macro-aggregates is determined with a gamma-camera, which produces multiple views of pulmonary perfusion. Significant perfusion defects are seen as 'cold' spots. Although a normal perfusion study essentially excludes pulmonary embolism, false positive scans are common, with defects produced by numerous conditions affecting pulmonary blood flow, including chronic obstructive airway disease, pneumonia and pleural effusions. In these cases, a ventilation scan is needed to clarify the diagnosis. During a ventilation scan, the patient inhales a radioactive gas such as krypton–81 m, or uses a technetium–99 m-labelled aerosol. The gamma-camera records the distribution of alveolar gas in a multiple view series, which is compared with the perfusion scan. Ventilation should be preserved in the areas of abnormal perfusion in cases of pulmonary embolism. This *ventilation/perfusion mismatch* is the hallmark of pulmonary embolism. If the area of hypoperfusion is due to primary lung disease, ventilation to the same area will be impaired, resulting in a *matched defect*. Lung scans are usually reported as representing a low, moderate or high likelihood of pulmonary embolism. When suggestive of pulmonary embolism, it is likely that the scan underestimates the size of the embolus.

Spiral CT angiography can demonstrate emboli directly as filling defects within the proximal pulmonary arteries following an injection of iodinated contrast medium. Small emboli may be missed. Computed tomography (CT) can also identify alternative causes for chest pain and breathlessness.

Bilateral leg ultrasound or venography, even in the absence of leg symptoms, may be helpful in showing thrombus if other tests have been normal, but the degree of suspicion remains high. CT of the leg veins immediately after spiral CT angiography can be used to identify thrombus without needing a separate examination (Cham et al, 2000).

Echocardiography

Transthoracic echocardiography cannot identify thrombus in the pulmonary vessels, but may show thrombus floating in the right heart. The finding of right ventricular dysfunction is not specific, but a dilated and overloaded right ventricle may be supportive of the diagnosis of large emboli. The echo may be normal, even in patients with large pulmonary emboli.

Other conditions, such as myocardial infarction, aortic dissection and pericardial tamponade, can be demonstrated by echocardiography.

Pulmonary arteriography

Pulmonary angiography is the 'gold standard' for making the diagnosis, although it is seldom required. It is indicated in severely ill patients where the diagnosis is not clear, particularly if pulmonary embolectomy or thrombolysis is being considered. It is also useful where clinical suspicion is high, but other investigations have been non-diagnostic.

Diagnosis

The accuracy of both ventilation/perfusion scintigraphy and spiral CT angiography depends on the pre-test likelihood of pulmonary embolism, so if selection criteria are weak the prevalence of pulmonary embolism will be low and overall accuracy will fall. D-dimer concentrations may be assessed as a measure of fibrinolytic activity. Elevated values are non-specific, so D-dimer assays can be used to help exclude rather than confirm venous thromboembolism, but may reduce the need for further investigation (British Thoracic Society, 1997). Because a negative result virtually excludes pulmonary embolism (Egermayer et al, 1998), definitive imaging can be reserved for patients with a positive result. If the chest radiograph is normal or near normal, a V/Q scan should be diagnostic, but if the chest X-ray is abnormal, or an urgent result is required, a spiral CT is the better first-line investigation (Dixon et al, 2001).

Management

The treatment of pulmonary embolism is determined by the symptoms and degree of haemo-

dynamic upset (Gray and Firoozan, 1992). Most emboli will break up spontaneously, and management should be directed towards sustaining life and preventing recurrence. Pain and anxiety should be treated with diamorphine, and 100% oxygen should be given. Vasodilators are contraindicated, and a high central venous pressure should be maintained.

There are three treatment options:

- Anticoagulation
- Thrombolysis
- Surgery.

Anticoagulation

Heparin accelerates the action of antithrombin III and prevents further fibrin deposition, allowing spontaneous endogenous thrombolysis. Unfractionated heparin is used with a loading dose of 5000–10 000 U, followed by a continuous intravenous infusion of 1000–2000 U/h. This requires frequent blood sampling to ensure that the APTT (activated partial prothrombin time) remains 2–3 times the control for at least 7 days, with warfarin overlapping for 5 days. Longer periods of heparin are needed for massive pulmonary emboli. Low molecular weight heparin has now mostly replaced standard heparin, and is as at least as effective (Anonymous, 1998).

Thrombolysis

Thrombolysis is indicated in massive pulmonary embolism with right ventricular overload and hypotension. In contrast to coronary thrombolysis, it may be effective for up to 14 days after the acute event. Streptokinase, urokinase, tPA (tissue plasminogen activator) and reteplase have all been used, and are equally effective if administered either by a pulmonary arterial catheter or peripherally. The usual precautions and contraindications apply, as for coronary thrombolysis. Complications are of course similar. Thrombolysis has not yet been shown to be superior to heparin with regard to mortality, although patients do become haemodynamically stable more quickly following thrombolysis.

Surgery

Embolectomy is very effective in selected cases, but requires cardiopulmonary bypass and is associated with a mortality of over 50%. Prior pulmonary angiography is mandatory. Those normally considered are patients who continue to deteriorate despite thrombolytic therapy, those in whom thrombolysis is contraindicated and those with respiratory failure and shock.

Prognosis

Most deaths from pulmonary emboli occur in the first hour, and the overall mortality is about 10%. Spontaneous endogenous thrombolysis starts within hours, and small emboli will not be detectable after 5 days. About 50% of lung scans will be normal by 2 weeks.

DISSECTING THORACIC AORTIC ANEURYSM

An acute dissecting aneurysm is the most frequent, and most lethal, disorder of the thoracic aorta. There is an incidence of 5–10 per million population, and it is thus twice as common as rupture of an abdominal aortic aneurysm. It is more common in men over the age of 60 years, and there is usually a previous history of hypertension. A combination of a high intraluminal pressure and/or degenerative medial arterial disease is usual. Inherited diseases such as Marfan's syndrome, Ehlers–Danlos syndrome and other familial forms of thoracic aneurysms are common, and a positive family history may be a useful diagnostic aid. Cocaine and amphetamine abuse associate with aneurysm formation.

The aneurysm is a sac that is filled with blood, which forms a pulsatile mass and usually presents with acute dissection, leakage or rupture. Most dissections (66%) arise in the ascending aorta, and the blood passes into the medial layer of the aortic wall. The dissection is usually spontaneous, initiated by a small tear in the aortic intima typically 1–3 cm distal to the coronary ostia, which is the site of maximal haemodynamic and torsional stress. The next most common

site is distal to the origin of left subclavian artery where the relatively mobile aortic arch is anchored to the chest wall by the *ligamentum arteriosum*. Blood is driven at high pressure into the aortic wall, which splits along planes of least resistance. The blood may then flow proximally into the pericardium causing tamponade, or distally to involve the aortic arch, descending and abdominal aorta and its branches. Antegrade dissection seems to be more common.

The De Bakey classification describes dissections as type 1 if they involve the whole aorta, type 2 if they involve the ascending aorta, and type 3 if they involve the descending aorta. The Stanford classification simply divides dissections into type A and type B. Type A is any dissection involving the aortic arch, regardless of the site of the intimal tear. Type B dissections are those restricted to the aorta distal to the left subclavian artery.

Clinical features

The presentation of dissecting thoracic aortic aneurysm is usually dramatic and dominated by pain. There is sudden, sharp and excruciating pain felt anywhere from the epigastrium to the neck. It radiates to the back and, sometimes, all four limbs. The patient is cold, clammy and paradoxically hypertensive, with a systolic blood pressure often in excess of 200 mmHg, particularly if the dissection is distal. Shortness of breath may be due to left ventricular failure, a haemothorax or pericardial tamponade. Leaking aneurysms may cause pleuritic chest pain. Peripheral pulses may be absent, reduced or asymmetrical. Subsequent signs and symptoms depend upon which branches of the aorta are involved in the dissection process. For example, there may be a hemiplegia due to involvement of a carotid artery, or inferior myocardial infarction when the right coronary artery is involved (occlusion of the left coronary artery is usually fatal). Blood in the pericardial sac may give rise to a pericardial friction rub, and aortic incompetence may develop secondary to dilatation of the aortic ring. Such presentations often serve to confuse the diagnosis, as may the ECG, which can show ST elevation, dysrhythmias, left ventricular hypertrophy or conduction defects. Thrombolytic therapy may be given in error (Blankenship and Almquist, 1989). The chest X-ray is diagnostic in two-thirds of cases, showing a widened superior mediastinum, and sometimes a left-sided pleural effusion caused by extravasated blood. Care must be taken in interpreting the emergency anteroposterior (portable) chest film; apparent mediastinal widening may be seen in a normal patient. Echocardiography, particularly transoesophageal echocardiography, is useful in confirming the diagnosis, and may be supplemented by MRI (magnetic resonance imaging) or spiral CT scanning. Aortography is the standard technique for guiding interventions, but coronary angiography is not required in all cases.

Management

The two leading problems are pain and shock. Large doses of diamorphine are often required to control the severe pain, and are best given by intravenous infusion. Shock is usually secondary to the severe pain, since there will be only slight blood loss unless there is aortic rupture.

After pain relief, the next vital step is to reduce the blood pressure. Beta-blockade is particularly useful, since it will reduce both systolic blood pressure and the pulse pressure. The reduced force of cardiac contraction may further limit intimal tearing. Atenolol and metoprolol are available for intravenous use, but have long half-lives. Propranolol or esmolol are shorter-acting alternatives. Labetalol may be particularly suited as the alpha-blocking activity of the drug helps to maintain peripheral vasodilatation. If beta-blockade alone does not control the blood pressure, vasodilators are ideal additional agents, but will increase the force of ventricular contraction unless co-prescribed with a beta-blocker. Sodium nitroprusside is a useful alternative in view of its short half-life. The antihypertensive therapy should be carefully titrated to keep the systolic blood pressure to 100–120 mmHg, whilst maintaining adequate renal perfusion. With successful hypotensive treatment, up to half the patients can survive, particularly those with small, distal dissections. If complications emerge, or the blood pressure cannot be controlled, surgical intervention is required, and this is always needed if the ascending aorta is involved.

The aim of surgery is the prevention of aortic rupture or cardiac tamponade (Erbel et al, 2001). It is also important to eliminate aortic regurgitation and to avoid myocardial ischaemia. For proximal dissections, the intimal tear or whole flap is excised, and a composite graft is set in, with or without implantation of the coronary arteries. For distal dissections, medical treatment is preferred, unless there are clinical signs of aortic expansion, persistent chest pain or peri-aortic haematomas. Treatment is directed primarily to alleviate the expansion process, and involves the replacement of the affected portion with a tubular graft.

Prognosis

Untreated, the mortality is 30% in the first day, increasing to 70% in 7 days and 90% by 3 months. With modern medical and surgical intervention, the 1-year survival is 52%, 69% and 70% for type 1, 2 and 3 dissections, respectively, falling to 48%, 50% and 60% after 2 years.

PERICARDITIS

Acute pericardial disease has many causes, the most common being acute viral pericarditis and post-infarction pericarditis. The pain may be severe, especially if the adjacent pleura is affected. Pericardial pain may radiate to the arms, back, upper abdomen, shoulder tip or neck. The diagnosis should be suspected if the pain is worse on lying flat, and may be confirmed by an audible pericardial friction rub. The rub is high-pitched, superficial and scratchy and is similar to the sound made by stroking the hair above the ear. It has a to-and-fro sound passing between diastole and systole as the ventricles fill. It may be missed since it is often soft, transient, localised and intermittent. Shoulder-tip pain is common if the inferior surface of the heart is involved. The ECG in acute pericarditis shows ST segment elevation, which is concave upwards (like a saddle) in many leads. Reciprocal ST depression is sometimes present. As the inflammation improves, T wave inversion may develop.

Post-infarction pericarditis

Up to 20% of transmural myocardial infarcts are complicated by pericarditis within the first week. Small effusions may be detectable on echocardiography. Pericarditis may also recur within 3 months, in association with plural effusions and systemic symptoms, including malaise and fever (Dressler's syndrome). It may associate with pleurisy and pleural effusions. Dysrhythmias are less common. The mechanism is thought to be autoimmune, triggered by a response to the products of myocardial damage. Antimyocardial antibodies can be found. A similar condition may rarely complicate cardiac surgery (postcardiotomy syndrome).

Viral pericarditis

Acute viral pericarditis affects young adults; the usual viruses are from the Coxsackie B group, echoviruses, influenza and infectious mononucleosis. Following a typical flu-like illness there is fever and chest pain, which is sharp, retrosternal and radiates to the left shoulder. The pain may be mild or excruciating. Atrial dysrhythmias are common, possibly caused by inflammation of the superficially located sinus node. The ECG may show sinus tachycardia and widespread ST elevation, which is concave upwards in the leads facing the affected cardiac surface (Fig. 12.2).

Treatment

Treatment depends on the severity of the symptoms. In most cases simple analgesia or nonsteroidal inflammatory agents are enough, with bedrest. More severe cases require steroids, which will quickly control pain, fever and any resistant atrial dysrhythmias. If there is an associated myocarditis, bedrest is important. A small number of patients will develop transient pericardial constriction or effusion following viral pericardi-

tis. Anticoagulation therapy should be reduced or stopped to avoid haemorrhagic pericarditis. It is obviously important that patients who present with viral pericarditis are not inadvertently thrombolysed, since fatal tamponade can result. Recurrence of pericardial pain may return weeks or months after the initial attack. These attacks are self-limiting and eventually settle within 6–12 months (Fowler and Harbin, 1986).

PNEUMOTHORAX

The pain from pneumothorax is sudden, often severe, and usually unilateral, although a mediastinal pneumothorax can present with central chest pain. Dyspnoea and hypotension may follow, sometime with cyanosis. Transient nonspecific ECG changes may be seen. Diagnosis is by X-ray, and treatment governed by the size of the pneumothorax. Most cases can be treated conservatively, but, for patients with respiratory difficulty, aspiration or a chest drain will be required.

OESOPHAGEAL PAIN

Oesophageal pain has many patterns. It may be described as burning, gripping, pressing or stabbing. *Reflux oesophagitis* can be demonstrated in about 40% of the general adult population, and related pain is often confused with angina because it often radiates to the jaw and may be relieved by nitrates. Unfortunately, because it is so common, it frequently co-exists with ischaemic chest pain, and the diagnosis of reflux oesophagitis does not exclude co-existent myocardial ischaemia. Oesophageal reflux lowers the threshold for anginal pain (Davies et al, 1985). Endoscopy should not be performed until acute cardiac ischaemia has been excluded.

Oesophageal rupture is an uncommon disorder, which may easily be confused with myocardial infarction. The pain is severe, central and often radiates to the back. The patient may be sweating, cyanosed or shocked. Chest pain follows rather than precedes the vomiting, as in myocardial infarction. If there is leakage of gastro-oesophageal contents into the mediastinum, the condition can be lethal if untreated.

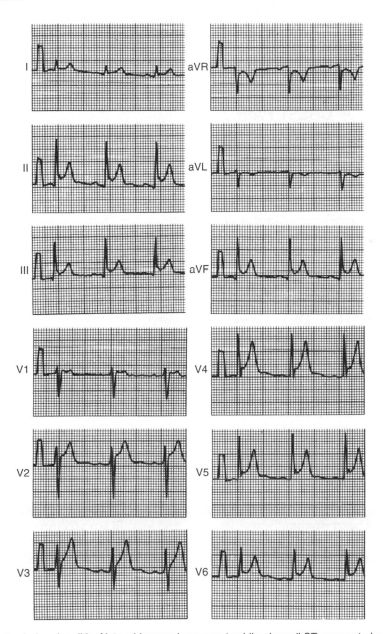

Figure 12.2 ECG: acute viral pericarditis. Note widespread concave 'saddle-shaped' ST segment elevation.

ABDOMINAL CAUSES OF CHEST PAIN

Peptic ulcer disease or gallbladder disease may present with lower chest/upper abdominal pain, which may be referred to the shoulders. Chronic cholecystitis may have many similarities to anginal pain. During acute cholecystitis, the ECG may show T wave inversion, especially in the inferior leads. A perforated peptic ulcer may mimic myocardial infarction.

Occult *gastrointestinal bleeding* may present with pain and shock and can be easily confused with acute myocardial infarction.

Acute pancreatitis may present with shock, hypoxia and severe upper abdominal/lower chest pain. Sitting forward may ease the pain forward, rather as in pericarditis. The common associates are alcohol misuse, hyperlipidaemia or gallstone disease.

OTHER CAUSES OF CHEST PAIN

There are many benign causes of chest pain that present on the coronary care unit, usually because the patient is anxious and hyperventilating, and particularly if the patient has an abnormal ECG. Musculoskeletal pain may produce localised chest pain, worse on movement or on moving the arms. Tietze's syndrome describes costochondritis.

DYSRHYTHMIAS

Dysrhythmias not associated with acute myocardial infarction often present to the coronary care unit. Coronary artery disease may or may not be an underlying cause. Supraventricular tachycardias may be regular (atrioventricular re-entry tachycardia, atrioventricular node re-entry tachycardia, atrial flutter, atrial tachycardia), or irregular (atrial fibrillation).

ATRIAL FIBRILLATION

Atrial fibrillation (AF) is the most common sustained disturbance of heart rhythm. Its incidence doubles for every decade after the age of 55 years, resulting in a prevalence of 11–17% in people over the age of 70 years (Psaty et al, 1997). Much of the morbidity and some of the mortality associated with AF is due to stroke. Patients at the highest risk of stroke associated with AF include those with long-standing hypertension, valvular heart disease (rheumatic), left ventricular hypertrophy, coronary artery disease (with or without depressed left ventricular function), or diabetes. The attributable risk of stroke from AF is estimated to be 1.5% for those aged 50–59 years and it approaches 30% for those aged 80–89 years. Many patients with new-onset AF and those with associated symptoms are often admitted to the coronary care unit to exclude an acute

ischaemic event or for cardioversion. Those who are stable may benefit from simple rate-control measures (e.g. intravenous beta-blockers); unstable patients with myocardial infarction and AF should be considered candidates for immediate cardioversion.

Lone AF is idiopathic, and is defined by the absence of any obvious underlying cause plus normal ventricular function by echocardiography. The majority are younger than 65 years. More frequently, AF is a marker for underlying cardiac pathology (coronary heart disease, sick sinus syndrome, cardiomyopathy, infiltrative heart disease). It may also indicate a systemic abnormality that predisposes the individual to the arrhythmia, such as thyrotoxicosis. Use of over-the-counter herbs (e.g. ephedra, ginseng) has been noted in some patients with new-onset AF. Ethanol use, both acutely (holiday heart) and chronically, is a common cause of AF.

When patients present, AF may be paroxysmal, persistent or permanent, although classification may be difficult, making management difficult. Paroxysmal AF is the most difficult form to manage, but fortunately most often occurs in normal hearts.

The development of AF requires both an underlying abnormality and a trigger (or triggers) to precipitate the onset. Prolonged AF produces myocyte degeneration and fibrosis, and significant electrophysiological changes so that AF begets AF. Triggers will vary between individuals and may include physical factors, such as atrial wall stress or metabolic factors such as ischaemia or acidosis. A focal area of ectopy has also been recognised in some cases, comprising sleeves of atrial myocardium extending into the pulmonary veins, which may be amenable to focal ablation (Thomas et al, 2000).

The dysrhythmia is easily recognised by ECG, but management may be difficult, as it is not a benign dysrhythmia. Its presence is associated with a doubling of mortality, mostly due to the marked increase in the rate of stroke. The loss of synchronised trial contraction also reduces cardiac efficiency, being most relevant when there is underlying cardiac pathology. There are three basic considerations in each patient:

- Whether to restore and maintain sinus rhythm
- Whether simply to control ventricular rate
- How to prevent stroke.

The decision of whether simply to control ventricular rate or to try and restore sinus rhythm is difficult. The Pharmacological Intervention in Atrial Fibrillation (PIAF) trial looked at patients with symptomatic atrial fibrillation of more than 1 week, but less than 1 year, duration (Hohnloser et al, 2000). Patients were randomised to either ventricular rate control with diltiazem, or attempted cardioversion to sinus rhythm using cardioversion and/or amiodarone. Amiodarone only restored sinus rhythm in 23% of patients, and the remainder needed cardioversion at least once. Neither treatment proved superior in terms of improvement in symptoms related to AF, but walking distance was better for those in whom sinus rhythm was restored, consistent with the haemodynamic improvement of establishing sinus rhythm. Hence, there are those in whom rate control may be considered as first-line treatment, such as those who are only mildly symptomatic. Rate control is also appropriate for those who have been in AF for more than 12 months, and where restoration of sinus rhythm would be unlikely. However, this strategy implies the need for lifelong anticoagulation to protect the patient from thromboembolism.

Ventricular rate control is usually straightforward with a beta-blocker or diltiazem, combined if necessary with digoxin. Beta-blockers are especially effective in the presence of thyrotoxicosis and hypertension.

Restoration and maintenance of sinus rhythm may be established chemically. Amiodarone is probably the most widely utilised drug, and has been shown to be superior to both sotalol and propafenone (Roy et al, 2000). Two new class III agents, dofetilide and ibutilide, have been introduced in Europe (but not yet in the UK). Oral dofetilide is more effective than amiodarone in restoring sinus rhythm, and maintaining normal rhythm. It is safe in those with abnormal left ventricular function. Ibutilide is used for the intravenous cardioversion of AF and atrial flutter, and, where it fails, it makes DC cardioversion more likely to succeed. Another class III drug, azimilide, is currently under investigation, as is dronedarone, a de-iodinated derivative of amiodarone that has none of the usual major toxicity of amiodarone.

Implantable atrial defibrillators can be programmed to restore sinus rhythm in paroxysmal AF, although their place is not yet established, as most patients cannot tolerate multiple shocks (Doaud et al, 2000). An 'ablate and pace' strategy involving AV node ablation with pacemaker implantation is sometimes used, which may improve ventricular function and quality of life (Wood et al, 2000). It is however, destructive and most would regard it as a last resort.

ATRIAL FLUTTER

Atrial flutter is much less common, and usually associates with underlying cardiac disease. In typical atrial flutter, an organised circular re-entry circuit depolarises in an anti-clockwise direction down the lateral border of the right atrium and back-up the interatrial septum at a rate of 300/min. The normal AV node cannot conduct at this rate, and 2:1 AV block usually occurs, giving rise to a regular narrow-complex tachycardia at a rate of 150 beats/min. Typical saw-tooth waves may be visible, especially in V1. These may be made more apparent with vagal manoeuvres that temporarily increase AV block.

Treatment depends upon the clinical situation. Urgent or elective cardioversion is usually the best therapy, because the rhythm is generally resistant to drug therapy. Class 1 antidysrhythmic agents may terminate the attack, but may paradoxically permit 1:1 conduction by transiently slowing the flutter rate. Amiodarone is therefore the drug of choice. It helps stabilise atrial activity, as well as blocking the AV node.

Patients are probably at similar risk of cardiac thromboembolism as patients with AF, and anticoagulation is required.

ATRIOVENTRICULAR NODAL RE-ENTRY TACHYCARDIAS

This is the most common type of regular supraventricular tachycardia, often presenting in early adult life when maturation of the AV node associates with development of two separate atrial inputs, one fast-conducting and one slow-conducting, predisposing to re-entry tachycardias. They share a final common pathway through the lower part of the AV node and bundle of His. The fast pathway has a long refractory period; the slow pathway has a short refractory period. During normal sinus rhythm, the impulse travels preferentially to the ventricles via the fast pathway. Impulses also travel down the slow pathway, but terminate because the common pathway is refractory. Episodes of tachycardia may be provoked by a premature atrial beat that occurs when the fast pathway is refractory. It then travels via the slow pathway, and is returned through the fast pathway back up to the atria, and circus movement through the AV node is initiated. Episodes of supraventricular tachycardia start suddenly, and may last for a few seconds to several days. Carotid massage or other vagal manoeuvres may terminate attacks. Adenosine, verapamil, flecainide and beta-blockers may all be useful for acute and chronic therapy. Recurrence on drugs is about 20%, and these patients should be referred for curative ablation (Schilling, 2002).

ATRIOVENTRICULAR RE-ENTRY TACHYCARDIAS

Accessory pathways are responsible for recurrent symptomatic regular supraventricular tachycardias in about 10% of cases. Patients are born with accessory pathways that connect atrial and ventricular myocardium, and related tachycardias may occur at any age. ECGs showing evidence of an accessory pathway are found in 0.15% of the general population, but less than half of these will ever develop symptomatic tachycardias. Typically, the resting ECG shows a short PR interval, often with a delta wave. Some AV connections only allow conduction from ventricles to atria, and cannot be detected on the resting ECG (concealed accessory pathway). Concealed accessory pathways account for 20% of regular paroxysmal supraventricular tachycardias. The resting ECG is normal, but, during episodes of tachycardia, P waves will be seen after the QRTS complex.

Although atrioventricular re-entry tachycardias are usually a benign phenomenon, a small number of patients have pathways capable of very rapid conduction. If the patient develops atrial fibrillation, fast AV conduction can precipitate ventricular fibrillation. Those with intermittent pre-excitation, or whose abnormal conduction disappears on exercise, are likely to have slow pathways, but electrophysiological studies are usual, with a view to ablation.

If the tachycardia is well tolerated, drug therapy can be used, but agents that block the AV node should be avoided (e.g. digoxin, verapamil, adenosine), as they can encourage rapid extranodal conduction, which may sometimes initiate ventricular fibrillation. Flecainide and amiodarone slow conduction in both the accessory pathway and the AV node and are preferable.

BROAD-COMPLEX TACHYCARDIAS

Almost any dysrhythmia can present as a broad-complex tachycardia. The majority will be (and should be assumed to be) of ventricular origin, but broad-complex supraventricular tachycardias may occur with rate-related or pre-existing bundle branch block. The Wolff–Parkinson–White syndrome may also present as a broad-complex tachycardia related to pre-excitation flutter or antidromic tachycardias.

ECG analysis may help differentiate the nature of the tachycardia, but has limitations. Access to an ECG in sinus rhythm is very helpful. Clinical signs of AV dissociation should be sought, such as variation in the venous pulse, loudness of the first heart sound and changes in the systolic blood pressure. The 12-lead ECG should then be examined systematically, bearing in mind that the majority of patients admitted to the coronary care unit with a broad-complex tachycardia have a tachycardia of ventricular origin, given the high prevalence of coronary heart disease, cardiomyopathy and electrolyte disturbances. The diagnosis of ventricular tachycardia (VT) is supported by:

- AV dissociation
- QRS duration >160 ms
- Left axis deviation (<−30°)
- Concordance of the QRS complex in the chest leads.

Characteristic patterns may also be seen in idiopathic VT. Those arising in the right ventricle will have a left bundle branch block type of QRS pattern, and those arising in the left ventricle will produce a right bundle branch block pattern. Other broad-complex tachycardias of ventricular origin include *torsade de pointes*, *right ventricular outflow tachycardia* and a *fascicular tachycardia*.

A *right ventricular outflow tachycardia* originates in the right ventricle, and produces ventricular complexes similar to those seen in left bundle branch block. Because it originates in the outflow tract, the impulse travels inferiorly, and produces a right axis pattern. The VT is non-sustained, and settles with beta-blockade. It usually does not associate with heart disease, but this should be distinguished from VT associated with right ventricular dysplasia.

A *fascicular tachycardia* is uncommon, and arises from round the posterior hemifascicle. The complexes are thus of a right bundle branch block appearance, and there is left axis deviation. The complexes are often only slightly widened to 0.12–0.14 s, and may resemble a supraventricular

tachycardia. Again, structural heart disease is unusual.

Confusion of VT with supraventricular tachycardia remains common, and, although misdiagnosis may put the patient in danger, treatments to terminate VT are unlikely to harm a patient in supraventricular tachycardia, but treating VT with verapamil may cause severe hypotension or cardiac arrest. Adenosine has a diagnostic role, and supraventricular tachycardia can be diagnosed if there is slowing of AV conduction or cardioversion occurs. If patients are haemodynamically compromised, the patient should undergo DC cardioversion as soon as possible and resuscitation guidelines followed as appropriate.

Episodes of broad-complex tachycardia are unlikely to be isolated, and recurrence may be anticipated unless a precipitant can be identified and eliminated. Tachycardias of ventricular origin require further investigation. Arguably, most should undergo coronary angiography, and, as a minimum, all should undergo echocardiography and exercise stress testing. Where there is no easily remediable cause, electrophysiological studies are usual, with drug therapy, ablation and implantation of automatic implantable cardiodefibrillators in selected cases.

BRADYCARDIAS

Symptomatic bradycardias are common secondary to age-related degenerative disease affecting the conducting tissues, often exacerbated by institution of AV node blocking drugs. Temporary or permanent pacing is often required.

REFERENCES

ACC/AHA (1999) Guidelines for coronary artery bypass graft surgery: executive summary and recommendations. *Circulation*, **100**: 1464–1480.

Anonymous (1998) Low molecular weight heparins for venous thromboembolism. *Drugs and Therapeutics Bulletin*, **36**: 25–29.

Blankenship JC, Almquist AK (1989) Cardiovascular complications of thrombolytic therapy in patients with a

mistaken diagnosis of acute myocardial infarction. *Journal of the American College of Cardiology*, **14**: 1579–1582.

British Thoracic Society (1997) Suspected acute pulmonary embolism: a practical approach. *Thorax*, **52** (suppl 4): S1–S24.

Bucher HC, Hengstler P, Schindler C et al (2000) Percutaneous transluminal coronary angioplasty versus medical treatment for non-acute coronary heart disease:

meta-analysis of randomised controlled trials. *BMJ,* **321:** 73–77.

Caruana L, Petrie MC, Davie AP et al (2000) Do patients with suspected heart failure and preserved left ventricular systolic function suffer from 'diastolic heart failure', or from misdiagnosis? A prospective description study. *BMJ,* **321:** 215–218.

Cham MD, Yankelevitz DF, Shaham D et al (2000) Deep venous thrombosis: detection by using indirect CT venography. *Radiology,* **216:** 744–751.

Cleland JGF, Clark A, Caplin JL (2000) Taking heart failure seriously. *BMJ,* **321:** 1095–1096.

Cowie MR (2000) BNP: soon to become a routine measure in the care of patients with heart failure? *Heart,* **83:** 617–618.

Cowie MR, Wood DA, Coats AJS et al (1999) Incidence and aetiology of heart failure. A population based study. *European Heart Journal,* **20:** 421–428.

Crilley JG, Farrer M (2001) Left ventricular remodeling and brain natriuretic peptide after first myocardial infarction. *Heart,* **86:** 638–642.

Davies HA, Rush EM, Lewis MJ et al (1985) Oesophageal stimulation lowers angina thresholds. *Lancet,* **i:** 1011–1014.

de Bono for the Joint Working Party of the British Cardiac Society and the Royal College of Physicians of London (1999) Investigation and management of stable angina: revised guidelines 1998. *Heart,* **81:** 546–555.

Digitalis Investigation (DIG) Group (1997) The effect of digoxin on mortality and morbidity in patients with heart failure. *New England Journal of Medicine,* **336:** 525–533.

Dixon AK, Coulden RAR, Peters AM (2001) The non-invasive diagnosis of pulmonary embolus. *BMJ,* **323:** 412–413.

Doaud EG, Timmermans C, Fellows C for the Metrix Investigators (2000) Initial clinical experience with ambulatory use of an implantable atrial defibrillator for cardioversion of atrial fibrillation. *Circulation,* **102:** 1407–1413.

Egermayer P, Town GI, Turner JG et al (1998) Usefulness of D-dimer, blood gas and respiratory rate measurements for excluding pulmonary embolism. *Thorax,* **53:** 830–834.

Erbel R, Alfonso F, Boileau C et al (2001) Diagnosis and management of aortic dissection. *European Heart Journal,* **22:** 1642–1681.

Felker GM, O'Connor CM (2001) Inotropic therapy for heart failure: an evidence-based approach. *American Heart Journal,* **142:** 393–401.

Fowler NO, Harbin AD (1986) Recurrent pericarditis; follow up of 31 patients. *Journal of the American College of Cardiology,* **7:** 300–305.

Gaasch WH (1994) Diagnosis and treatment of heart failure based on left ventricular systolic or diastolic dysfunction. *JAMA,* **271:** 1276–1280.

Gray HH, Firoozan S (1992) Management of pulmonary embolism. *Thorax,* **47:** 825–832.

Heberden W (1772) Some account of a disorder of the breast. *Medical Transactions of the Royal College of Physicians of London,* **2:** 59.

Hohnloser SH, Kuck KH, Lilienthal J for the PIAF Investigators (2000) Rhythm versus rate control in atrial fibrillation. Pharmacological Intervention in Atrial Fibrillation (PIAF): a randomised trial. *Lancet,* **356:** 1789–1794.

Kramer K, Kirkman P, Kitzman D et al (2000) Flash pulmonary edema: association with hypertension and re-occurrence despite coronary revascularisation. *American Heart Journal,* **140:** 451–455.

Latini R, Maggioni AP, Masson S (2001) What does the future hold for BNP in cardiology? *Heart,* **86:** 601–602.

McMurray JJ, Stewart S (2000) Epidemiology, aetiology and progress of heart failure. *Heart,* **83:** 596–602.

Miller AB, Srivastava P (2001) Angiotensin receptor blockers and aldosterone antagonists in chronic heart failure. *Cardiology Clinics,* **19:** 195–202.

Nidorf SM, Thompson PL, Jamrozik KD et al (1990) Reduced risk of death at 28 days in patients taking beta-blockers before admission to hospital with myocardial infarction. *BMJ,* **300:** 71–74.

Nony P, Boissel JP, Lievre M et al (1994) Evaluation of the effect of phosphodiesterase inhibitors on mortality in chronic heart failure patients. A meta-analysis. *European Journal of Clinical Pharmacology,* **46:** 191–196.

Northridge D (1996) Furosemide or nitrates for acute heart failure? Lancet, **347:** 667–668.

Packer M (1992) Patho-physiology of chronic heart failure and treatment of heart failure. *Lancet,* **340:** 88–95.

Pitt B, Zannad, Remme WJ et al for the RALES Investigators (1999) The effects of spironolactone on morbidity and mortality in patients with severe heart failure. *New England Journal of Medicine,* **341:** 709–717.

Psaty BM, Manolio TA, Kuller LH et al (1997) Incidence and risk factors or atrial fibrillation in older adults. *Circulation,* **96:** 2455–2461.

Remme WJ, Swedberg K (2001) Guidelines for the diagnosis and treatment of chronic heart failure. *European Heart Journal,* **22:** 1527–1560.

Roy D, Talajic M, Dorian P et al (2000) Amiodarone to prevent recurrences of atrial fibrillation. *New England Journal of Medicine,* **342:** 913–920.

Schilling RJ (2002) Which patients should be referred to an electrophysiologist: supraventricular tachycardia. *Heart,* **87:** 299–304.

Spargias KS, Hall AS, Ball SG (1999) Safety concerns about digoxin after acute myocardial infarction. *Lancet,* **354:** 391–392.

Tendera M, Ochala A (2001) Overview of the results of recent beta-blocker trials. *Current Opinion in Cardiology,* **16:** 180–185.

Thomas SP, Nunn GR, Nicholson IA et al (2000) Mechanism, localisation and cure of atrial arrhythmias occurring after a new intra-operative endocardial radio-frequency ablation procedure for atrial fibrillation. *Journal of the American College of Cardiology,* **35:** 442–450.

Vasan RS, Larson MG, Benjamin EJ et al (1999) Congestive heart failure in subjects with normal versus reduced left ventricular ejection fraction: prevalence and mortality in a population based cohort. *Journal of the American College of Cardiology,* **33:** 1948–1955.

Wood MA, Brown-Maloney C, Kay GN et al (2000) Clinical outcomes after ablation and pacing therapy for atrial fibrillation. A meta-analysis. *Circulation,* **101:** 1138–1144.

Yellon D (1995) Ischaemic pre-conditioning. *British Journal of Cardiology,* **2:** 39–42.

13

Cardiac pacing and implantable defibrillators

Control over the electrical activity of the heart may be made by means of an artificial pacemaker. Temporary cardiac pacing is often used in coronary care and intensive care units to treat transient conduction problems, or sometimes to terminate abnormal tachycardias. If pacing is for a short time only, an external power source is used to deliver electricity to the heart, either internally (endocardial pacing), via the skin (transcutaneous pacing), or via the oesophagus (oesophageal pacing). However, when long-term control is required, a permanent pacemaker is implanted. The first implant was reported in 1958, and now over 200 000 permanent pacemakers are implanted worldwide every year.

INDICATIONS FOR PACING

Indications for pacing vary widely, both nationally and internationally. There is no consensus, and recommendations come from clinical experience rather than from scientific trials. The two main indications for pacing are where there is failure of impulse generation, or where there is failure of atrioventricular (AV) conduction. The American College of Cardiology and American Heart Association have produced pacing guidelines (ACC/AHA, 1998); some of the indications for temporary and permanent pacing are summarised in Boxes 13.1 and 13.2.

STOKES–ADAMS ATTACKS

Stokes-Adams attacks are often associated with second- and third-degree heart block, and require

---

Box 13.1   Some indications for temporary pacing

Acute myocardial infarction
1. Anterior myocardial infarction accompanied by:
   Complete heart block
   Second-degree heart block
   First-degree heart block with bifascicular block
   Newly acquired left bundle branch block
2. Inferior myocardial infarction accompanied by:
   Any of the above, accompanied by actual or
   threatened haemodynamic decompensation

Prior to permanent pacing
When patients are symptomatic and immediate
permanent pacing facilities are not available

Prophylactic peri-operatively
1. During general anaesthesia or cardiac
   catheterisation in patients with:
   Intermittent heart block
   Bifascicular block with first-degree heart block
2. During cardiac surgery
   Especially for aortic and tricuspid surgery
   Septal defect closure

Treatment of tachycardias
Overdrive pacing (rare)

Box 13.2   Some indications for permanent pacing

General agreement
Acquired symptomatic complete heart block
Symptomatic second-degree heart block
Symptomatic sinus bradycardia
Sinus node dysfunction
Carotid sinus syndrome

Frequent indications
Asymptomatic complete heart block
Asymptomatic second-degree heart block
Transient Möbitz type II heart block following acute
myocardial infarction
Bifascicular block in patients with syncope
Overdrive pacing for recurrent ventricular tachycardia

Generally not indicated
Syncope of unknown cause
Asymptomatic bradycardia
Sinus bradycardia with non-specific symptoms
Asymptomatic sinus arrest
Nocturnal bradycardia

---

pacing without the need for further investigation. The underlying disease in most of these cases is *Lenegre's disease* (AV fibrosis), and only a small number are due to ischaemic damage. As such, left ventricular function is usually normal, and the outcome following pacing is good. Less frequently, the aetiology is the sick sinus syndrome or paroxysmal tachycardias, which are usually evaluated by electrophysiological testing.

LOW-OUTPUT STATES ASSOCIATED WITH BRADYCARDIA

Raising the heart rate to between 70 and 80 beats/min by inserting a temporary pacemaker can improve cardiac failure or other symptoms, if these have been associated with bradycardia. Progressively raising the heart rate, however, may be detrimental, and associated with a fall of the cardiac output. In these circumstances, it is preferable to insert an atrial pacing wire and synchronise atrial and ventricular emptying in physiological sequence.

CONDUCTION DEFECTS FOLLOWING ACUTE MYOCARDIAL INFARCTION

Pacing is usually not indicated following inferior myocardial infarction, unless there are symptoms or signs attributable to low-output cardiac failure. Most bradycardias are responsive to atropine. The prognosis for conduction defects following anterior myocardial infarction is poor, with mortality relating to the extent of myocardial damage rather than to the conduction defects. Temporary pacing is often carried out, but seldom influences outcome. There is little doubt that pacing may be life-saving acutely, but its long-term value is a little more difficult to assess. Prognosis is influenced, not only by complications of the procedure (dysrhythmias, cardiac perforation and septicaemia), but also by the degree of underlying myocardial damage that originally led to the conduction defect. Many patients effectively treated acutely by temporary pacing die later while still in hospital from heart failure due to extensive myocardial infarction.

REFRACTORY TACHYCARDIAS

Where tachydysrhythmias are not controlled by medical therapy, permanent pacing may have a beneficial role. Ectopic foci can be suppressed by ventricular pacing at a higher rate than sinus rhythm (*overpacing*). Alternatively, fixed-rate pacing in short bursts either slower (*underdrive*) or faster (*overdrive*) than the sinus rate may be effective in preventing dysrhythmias. In the 'brady–tachy' syndrome, where the patient has both fast and slow dysrhythmias, drugs such as beta-adrenergic blocking agents and digoxin can be given to control the faster rates, using a pacemaker to prevent very slow heart rates.

PERI-OPERATIVE HEART BLOCK

Patients with sino-atrial (SA) disease or incomplete heart block may be at risk of developing complete heart block during drug therapy or surgery. General anaesthesia with fluorinated hydrocarbons (e.g. halothane) may adversely affect AV conduction. A pacing wire may need to be inserted peri-operatively for prophylactic reasons.

MISCELLANEOUS

Temporary pacing may be required in cases of permanent pacemaker failure, or for extreme bradycardias caused by drugs (e.g. digoxin or beta-adrenergic blocking agents) or electrolyte disturbances.

TEMPORARY CARDIAC PACING

Temporary endocardial pacing has been used since the early 1960s to maintain cardiac output during episodes of extreme bradycardia, heart block and asystole, particularly in association with acute myocardial infarction. Before the advent of cardiac pacemakers, the combination of acute myocardial infarction and complete heart block was usually fatal (Cohen et al, 1958). Pacing electrodes are now easily passed percutaneously into the right ventricle under local anaesthesia, and, in experienced hands, this is a safe and simple procedure (Gammage, 2000). Thrombolysis and other acute perfusional strategies have resulted in a decline in the number of patients requiring temporary pacing (Petch, 1999), so experience of the procedure is much less widespread than in the past, which may increase the morbidity of the procedure (Murphy, 2001). The wider availability of transcutaneous and transoesophageal pacing provides safe alternatives, and the beneficial effects of atropine and adrenaline (epinephrine) should not be forgotten.

ACUTE MYOCARDIAL INFARCTION, HEART BLOCK AND PACING
Pathophysiology

Inferior myocardial infarction (Table 13.1) is usually caused by occlusion of the right coronary artery, which supplies the inferior wall of the heart. The AV node is supplied by the right coronary artery in 90% of cases, and by the circumflex artery in the remainder. As a result, conduction disturbances commonly occur following acute inferior myocardial infarction, caused by ischaemia or oedema of the AV node. These

Table 13.1 Characteristics of complete heart block complicating inferior and anterior myocardial infarction

	Anterior infarction	Inferior infarction
Incidence	25–40%	60–75%
Pathology	Septal necrosis and infarction of the AV node and bundle branches	Ischaemia of the bundle branches
Timing	Usually sudden, following sinus rhythm or second-degree heart block	Normally slow, following first- and second-degree heart block
Ventricular response	30–40, unstable	40–60, stable
QRS morphology	Widened	Narrow
Risk of asystole	High	Low
Mortality	60–75%	25–40%
Prognosis	Often permanent	Most reverse within 14 days

effects will be exacerbated if there is pre-existing damage to the conducting tissues, such as ischaemia or fibrosis of the AV node and bundle branches. For unknown reasons, ischaemic injury to the AV node following inferior myocardial infarction is rarely permanent. Complete heart block usually develops slowly, and the escape rhythm usually has a high, junctional origin at 40–60 beats/min. This is generally haemodynamically stable, and pacing is not usually necessary, providing blood pressure and renal perfusion are maintained (Jowett et al, 1989). Conduction disturbances can occur at any time in the first 2 weeks, but are usually transient, with normal conduction returning in hours or days.

Anterior myocardial infarction (Table 13.1) is caused by occlusion of the left anterior descending coronary artery, which provides the major blood supply to the bundle of His and bundle branches. Proximal occlusion of the left coronary artery leads to extensive myocardial damage, often resulting in heart failure and cardiogenic shock. Heart block is a sinister and sudden complication, and is due to ischaemic destruction of the conducting tissues below the AV node. Emergent ventricular escape rhythms are unreliable, slow and irregular; there is a marked tendency to develop asystole. Insertion of a temporary pacing wire under these circumstances probably has little influence on the outcome, although it is usual practice. Mortality is high, and late deaths are common.

Hypertension, pre-existing diabetes mellitus and high blood glucose concentrations on admission to hospital are common risk factors for those requiring temporary pacing following acute myocardial infarction. Disorders of AV and intraventricular conduction are significantly more common in diabetic patients with acute myocardial infarction than in those who are not diabetic, and this may be due to pre-existing microangiopathic damage of the conducting system (Blandford and Burden, 1984). The higher incidence of previous myocardial infarctions and hypertension in those patients requiring pacing is probably an indication of underlying myocardial damage.

Prophylactic pacing

The potential complications of temporary pacing (especially bleeding following thrombolysis) should be considered before prophylactic wires are inserted following acute myocardial infarction. The more important indications are bifascicular block with AV block or left bundle branch block acquired during the infarct.

TEMPORARY PACING

There are three main forms of temporary pacing:

- Transcutaneous
- Transoesophageal
- Transvenous.

Transcutaneous pacing

External temporary cardiac pacing was first introduced in 1952, and was used widely as a temporary measure for the treatment of profound bradycardia and asystole until superseded by transvenous pacing in 1959. Contemporary temporary pacing guidelines place more emphasis on transcutaneous pacing, since invasive techniques involved in endocardial pacing are particularly hazardous following thrombolysis. Active (demand) pacing patches can be placed for those not requiring immediate pacing, but who are at risk of progression to AV block (ACC/AHA, 1999), and transcutaneous pacing is simple to institute following minimal training. Some indications for placement of transcutaneous patches are shown in Box 13.3.

Box 13.3 Demand transcutaneous pacing: some indications for placement of transcutaneous pacing patches following acute myocardial infarction

- Sinus bradycardia less than 50 beats/min, with hypotension
- Möbitz type II heart block
- Inferior myocardial infarction with complete heart block
- Newly acquired bifascicular block
- Bundle branch block with first-degree heart block

Two large pad electrodes are attached to the chest (preferably in the anteroposterior position). The positive electrode is located beneath the left scapula and the negative electrode under the left breast. Multifunctional electrode pads may allow both pacing and defibrillation if required. When temporary pacing is required, the output from the unit is then increased, until the pacing impulse 'captures' the heart. Modern units use longer pulse duration, allowing lower pulse amplitude, so that pacing is usually well tolerated with little more than slight cutaneous discomfort (tingling or tapping) and occasional muscle twitching (Zoll and Zoll, 1985). The pacing system is set in either active or standby mode to allow immediate use on demand. Clinical studies have shown efficacy for up to 14 h, although long-term transcutaneous pacing is unpleasant, and high-risk patients or those who will require long periods of pacing should be taken for insertion of a temporary endocardial wire.

Transoesophageal pacing

The technique of transoesophageal pacing was originally described in the late 1960s in New York (Burack and Furman, 1969). Unfortunately, the method is not very reliable, but it may act as a holding measure until transcutaneous pacing can take over, or a percutaneous wire can be inserted. The pacing electrode is passed transnasally into the oesophagus (rather like a nasogastric tube) and the current switched on, initially at about 30 V. When the diaphragm is reached (producing diaphragmatic twitching), the electrode is slowly withdrawn, until ventricular capture is seen on the ECG monitor, and the threshold is then determined.

Transvenous pacing

Transvenous endocardial pacing is the most common pacing method employed and involves the passage of a bipolar electrode into the apex of the right ventricle. The wire is best positioned with the aid of fluoroscopy, but may be located 'blindly' using a balloon-tipped 'flotation' pacing wire in patients who cannot be screened. Wires posi-

tioned in this way are often unstable, and transthoracic (external) pacing is probably a better emergency alternative.

It is usual for a special room to be set aside for pacing, so that there are facilities for sterility, fluoroscopy and resuscitation. The use of fluoroscopy is governed by a European Economic Community Directive (EEC, 1988). Those operating such equipment are required to be certified for proficiency, with an awareness of the safety aspects of radiation to the patient, the operator and others present.

CHOICE OF ROUTE FOR INSERTION OF TEMPORARY PACING WIRES

The choice of site of insertion of temporary pacing wires depends upon the expertise of the operator and the problems with the wire in the chosen location. Of the usual insertion sites (internal jugular, subclavian, femoral, brachial), the least skill is required for the femoral and brachial approaches. The subclavian route is the most hazardous, largely because of the dangers of pneumothorax and subclavian arterial puncture. The jugular line is much more stable, is the most comfortable for the patient, and does not inhibit mobility.

The right internal jugular approach is the most direct to the right ventricle if there is difficulty entering the heart, particularly if a balloon flotation catheter is used. The British Cardiac Society recommends the right internal jugular route, particularly for those with limited experience of central venous catheterisation (Parker and Cleland, 1993). Central venous cannulation could become less hazardous with the advent of ultrasound guides, although these are expensive.

METHODS OF CATHETERISATION

- Percutaneous needle and sheath techniques
- Percutaneous Seldinger technique, using a guide-wire
- Cut-down (suitable for the arm veins).

The method of choice is probably the Seldinger technique, although, once again, experience of the technique is desirable. The advantage is that a long cannula is passed into the superior vena cava, which helps the passage of the pacing wire into the heart. In addition, unlike shorter cannulae, it will not become displaced if external cardiac massage is required during the insertion procedure. If there is a cardiac arrest, it can be occluded and pacing resumed following resuscitation. The cannula can also be conveniently used for infusing drugs and other fluids as required.

The pacing wire becomes more pliable as it warms to body temperature, so should be inserted as quickly as possible. Sometimes, there is difficulty in passing the electrode into the superior vena cava; this can be made easier by moving the patient's shoulders or rotating the arm across the body. Passage through the heart requires experience and the ability to judge position from the fluoroscopic image. Traversing the tricuspid valve is a frequent problem, particularly if the heart rate is fast, or if the myocardium is irritable. Gently manipulating the tip downwards and towards the left heart border is often the best way to cross the valve. Occasionally it is necessary to loop the wire in the right atrium, and allow it to prolapse into the right ventricle. Gentle withdrawal then allows the tip to flick through the valve. Passage into the right ventricle can be confirmed by observing the characteristic 'bucking' of the catheter by the tricuspid valve about 5 cm from the tip. Wedging the electrode is sometimes made easier by passing it directly into the pulmonary artery (especially if a balloon flotation-type catheter has been used) and then letting it fall back into the apex. This can be seen just medial to the apex on the cardiac silhouette, and the tip of the electrode should point slightly inferiorly. Once wedged, verification of pacing and threshold measurements is necessary. The former is judged from the appearance of a pacing 'spike' preceding the QRS complex on the ECG. Each spike should capture a QRS complex (Fig. 13.1). The pacing threshold is obtained by determining the lowest pacing voltage that produces a paced beat. This threshold should be less than 1 V and preferably below 0.5 V. The wire can then be fixed to the skin with a

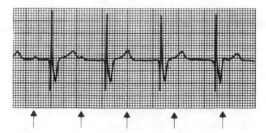

Figure 13.1 ECG: trace obtained when the cardiac pacing wire is correctly positioned. The pacing spike can be seen preceding each QRS complex. Independent atrial P waves are indicated.

suture. The pacing mode is then selected (usually 'demand') and the voltage set at about twice the threshold.

PROBLEMS DURING TRANSVENOUS PACING

Pacing and thrombolysis

The presence of complete heart block following acute myocardial infarction should not contraindicate thrombolysis. As for other cases of myocardial infarction, thrombolysis (preferably with tissue plasminogen activator, tPA) should be given immediately, along with atropine. In the majority of cases, AV conduction improves, and many cases of complete heart block may be tolerated without the need to insert a temporary pacemaker (Jowett et al, 1989). Anterior myocardial infarction complicated by complete heart block always warrants temporary pacing, but thrombolysis should still be given first. An insertion site that may be easily compressed should be chosen, and thus the femoral, brachial or external jugular routes are preferred.

Dysrhythmias

The major complications of temporary pacing are ventricular tachycardia and fibrillation, which are probably produced by mechanical irritation of the endocardium. The appearance of ventricular ectopics is usually a good sign that the catheter has entered the right ventricle, but the wire should be moved if these are frequent or occur in runs. This complication may also be caused electrically if the 'fixed' rather than the 'demand' mode is selected on the pacing box, or if an inappropriately high pacing threshold is used. Standard resuscitation is required during ventricular fibrillation, although overpacing can sometimes be used to restore a more stable rhythm in ventricular tachycardia. Recurrent ventricular dysrhythmias may require repositioning or even removal of the wire.

Patients with temporary wires should have the wire disconnected during the defibrillatory shock, to prevent damage to the external generator, although many have protective circuitry.

Perforation of the heart or septum

This may be an early or late complication, and may be indicated by:

- Failure to pace despite good radiological position
- Signs of pericarditis or tamponade
- Diaphragmatic twitching.

The lead can usually be withdrawn back into the ventricle and repositioned without any problem. Tamponade is very uncommon.

A change of the ECG pacing pattern from the usual left bundle branch block to right bundle branch block indicates that the wire has perforated the septum. This is usually insignificant, but the wire should be moved.

Failure to pace

Pacing failure may be evident from absence of a pacing spike (implying failure of pulse generation), or the spikes failing to capture (implying a displaced electrode or change in threshold). The box or the wire will then need replacing or repositioning.

Pacemaker dependence

Pacing wires often need repositioning, because they have moved, because of increasing pacing thresholds, or because of dysrhythmias. Unfortunately, pre-existing rhythms are often abolished after pacing for a while, leaving complete asystole as the underlying 'rhythm' (seen if the pacing box is momentarily turned off). Movement of the wire or transient rises in the threshold may then be associated with Stokes–Adams attacks, because the heart has become 'pacemaker-dependent'. This problem may need the passage of a second pacing wire, to take over while the other is relocated or removed.

Infection

Infection is more common when the temporary wire is left in for several days, or has been introduced via the femoral vein, when antibiotic prophylaxis should be considered. Most infections are with *Staphylococcus epidermidis*, but coliforms may complicate the femoral approach. Because of the problem of infection, temporary pacing should be avoided if permanent pacing is going to be required.

WHEN TO STOP TEMPORARY PACING

Following acute myocardial infarction, it is usual to leave pacing wires *in situ* for 24–48 h after reliable AV conduction has recovered.

Patients with inferior myocardial infarction usually develop AV nodal dysfunction because of oedema rather than necrosis. The recovery period is usually short but may be up to 14 days. Those with anterior myocardial infarction will usually have infarcted conduction tissue and will need permanent pacing. These patients often have severe left ventricular damage, and a poor prognosis. Dual chamber pacing is often used to maximise cardiac output.

CARE OF PATIENTS WITH TEMPORARY PACING WIRES

Patients often feel much better following temporary pacing, and are in a much better physical and psychological state for discussion about the pacemaker and its implications. Mobility will necessarily be restricted, but if the jugular approach has been used, this will be minimal. However, the wire should be secured to the body to prevent accidental pulling. Many pacing boxes are now small and portable, thus enabling early mobilisation of the patient. There is usually not much pain at the site of wire insertion, but this should be routinely observed for signs of bleeding and infection. Routine checks are also required on the equipment, with attention to connections and performance. The threshold and underlying rhythm need charting on a twice-daily basis and settings discussed for the following 12-h period. This should be documented in the patient's notes and the nursing notes, as well as on the charts beside the bed. Although many pacing units are protected, it is advisable to turn off the pacemaker to prevent electrical damage if the patient needs defibrillation.

Removal of the pacing wire is a simple and straightforward procedure carried out at the patient's bedside. The unit should be turned off and the dressing and retaining sutures removed. While observing the ECG monitor for ectopic activity, the wire should be slowly withdrawn and a sterile pad held firmly over the puncture site for a few minutes, to prevent bleeding. It may be advisable to remove the tip of the disposable pacing wire aseptically, for sending to the bacteriology laboratory if the patient has been pyrexial.

PERMANENT PACEMAKERS

The development of implantable cardiac pacemakers has made the selection of the correct unit required for permanent pacing very difficult, and recommendations are changing rapidly. Generator choices include single-versus dual-chamber devices, unipolar or bipolar configuration, sizes, battery capacity and cost. There are many different types of lead and programmable features. With the ever-increasing demand for specialist assessment, pacemaker implantation may soon be established as a subspecialty. About 200 new pacemakers are inserted annually for every million people in Britain, and this number is increasing. The cost of the systems increases with the degree of complexity and sophistication, and trials are needed to evaluate the incremental cost-effectiveness of additional features. About 16% of pacemaker implantations are for replacement of the generator, mostly because of battery failure.

The indications for pacing are based upon careful evaluation of symptoms, ECGs, Holter tapes and, sometimes, electrophysiological tests. Additionally, long-term prognosis and general medical and psychological health need to be taken into account before any decision is made to implant a permanent pacemaker.

THE PERMANENT PACEMAKER

The modern pacemaker is a small metal box weighing 30–130 g, and powered by a lithium battery that lasts up to 15 years. Two types of pulse generator are currently available for permanent implantation: single-chamber pacemakers have the electrode placed in either the atrium or the ventricle; dual-chamber pacemakers have electrodes situated in both chambers. Although non-programmable pacemakers are still in use, new implants are now programmable. These enable greater flexibility in pacemaker function (e.g. rate, output, sensitivity and inhibitory functions, which can be altered to meet the specific requirements of the individual patient). Changes are needed in about 20% of patients following implantation and can be undertaken without need for a second operation or implantation of a different pacemaker.

INDICATIONS FOR PERMANENT PACING

Pacing may be considered for either symptomatic benefit or to improve prognosis. For example, untreated complete heart block has a poor prognosis, with a mortality of up to 30% per year, even in asymptomatic patients. Treatment by cardiac pacing restores normal life expectancy.

The British Pacing and Electrophysiology Group (BPEG) (1991) and the North American Task Force (ACC/AHA, 1998) have produced similar recommendations for the selection of pacemakers for particular patients. The essential elements are that the ventricle should be paced if there is threatened or actual AV block, and the atrium should be sensed and/or paced unless contraindicated. Wherever possible, a pacing mode that produces the best equivalent of sinus rhythm should be adopted, and for most purposes this is best produced by dual-chamber systems.

SINGLE- AND DUAL-CHAMBER PACING

The original permanent pacemakers were single-chamber pacemakers (VVI units; see Table 13.2), the electrode being located in the right ventricular apex. However, ventricular pacing results in the reduction of about 20% of the cardiac output because of the loss of the haemodynamic contribution of atrial systole. This may be critical in patients with poor left ventricular function, who would benefit from synchronised sequential AV activity. Atrial pacemakers will obviously overcome this problem, provided there is no AV nodal conduction block. These simple pacemakers are useful for those patients with symptomatic SA disease and require a single electrode in the right atrial appendage. A second, and often distressing, problem with ventricular pacemakers is the *pacemaker syndrome*, again caused by impairment of cardiac output. Although the pacemaker may be functioning correctly, the patient continues to complain of dizzy spells, syncope, exercise limitation and postural hypotension. This is a consequence of episodic mechanical AV dissociation, when the atria contract during ventricular systole. Retrograde conduction from the ventricles to the atria causes them to contract against closed AV valves, result-

ing in raised left and right atrial pressures. A fall in cardiac output and systemic blood pressure then follows, which is often symptomatic. Drugs, such as flecainide and disopyramide, can be used to prevent this abnormal conduction, often with complete resolution of these distressing symptoms. However, what is required and preferred is sequential AV contraction, as occurs physiologically. This may be achieved with dual-chamber pacemakers. Pacing of the atrium to improve symptoms and exercise tolerance is becoming routine. Restoring atrial transport improves cardiac output and reduces the risk of atrial fibrillation, emboli, stroke and heart failure. In addition, symptoms attributable to the pacemaker syndrome are abolished (Traville and Sutton, 1992).

PACEMAKER CODES

An international identification code, universally referred to as the 'NBG code', has been produced jointly by the British Pacing and Electrophysiology Group (BPEG) and the North American Society for Pacing and Electrophysiology (NASPE), and is shown in Table 13.2. The five-letter code provides a standardised means of identifying the functional operation of a cardiac pacemaker, regardless of its make or model (Bernstein et al, 1987). The minimum code length is three letters (I–III), 0 being used if a function is not present. Code letters IV and V are often omitted.

The first two code letters indicate the chambers in which the pacemaker operates. *Position I* represents the chamber paced, *position II* indicates the chamber sensed. If the pacemaker can sense and pace the same chamber, it is designated D (dual).

Table 13.2 Permanent pacemaker coding of modes and functions

I: chamber(s) paced	II: chamber(s) sensed	III: mode(s) of response	IV: programmable functions	V: anti-tachycardia functions
V = ventricle	V = ventricle	T = triggered	R = rate-modulated	P = paced
A = atrium	A = atrium	I = inhibited	M = multiprogrammable	S = shocks
D = dual	D = dual	D = dual	C = communicating	D = dual
0 = none	0 = none	0 = none	0 = none	0 = none

Position III describes the mode of response to sensing, such as I for 'inhibited' (when the presence of sensed electrical activity from the heart inhibits the pacemaker), or T for pacemakers that are 'triggered' by spontaneous cardiac electrical activity. D in position III indicates a double response: an atrial-triggered and ventricular-inhibited pacemaker. Reverse-pulse generators come into action only during abnormally fast rates, to terminate the dysrhythmia. Placing a pacemaker magnet over most pacemakers will temporarily turn the sensing function off, and the pacemaker functions in asynchronous mode (A00, V00, D00).

Position IV describes the programmable features, such as rate and/or output, which may be altered non-invasively. Details of programming are transmitted using strings of electronic impulses from an external programming head, which also permits reprogramming if required. An increasing number of pacemakers incorporate some kind of sensor, which can be programmed to modify the pacing rate in response to exercise or emotion, thus improving functional capacity (rate-responsive pacemakers). These sensors are piezo-electric crystals or accelerometers that detect motion, vibration, pressure or acceleration, and modify the pacing rate accordingly. Position IV may be used to identify the presence of a rate-responsive pacemaker, denoted by the letter 'R'. The letter 'C' in position IV indicates a communicating pacemaker. This letter is mostly redundant now as virtually all modern units can be 'interrogated', allowing information such as pacemaker type, clinical function and performance to be extracted from the unit. Any physician can access the data from the implanted pacemaker to determine unit programming, battery life, patient medication and physiological data, such as ectopic activity, heart rate variability, conduction patterns and other parameters.

Position V is used to indicate antidysrhythmic function, the pacemaker being employed to prevent or terminate tachydysrhythmias by inducing changes in heart rate and rhythm using single or multiple stimuli. These pacemakers must be able to differentiate simple physiological sinus tachycardias from abnormal rhythms. The

unit is designed to break the re-entrant circuit by making any myocardial cells in the path of the circuit refractory.

The most sophisticated pacemaker system is the DDD ('universal'), where both atria and ventricles can sense and pace. Hence, they can pace atria on demand in patients with sinus bradycardia and intact AV nodes, ventricles in response to sensed atrial activity, and atria and ventricles sequentially in patients with sinus bradycardia and AV block. All DDD pacemakers are multi-programmable, and many are rate-responsive (DDDR).

Cardiac resynchronisation is used in patients with major conduction disorders to improve the timing of atrial and ventricular contraction (Barold, 2001). Biventricular pacing has been used to improve cardiac output in patients with heart failure and left bundle branch block, and bi-atrial pacing may be used in patients with bradycardia to prevent atrial fibrillation. Patients at high risk from sudden death may benefit from a combined approach of bi-ventricular pacing and automatic defibrillation (see below).

PERMANENT PACING FOLLOWING ACUTE MYOCARDIAL INFARCTION

The long-term prognosis of survivors of acute myocardial infarction who develop AV block is mostly related to the extent of myocardial damage, rather than to the AV block itself. Permanent pacing is seldom required following inferior myocardial infarction; those patients who do not regain normal conduction usually do not survive the acute infarct. The prognosis in terms of conduction is excellent for those who survive. However, following acute anterior myocardial infarction, the mortality in patients who develop heart block is very high, and conduction defects are often permanent in those who survive. It is likely that all these patients are at risk of further symptomatic rhythm disturbances, and indications for permanent pacing do not necessarily depend upon symptoms. Possible indications for permanent pacing in this group are shown in Table 13.3.

Table 13.3 Possible indications for permanent pacing in patients recovering from acute myocardial infarction with AV block

Infarct/block	Pace?
Inferior with transient AV block	No
Inferior with permanent second/third-degree block	Yes
Anterior with fascicular block	No?
Anterior with transient second/third-degree block	Yes?
Anterior with permanent second/third-degree block	Yes

For those who recover normal AV conduction, exercise testing and 24-h Holter monitoring are useful for post-infarction assessment. Electrophysiological testing, if available, may give an early indication of impaired infranodal conduction, allowing consideration for permanent pacing before problems arise (Cobbe, 1986).

IMPLANTABLE CARDIOVERTER-DEFIBRILLATORS

Sudden cardiac death (SCD) is a common problem, representing 25–30% of all cardiovascular deaths, and may be responsible for up to 100 000 deaths in the UK each year. About 80% of episodes of SCD are due to ventricular tachycardia or ventricular fibrillation, usually associated with coronary heart disease, where there has already been a myocardial infarction and in association with poor left ventricular function. In some, SCD will be the presentation of acute ischaemia, which may need reperfusion (thrombolysis or primary angioplasty). In the absence of an acute myocardial infarction, patients who survive SCD have a 15% risk of further episodes, which may be fatal. Although it is usual for patients with malignant ventricular dysrhythmias to be initiated on drugs, recurrence of SCD may still affect half of these patients within 5 years. Alternative prophylaxis is often required, and this may now be provided by an automatic implantable cardioverter-defibrillator (AICD). A meta-analysis involving 934 patients treated with an AICD and 932 treated with amiodarone showed a relative risk reduction of 27% for total mortality and 52% for dysrhythmic deaths in those treated with an AICD (Connolly et al,

2000). This equates with 1 death averted per 10 patients treated by implanting an AICD.

Dr Michel Mirowski developed AICDs in the 1970s, and the first human implant was undertaken at the Johns Hopkins Hospital in 1980 (Mirowski et al, 1980). There are now more than 50 000 new units implanted throughout the world each year. The total cost of the hardware for an implant is about £20 000, and although expensive, it may be more cost-effective than lifelong treatment with drug therapy (Wever et al, 1996).

The equipment

The original AICDs were implanted in the abdomen, with a thoracotomy needed for electrode placement. With advances in technology, the units have become smaller, so they resemble and can be inserted like normal cardiac pacemakers. All current AICD functions can be mediated through a single ventricular lead, although atrial wires may sometimes be needed as well. Changing the shock to a biphasic waveform has been the major improvement, and allows a reduction in the strength of the defibrillatory shock to 20 J or less in most cases. This has also helped extend battery life to about 9 years, depending upon defibrillator use. In addition to high-energy defibrillation shocks, modern devices now have the capability of low-energy synchronised cardioversion, VVI and antitachycardia pacing. The use of synchronised cardioversion of ventricular tachycardia requires lower-energy shocks that are quicker to deliver, and conserve battery life. Antitachycardia pacing (burst and ramp adaptive pacing) can also be used to terminate ventricular tachycardia. Normal back-up pacemaker function is important, as some patients require antidysrhythmic medication to suppress the development of VT/VF that may induce clinically significant bradycardia.

Holter function by the units can be used to capture long rhythm strips. The information may be useful diagnostically, or to provide evidence of correct and efficient device functioning. Dynamic electrocardiography has the great advantage in being able to show what happened to the patient's heart rhythm before and after administration of the shock, and greater storage facilities are being developed.

Implantation

In the past, AICD implantation was performed under general anaesthesia, but most units are now implanted under local anaesthesia with intravenous sedation, the procedure being only a little more complicated than for implantation of a standard permanent pacemaker.

An incision is made below the left clavicle and a pocket made either subcutaneously or deep to the pectoralis major muscle. The ventricular lead is then inserted into the right ventricle via the subclavian vein, and standard tests of pacing and sensing are performed. The unit is then tested by delivering a small shock synchronous with the T wave on the ECG to induce ventricular fibrillation. The device should be able to sense the abnormal rhythm and deliver a defibrillatory shock on three occasions before implantation is viewed as complete. The device may also be programmed to detect and treat episodes of ventricular tachycardia by antitachycardia pacing, low-energy cardioversion or high-energy defibrillation.

Pre-discharge management

Most patients are in hospital for 2–4 days, with pacing and sensing functions of the device being re-tested before discharge home. The patient should be provided with an AICD identity card, which should be carried at all times, and shown to relevant people as appropriate (e.g. hospital personnel, airline security).

Lifting should be avoided for the first 4–6 weeks, and the arm on the implant side should not be elevated above shoulder height. Patients are usually followed up at 3–6-month intervals, when the device memory is interrogated and standard pacing and sensing tests are performed. Any stored dysrhythmic events may be correlated with the patient's symptoms, and appropriate programming changes or alterations in the

patient's medication can be made. Many of the patients have coronary heart disease and heart failure, and need usual treatment and follow-up as for other similar cardiac patients.

Pre- and post-implantation counselling is important. The main problem is that syncopal or pre-syncopal attacks may still occur, if only for a few seconds before a shock is delivered. Many patients face significant life-style restrictions, particularly related to driving and occupation. Fears also arise from living with the device, including practical aspects of efficacy, malfunction and battery failure. There is also fear of the shock itself. Many patients tolerate defibrillation shocks very poorly, particularly multiple shocks, although recipients are generally happy to have the device, and feel more optimistic and confident. Fear, anxiety and depression are common, and are worsened by the unpredictability of the shocks (Gallagher et al, 1997). For this reason, anti-arrhythmic drugs may have a role in reducing the incidence of both ventricular and supraventricular arrhythmias in patients with AICDs.

Some patients have had to have their units removed because of worry. Adjustment disorders include anxiety with panic, and imaginary shocks are not uncommonly experienced. Recipients are also affected by intellectual changes. Both recipient and families may be affected by these psychological problems, and, although professional support tends to focus on the patient, family involvement is important (James, 1997). Adverse psychological reactions to AICD implantation often improve with time as the patient becomes accustomed to having the device and adapts to his physical and social limitations.

Current regulations allow driving, provided the device has been implanted for at least 6 months and has not delivered a therapeutic shock. Driving is also permitted if previous discharges have not been accompanied by incapacity, and provided there has not been any symptomatic antitachycardia pacing therapy for 6 months. Patients must stop driving for 1 month if the lead or generator has been revised, or if any change is made in anti-arrhythmic treatment.

Licensing is reviewed annually. Patients with AICDs lose any class 2 driving privileges (HGV licence).

Complications of AICDs

All the common complications of cardiac pacing may complicate AICD implantation, and many of these complications may require operative revision or even replacement of the system (Kumar and Jowett, 1999). Inappropriate shocking, usually provoked by atrial fibrillation, may be problematical. Patients require evaluation and the unit deactivating if inappropriate firing is documented.

Which patients should be offered an AICD?

Assessment for AICD therapy should be made by a cardiologist trained in electrophysiology, who be involved in implantation, testing, programming and follow-up. The National Institute for Clinical Excellence (2000) has published guidance on who should be considered for AICDs. There are two groups of patients normally considered (Box 13.4):

- The *primary prevention group* are those at high risk of sudden cardiac death
- The *secondary intervention group* who are those have been resuscitated from a sudden cardiac death, and in whom further investigation has not found any treatable cause.

Better techniques are required to identify the primary intervention group, who might benefit from this invasive treatment. Any patient who has had sustained ventricular tachycardia or who has been resuscitated from ventricular fib-

---

Box 13.4   Patient groups suitable for implantation of AICDs

a) **Primary prevention**
- Patients with a history of previous myocardial infarction plus:
  - Non-sustained ventricular tachycardia of Holter monitoring
  - Inducible ventricular tachycardia on electrophysiological testing
  - Left ventricular dysfunction (ejection fraction less than 35%)
- Family history of sudden cardiac death
- Hypertrophic obstructive cardiomyopathy
- Other patients at high risk for sudden death (e.g. long QT syndrome, Brugada syndrome)

b) **Secondary prevention**
- Cardiac arrest due to ventricular tachycardia or ventricular fibrillation
- Spontaneous ventricular tachycardia producing syncope or pre-syncope
- Sustained ventricular tachycardia with left ventricular dysfunction (ejection fraction less than 35%)

---

rillation should be considered for an AICD as first-line treatment (Winters et al, 2001).

Although AICD therapy has a small, but nevertheless important, impact on overall survival of the post-infarct patient, more lives may be saved by evidence-based secondary prevention measures, such as use of beta-blockade in patients who have suffered a myocardial infarction. A meta-analysis of 25 trials of beta-blockers showed a relative risk reduction for total mortality of 23% and for sudden death by 32% (Held and Yusuf, 1993). Mortality is known to be particularly high in those with heart failure, and, in the United States Carvedilol Heart Failure Study, MERIT-CHF and CIBIS II heart failure studies, beta-blocker therapy reduced sudden deaths by half (Priori et al, 2001).

REFERENCES

ACC/AHA (1998) Guidelines for implantation of cardiac pacemakers and anti-arrhythmia devices. Executive summary. *Circulation*, **97:** 1325–1335.

ACC/AHA (1999) Guidelines for the management of patients with acute myocardial infarction: executive summary and recommendations. *Circulation*, **100:** 1016–1030.

Barold SS (2001) What is cardiac resynchronisation therapy? *American Journal of Medicine*, **111:** 224–232.

Bernstein AD, Camm AJ, Fletcher RD et al (1987) The NASPE/BPEG generic pacemaker code for anti-bradyarrhythmia and adaptive-rate pacing and anti-tachyarrhythmia devices. *PACE*, **10**: 794–799.

Blandford RL, Burden AC (1984) Abnormalities of cardiac conduction in diabetics. *BMJ*, **289**: 1659.

British Pacing and Electrophysiology Group (1991) Recommendations for pacemaker prescriptions for symptomatic bradycardia. Report of a Working Party. *British Heart Journal*, **66**: 185–191.

Burack B, Furman S (1969) Trans-oesophageal cardiac pacing. *American Journal of Cardiology*, **23**: 469–472.

Cobbe SM (1986) Electrophysiological testing after acute myocardial infarction. *BMJ*, **292**: 1290–1291.

Cohen DB, Doctor L, Pick A (1958) The significance of atrioventricular block complicating myocardial infarction. *American Heart Journal*, **55**: 215–219.

Connolly SJ, Hallstrom AP, Cappato R et al (2000) Meta-analysis of the implantable cardioverter defibrillator secondary prevention trials. AVID, CASH and CIDS studies. *European Heart Journal*, **21**: 2071–2078.

EEC (1988) *Ionising Radiation Regulations*. Brussels: EEC.

Gallagher RD, McKinley S, Mangan B et al (1997) The impact of the implantable defibrillator on quality of life. *American Journal of Critical Care*, **6**: 16–24.

Gammage MD (2000) Temporary cardiac pacing. *Heart*, **83**: 715–720.

Held PH, Yusuf S (1993) Effects of beta-blockers and calcium channel blockers in acute myocardial infarction. *European Heart Journal*, **14** (suppl F): 18–25.

James JE (1997) The psychological and emotional impact of living with an automatic internal cardioverter defibrillator (AICD): how can nurses help? *Intensive and Critical Care Nursing*, **13**: 316–323.

Jowett NI, Thompson DR, Pohl JEF (1989) Temporary transvenous endocardial pacing: six years experience in one coronary care unit. *Postgraduate Medical Journal*, **65**: 211–215.

Kumar S, Jowett NI (1999) Twiddler's twitch: symptomatic failure of an automatic implantable cardio-defibrillator. *British Journal of Cardiology*, **6**: 42–44.

Mirowski M, Reid PR, Mower MM et al (1980) Termination of malignant ventricular arrhythmias with an implanted automatic defibrillator in human beings. *New England Journal of Medicine*, **303**: 322–324.

Murphy JJ (2001) Problems with temporary cardiac pacing. *BMJ*, **323**: 527.

National Institute for Clinical Excellence (2000) Guidance on the use of implantable cardioverter defibrillators for arrhythmias. http://www.nice.org.uk.

Parker J, Cleland JGF (1993) Choice of route for insertion of temporary pacing wires: recommendations of the medical practice committee and council of the British Cardiac Society. *British Heart Journal*, **70**: 294–296.

Petch MC (1999) Temporary cardiac pacing. *Postgraduate Medical Journal*, **3**: 577–578.

Priori SG, Aliot E, Blomstrom-Lundqvist C et al (2001) Task force on sudden cardiac death of the European Society of Cardiology. *European Heart Journal*, **22**: 1374–1450.

Traville CM, Sutton M (1992) Pacemaker syndrome: an iatrogenic condition. *British Heart Journal*, **68**: 163–166.

Wever EFD, Hauer RNW, Schrivers G et al (1996) Cost-effectiveness of implantable defibrillators as first-choice therapy versus electrophysiologically guided, tiered strategy in post-infarction sudden death survivors. *Circulation*, **93**: 489–496.

Winters SL, Packer DL, Marchlinski FE et al (2001) Consensus statement on indications, guidelines for use, and recommendations for follow-up of implantable cardioverter defibrillators. *PACE*, **24**: 262–269.

Zoll PM, Zoll RH (1985) Non-invasive temporary cardiac stimulation. *Critical Care Medicine*, **13**: 925–926.

14

Cardiac rehabilitation

Cardiac rehabilitation is the process by which patients with coronary heart disease are helped to achieve their optimal physical, psychological, social, vocational and economic status. Rehabilitation cannot be regarded as an isolated form of therapy, but must be integrated with the whole treatment (World Health Organization, 1993). Standards for cardiac rehabilitation are documented in the National Service Framework for Coronary Heart Disease (Department of Health, 2000). Protocols and systems of care are needed to ensure that those admitted to hospital suffering from coronary heart disease are invited to participate in a multidisciplinary programme of cardiac rehabilitation and secondary prevention. The aim of the programme is to reduce their risk of subsequent cardiac problems and to promote their return to a full and normal life. The National Service Framework target is that more than 85% of eligible patients should be offered cardiac rehabilitation, and that 1 year after discharge at least 50% of people are non-smokers, exercise regularly and have a body mass index under 30 kg/m^2.

Cardiac rehabilitation is a multidisciplinary and multifaceted activity that requires a range of skills to bring together medical treatment, education, exercise, sexual and vocational counselling and behaviour change (American Association of Cardiovascular and Pulmonary Rehabilitation, 1999). It should be regarded as an integral part of cardiac care and the process should start at the time of the cardiac event, continue through the hospital stay and transfer seamlessly to rehabilitation and aftercare in the community

(Thompson et al, 1996). It should be offered to all who are likely to benefit, including those with even more potential for health gain, such as individuals with stable angina, heart failure and hypertension (Thompson and de Bono, 1999).

EVIDENCE BASE

There is good evidence attesting to the benefits of cardiac rehabilitation (Ades, 2001). Evidence base from primary and secondary studies (Wenger et al, 1995; NHS Centre for Reviews and Dissemination, 1998; Dinnes et al, 1999) demonstrates that rehabilitation can promote recovery, enable patients to achieve and maintain better health and reduce the risk of death in people who have heart disease. A combination of exercise, education and psychological interventions appears to be the most effective form of rehabilitation (NHS Centre for Reviews and Dissemination, 1998). Benefits include:

- Improvements in exercise tolerance
- Improvements in psychosocial well-being
- Improvements in blood lipid levels
- Reduction in symptoms
- Reduction in cigarette smoking
- Reduction of stress.

Despite the evidence, referral to and uptake of cardiac rehabilitation services is variable, and only about a quarter of patients with myocardial infarction are enrolled into rehabilitation programmes (Bethell et al, 2001). Most centres tend to restrict access to young, male, white patients who have suffered a (usually first, uncomplicated) myocardial infarction (Thompson et al, 1997a; Lewin et al, 1998), and certain groups are under-represented, including women, elderly people, ethnic minority groups and individuals who live in rural areas.

GUIDELINES

UK national guidelines have been developed to ensure that cardiac rehabilitation is offered to all who are likely to benefit, based on an individual assessment of need, and followed by a later menu of options (Thompson et al, 1996, 1997b). It should be accompanied by audit and individual monitoring of progress (Thompson et al, 1997c).

Interventions that should be offered at each stage of the rehabilitation process include:

- A comprehensive assessment of physical, psychological and social risk
- A written, individualised plan
- Life-style advice
- Psychological interventions
- Use of effective medications
- Involvement of carers
- Access to cardiac support groups
- Long-term follow-up.

Other interventions may include:

- Health promotion
- Vocational advice
- Structured exercise sessions
- Referral to specialist services as appropriate.

PHASES OF REHABILITATION

A systematic and structured framework can be useful to guide service provision at the right time and in the right place. Many programmes use a framework consisting of four phases, though this can be mechanistic, impose artificial boundaries and fragment care:

- *Phase 1 (in-patient stay)*: includes explanation of the disease, the prognosis and a positive approach to recovery, early mobilisation and discharge planning
- *Phase 2 (immediate post-discharge period, up to 6 weeks)*: includes further investigations, liaison with community-based healthcare professionals, assessment and health education as appropriate
- *Phase 3 (intermediate post-discharge period, 6–12 weeks)*: includes rehabilitation interventions, such as a tailored/supervised exercise programme
- *Phase 4 (long-term maintenance period, indefinite)*: includes chronic disease management, monitoring of secondary prevention, maintenance of life-style change.

PROCESS OF REHABILITATION

The process of rehabilitation should contain the following elements (Thompson et al, 1996):

- Process of explanation and understanding
- Specific rehabilitation interventions
- Process of re-adaptation.

The phases and the elements contained within them should be flexible and tailored to suit the individual needs of the patient and his partner and family. This means that the timing and location of sessions need to be flexible and the length of participation in a programme sufficient to cater for the patient.

COORDINATION

Cardiac rehabilitation involves the use of a wide range of skills from different health professionals, including the nurse, doctor, physiotherapist, occupational therapist, clinical psychologist, dietitian and social worker. The nurse assumes a central role by being responsible, directly or indirectly, for controlling the many factors that influence the patient's recovery; she is in most frequent contact with the patient and family and is responsible for planning and coordinating the amount of activity the patient is expected to undertake. The nurse can assist the patient and family to understand, accept and adapt to the illness, and may be able to stimulate them to take an active part in recovery and rehabilitation. In addition, the nurse can assist them in making realistic plans for the future. In order to achieve this, attainable goals need to be defined, plans being jointly agreed by the patient, the family and other members of the healthcare team. An attitude of optimism should be adopted by staff, remembering that most patients who are going to die from acute myocardial infarction do so before reaching hospital.

From early convalescence in hospital, the patient and partner should understand that a return to normality within a matter of a few weeks is not only expected, but is also safe and beneficial, given that the patient's condition warrants it. It is the success of coping and support that often ultimately determines the outcome of the patient's illness; the heart may recover more rapidly than the patient's often depressed mental state.

Individualised cardiac rehabilitation that starts early and is based on national guidelines for patients with myocardial infarction seems to be effective, with improvements in quality of life, more confidence about returning to activities and fewer further treatment needs (Thompson et al, 1996; Mayou et al, 2002).

Successful rehabilitation should not be viewed narrowly in terms of economic or vocational outcomes, but rather as the achievement of a lifestyle that enables the patient and family to enjoy a full and active life (with some allowance for physical limitations).

EDUCATION

Education and counselling involve teaching patients and their families to understand the illness and its management. Understanding the factors that may have caused it may also help them assume a large degree of responsibility for their care.

Information provided to patients and their partners during their stay in hospital is often poor, and, although patient teaching is recognised as an important nursing function, there is little evidence to show that it is being effectively and consistently accomplished. It is the responsibility of the healthcare team to ensure that the patient and family understand the illness, the purpose of treatment and how to cope both within and outside the hospital. Nurses are in an ideal position to teach, because they frequently become the most familiar person to the patient and are thus often in the best position to communicate with the patient and family.

Teaching programmes during the patient's stay in hospital are designed to decrease the patient's feeling of helplessness, to help restore self-esteem and to bolster the patient's confidence in terms of a successful outcome. Those who understand the cause and significance of their illness and its management are likely to have improved motivation to comply with therapy and cope with the consequences of their illness (Thompson, 1990). Patients particularly need information about potential events that may occur after their return home, when professional help is not immediately available.

Teaching and learning is a two-way process, and the individual patient's requirements will vary with his general educational background and intellectual capabilities. Assessment should include:

- Demographic variables, such as family composition, ethnic, cultural and religious background and educational level
- Pre-existing knowledge and misconceptions of coronary heart disease
- Life-style and habits
- Readiness to learn.

Simple language should be used, and earlier communication is remembered better than later on. Repetition increases recall, as does specific, rather than general, advice.

Contemporary approaches to patient teaching are numerous and varied, but information should be tailored to individual needs and given in a consistent and structured fashion. The comprehension of new information will be at its best when the patient is motivated and when the information is presented clearly, concisely and in small doses. There is no substitute for personal advice, and its value depends upon the attending medical and nursing staff adopting an informed, committed and uniform approach. Similar education of the patient's family is equally important, and giving this at the bedside (when the patient is surrounded by high technology and obvious intensive care) may reinforce the importance of such advice.

Instructional aids (physical, printed and audiovisual) are very useful as part of the educational process. Vocabulary, sentence length, illustrations, type size and style, as well as readability and accuracy of the information presented should be carefully considered. Visual information is usually assimilated better than the spoken word, so illustrations, pamphlets and models are a helpful and useful adjunct. A plastic model of the heart can be used to demonstrate cardiac anatomy and the coronary arteries, and explain about the blood supply to the heart. This helps to correct the common myth that the heart receives its nourishment by blood flowing through the chambers. The atherosclerotic process may then be described, including plaque formation, progressive narrowing and obstruction of the coronary arteries and myocardial infarction. The discussion should include an explanation of other symptoms that the patient may have experienced, such as sweating and palpitations. The role of coronary artery spasm can be discussed if the patient has a history of variant angina. The healing process of the heart and the meanings of ECG and laboratory findings should also be briefly explained. It is important to stress that coronary heart disease is a chronic health problem and that there is no 'cure', but that some medical intervention and modification of life-style may be necessary to alleviate symptoms and reduce the risk of further problems.

Nurses, doctors and patients generally agree upon certain topics that should be included for discussion, including the recognition of signs and symptoms of myocardial infarction, the names, dosages and side-effects of medications, and knowledge of personal risk factors and how to modify them. Other aspects that need to be covered are the nature of the disease, emergency treatment, resumption of activities, and physical, psychosocial and financial problems encountered on return to home and work. Aspects frequently neglected include how to take the pulse, sexual activity and instruction on the normal convalescence. It is important to try to avoid presenting information in a standardised fashion, and the nurse needs to find out what the patient's needs are. However, information should be presented clearly and taking care to avoid vague or meaningless comments such as 'do what you can manage'. Advice should be realistic, practical and accurate (Thompson and Lewin, 2000). It should be based on evidence and imparted in clear, unambiguous ways, such as 'eat five portions of fresh fruit and vegetables every day' (Department of Health, 1994), instead of 'try and eat more fruit'.

As half of the advice in a 5-min consultation is forgotten within the next 5 min, it is helpful if written or tape-recorded advice is provided.

Written information should be produced following the empirically determined guidelines for maximising comprehension and adherence.

Questionnaires may be useful for evaluating the patient's needs and level of comprehension. However, when assessing the efficacy of the education programme, it is important to differentiate between what patients learn and what they are actually going to do about it; the acquisition of new information does not necessarily result in a change of behaviour.

Involvement of the family

The family can have a direct influence on the rehabilitation process by understanding the illness and helping the patient adapt. They can also assist in life-style modification, and should therefore be included in most, if not all, teaching. Partner involvement has been minimal in rehabilitation, despite the widespread opinion that success generally depends upon their support (Thompson, 2002). A programme that involves both patients and partners provides an ideal opportunity for giving information, instilling hope and redefining health (Thompson and Meddis, 1990a,b; Johnston et al, 1999). The rest of the family also need information in order to feel useful to the patient, and to understand that he is receiving appropriate care.

Information provided on the coronary care unit and ward

Education initiated on the coronary care unit helps the patient to understand what has happened, what is immediately being done and what is likely to happen over the ensuing days. Teaching needs to be relevant to the individual concerned; vagueness and ambiguity will only result in increased fear and anxiety. A programme centred upon these principles is likely to improve the patient's attitudes, behaviour and understanding of the illness and improve his recovery.

At an early stage, brief explanations of the staff, equipment, procedures and routines of the coronary care unit will reduce anxiety and misunderstanding. The nurse should avoid bombarding patients with too much information during the early phase, as they invariably retain very few facts during this acute stage. Capacity for learning is impaired by fear, anxiety, pain and fatigue. Patients will, however, benefit from answers to specific questions, and answers should be clear, simple and repeated frequently.

If the patient has to undergo a painful or invasive procedure, information on the patient's likely experiences and sensations will be more effective in alleviating anxiety than will details about the procedure alone. When the patient's mental and physical condition permits the assimilation of more detailed and complex information, the nurse can provide information about his condition, probable limitations, possible problems and likely outcome.

EXERCISE

Exercise involves a graduated programme, beginning with early ambulation, both to avoid the complications of bedrest and to encourage a positive approach to recovery, passive and low-level activities and aiming for a full return to normal activities.

Originally, cardiac rehabilitation was focused almost exclusively on exercise, and, although exercise-based cardiac rehabilitation is effective in reducing cardiac deaths, a systematic review questioned whether it is exercise only, or the multifactorial, multidisciplinary cardiac rehabilitation intervention, that is more beneficial (Jolliffe et al, 2001).

Emphasising physical exercise following acute myocardial infarction usually represents a major change to the typical patient's sedentary life-style, involving the car, labour-saving devices and long hours in front of the television. However, exercise improves mood and morale, and physical fitness allows an earlier return to normal life-style and work. Regular exercise also helps cardiovascular performance, keeps the body supple and helps to control body weight. To produce the maximum benefit, the activity needs to be regular and aerobic. This involves using the large muscle groups in the arms, legs and back steadily and rhythmically so that breathing and heart rate are significantly increased (British Heart Foundation, 2002).

Regular moderate exercise (30 min on 5 or more days per week) at a level of 75–85% of maximal capacity is an ideal way of achieving physical fitness. Vigorous physical activity may be employed later and is recognised as an important factor in protection against the development of coronary heart disease. However, care is required in those with pre-existing heart disease; exercise is not without hazard, and low-level activities are preferable in older and less fit patients.

Formal exercise programmes are very useful following acute myocardial infarction. Early graduated physical activity, starting with gentle passive exertion, has been designed to avert or minimise the risk of venous stasis and its complications (deep vein thrombosis and pulmonary emboli). When the patient is first allowed out of bed, he is often shocked at the tremendous feeling of physical weakness, which is usually not expected or easily explicable in terms of the short period of bedrest and inactivity. The patient will need reassuring and encouragement to gradually increase the level of activity. Any restrictions thought necessary should be carefully explained in a positive fashion, so that the patient does not become frustrated.

Information regarding physical activity will depend on the stage of recovery the patient has reached. Initially, the reasons for temporary restriction of activity will need to be explained, and that the resumption of activity will be gradual to allow the myocardium to heal.

ACTIVITY PLANNING

The functional classification of the New York Heart Association provides a crude guide for determining appropriate activities, as well as expected symptoms, in patients following acute myocardial infarction (Table 14.1). Advice about specific activities should be individualised, and take into account the extent and severity of the myocardial infarction, the patient's previous level of activity, the extent of recovery and the stability of the current condition.

Progress in early rehabilitation can be assisted by the use of *metabolic equivalents* (METs) for prescribing specific physical activities. One MET is defined as the oxygen consumption by the patient at rest and is roughly equivalent to 3.5 ml of oxygen consumed per kilogram of body weight per minute.

Three months or more after an uncomplicated myocardial infarction, the average post-infarction patient is capable of performing at a level of up to 9 METs. This is equivalent to running at about 5 miles/h, cycling at 12 miles/h or playing 'non-competitive' squash. If less than ordinary activity produces symptoms, it may be necessary for a more suitable level of activity to be planned. Patients who have had congestive heart failure, for example, are often limited to 3–5 METs at 3 months.

PHYSICAL ACTIVITY ON THE CORONARY CARE UNIT

Early ambulation in uncomplicated myocardial infarction is essential to avert or minimise the deleterious effects of prolonged bedrest, including decreased physical work capacity. It also reduces the anxiety and depression that often follow acute myocardial infarction. In some coronary care units, patients are encouraged to sit out of bed on the day of admission, provided they are free from pain and significant dysrhythmias.

Table 14.1 Functional classification of patients with heart disease (Criteria Committee of the New York Heart Association, 1973)

Class	
I	Heart disease with no limitation on ordinary physical activity
II	Slight limitation. Ordinary physical activity (e.g. walking) produces symptoms
III	Marked limitation. Unable to walk on the level without disability. Less than ordinary activity produces symptoms
IV	Dyspnoea at rest. Inability to carry out any physical activity

If there has been a prolonged period of bedrest, resumption of activity often results in a moderate tachycardia and orthostatic hypotension. Physical activities should, therefore, be at a low level of intensity (1–2 METs), such as eating, dressing and undressing, washing the hands and face, use of a bedside commode, simple arm and leg exercises, or sitting in a bedside chair. Observation of patients as they perform these activities is useful to ensure that they can cope and that an inappropriate tachycardia is not provoked. Early rehabilitation should not be associated with chest pain, dyspnoea, sweating, palpitations or excessive fatigue. Dysrhythmias and ST segment displacement on the cardiac monitor should not occur, and systolic blood pressure should not fall more than 10–15 mmHg.

Patients are usually the best judge of how much they can do, but they should be warned of the feelings of weakness that may accompany increases in activity.

PHYSICAL ACTIVITY ON THE WARD

Once patients leave the coronary care unit, the aim is for them to attain a level of activity that permits personal care and independence (or at least semi-independence) by the time of discharge from hospital. In these days of early discharge following uncomplicated myocardial infarction, patients usually return home after 5–7 days.

The ward activity plan should consist of 'warm-up' isotonic (dynamic) exercises, which allow the heart rate to increase proportionally to the intensity of the activity. The systolic blood pressure increases slowly, and the diastolic blood pressure remains unchanged or decreases slightly. Isometric exercises should be avoided. These result in a minimal increase in heart rate, but a significant and steep increase in the systolic blood pressure. This causes a sudden increase in cardiac afterload, which may be poorly tolerated by an ischaemic left ventricle, resulting in angina or malignant tachydysrhythmias.

Walking with a gradual and progressive increase in speed and distance should be the major component of the activity plan. It is advisable for most patients who will have to climb stairs at home to try stairs in hospital under supervision. This results in increased confidence and reduced worry for the patient and family. At the time of discharge from hospital, patients should be able to perform activities at peak levels of 3.5–4.0 METs for short periods, to simulate usual activities at home.

EXERCISE STRESS TESTING

Exercise stress testing is widely recommended to establish safe and appropriate guidelines for physical activity, especially for patients with heart disease. The current practice of early ambulation and exercise training soon after myocardial infarction has resulted in the more widespread use of exercise testing earlier in the course of the illness, and often before discharge home. A normal response to an early exercise test reliably identifies patients at low risk of future cardiac events. Partners who observe and even participate in stress testing are likely to gain more confidence in the patient's physical and cardiac capability.

PHYSICAL ACTIVITY DURING CONVALESCENCE

When the patient returns home, progressive increases in physical activity are used to achieve a level of activity that allows normal daily activities and will later permit a return to work. The activity plan within hospital will usually have helped to allay the patient's and family's fears of a further heart attack or sudden death resulting from physical exertion. Patients should be encouraged to exercise daily, and it should be stressed that a lack of exercise may be harmful rather than beneficial. The best form of exercise is walking, but golf, swimming, jogging and cycling can be encouraged when the patient feels well enough. Exercises that use less than half of the patient's working capacity will not help to increase fitness.

The benefits of exercise, including weight control, improvement of respiratory function and a general feeling of well-being, should be stressed.

Practical advice is helpful too, such as only exercising in warm environments and not after heavy meals, by the fireside in winter, or in the midday sun in summer. Competitive sports are not advisable in the early months following infarction, for obvious reasons.

The levels of activity performed at the end of the hospital stay should be maintained and gradually increased. Walking speed and distance should be increased, so that by the end of 4–6 weeks the patient may walk up to 5 miles per day. The patient and family will usually gain confidence, and the patient more independence, when accomplishing each objective.

FORMAL EXERCISE PROGRAMMES FOR OUTPATIENTS

The main emphasis for rehabilitation has been early programmes of hospital-based exercise training, but it is now widely accepted that there is need for a wider and more flexible range of methods, greater individual prescription of care and closer cooperation with on-going medical care. Exercise is popular with many patients and appears effective in the early stages in improving exercise capacity, reducing anxiety and encouraging a rapid return to activities. Both light and heavy exercise have been shown to be of benefit in improving physical conditioning, and, although these can easily be provided in a hospital gym, they can just as successfully be provided in the community.

During exercise sessions, direct observation, including ECG monitoring by telemetry, is recommended. A warm-up period of 5 min is needed to gradually increase the pulse rate and blood pressure and to help joint flexibility. Maintaining a target heart rate is a useful guide for achieving the correct intensity of exertion. The level of activity is altered until the desired heart rate is achieved, and the exercise is maintained for the duration of the session (continuous training) or interspersed with brief rest periods (intermittent training). The exercise devices used include the treadmill, arm/leg ergometer, rowing machine and wall pulleys. The ECG is observed for dysrhythmias or ST segment displacement. Heart rate and adverse signs or symptoms need to be recorded. At the conclusion of the exercise session, it is important to taper the activity down gradually (a 'cool down'), rather than to stop it abruptly.

Home-based exercise programmes are probably as effective as group training (Miller and Taylor, 1995), although a rehabilitation programme that is community based may be more beneficial in terms of social contact and support.

PREPARATION FOR DISCHARGE

Exercise sessions may usefully be combined with education and counselling of the patient and family and providing information for convalescence.

It is not uncommon for the patient and family to be left to cope by themselves with only vague instructions about discharge and rehabilitation, which results in uncertainty, distress and failure to adjust. A well-planned programme is desirable, to anticipate the patient's home-coming and return to work. Patients and spouses often have specific questions about convalescence, medication, diet, drinking, driving and smoking, as well as resumption of leisure, and sexual and work activities.

Group discussions after the exercise session provide a means of asking questions, sharing feelings and concerns, and learning from others who have similar problems. General health recommendations, where appropriate, to patients and their families should include:

- *Diet*: a reduction in fat intake, particularly of saturated fats, a reduction in salt intake and an increase in carbohydrate intake, and the consumption of at least five portions of fruit and vegetables each day, with appropriate calorific intake to achieve or maintain an ideal body weight (Department of Health, 1994).
- *Alcohol*: avoiding consumption of more than four units a day by men and three by women (Department of Health, 1995).
- *Smoking*: stopping smoking, teaching behavioural skills for coping with high-risk situations, providing relaxation training,

maintaining periodic telephone contact and, where necessary, referring the patient to a smoking cessation programme (Miller and Taylor, 1995).

- *Physical activity*: participating in a graded exercise programme with the long-term aim of achieving a minimum of 30 min of at least moderate intensity activity (such as brisk walking, cycling or climbing the stairs) on 5 or more days of the week (Department of Health, 1996).
- *Health*: undergoing regular health examination, including testing of the urine for sugar and protein, measurement of blood pressure and assessment of lipids.

LIFE-STYLE CHANGE

In practice, changing an individual's behaviour is notoriously difficult and is fraught with problems. Efforts are more likely to be successful in those patients who are able and willing to make changes to their life-style. However, there are numerous factors that inhibit them from making such changes, or result in lapses. It is difficult to change behaviour through advice alone; there must be an incentive for change. Patient adherence to any measures instituted is more likely to be accomplished if staff understand behaviour change, and apply, where appropriate, such strategies. There are good examples of where this has been successful, notably the MULTIFIT (multiple risk factor intervention) programme at Stanford University (Miller and Taylor, 1995), which is designed to facilitate recovery in the first year following a myocardial infarction.

Individuals are more likely to change behaviour when they believe they are at risk of developing a problem, when they believe the recommended change will improve their condition or reduce their risk, and when they believe they have the ability to accomplish the desired changes (Becker, 1974). It is important, therefore, to discuss the following with each patient (and carer) for each behaviour to be changed (Miller and Taylor, 1995):

- Why the patient is at risk

- How the recommended changes will improve the patient's condition or reduce his risk
- Whether the patient has the confidence and resources to accomplish the change.

Individuals may be at different stages of readiness to change (Prochaska and Di Clemente, 1983). Many will consider change, but are not strongly committed; others can be influenced to do so, but the minority are highly committed to change and have begun the process of change. It is usually easy to assess commitment by simply asking the patient if he intends to adopt a particular behaviour.

The following principles are adopted in the Stanford programme.

- Build positive and accurate expectations
- Define the behaviour to be changed
- Set realistic goals
- Use contracts to enhance commitment
- Prepare for lapses/relapses
- Model the desired behaviour
- Use prompts to remind the patient of the desired behaviour
- Provide feedback about the patient's progress
- Teach problem-solving
- Reward achievement
- Enlist appropriate social support as needed.

Accomplishing life-style change is difficult, but maintaining it is even more difficult. Behaviour strategies that are likely to affect this include social support from a partner, family, friend or healthcare professional, which will help and also aid recognition of warning signals indicating that relapse might occur.

The two major life-style changes are usually weight control (diet) and smoking. Stopping patients smoking is not easy, and the best approach is encouragement with support (Van Berkel et al, 1999). Simple advice has a small effect on cessation rates, and more intensive interventions are marginally more effective than minimal interventions (Silagy and Stead, 2001).

There is good systematic review evidence that dietary advice to cardiac patients can reduce mortality and morbidity as well as modify risk factors. For those individuals who are overweight, the priority is weight control plus risk factor reduction, not major weight loss (Hooper, 2001).

PSYCHOLOGICAL CARE

Patients with myocardial infarction who are distressed in hospital are at high risk of adverse psychological and quality of life outcomes during the ensuing year (Mayou et al, 2000). Many of these patients are confronted by fear and uncertainty when they arrive back home, which, when combined with minor physical symptoms, result in increased anxiety and depression, thus compounding the situation. Anxiety reduces post-infarct physical function independently from the extent of coronary disease (Sullivan et al, 1997). Depression increases the risk of death in post-infarct patients in the following 18 months, as well as re-admission to hospital in the following 6 months (Frasure-Smith et al, 1995; Levine et al, 1996). Depressed post-infarct patients are more likely to smoke, to suffer from angina and are less likely to return to work (Ladwig et al, 1994). Cardiac rehabilitation reduces both anxiety and depression in coronary patients (Kugler et al, 1994; Milani et al, 1996). Thus, there is a need to identify psychological distress and manage it appropriately, including referral for treatment if necessary.

Psychological assessment should include the measurement of anxiety and depression, which are common precursors and reactions to heart disease (Lane et al, 2002). The recommended instrument for routine use is the Hospital Anxiety and Depression Scale (Zigmond and Snaith, 1983). It has been shown to be an acceptable, reliable and valid measure with good sensitivity and specificity for detecting anxiety and depression (Herrman, 1997), and it is quick and easy to use and score.

Pre-discharge counselling is useful in improving morale and aiding a successful return to home and work. Preparation should include discussions of potential problems, such as anxiety, depression, poor concentration, irritability, sleeplessness and fear of complications (especially death) that may occur on the return home.

'Home-coming depression' is almost universal, and patients and partners should be warned that it is likely to happen. The partner often experiences a greater degree of anxiety than the patient and may need careful and supportive counselling (Thompson, 1990). The family particularly needs to be cautioned against overprotectiveness towards the patient.

Such interventions have generally shown significant improvements in psychosocial and physical functioning for at least a year after the infarct (Thompson, 1990; Johnston et al, 1999). Whether these improvements can be sustained over a longer period remains to be seen.

Because the transition from hospital to home is frequently a traumatic and neglected aspect of post-myocardial infarction management, it may be appropriate to make arrangements that will ensure continuity of care. Periodic checks (e.g. telephoning the patient and partner, or home visits) may be useful, in some instances, to bridge this gap, and this is probably best achieved by close liaison between hospital and community nurses. The community nurse can play an important role in teaching, counselling and evaluating the care that has been initiated within the hospital, and is also ideally placed for informing the patient and partner about community resources, including counselling services, home-helps and rehabilitation facilities.

The multidisciplinary health team approach is advantageous as it combines the skills of different professionals, provides continuity between hospital and community care and thus maximises the resources available to the patient and family. Nevertheless, it is important to avoid encouraging patient and family dependence; ultimately, each individual is responsible for his own health and must be encouraged to assume overall responsibility and control.

Impressive improvements in mood have been claimed for a self-help behavioural programme, and are especially suitable for low-risk patients (Lewin et al, 1992). It is estimated that up to 30% of subjects might benefit from individually planned help in later convalescence, even if they have attended early rehabilitation programmes (Lewin et al, 1992).

SEXUAL COUNSELLING

Sexual needs cannot be ignored. Although discussion of this intimate aspect of the patient's life is difficult for both patient and healthcare staff, sexual counselling should be viewed as an integral part of the cardiac rehabilitation programme. Sexual problems are common, and many patients have concerns about erectile dysfunction and about the resumption of sexual activity (Taylor, 1999). The complicated association between psychological distress, previous sexual adjustment, organic factors and existing family support should be considered in cardiac rehabilitation (Friedman, 2000). The subject of sex should be approached as a matter of routine in the rehabilitation of all coronary patients and their partners.

The energy expenditure during intercourse is not as great as is popularly believed, being equivalent to that of climbing about two flights of stairs (4 METs). Experimental data have demonstrated that peak heart rates occur during orgasm, and adequate foreplay will allow the pulse rate to increase gradually from resting levels to a transient peak of about 180 beats/min. Blood pressure also rises gradually, to peak just before or during orgasm, with increases of 20–100 mmHg systolic and 20–40 mmHg diastolic. Hyperventilation occurs, with respiratory rates recorded of up to 60/min. These physiological variables rapidly return to pre-coital levels after orgasm. Extramarital and other illicit encounters may, however, expend much more energy, and are often associated with faster heart rates, higher blood pressures and an increased risk of sudden death.

Sexual problems

Patients recovering from acute myocardial infarction often suffer from a depressed libido, which may result in sexual disharmony. Interestingly, impotence is rarely a problem. The partner is often more concerned than the patient and may be frightened of resuming sexual activity because of precipitating a heart attack or sudden death. The severity of the infarct and the extent of cardiac decompensation are much less important causes of sexual debility than is the psychological condition of the patient. Many factors, including normal age-related changes in sexual response, medication-induced dysfunction, diabetes and the emotional impact of heart disease may influence sexual function in these patients.

Patients and staff are often anxious about broaching this topic. A useful way to introduce it is by saying: 'Many people are worried about when they can resume normal sexual relations. I wonder whether there are any questions or concerns that either of you may have regarding your sex life?' Many patients lack sufficient information, which results in unnecessary worry. For instance, the most common fear is that of re-infarction or death occurring during intercourse. This is, in fact, an extremely rare occurrence, with most of these fatalities occurring during extramarital sex. Fear of resuming sexual activity is more harmful than the actual activity, and sexual frustration should be avoided at all costs. In general, most patients can resume sexual intercourse about 2–4 weeks after discharge home. Typical advice may be: 'If you can make it up the stairs to the bedroom in one go, you can resume sexual activity'. This may be hazardous, though, if they live in a lighthouse! Good sex need not be an athletic feat.

There may be a need to advise patients on how to minimise symptoms that may accompany intercourse. A warm bedroom and warm sheets are desirable. If chest pain, breathlessness or palpitations occur during or after sexual activity, the couple should stop and seek medical advice. Often, all that is required is for prophylactic glyceryl trinitrate to be taken immediately before coitus, as the patient might do before any form of physical activity. Beta-blockers are also very useful for limiting heart rate and myocardial work. It should be noted that patients using cutaneous nitrates may deposit some of their medication on their partner, imparting typical nitrate side-effects of them ('Not now, I've got a headache!').

If psychological problems remain unresolved, it may be necessary to refer the patient for specialised sexual counselling by a clinical psychologist, often within a sexual dysfunction clinic;

intensive therapy may be indicated in resistant cases. There are detailed guidelines available for the management of sexual dysfunction in cardiac patients (De Busk et al, 2000) cases.

MEDICATION

Adherence to drug therapy varies from patient to patient, but often remains unacceptably poor. Difficulty in understanding and complying with drug therapy may occur for a variety of reasons, including fear of dependency or of side-effects. The more complex the drug regimen, the less likely compliance seems to be, and careful review of the patient's medication is necessary before discharge. Many patients will not have taken tablets before their heart attack, and the habit of taking regular medication may be unfamiliar.

Information should include correct identification of the drug, what it is for, the dosage and other special instructions (e.g. the storage and limited life of glyceryl trinitrate). Re-issue of prescriptions needs to be covered. Patients often stop what is intended to be continuous therapy when they have finished 'the course'. In addition, they should be warned that they should not allow themselves to run out of tablets or go away on holiday with insufficient supplies. Sudden withdrawal of certain drugs (e.g. beta-blockers) may be associated with sudden cardiac events, including unstable angina, myocardial infarction and sudden death. Patients should enquire about whether or not it would be cheaper to obtain an annual prescription ('season ticket'), rather than paying for individual medications.

It may be useful to issue a small record card listing the patient's medications, with dose, time to be taken, action and possible side-effects written on the card. This may be kept with the medication at home, thus serving as a reminder and providing important information about the drugs. The cards are also useful to summarise therapy when the patient's family doctor is re-issuing prescriptions, and they can be taken to hospital appointments so that all concerned know what medication is actually being taken.

Family participation in teaching about drugs may exert a strong influence on the patient's understanding and thus improve compliance with therapy.

DRIVING

Patients can usually resume driving 4 weeks after an uncomplicated myocardial infarction. However, they should initially avoid rush-hour traffic and long journeys, as well as aggressive or competitive driving. Patients may be precluded from holding licences to drive large goods vehicles or passenger-carrying vehicles after they have had a myocardial infarction. If recovery is satisfactory, driving may be permitted without notifying the licensing authority. However, motor insurance companies normally require formal notification about changes in health circumstances (Petch, 1998).

FLYING

Patients are usually safe to travel by air as soon as the period of convalescence is over, although long flights are probably initially inadvisable.

RETURN TO WORK

The importance of vocational assessment and counselling cannot be overestimated. For many individuals, return to work usually increases self-satisfaction, restores self-respect and relieves financial worries. Many consider return to work to be the goal of cardiac rehabilitation, although in the current employment climate the use of return to work as a valid outcome of post-infarction rehabilitation is questionable. In addition, return to work can be influenced by demographic, clinical, psychosocial and work-place-related factors.

At about 6 weeks after acute myocardial infarction, the greater part of the affected heart muscle should be healed by the formation of a firm scar, and any collateral circulation should also be well developed. As a consequence, most patients should be ready to resume work, provided it is not physically or mentally too demanding. It is important that the myocardial infarction is not seen as an absolute deterrent to returning to work.

In general, the rates of return to work for post-infarction patients are not as good as might be anticipated. Only about one-half to three-quarters of patients return to their former employment. About 25 million working days are lost annually from coronary heart disease in the UK.

Several factors influence the return to work, including:

- The severity of myocardial infarction
- Complications and symptoms (especially breathlessness and angina)
- Advanced working age
- Stressful work environment
- A sporadic pre-coronary work record
- Family instability.

It can be seen from these factors that non-cardiac causes of invalidity are just as important as cardiac causes in failure to return to work. It is important, therefore, for rehabilitation staff to explore the physical and psychosocial dimensions of the job, the receptivity of the employer and other issues needed to promote a safe and timely return to work (Shrey and Mital, 2000). There is some evidence that a low-intensity cardiac rehabilitation programme that simulates elements of work results in better return to work rates (Mital et al, 2000).

Discouragement by the family is a major cause of the patient not returning to work. This may be because of shared fear of further cardiac problems, although possible early retirement and social security payments may sometimes create a disincentive to return. Ill-considered advice from the patient's medical advisor to 'lay off work and take things easy for a few months' will not help, and some employers seem to believe that coronary patients cannot, or should not, work at all.

The patients likely to do best are those given encouragement from the start of the illness, particularly from their family. It is likely that the better a patient perceives his health to be, the more likely he is to return to work. A multidisciplinary approach is often required, involving the social worker, disability employment advisor and employer. Initially, the patient may be advised to return to work on a part-time basis, occasionally with lighter work. A few patients involved in heavy manual work may need to change their occupation, although this is not always acceptable or practical. When patients do return to work, their level of activity may need to be closely monitored. Many manual workers continue to try to carry out heavy duties, which may be harmful. The patient may dispute this and feel fully capable or not wish to show weakness.

The daily workload of the female patient who is a housewife also needs careful consideration. She has often played a central role in home life and feels a tremendous responsibility to her family, both while she is in hospital and on her return home. Such patients often feel that the house has been neglected, shopping for essential items has been forgotten and the house has not been cleaned adequately. They worry about being unable to look after their family, including cleaning, shopping and cooking. The family will need careful counselling about the psychological stresses on such women and must provide both moral and physical support. Patients should not initially be left at home alone and will need help in performing the household chores, particularly physically taxing jobs such as making the beds and hanging out the washing. Careful consideration should be given to those individuals who live alone.

SICKNESS BENEFIT

Many patients and partners are anxious about how and when to claim sickness benefit. It is helpful to provide them with brief details.

In the UK, sickness benefit is paid by the employer, providing that sufficient national insurance contributions have been paid during the relevant tax year. Sickness benefit will be paid for up to 28 weeks, and thereafter an invalidity benefit may be paid. Supplementary benefit (for items such as the mortgage) may additionally be payable from the Department of Social Security. The old-age pension is payable at the age of 65 years for men and 60 for women, the amount being dependent on the length of working life and the contributions paid.

QUALITY OF LIFE

Cardiac rehabilitation aims to prolong life, relieve symptoms and improve function in patients, and it is imperative that valid and reliable measures of outcome are utilised to assess the impact on functioning and well-being. Thus, measurement of quality of life is important in evaluating the efficacy of cardiac interventions and treatments, including rehabilitation (Dempster and Donnelly, 2000; Smith et al, 2000). Despite the widespread use of the phrase, there is vagueness and little agreement as to the precise definition of quality of life, though health, defined as physical, mental and social well-being, is an important aspect. The assessment of physical outcomes alone is not sufficient and, as a consequence, assessment of well-being and health-related quality of life is considered to be important (Thompson et al, 1998).

There has been a rapid and significant growth in the measurement of quality of life as an indicator of health outcome. A number of measures have evolved which provide an assessment of the patient's experience of his health problems in areas such as physical function, emotional function, social function, role performance, pain and fatigue.

Health-related quality of life measures include generic instruments, which address multiple aspects of quality of life across a range of different patient or illness groups, and disease-specific instruments, which comprise content specific to the disease in question and thus are more clinically sensitive and potentially more responsive in detecting change (Thompson and Roebuck, 2001). An example of the former is the Medical Outcomes Study Short-Form 36-Item (SF–36) Health Survey (Ware and Sherbourne, 1992) and the Quality of Life after Myocardial Infarction (QLMI) questionnaire (Oldridge et al, 1991). Each of these measures has its particular strengths and weaknesses and there is some merit in combining both types. However, it should be emphasized that many of these instruments are rather cumbersome and time-consuming for routine application in clinical settings. What is required are simple tools that are responsive, easily applied and rapidly interpreted.

A new disease-specific measure, the Myocardial Infarction Dimensional Assessment Scale (MIDAS), has just been developed and validated in the UK (Thompson et al, 2002). Also, the National Service Framework for Coronary Heart Disease makes reference to the Cardiovascular Limitations and Symptoms Profile (CLASP), which appears potentially useful across cardiac patient groups (Lewin et al, 2002b).

AUDIT AND EVALUATION

The routine audit and evaluation of cardiac rehabilitation provision has been generally poor. Part of the reason has been the lack of common audit data. An audit tool was developed for use alongside the clinical guidelines for cardiac rehabilitation (Thompson et al, 1996, 1997b) and has been included in the National Service Framework. What is required, however, is an agreed national minimum dataset for routine collection using a standard computerised package. This will facilitate bench-marking of programmes and aid quality improvement.

REFERENCES

Ades PA (2001) Cardiac rehabilitation and secondary prevention of coronary heart disease. *New England Journal of Medicine*, **345**: 892–902.

American Association of Cardiovascular and Pulmonary Rehabilitation (1999) *Guidelines for Cardiac Rehabilitation Programs*, 3rd edn. Champaign, IL: Human Kinetics.

Becker MH (1974) The Health Belief Model and personal health behavior. *Health Education Monographs*, **2**: 236–508.

Bethell HJN, Turner SC, Evans JA et al (2001) Cardiac rehabilitation in the United Kingdom. How complete is the provision? *Journal of Cardiopulmonary Rehabilitation*, **21**(2): 111–115.

British Heat Foundation (2002) *Coronary Heart Disease Statistics*. London: British Heart Foundation.

Criteria Committee of the New York Heart Association (1973) *Nomenclature and Criteria for the Diagnosis of the Heart and Great Vessels*. Boston: Little, Brown.

De Busk RF, Drory Y, Goldstein I et al (2000) Management of sexual dysfunction in patients with cardiovascular disease: recommendations of the Princeton Consensus Panel. *American Journal of Cardiology*, **86:** 175–181.

Dempster M, Donnelly M (2000) Measuring the health related quality of life of people with ischaemic heart disease. *Heart*, **83:** 641–644.

Department of Health (1994) *Nutritional Aspects of Cardiovascular Disease*. Report of the Cardiovascular Review Group of the Committee on Medical Aspects of Food Policy. London: HMSO.

Department of Health (1995) *Sensible Drinking*. The report of an interdisciplinary working group. London: Department of Health.

Department of Health (1996) *Strategy Statement of Physical Activity*. London: Department of Health.

Department of Health (2000) *National Service Framework for Coronary Heart Disease*. London: The Stationery Office.

Dinnes J, Kleijnen J, Leitner M et al (1999) Cardiac rehabilitation. *Quality in Health Care*, **8:** 65–71.

Frasure-Smith N, Lesperance F, Talajic M (1995) Depression and 18-month prognosis after myocardial infarction. *Circulation*, **91:** 999–1005.

Friedman S (2000) Cardiac disease, anxiety, and sexual functioning. *American Journal of Cardiology*, 86 (suppl F): 46F–50F.

Herrman C (1997) International experiences with the Hospital Anxiety and Depression Scale: a review of validation data and clinical results. *Journal of Psychosomatic Research*, **42:** 17–41.

Hooper L (2001) Dietetic guidelines: diet in secondary prevention of cardiovascular disease. *Journal of Human Nutrition and Dietetics*, **14:** 297–305.

Johnston M, Floukes J, Johnston D et al (1999) Impact on patients and partners of inpatient and extended cardiac counseling and rehabilitation: a controlled trial. *Psychosomatic Medicine*, **61:** 225–233.

Jolliffe JA, Rees K, Taylor RS et al (2001) Exercise-based rehabilitation for coronary heart disease. *Cochrane Library Issue 4*. Oxford: Update Software.

Kugler J, Seelbach H, Kruskemper GM (1994) Effects of rehabilitation exercise on anxiety and depression in coronary patients: a meta-analysis. *British Journal of Clinical Psychology*, **33:** 401–410.

Ladwig KH, Roll G, Budde T et al (1994) Post-infarction depression and incomplete recovery 6 months after acute myocardial infarction. *Lancet*, **343:** 20–23.

Lane D, Carroll D, Ring C et al (2002) The prevalence and persistence of depression and anxiety following myocardial infarction. *British Journal of Health Psychology*, **7:** 11–21.

Levine JB, Covino NA, Slack WV et al (1996) Psychological predictors of subsequent medical care among patients hospitalized with cardiac disease. *Journal of Cardiopulmonary Rehabilitation*, **16:** 109–116.

Lewin B, Robertson IH, Cay EL et al (1992) Effects of self-help post-myocardial-infarction rehabilitation on psychological adjustment and use of health services. *Lancet*, **339:** 1036–1040.

Lewin RJP, Ingleton R, Newens A et al (1998) Adherence to cardiac rehabilitation guidelines: a survey of rehabilitation programmes in the United Kingdom. *BMJ*, **316:** 1354–1355.

Lewin RJP, Thompson DR, Elton RA (2002a) Trial of the effects of an advice and relaxation tape given within the first 24 h of admission to hospital with acute myocardial infarction. *International Journal of Cardiology*, **82:** 107–114.

Lewin RJP, Thompson DR, Martin CR et al (2002b) Validation of the Cardiovascular Limitations and Symptoms Profile (CLASP) in chronic stable angina. *Journal of Cardiopulmonary Rehabilitation*, **22:** 184–191.

Mayou RA, Gill D, Thompson DR et al (2000) Depression and anxiety as predictors of outcome after myocardial infarction. *Psychosomatic Medicine*, **62:** 212–219.

Mayou RA, Thompson DR, Clements A et al (2002) Guideline-based early rehabilitation after myocardial infarction. A pragmatic randomized controlled trial. *Journal of Psychosomatic Research*, **52:** 89–95.

Milani RV, Lavie CJ, Cassidy MM (1996) Effects of cardiac rehabilitation and exercise training programmes on depression in patients after major coronary events. *American Heart Journal*, **132:** 726–732.

Miller NH, Taylor CB (1995) *Life-style Management for Patients with Coronary Heart Disease*. Champaign, IL: Human Kinetics.

Mital A, Shrey DE, Govindaraja M et al (2000) Accelerating the return to work (RTW) chances of coronary heart disease (CHD) patients. Part 1: Development and validation of a training programme. *Disability and Rehabilitation*, **22:** 604–620.

NHS Centre for Reviews and Dissemination (1998) Cardiac rehabilitation. *Effective Health Care*, **4:** 1–12.

Oldridge N, Guyatt G, Jones N et al (1991) Effects on quality of life with comprehensive cardiac rehabilitation after acute myocardial infarction. *American Journal of Cardiology*, **74:** 1240–1244.

Petch MC (1998) Driving and heart disease. *European Heart Journal*, **19:** 1165–1177.

Prochaska JO, Di Clemente CC (1983) Stages and processes of self-change of smoking: towards an integrative model of change. *Journal of Consulting and Clinical Psychology*, **51:** 390–395.

Shrey DE, Mital A (2000) Accelerating the return to work (RTW) chances of coronary heart disease (CHD) patients. Part 2: Development and validation of a vocational rehabilitation programme. *Disability and Rehabilitation*, **22:** 621–626.

Silagy C, Stead LF (2001) Physician advice for smoking cessation. *Cochrane Library Issue 4*. Oxford: Update Software.

Smith HJ, Taylor R, Mitchell A (2000) A comparison of four quality of life instruments in cardiac patients: SF–36, QLI, QLMI, and SEIQoL. *Heart*, **84:** 390–394.

Sullivan MD, LaCroix AZ, Baum C et al (1997) Functional status in coronary artery disease: a one-year prospective study of the role of anxiety and depression. *American Journal of Medicine*, **103:** 348–356.

Taylor HA Jr (1999) Sexual activity and the cardiovascular patient: guidelines. *American Journal of Cardiology*, **84** (5B): 6N–10N.

Thompson DR (1990) *Counselling the Coronary Patient and Partner*. London: Scutari.

Thompson DR (2002) Involvement of the partner in rehabilitation. In: Jobin J, Maltais F, Poirier P et al (eds.)

Advancing the Frontiers of Cardiopulmonary Rehabilitation. Champaign, IL: Human Kinetics.

Thompson DR, de Bono DP (1999) How valuable is cardiac rehabilitation and who should get it? *Heart,* **82:** 545–546.

Thompson DR, Lewin RJP (2000) Management of the post-myocardial infarction patient: rehabilitation and cardiac neurosis. *Heart,* **84:** 101–105.

Thompson DR, Meddis R (1990a) A prospective evaluation of in-hospital counselling for first time myocardial infarction men. *Journal of Psychosomatic Research,* **34:** 237–248.

Thompson DR, Meddis R (1990b) Wives responses to counselling early after myocardial infarction. *Journal of Psychosomatic Research,* **34:** 249–258.

Thompson DR, Roebuck A (2001) The measurement of health-related quality of life in patients with coronary heart disease. *Journal of Cardiovascular Nursing,* **16:** 28–33.

Thompson DR, Bowman GS, Kitson AL et al (1996) Cardiac rehabilitation in the United Kingdom: guidelines and audit standards. *Heart,* **75:** 89–93.

Thompson DR, Bowman GS, Kitson AL et al (1997a) Cardiac rehabilitation services in England and Wales: a national survey. *International Journal of Cardiology,* **59:** 299–304.

Thompson DR, Bowman GS, de Bono DP et al (1997b) *Cardiac Rehabilitation: Guidelines and Audit Standards.* London: Royal College of Physicians.

Thompson DR, Bowman GS, de Bono DP et al (1997c) The development and testing of a cardiac rehabilitation audit tool. *Journal of the Royal College of Physicians,* **31:** 317–320.

Thompson DR, Meadows KA, Lewin RJP (1998) Measuring quality of life in patients with coronary heart disease. *European Heart Journal,* **19:** 693–695.

Thompson DR, Roebuck A, Jenkinson C et al (2002) The development and validation of a new measure of quality of life: the myocardial infarction dimensional assessment scale (MIDAS). *Quality of Life Research,* **11:** 535–543.

Van Berkel TF, Boersma H, Roos-Hesselink JW et al (1999) Impact of smoking cessation and smoking interventions with coronary heart disease. *European Heart Journal,* **20:** 1773–1782.

Ware JE Jr, Sherbourne CD (1992) The MOS 36-item short-form health survey (SF-36) I: conceptual framework and item selection. *Medical Care,* **30:** 473–483.

Wenger NK, Froelicher ES, Smith LK et al (1995) *Cardiac Rehabilitation.* Clinical practice guideline no. 17. Rockville, MD: Agency for Health Care Policy and Research and National Heart, Lung and Blood Institute.

World Health Organization (1993) *Needs and Action Priorities in Cardiac Rehabilitation and Secondary Prevention in Patients with Coronary Heart Disease.* Copenhagen: WHO Regional Office for Europe.

Zigmond AS, Snaith RP (1983) The hospital anxiety and depression scale. *Acta Psychiatrica Scandinavica,* **67:** 361–370.

15

Assessing prognosis and reducing risk in patients with acute coronary syndromes

Approximately half of all cases of myocardial infarction and three-quarters of sudden cardiac deaths occur in patients already known to have cardiovascular disease. In the UK, there are about 1.3 million survivors of myocardial infarction who remain at increased risk of angina, another myocardial infarct or sudden death. The three main independent predictors of morbidity and mortality in patients following myocardial infarction are the degree of left ventricular dysfunction, the extent of residual ischaemia and vulnerability to ventricular dysrhythmias. Episodes of unstable angina and re-infarction are also most likely to occur in the early post-infarction period, and more than half the deaths occur within 3 months. The 12-month mortality for those leaving hospital is 10%, after which the annual mortality falls to 5%, which is still 6 times the expected death rate.

The results of various clinical trials support an intensified approach to secondary prevention and rehabilitation following an acute coronary syndrome (AHA/ACC, 2001). This usually involves a major change in the patient's life-style, and specific drug treatment will dramatically reduce subsequent cardiac events (Hennekens et al, 1996). Life-style changes include stopping smoking, making healthier food choices and increasing anaerobic exercise to increase physical fitness and reduce obesity. However, life-style modification is not easy. Habits are hard to change, and denial has to be overcome. Modifying behaviour is often a difficult and long-term process, and allowing time for the patient to consider and reappraise the situation is valuable. Rehabilitation programmes should include changes relevant to the patient, and it is important to explain that changing any life-long habit, whether it is smoking, diet or exercise, will never guarantee freedom from heart disease, or from any other ailment for that matter.

Although the hospital setting provides an ideal environment for discussion and motivation towards a healthier way of life, educational opportunities are often constrained by the acute illness and rapid hospital discharge. Nevertheless, inpatient counselling provides an ideal foundation for patient and family education while the severity of the illness is still in their minds.

Box 15.1 Factors associated with a poor prognosis following acute myocardial infarction

- Age over 60 years
- Male sex
- Poor left ventricular function (heart failure, hypotension)
- Post-infarction angina
- Cardiomegaly on the chest X-ray
- Previous evidence of coronary heart disease
- ECG:
  - Persistent ST–T wave changes
  - Ventricular ectopic activity
  - Atrial fibrillation
  - Conduction defects
  - Left ventricular hypertrophy
- Other co-existing diseases:
  - Hypertension
  - Diabetes

ASSESSING PROGNOSIS FOLLOWING MYOCARDIAL INFARCTION

Risk stratification of patients who survive a myocardial infarction aims to identify those at increased risk of major adverse cardiovascular events, so that therapy may be optimised and new treatments evaluated. Stratification of risk is a continuous process and should not be based upon a single assessment, since prognosis may change with various interventions (Krone, 1992). The response to exercise stress testing is of particular value in determining those at low risk who require less intensive evaluation, and who are candidates for early rehabilitation and return to work (Campbell et al, 1988). It is often easy to recognise patients at high risk without exercise testing (Box 15.1), and most will have shown problems in the early days following acute myocardial infarction (Glover and Littler, 1987). These patients should undergo coronary angiography without any further assessment. Unfortunately, effective strategies for identifying and treating all high-risk patients have not yet been developed.

FACTORS DETERMINING PROGNOSIS

There is a strong relationship between age and prognosis. This seems to be independent of the extent of coronary disease, and it may be simply that the ageing myocardium is less able to withstand the effects of infarction. Following thrombolysis, mortality is about 4% for patients under 55 years of age, but 25% for those over 75 years. Female mortality is double that of men. Diabetic patients have a very poor long- and short-term prognosis. Overall the most important determinants of prognosis seem to be:

- The extent of myocardial damage (and thus residual left ventricular function)
- The extent of coronary arterial disease (and thus myocardium in jeopardy).

The extent of myocardial damage

The magnitude of the myocardial infarction influences outcome, and loss of more than 40% of the left ventricular myocardium usually associates with cardiogenic shock and death. This may be the result of a single extensive infarct, or may accumulate with several episodes of myocardial infarction. A history of a previous myocardial infarction has a major adverse effect on outcome. The degree of damage may be assessed clinically, by ECG or by imaging techniques (echocardiography or nuclear ventriculography). The prognosis is best in patients with left ventricular ejection fractions of 50% or more at rest; those with ejection fractions of less than 35% are at greatest risk.

Early indications of risk may come from cardiac marker concentrations in the blood. For example, there is a strong correlation between the peak creatine kinase level and 4-year mortality (Thompson et al, 1979). Troponin concentrations have been shown to have particular value in risk stratification in acute coronary syndromes (Antman et al, 1996; Stubbs et al, 1996).

The location of the infarct is of prognostic importance. Mortality is lower with inferior, as opposed to anterior, infarction, even when estimates of infarct size are identical. This may be because infarct extension, mural thrombus, left ventricular aneurysm and cardiac rupture are more common with anterior myocardial infarction (Stone et al, 1988). Following thrombolysis, fatality at 28 days is 1.5 times greater with anterior infarctions than with inferior infarctions (Lee et al, 1995).

As might be expected, short-term prognosis is better with non-transmural, as opposed to full-thickness, infarcts. However, even non-transmural infarcts do not seem to have a good long-term prognosis, probably because of residual myocardial ischaemia (de Wood et al, 1986). Since reperfusional therapy is usual, aborted myocardial infarction is now more common, and the underlying vulnerable plaque remains. However, a meta-analysis of randomised trials found that routine angiography with percutaneous coronary intervention in unselected patients did not improve the 6-week and 1-year mortality, or the re-infarction rate in comparison with thrombolysis alone (Michels and Yusuf, 1995). Identifying those with important coronary disease is needed while still in hospital, with selective referral for coronary angiography and revascularisation to improve outcome.

The extent of co-existing coronary artery disease

Peri-infarction angina is associated with a poor prognosis, and is usually a marker of extensive coronary artery disease. Most patients who present with acute myocardial infarction have multi-vessel coronary disease, and, if there is poor perfusion of the surviving myocardium following the infarct, not only will left ventricular function be impaired, but the surviving myocardium will also be placed in jeopardy from further coronary events, unless revascularisation is possible. An initial clue to extensive coronary artery disease is ST segment depression on the presenting ECG. Others likely to have prognostically important coronary disease include those with heart failure, previous infarctions, the elderly and those with diabetes. These patients should undergo coronary angiography without further investigation. Exercise stress testing helps select other high-risk patients who will benefit from early angiography and revascularisation.

Ideally, a submaximal treadmill stress test should be performed in all patients before hospital discharge (70% predicted heart rate or a maximum of 120 beats/min). Low-level stress testing is safe, provided there is no heart failure, hypotension, recurrent ventricular dysrhythmia or post-infarct angina. Those with negative tests may be treated medically, and those with mildly abnormal pre-discharge submaximal stress tests should be considered for perfusion scanning to look for areas of reversible ischaemia. Alternatively, these patients and those returning to work in strenuous occupations, or those who engage in strenuous leisure activities, should undergo a further symptom-limited stress test at 4 weeks.

The Coronary Artery Surgery Study registry (CASS, 1983) suggested risk stratification with the Bruce protocol testing as follows:

- Low risk: able to exercise to stage III with <1 mm ST depression
- Moderate risk: able to exercise to stage II or stage III, but with >1 mm ST depression
- High risk: unable to exercise beyond Stage I with >1 mm ST depression.

All high-risk, and most moderate-risk, patients will need coronary angiography to define coronary anatomy, where the number and distribution of coronary vessels stenosed affects prognosis (Table 15.1). A significant stenosis is usually defined as one that occludes 70% or more of the internal diameter of the coronary vessel (50% for the left main stem artery). Involvement

Table 15.1 Survival and coronary artery stenosis (CASS, 1983)

	1-year survival (%)	5-year survival (%)
Number of vessels stenosed >70%		
1	98	89
2	96	88
3	89	67
Left main stem > 50% stenosis	71	57

of the right coronary artery is generally less serious than involvement of the left coronary artery, but stenosis of the left anterior descending artery proximal to the first septal branch is particularly unfavourable.

Perfusion scanning is needed in those where the baseline ECG makes exercise-induced changes difficult to interpret, such as bundle branch block, left ventricular hypertrophy, or those taking digoxin. Stress echocardiography is an alternative, but is labour-intensive and requires expertise. Pharmacological stress testing with dipyridamole or dobutamine is helpful in the 20% of patients who are unable to exercise, although such patients are usually high-risk, and should perhaps proceed directly to coronary angiography.

Dysrhythmias and prognosis

Early dysrhythmias following acute myocardial infarction reflect short-lived electrical instability and are without any prognostic significance. Atrial fibrillation, however, developing in the first 72 h following infarction is associated with a higher mortality, often reflecting post-infarction complications, such as heart failure. Ventricular dysrhythmias are very common in the first 48 h and are usually transient. Asymptomatic, but frequent, ventricular ectopic beats indicate an adverse prognosis, but treatment may not influence outcome. After 48 h, the presence of ventricular dysrhythmias is a poor prognostic indicator, often signifying poor cardiac function, and many of these patients die before discharge.

Latent dysrhythmias

There are a number of methods of assessing patients with myocardial irritability that associates with sudden cardiovascular death in the first year following myocardial infarction (Mattioni, 1992). Pre-discharge Holter monitoring or exercise stress testing may reveal complex ventricular dysrhythmias, and are an indication for early angiography, and sometimes electrophysiological testing. Inducible ventricular tachycardia is the best indicator of the likelihood of spontaneous ventricular tachycardia after acute myocardial infarction, and prognosis may be improved by implantation of an automatic implantable cardioverter defibrillator (see Ch. 13).

Beta blockers will reduce all-cause mortality and risk of sudden death following acute myocardial infarction by 20–30% (Freemantle et al, 1999).

ASSESSING OVERALL RISK

Assessing global risk in individual patients is important, so that resources are targeted towards those who will benefit most, and to enable closer surveillance of those who most need it. The therapeutic goals defined by the Joint British Recommendations for the Prevention of Coronary Heart Disease in Clinical Practice (Wood et al, 1998) emphasise that individual cardiovascular risk factors should not be considered in isolation, and an integrated approach should be adopted for prevention of further events in patients following an acute coronary syndrome. This includes:

- Life-style changes (exercise, smoking, diet)
- Blood pressure control
- Modification of serum lipids
- Control of hyperglycaemia
- Use of cardioprotective drugs (aspirin, beta-blockers, ACE inhibitors, etc.).

LIFE-STYLE CHANGES

There is considerable scope for life-style modification in most patients following myocardial infarction. Two-thirds of patients with symptomatic atherosclerotic disease are overweight; one-half take little or no exercise, and most ingest large quantities of dietary fat. Despite suffering an acute coronary syndrome, nearly 20% will continue to smoke (Campbell et al, 1998). For married couples, there is concordance for these modifiable risk factors, so encouraging the family rather than the individual to change is more likely to be effective.

ADVICE ON DIET

Apart from providing essential nutrients to the body, eating and drinking are pleasurable experiences, a fact that seems to be forgotten by many of those giving advice. Misconceptions regarding diet clutter the popular press, compounded by conflicting and unsubstantiated information given by friends, relatives and even some health professionals. Dietary modifications often require major change in the patient's normal eating habits, and it is important that factual information is presented objectively and consistently, in a way that can be readily understood by the patient and his family. For most, it is better to emphasise an alteration in general eating habits, rather than the necessity of adhering to a specific dietary plan. Patients are not going to change the habits of a lifetime based on a 10-min chat with a doctor, nurse or dietitian. Involvement of the patient's family is very important. Eating is usually a family or communal activity, and it is important to educate not only those who eat the food, but also those who buy and prepare it.

Population data suggest that a diet high in saturated fat, low in fruit and vegetables and high in salt associates with increased risk of atherosclerotic disease. Accordingly, the Department of Health Committee on Medical Aspects of Food Policy (COMA, 1994) recommend less fat in the diet (particularly saturated fat), at least five portions of fruit and vegetables per day, a third less sodium (9 g to 6 g) and at least two portions of fish (one oily) each week (Table 15.2). Sugar should be avoided, and foods high in starch and fibre are to be encouraged. In general, individuals should eat a wide variety of foods and in the right amounts to prevent obesity.

Table 15.2 Dietary goals for a healthy population

Food type	Total calories
Total fat	< 30% (but more monounsaturated and polyunsaturated)
Carbohydrate	> 50%
Protein	10–20%
Fibre	> 35 mg/day
Cholesterol	< 300 mg/day
At least five portions of fruit and vegetables per day	
Less salt (under 6 g/day)	
Less alcohol (21 units for men, 14 units for women per week)	
Two or more portions of fish each week (preferably oily)	

Weight control

Probably the most important dietary intervention is to achieve weight control. Being overweight (body mass index of more than 25 kg/m^2) is associated with elevated plasma lipids, glucose intolerance and hypertension. The cardiovascular dysmetabolic syndrome describes patients at high risk of cardiovascular events because of insulin resistance, central obesity, glucose intolerance, hypertension, hypertriglyceridaemia and depressed HDL-cholesterol levels (Fagan and Deedwania, 1998). Weight loss reduces triglyceride concentrations, blood pressure, insulin levels, and increased HDL-cholesterol concentrations (James et al, 2000). However, there are no trials demonstrating that weight loss alone affects cardiovascular morbidity or mortality (Drugs and Therapeutics Bulletin, 1998).

Body weight is essentially controlled by food intake, and it is always possible to lose weight by eating less than the body requires, despite what our obese patients tell us. Long-established Western dietary habits are hard to break, and we generally eat and drink more than is good for us, particularly saturated fats, simple sugars and alcohol. Combining exercise with behavioural therapy or drug treatment (such as orlistat or sibutramine) appears to help maintain weight loss better than diet alone (Despres, 2001). Attending 'Weight Watchers' or other slimming clubs may be helpful, but it will be more difficult to influence the individual if other family members, and those counselling the patient, are overweight.

A mutually agreed goal for weight reduction should be established, and a record kept, such as a graph that gives a quick visual indication of how the patient is progressing. Practical advice should include explanation of calorific intake versus expenditure, the regular and slow eating

of smaller amounts of food and the participation in regular physical activity. The ultimate goal is to achieve a body weight appropriate for age, height and sex (Fig. 15.1). The potential health benefits of a 10% body weight reduction for secondary prevention have been summarised by Jung (1997) as:

1. Mortality
   - 20–25% reduction in total mortality
   - 40–50% fall in obesity-related cancer deaths

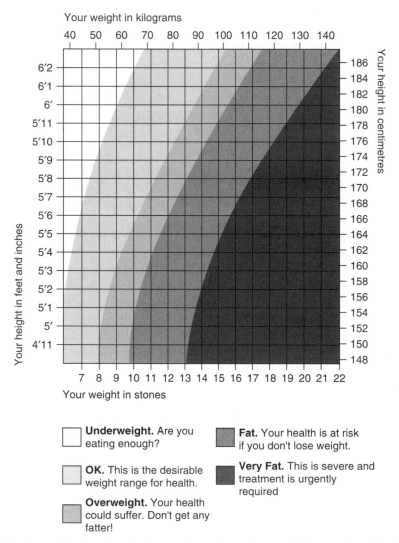

Figure 15.1 Desirable body weights based on body mass index. (From Garrow, 1981; reproduced by kind permission from Churchill Livingstone, with acknowledgement to the Health Education Council and E Fullard, Oxford.)

2. Lipids
   - 10% reduction in total cholesterol
   - 15% reduction in LDL-cholesterol
   - 30% reduction in triglycerides
   - 8% increase in HDL-cholesterol
3. Blood pressure
   - 10 mmHg reduction in systolic and diastolic blood pressures
4. Glucose tolerance
   - Over 50% reduction in risk of developing diabetes
   - Fasting blood glucose reduced by 30–50%
   - HbA_{1c} reduced by 15%.

Making a direct relationship between body mass index and associated health hazards is probably too simplistic, and the regional distribution of body fat is well recognised as a very important consideration. For example, abdominal obesity is a better predictor of type II diabetes and cardiovascular disease. Highly atherogenic metabolic changes are seen in patients with this obesity pattern, including hyperinsulinaemia and dyslipidaemia. Definitions of abdominal obesity are age-, sex- and race-dependent, and the conferred risk is not uniform for all groups. In general, a suggested target waist measurement should be:

- Less than 94 cm (36 inches) in men
- Less than 80 cm (31 inches) in women.

The simple assessment of waist circumference is quicker and easier than other more complex assessments, such as waist:hip ratio and skinfold thickness. Advice on controlling the waistline may prove a very useful strategy for reducing cardiovascular risk (Lamarche, 1998).

Dieting alone is largely ineffective in maintaining any initial weight loss, with most individuals regaining their original weight within 3–5 years. Regular exercise has been shown to be one of the best interventions for successful weight maintenance, and cardiovascular morbidity and mortality are reduced, even without weight loss. Prescribing exercise rather than issuing a simple instruction to 'diet' is likely to be the key to ensuring long-term weight loss and improved health (McInnis, 2000).

Dietary fat

The two main categories of fat in the diet are saturated fats (which tend to raise serum cholesterol levels) and unsaturated fats (which tend to lower blood cholesterol). The major dietary sources of fats are spreading fats (butter and margarine), cooking fats, meat and dairy produce. Much of fat intake is hidden in foods such as cakes and biscuits. Offal (liver, kidney and pâté), shellfish and eggs all contain large amounts of cholesterol, although these foods only have a small effect on serum cholesterol.

Simple low-fat diets do not significantly reduce serum cholesterol unless combined with an increase in polyunsaturated fats (Oliver, 1996), so total fat intake should be reduced to less than 30% of the total food energy intake, with two-thirds of this as vegetable fat. Not all vegetable fats are acceptable; palm and coconut oil, for example, are high in saturated fat, and olive oil (a monounsaturated fat) is a better source of vegetable fat. Unlike polyunsaturated fat, it does not reduce HDL-cholesterol levels, which may explain the negative correlation between olive oil consumption and coronary deaths.

Fish oils have notable antithrombotic activity, and a high intake reduces blood fibrinogen levels, as well as blood pressure. Eating oily fish (such as mackerel and sardines) has therefore been emphasised in cardioprotective diets. In the Diet And Re-infarction Trial (DART) of 2033 men recovering from myocardial infarction, advice on eating oily fish on a daily basis reduced all-cause mortality by 29% in the first 2 years, compared with those who were not advised (Burr, 1989). Interestingly, there was no significant effect on serum cholesterol in those eating oily fish. The 'Mediterranean'-type diet is also rich in omega-3 fatty acids, and in the Lyon trial (de Lorgeril et al, 1994) there was a 70% reduction in cardiac events in post-infarct patients adopting such a diet, independent of changes in cholesterol concentrations. This suggests that the beneficial effects of omega-3 fatty acids are possibly due to a direct antithrombotic effect, rather than mediated through changes in serum cholesterol.

Dietary fibre

An increased fibre intake is recommended, because high consumption of bread and cereal products, particularly oats, may help reduce cholesterol levels and has been associated with a reduced rate of coronary death. Viscous fibre (e.g. guar or pectin) will help modulate plasma lipid and glucose concentrations.

Fruit, vegetables and vitamins

Fresh vegetables and fruit provide excellent sources of antioxidants such as beta-carotene and vitamins C and E. They also contain other bioactive factors, such as potassium and folic acid, that help protect against cardiovascular disease. Increasing folic acid, vitamin B_6 and B_{12} intake reduces homocysteine concentrations.

Salt

The amount of salt ingested in Western countries is greatly in excess of nutritional requirements, but why reducing intake improves cardiovascular outcome is not known. The association of dietary salt and hypertension is not resolved, but avoiding obviously salty foods such as crisps, peanuts and Marmite, and not adding salt to food after cooking, may be particularly important in those with high or borderline blood pressure, and patients with heart failure.

Sugar

Countries with a high per capita intake of sugar have high rates of coronary heart disease (Keys, 1980). However, there is a close link between sugar and fat intake in the poorer countries, and it is unlikely that sugar is an independent risk factor. However, a reduction in simple sugars and other refined carbohydrates is helpful in preventing obesity, treating glucose intolerance and reducing the incidence of dental caries.

Alcohol

The relationship between alcohol intake and coronary heart disease is complex, mainly due to concomitant smoking and overeating that often accompany drinking. Alcohol may damage the myocardium directly, as well as aggravating hypertension and hyperlipidaemia. Despite this, moderate intake of alcohol is probably protective against coronary heart disease, and even light drinkers derive more cardioprotection than those who drink no alcohol. The Framingham Study found that coronary risk was diminished by one-third in those who consumed more than 30 g of alcohol per month (8 g = 1 unit of alcohol). This effect probably derives from the beneficial influence on coagulation factors and from an increase in HDL-cholesterol.

Garlic

Garlic has been used for hundreds of years for its medicinal purposes, and may have a beneficial action on many cardiovascular risk factors, such as lipids and blood pressure, as well as advantageous effects on coagulation factors and platelets. The active ingredients, allicin and ajoene, may be destroyed by cooking or processing. Carefully dried slices retain their active ingredients, but a daily intake of 1 g or more is probably needed for beneficial effect.

Electrolytes and trace elements

The myocardium is more susceptible to damage, dysrhythmias and digoxin in the presence of hypokalaemia. Blood potassium is a poor indicator of total body potassium, and many cases of chronic hypokalaemia are due to use of diuretics. A high intake of potassium is desirable for cardiac patients, particularly those with heart failure. Fresh fruit and vegetables are excellent sources of potassium (1 inch of banana = 1 mmol of potassium). Magnesium depletion often accompanies hypokalaemia.

Vegetarian and Mediterranean diets

Communities in which vegetarianism is common have generally lower rates of cardiovascular disease, and individuals seem to live longer. This probably derives from avoidance of obesity and a higher intake of unsaturated fats, fresh fruit and vegetables that are often rich in vitamins A and C (antioxidant vitamins). The diet in many Mediterranean countries has these benefits, combined with a higher intake of olive oil, garlic and regular moderate alcohol (Ulbricht and Southgate, 1991).

The potential benefits of a healthy diet

Many dietary recommendations have been advanced on the basis that they will prevent or minimise the risk of heart disease, and detailed and complicated dietary modifications are to be found in abundance in the glossy magazines (Thompson, 1983). Although modifying the diet is vital in the management of obesity and diabetes, and is probably helpful in the treatment of hyperlipidaemia, hypertension and congestive heart failure, dietary modification alone has not been shown to prevent heart disease. Many patients become distressed when, having made major alterations in their diet, they find they have cardiovascular disease.

SMOKING

The habit of smoking is a complex addiction with strong dependence. It exerts its addictive influence by satisfying a physical need, providing stimulation and pleasure, as well as relieving anxiety and tension.

Smoking is the most important risk factor for first and subsequent heart attacks, and even passive smoking increases this risk by as much as 20% (Law et al, 1997). Patients with angina are twice as likely to have a myocardial infarction if they continue to smoke, but the risk of a first heart attack is halved within 5 years of stopping smoking (Doll and Peto, 1976). Stopping smoking after myocardial infarction is associated with a substantial reduction in major adverse cardiovascular events and death, in both the long and the short term (Wilhelmsen, 1998), as well as, of course, reducing the extra risk of chronic bronchitis and lung cancer. Observational studies suggest that for every 1000 patients who stop

smoking, there will be 15 deaths and 46 re-infarctions prevented. A 20% reduction in cigarette smokers could result in 8000 fewer deaths in the UK every year.

Surveys show that about 70% of smokers say they want to stop, but only a minority succeed. Only 20% give up smoking as a result of suffering an acute myocardial infarction. Others will try and many will need support. Advice on smoking should start on the coronary care unit, and non-smokers are more credible role models. Like all rehabilitation advice, its value depends heavily upon an informed, committed and uniform approach. Similar education of the patient's family is equally important, and giving such information in coronary care reinforces the importance of such advice.

A realistic plan can be drawn up, with the aim of complete cessation of smoking. Cutting down is not the answer, nor is switching to low-tar cigarettes, cigars or a pipe (Kaufman et al, 1987). This is because the smoking pattern will change to extract the same amount of nicotine from weaker or fewer cigarettes by automatically puffing harder to extract the same amount of nicotine (Woodward and Tunstall-Pedoe, 1993). With this come other harmful constituents of tobacco smoke, including carbon monoxide, thiocyanates and tar.

The benefits of cessation of smoking include improved health and finances, improvement of the senses of taste and smell, and a greater physical attraction when freed from the smell of smoke, and should be stressed. Many smokers advance the excuse that they will put on weight if they stop smoking. This is not an inevitable consequence, and a weight gain of 10–15 kg would be required to nullify the benefits of stopping smoking.

For many smokers, particularly heavy smokers, nicotine addiction is a major factor in persistence of the habit and the high relapse rate on attempts to stop. Nicotine-withdrawal symptoms include anxiety, restlessness and craving, and patients (and their relatives) should be warned that, during the initial period of withdrawal, they might become irritable and unable to concentrate. There may be mood swings, gastrointestinal upsets, or even an initial worsening of their 'smoker's' cough. These effects are temporary, and it is important that the patient does not succumb to 'just one more'.

Nicotine replacement therapy doubles sustained cessation rates and can achieve success rates of about 10% in a medical care setting provided the smoker is sufficiently motivated (Tang et al, 1994; Silagy et al, 1999). Transdermal nicotine patches, nicotine gum and nicotine lozenges are all available without prescription. Although particular caution is advised in the peri-infarction period, it seems unlikely that the effects of nicotine replacement could be any worse than a return to smoking. Other smoking cessation interventions (e.g. acupuncture, hypnotherapy) have not been shown to be of benefit in most cases, but the antidepressant bupropion (Zyban) is an effective aid to smoking cessation (Jorenby et al, 1999). However, due to its complex pharmacology, there is potential for many drug interactions, and its safety is under close scrutiny.

STRESS

Type A behaviour may be reduced in patients undergoing regular counselling, at least in the short term, and can lead to a sustained fall in cardiovascular mortality (Friedman et al, 1986). Some would suggest that counselling should be a routine component of post-infarction rehabilitation for all patients (Lloyd, 1991). Polyphasic activities during everyday life (e.g. watching television, eating and reading simultaneously) must be avoided. The role of frequent, moderate exercise is often underplayed. Jogging, for example, is ideal for reducing muscular tension and giving the patient an opportunity for privacy and self-appraisal while running. The risk of developing persistent psychological disturbance is greater for those patients who were psychiatrically ill before their myocardial infarction. Drug therapy needs careful consideration in view of the frequent cardiovascular side-effects of antidepressant medication. Serotonin re-uptake inhibitors are better than the traditional tricyclic drugs.

EXERCISE

Exercise training programmes are recommended to aid recovery from myocardial infarction, although these need not be of very high intensity (Worcester et al, 1993). Approximately 30 min of moderate aerobic exercise on alternate days, or 20 min daily, is the usual advice, although this should be related to individual capacity. For those with physical impairment, light physical activities, such as walking, gardening and swimming, are beneficial too. A meta-analysis of rehabilitation trials based on exercise showed that, at 3 years following myocardial infarction, total mortality was reduced by 20%, cardiovascular mortality by 22%, and fatal re-infarction by 25% (O'Connor et al, 1989). Data from the British Regional Heart Study in men with cardiovascular disease showed that light and moderate amounts of physical activity were associated with a significant reduction in all-cause mortality when compared with men who remained inactive. Men who become inactive following myocardial infarction have the highest all-cause and cardiovascular mortality (Wannamethee et al, 1998).

Physical fitness is psychologically beneficial, and exercise favourably influences lipid profiles, glucose tolerance, fibrinolytic activity and blood pressure, as well as helping to combat obesity.

HYPERLIPIDAEMIA

There is a strong, positive, graded relationship between serum cholesterol and death from coronary heart disease (Neaton and Wentworth, 1992). A raised serum cholesterol and low HDL-cholesterol continue to be risk factors for recurrent cardiac events after acute myocardial infarction. The evidence for reducing cholesterol in patients with coronary heart disease is exceptionally strong, and has been demonstrated in many clinical trials using diet, drugs and surgery (Law et al, 1994). The most compelling evidence has come from large clinical trials using 3-hydroxy-3-methylglutaryl coenzyme A reductase inhibitors (statins). These trials have demonstrated unequivocally that reducing the serum cholesterol with certain statins reduces cardiovascular morbidity and mortality in patients either with or without established coronary heart disease (Packard, 1999). These benefits are independent of gender, and other treatments such as aspirin or antihypertensive agents. An unexpected further benefit is a reduced risk of stroke. The Medical Research Council/British Heart Foundation Heart Protection Study has provided additional evidence for the use of simvastatin in both men and women aged 40–80 years with cardiovascular disease, diabetes mellitus and treated hypertension. The National Service Framework for Coronary Heart Disease (2000), published prior to the HPS, advises: 'statins and dietary advice should be given to lower the total serum cholesterol concentrations either to less than 5 mmol/l (LDL-cholesterol to below 3 mmol/l) or by 30% (whichever is greater)'. This recommendation will need revision given that benefits in the Heart Protection Study were seen in those with total blood cholesterol levels of as little as 3.5 mmol/l prior to treatment with simvastatin 40 mg.

TREATMENT OF HYPERLIPIDAEMIA

The main dietary influence on plasma cholesterol levels is ingestion of saturated fats, and eating cholesterol is generally less influential. The average daily British diet only contains about 500 mg of cholesterol, and reducing this to the recommended level of less than 300 mg a day will only have a small effect on the serum cholesterol. The general dietary recommendations shown in Table 15.2 are appropriate, but will probably only reduce the cholesterol by 5–10%, and few will achieve the currently recommended target cholesterol concentrations with diet alone (Jowett and Galton, 1987). It has been usual to wait 6–12 weeks following myocardial infarction to see the effect of diet before initiating drug therapy. However, given that diet alone is unlikely to achieve target cholesterol concentrations, a pragmatic approach is recommended, with all patients suffering an acute coronary syndrome being prescribed hypolipidaemic therapy before

discharge from hospital. Statins are the preferred drugs for secondary prevention, but the choice of statin and starting dose is an area of contention between those who use an evidence-based approach and those who prefer a cost-effectiveness approach. The controlled trials of secondary prevention following myocardial infarction used pravastatin and simvastatin, and have evidence of efficacy and safety (Table 15.3). These 'natural' statins are fermentation-derived and differ structurally from the 'synthetic' statins (atorvastatin and fluvastatin), which are more potent and may be more cost-effective in terms of cholesterol-lowering. However, relying on reductions in total cholesterol alone as a surrogate for efficacy in terms of reduction in mortality may lead to unproven statins being prescribed in place of evidence-based drugs. This exposes the patient to the unnecessary risk of drug side-effects, as well as not benefiting from the desired intervention. The recent withdrawal of cerivastatin (Lipobay) because of deaths from rhabdomyolysis has emphasised this fact. Despite paucity of outcome data, this drug was widely prescribed because it was cheap.

The natural statins should be used as first-line drugs in the prevention of cardiovascular disease, and other cholesterol-lowering agents should be only be considered for patients who do not respond until alternatives are proven to be superior or equivalent. Statins are most effective if taken in the evening, and the trial data support starting either simvastatin 40 mg or pravastatin 40 mg daily without titration. If other statins or smaller doses are used, it is essential to increase the dose every 4–6 weeks to achieve the target cholesterol. Beyond the age of 80 years, there are limited data on the value of cholesterol lowering, and prescribing statins in the very elderly may not be justified (Oliver, 1999). However, statins should be continued in those already taking them, and should be utilised in those undergoing coronary intervention.

The use of fibric acid derivatives, such as bezafibrate, suggests that these agents decrease cardiovascular mortality, but may increase overall mortality (Gould et al, 1995). Although fibrates are generally suitable for patients with

Table 15.3 Evidence-based trials for the statins

	Simvastatin	Pravastatin	Fluvastatin	Lovastatin[a]
Mortality post-MI[b]	4S	CARE, LIPID	–	–
Events post-MI	4S	CARE, LIPID	LISA	–
Mortality pre-MI	HPS	WOSCOPS	–	–
Events pre-MI	HPS	WOSCOPS	–	AFCAPS/TexCAPS
Angiographic studies	MAAS	PLAC I & II REGRESS	FLARE, LCAS	Post-CABG ACAPS
Diabetes	4S, HPS	CARE, LIPID	–	–
Stroke	4S, HPS	CARE	–	–

[a] Not licensed in the UK.
[b] MI, myocardial infarction.
4S = Scandinavian Simvastatin Survival Study (1994) *Lancet,* **344:** 1383–1389.
CARE = Cholesterol And Recurrent Events (1996) *New England Journal of Medicine,* **335:** 1001–1009.
WOSCOPS = West of Scotland Coronary Prevention Study (1995) *New England Journal of Medicine,* **333:** 1301–1307.
LIPID = Long-term Intervention with Pravastatin in Ischaemic Disease (1998) *New England Journal of Medicine,* **339:** 1349–1357.
AFCAPS/TexCAPS = Air Force/Texas Coronary Atherosclerosis Prevention Study (1998) *JAMA,* **279:** 1615–1622.
HPS = Heart Protection Study (2002) *Lancet,* **360:** 7–22
Post-CABG = Post-Coronary Bypass Graft Trial (1997) *New England Journal of Medicine,* **336:** 332–336.
ACAPS = Asymptomatic Carotid Artery Progression Study (1995) *Circulation,* **90:** 1679–1687.
LISA = Lescol In Severe Atherosclerosis (1999) *Atherosclerosis,* **144:** 263–270.
LCAS Lipoprotein and Coronary Atherosclerosis Study (1997) *American Journal of Cardiology,* **80:** 278–286.
FLARE = Fluvastatin Angiographic Restenosis Trial (1999) *European Heart Journal,* **20:** 58–69.
MAAS = Multi-centre Anti-Atheroma Study (1994) *Lancet,* **344:** 633–638.
PLAC I and II = Pravastatin Limitation of Atherosclerosis in the Coronary Arteries (1995) *American Journal of Cardiology,* **76:** 60c–63c.
REGRESS = Regression Growth Evaluation Statin Study (1995) *Circulation,* **91:** 2528–2540.

both raised cholesterol and triglycerides, statins should still be used as first-line therapy, and in most cases will be effective.

Despite excellent evidence of cholesterol-lowering in post-infarct patients, a national survey (ASPIRE) by the British Cardiac Society in 1996 showed that 78% of men and 86% of women still had a cholesterol of 5 mmol/l or more following myocardial infarction (Bowker et al, 1996).

HYPERTENSION

Although the link between hypertension and stroke is well recognised, the most common cause of death in patients with hypertension is myocardial infarction, which occurs 2–3 times more commonly than stroke. Nearly a quarter of patients with hypertension have a past history of coronary heart disease, and a raised blood pressure continues to be a risk factor for subsequent cardiovascular events in patients following acute myocardial infarction. Although there is little evidence to support secondary intervention fol-

lowing myocardial infarction, treatment targets have been extrapolated from primary prevention trials to help prevent heart failure and stroke. Those with systolic blood pressure of 140 mmHg and/or diastolic of 85 mmHg or above should be offered antihypertensive advice and drug therapy (Ramsey et al, 1999). Non-pharmacological intervention is helpful regardless of the need for medication, and includes advice on exercise, weight reduction and dietary restriction of salt and alcohol. Vegetarian diets and foods high in potassium may also help reduce blood pressure.

If drug therapy is required, it must be made clear that it is usually permanent. Patients should not just complete the 'course' of tablets, and doses may also need titration to achieve target blood pressure reductions. In the ASPIRE trial (Bowker et al, 1996), when blood pressure was measured in patients 6 months after myocardial infarction, 56% of patients had a blood pressure greater than 140/85 mmHg.

No direct comparisons of the different antihypertensive agents have been made following myocardial infarction, but, given their cardioprotective role, beta-blockers or ACE inhibitors should perhaps be the first choice. Rate-limiting calcium antagonists such as verapamil and diltiazem may be used if there is no evidence of left ventricular dysfunction.

DRUG THERAPY

ASPIRIN

Administration of aspirin acutely and long term greatly reduces the risk of death by 12%, re-infarction by 31% and non-fatal stroke by 42% (Antiplatelet Trialists' Collaboration, 1994). For every 1000 patients treated, there are 18 non-fatal infarcts prevented, as well as 13 vascular deaths and 6 non-fatal strokes. The beneficial dose of aspirin is unknown, but is probably in the range of 75–325 mg daily. There are few proven alternatives, but clopidogrel should be substituted where aspirin is contraindicated (CAPRIE Steering Group, 1996).

BETA-BLOCKERS

The use of timolol, metoprolol or propranolol following myocardial infarction has been shown to reduce the risk of sudden death, non-fatal re-infarction and all-cause mortality by 20–30% (Yusuf et al, 1985). Reduction in heart rate seems important, which is possibly why using beta-blockers with intrinsic sympathomimetic activity (e.g. pindolol and oxprenolol) does not confer benefit. Patients at highest risk benefit most from beta-blockade, particularly the elderly, diabetics, those with large and anterior infarcts, and those with heart failure. These patients are often denied beta-blocker therapy. Treatment should be started within 24 h and continued for at least 2–3 years if tolerated (Freemantle et al, 1999). Most physicians would continue the drug indefinitely unless there were problems.

CALCIUM ANTAGONISTS

In general, these agents have not been shown to have any benefit following myocardial infarc-

tion, and their use may be hazardous in patients with heart failure. Verapamil and diltiazem slow the pulse, and have been used where beta-blockers are contraindicated. Verapamil reduces the re-infarction rate in patients with good left ventricular function (DAVIT II, 1990), and diltiazem helps prevent re-infarction in the 6 months following non-transmural myocardial infarction (Gibson et al, 1986), although late re-infarction rates are similar to those treated with placebo.

ACE INHIBITORS

The routine use of ACE inhibitors in unselected patients following acute myocardial infarction was addressed in the ISIS-4 (ISIS-4 Collaborative Group, 1995) and GISSI-3 (1994) studies, which showed a small benefit with early administration. This has been confirmed in a large meta-analysis of over 100 000 patients (ACE Inhibitor Myocardial Infarction Collaborative Group, 1998). A greater reduction in mortality is seen in those patients with symptomatic and asymptomatic left ventricular dysfunction (Pfeffer et al, 1992; AIRE Investigators, 1993; Vannan et al, 1993), and ACE inhibitors should be prescribed to all patients with evidence of left ventricular dysfunction following acute myocardial infarction.

The duration of therapy is not yet established. Low-risk patients with normal or near normal left ventricular function on a pre-discharge echocardiogram could probably have therapy stopped at 6 weeks, and, since no further left ventricular remodelling occurs after a year, this might be another time to consider discontinuation of therapy. However, the effect of ACE inhibitors on factors other than remodelling may explain why survival curves of those treated and not treated in all trials remain permanently separated, and would endorse lifelong treatment. The HOPE study (Heart Outcomes Prevention Evaluation Study Investigators, 2000) supports indefinite use of ramipril in high-risk patients over the age of 55 years, even in the absence of left ventricular dysfunction.

The doses of ACE inhibitors currently prescribed in the UK are significantly lower than those shown to improve survival, and there is no evidence that lower doses are of prognostic benefit. Large doses of ACE inhibitors are more effective than small doses, and are not associated with increased toxicity. Asymptomatic hypotension or a modest creatinine change should not impede this concept, but these patients will require close monitoring during the titration phase. Target doses of the recommended ACE inhibitors are:

- Captopril 50 mg three times a day
- Enalapril 20 mg twice daily
- Ramipril 5 mg twice daily
- Lisinopril 40 mg once daily
- Trandolapril 4 mg once daily.

The dosage schedule as shown above is necessary to cover the full 24-h period, because if the renin–angiotensin system kicks in during the early morning, the diseased left ventricle will not be able to cope with the extra burden, and fails (early morning heart failure).

ANTICOAGULANTS

Studies of anticoagulant treatment after myocardial infarction indicate reduction in death, recurrent infarction and thromboembolic complications, but there is no major difference between aspirin and warfarin, and no benefit from using both. Warfarin is indicated for those who are aspirin-intolerant, and for those at high risk of cardiac thromboembolism (e.g. large left ventricle, ventricular aneurysm, atrial fibrillation). The suggested target INR is 2.5.

The incidence of left ventricular thrombus is now much lower than previously due to routine treatment with heparin, thrombolysis and ACE inhibitors which attenuate ventricular dilatation and aneurysm formation. High-risk patients can be identified by pre-discharge echocardiography, and those with large anterior dyskinetic areas should receive warfarin. The SOLVD and SAVE trials showed benefits of long-term anticoagulation in those with ejection fractions under 35% (Weigers and St John Sutton, 2000).

Risk/benefits must be assessed and discussed with the patient. In some patients, particularly

the elderly, the risks of bleeding, compliance and poor anticoagulant control may make warfarin dangerous.

HORMONE REPLACEMENT THERAPY

Ovarian hormones are cardioprotective in post-menopausal women, attributed to beneficial effects on lipid levels, insulin resistance and endothelial function. Post-menopausal oestrogen replacement is associated with a 35–50% lower risk of cardiovascular disease (Grady et al, 1992), but less is known about the effects of progestogens. Administration of a progestogen is necessary in women with a uterus because of the carcinogenic effect of unopposed oestrogen, and combined hormone replacement therapy (HRT) is not currently recommended for cardioprotection (Barrett-Connor et al, 1998). The Heart and Estrogen/progestin Replacement Study (HERS) showed no benefit of hormone replacement in post-menopausal women with coronary disease. In fact, there was a slight increase in cardiac events in the first year of therapy (perhaps due to an immediate prothrombotic effect), but a subsequent decreased risk (Hulley et al, 1998). Decisions regarding HRT must be individualised, depending on the competing risks of coronary heart disease, osteoporosis, menopausal symptoms and endometrial and breast cancer. Current advice for post-menopausal women following acute myocardial infarction is that HRT should not be started for cardioprotection, but may be continued if they were already taking it (Grodstein et al, 2001).

BENEFITS OF SECONDARY PREVENTION

The relative benefits of treatment following acute myocardial infarctions are shown in Table 15.4. Despite the clear benefits of secondary prevention, many patients in Europe remain on inadequate therapy (Table 15.5) The Action on Secondary Prevention through Intervention to Reduce Events (ASPIRE) study (Bowker et al,

Table 15.4 Relative benefits of secondary intervention following myocardial infarction

Treatment	Events prevented per 1000 treated
Aspirin	16 deaths/myocardial infarcts/strokes
Stopping smoking	27 deaths
Beta-blockers	13 deaths
	5 myocardial infarcts
Reducing cholesterol by 10%	7 deaths/myocardial infarcts
ACE inhibitors	12 deaths
	9 myocardial infarcts
	16 cases of heart failure

Box 15.2 Medical interventions for patients following an acute coronary syndrome

- Advice on smoking cessation and use of nicotine replacement therapy
- Advice on weight control, diet, alcohol and exercise
- Treat blood pressure to target of under 140/85 mmHg (especially with beta-blockers/ACE inhibitors)
- Aspirin (plus clopidogrel following unstable coronary syndromes)
- Simvastatin or pravastatin to lower total cholesterol concentrations EITHER to less than 5 mmol/l (LDL-cholesterol to below 3 mmol/l) OR by 30% (whichever is greater)
- ACE inhibitors for those with left ventricular dysfunction
- Beta-blockade (especially propranolol, metoprolol, pindolol)
- Warfarin or aspirin for those in atrial fibrillation
- Meticulous blood pressure and glycaemic control in those with diabetes.

1996) also demonstrated failure to achieve targets in those recently discharged from hospital. At a 6-month review following a coronary event:

- 27% of patients were still smoking
- 75% were still overweight
- 25% were still hypertensive
- 75% had a cholesterol over 5.2 mmol/l
- 20% were not taking aspirin
- 66% were not taking a beta-blocker.

Supervision and follow-up often fail because of breakdown in the link between primary and secondary care, and there is considerable scope for risk-factor clinics and nurse-led intervention (Jolly, 1999; Brady et al, 2000). Interventional targets are shown in Box 15.2.

Delivery of secondary prevention is not cheap, and guidelines for intervention must take cost-effectiveness into consideration. Estimated costs of 5 years' therapy per life-year saved following acute myocardial infarction are:

- Aspirin: £35
- Metoprolol: £500
- Ramipril: £4000
- Simvastatin: £4410.

The cardiac rehabilitation programme adds about £7500 per life-year saved. These figures do not account for changes in drug costs, or improvements in non-fatal outcomes, and reduced need for further medical interventions.

SURGICAL THERAPY

The role of cardiac surgery and other reperfusional strategies following myocardial infarction

Table 15.5 Percentage of patients receiving adequate therapy for secondary prevention in Europe

STUDY[a]	Where, when	Percentage of patients treated			
		Aspirin	Statin	Beta-blocker	ACE inhibitor
ASPIRE	UK, 1994	86	16	36	18
EUROASPIRE I	Europe, 1995	81	32	54	30
HEALTHWISE	UK, 1997–1998	50	16	21	13
PRAIS-UK	UK, 1998	78	44	41	–
PREVENIR	France, 1998	90	52	68	42
EUROASPIRE II	Europe, 1999	84	63	66	43

[a]References: Bowker et al, 1996; Collinson et al, 2000; EUROASPIRE I and II Groups, 2001; Marques-Vidal et al, 2001.

is discussed in Ch. 16. Both coronary bypass surgery and percutaneous transvenous coronary angioplasty are widely utilised to relieve symptoms and prolong survival following myocardial infarction. In the absence of diabetes, the benefits are now almost identical among patients with multivessel disease assigned to percutaneous coronary intervention versus those assigned to bypass surgery, although additional intervention is 2–4 times more likely in those initially treated by percutaneous coronary intervention (Bourassa, 2000).

REFERENCES

ACE Inhibitor Myocardial Infarction Collaborative Group (1998) Indications for ACE inhibitors in the early treatment of acute myocardial infarction: systematic overview of individual data from 100,000 patients in randomised trials. *Circulation*, **97**: 2202–2212.

AHA/ACC (2001) Guidelines for preventing heart attack and death in patients with atherosclerotic cardiovascular disease: 2001 update. *Circulation*, **104**: 1577–1579.

AIRE (Acute Infarction Ramipril Efficacy) Investigators (1993) Effect of ramipril on mortality and morbidity of survivors of acute myocardial infarction with clinical evidence of heart failure. *Lancet*, **342**: 821–828.

Antiplatelet Trialists' Collaboration (1994) Overview I. Prevention of death, myocardial infarction and stroke by prolonged antiplatelet therapy in various categories of patients. *BMJ*, **308**: 81–106.

Antman EM, Tanasijevic MJ, Thompson B et al (1996) Cardiac specific troponin I levels to predict the risk of mortality in patients with acute coronary syndromes. *New England Journal of Medicine*, **335**: 1342–1349.

Barrett-Connor E, Wenger NK, Grady D et al (1998) Coronary heart disease in women, randomised trials, HERS and RUTH. *Maturitas*, **31**: 1–7.

Bourassa MG (2000) Clinical trials of coronary re-vascularisation: coronary angioplasty versus coronary bypass grafting. *Current Opinion in Cardiology*, **15**: 281–286.

Bowker TJ, Clayton TC, Ingham J (1996) A British Cardiac Society survey of potential for the secondary prevention of coronary disease ASPIRE (Action on Secondary Prevention through Intervention to Reduce Events). *Heart*, **4**: 334–342.

Brady AJB, Oliver MA, Pittard JB (2001) Secondary prevention in 24,431 patients with coronary heart disease. Survey in primary care. *BMJ*, **322**: 1463.

Burr ML, Fehily AM, Holliday RM et al (1989) Effects of changes in fat, fish and fibre intakes on death and myocardial re-infarction: diet and re-infarction trial (DART). *Lancet*, **343**: 1454–1459.

Campbell S, A'Hern R, Quigley P et al (1988) Identification of patients who are at low risk of dying after acute myocardial infarction by simple clinical and sub-maximal exercise test criteria. *European Heart Journal*, **9**: 938–947.

Campbell NC, Thain J, Deans HG et al (1998) Secondary prevention in coronary heart disease: baseline survey of provision in general practice. *BMJ*, **316**: 1430–1434.

CAPRIE Steering Group (1996) A randomised blinded trial of clopidogrel versus aspirin in patients at risk of ischaemic events (CAPRIE). *Lancet*, **348**: 1329–1339.

CASS. The Coronary Artery Surgery Study (1983) A randomised trial of coronary artery bypass surgery: survival data. *Circulation*, **68**: 939–950.

Collinson J, Flather M, Fox KA et al (2000) Clinical outcomes, risk stratification and practice patterns of unstable angina and myocardial infarction without ST elevation: Prospective Registry of Acute Ischaemic Syndromes in the UK (PRAIS-UK). *European Heart Journal*, **21**: 1450–1457.

COMA (1994) *Diet and Risk*. Report of the Committee on Medical Aspects of Food Policy. London: HMSO.

DAVIT II (1990) The Danish Study Group on Verapamil in Myocardial Infarction. Effect of verapamil on mortality and major events after acute myocardial infarction. *American Journal of Cardiology*, **66**: 779.

de Lorgeril M, Renaud S, Mamelle N et al (1994) Mediterranean alpha-linoleic acid-rich diet in the secondary prevention of coronary heart disease. *Lancet*, **343**: 1454.

Department of Health (2000) *National Service Framework for Coronary Heart Disease*. London: The Stationery Office. ch. 2.

Despres J-P (2001) Drug treatment for obesity. *BMJ*, **322**: 1379–1380.

de Wood M, Stifter WF, Simpson CS et al (1986) Coronary angiographic findings soon after non-Q-wave myocardial infarction. *New England Journal of Medicine*, **315**: 412–422.

Doll R, Peto R (1976) Mortality in relation to smoking: 20 years' observations on male British doctors. *BMJ*, **2**: 1525–1536.

Downs JR, Clearfield M, Wies S et al (1998) Primary prevention of acute coronary events with lovastatin in men and women with average cholesterol levels: results of AFCAPS/TexCAPS. Air Force/Texas Coronary Atherosclerosis Prevention Study. *JAMA*, **279**: 1615–1622.

Drugs and Therapeutics Bulletin (1998) Why and how should adults lose weight? *Drugs and Therapeutics Bulletin*, **36**: 89–92.

EUROASPIRE I and II Groups (2001) Clinical reality of coronary prevention guidelines. A comparison of EUROASPIRE I and II in nine countries. *Lancet*, **357**: 995–1001.

Fagan TC, Deedwania PC (1998) The cardiovascular dysmetabolic syndrome. *American Journal of Medicine*, **105**: 77S–82S.

Freemantle N, Cleland J, Young P et al (1999) Beta-blockade after myocardial infarction: systematic review and meta-regression analysis. *BMJ*, **318**: 1730–1737.

Friedman M, Thorensen CE, Gill JJ (1986) Alteration of type A behavior and its effect on cardiac recurrences in post-myocardial infarct patients: summary results in the

Recurrent Coronary Prevention Project. *American Heart Journal,* **112:** 653–665.

Gibson RS, Boden WE, Theroux P et al (1986) Diltiazem and re-infarction in patients with non-Q-wave myocardial infarction. *New England Journal of Medicine,* **315:** 423–429.

GISSI-3 (1994) Effects of lisinopril and transdermal glyceryl trinitrate singly and together on 6-week mortality and ventricular function after acute myocardial infarction. Gruppo Italiano per lo Studio della Sopravivenza nell'Infarto Miocardico. *Lancet,* **343:** 1115–1122.

Glover DR, Littler WA (1987) Factors influencing the survival and mode of death in severe ischaemic heart disease. *British Heart Journal,* **57:** 125–132.

Gould AL, Rossouw JE, Santanello NC et al (1995) Cholesterol reduction yields clinical benefit: a new look at old data. *Circulation,* **91:** 2274–2282.

Grady D, Ribin SM, Petitti DB et al (1992) Hormone therapy to prevent disease and prolong life in post-menopausal women. *Annals of Internal Medicine,* **117:** 1016–1037.

Grodstein F, Manson JE, Stampfer MJ(2001) Postmenopausal hormone use and secondary prevention of coronary events in the nurses' health study: a prospective observational study. *Annals of Internal Medicine,* **135:** 1–8.

Heart Outcomes Prevention Evaluation Study Investigators (2000) Effects of angiotensin-converting-enzyme inhibitor, ramipril, on cardiovascular events in high risk patients. *New England Journal of Medicine,* **342:** 145–153.

Heart Protection Study Group (2002) MRC/BHF heart protection study of cholesterol lowering with simvastatin in 20 536 high-risk individuals: a randomised placebo-controlled trial. *Lancet,* **360:** 7–22.

Hennekens CH, Albert CM, Godfried SL et al (1996) Adjunctive drug therapy of acute myocardial infarction: evidence from the clinical trials. *New England Journal of Medicine,* **335:** 1660–1667.

Hulley S, Grady D, Bush T et al (1998) Randomised trial of estrogen plus progestin for secondary prevention of coronary heart disease in post-menopausal women. *JAMA,* **280:** 605–613.

ISIS-4 Collaborative Group (1995) A randomised factorial trial assessing early oral captopril, oral mononitrate, and intravenous magnesium sulphate in 58,050 patients with suspected acute myocardial infarction. *Lancet,* **345:** 669–685.

James WPT, Astrup A, Finer H et al (2000) Effect of sibutramine on weight maintenance after weight loss: a randomised trial. *Lancet,* **356:** 119–125.

Jolly K for the SHIP Collaborative Group (1999) Randomised controlled trial of follow up care in general practice of patients with myocardial infarction and angina: final results of the Southampton Heart Integrated Care Project (SHIP). *BMJ,* **318:** 706–711.

Jorenby DE, Leischow SJ, Nides MA et al (1999) A controlled trial of sustained-release bupropion, a nicotine patch, or both for smoking cessation. *New England Journal of Medicine,* **340:** 685–691.

Jowett NI, Galton DJ (1987) The management of the hyperlipidaemias. In: Hamer J (ed.). *Drugs for Heart Disease,* 2nd edn. London: Chapman and Hall.

Jung RT (1997) Obesity as a disease. *British Medical Bulletin,* **53:** 307–321.

Kaufman DW, Palmer JR, Rosenberg L et al (1987) Cigar and pipe smoking and myocardial infarction in young men. *BMJ,* **294:** 1315–1316.

Keys A (1980) *Seven Countries.* London: Harvard University Press.

Krone RJ (1992) The role of risk stratification in the early management of a myocardial infarction. *Annals of Internal Medicine,* **116:** 223–237.

Lamarche B (1998) Abdominal obesity and its metabolic complications: implications for the risk of ischaemic heart disease. *Coronary Artery Disease,* **9:** 473–481.

Law MR, Wald NJ, Thompson SG (1994) By how much and how quickly does reduction in serum cholesterol concentration lower risk of ischaemic heart disease? *BMJ,* **308:** 367–373.

Law MR, Morris JK, Wald N (1997) Environmental tobacco smoke exposure and ischaemic heart disease: an evaluation of the evidence. *BMJ,* **315:** 937–980.

Lee KL, Woodlieff LH, Topol EJ et al (1995) Predictors of 30-day mortality in the era of reperfusion for acute myocardial infarction. Results from an International trial of 41,021 patients. *Circulation,* **91:** 1659–1668.

Lloyd GG (1991) Myocardial infarction and the mind. *Hospital Update,* December: 943–944.

Marques-Vidal P, Cambou JP, Ferrieres J et al (2001) Etude PREVENIR. Distribution and treatment of cardiovascular risk factors in coronary patients: the PREVENIR study. *Archives des Maladies du Coeur et des Vaisseaux,* **94:** 673–680.

Mattioni TA (1992) Long-term prognosis after myocardial infarction. Who is at risk for sudden death? *Postgraduate Medicine,* **92:** 107–108, 111–114.

McInnis KJ (2000) Exercise and obesity. *Coronary Artery Disease,* **11:** 111–116.

Michels KB, Yusuf S (1995) Does PTCA in acute myocardial infarction affect mortality and re-infarction rates? A quantitative overview (meta-analysis) of the randomised clinical trials. *Circulation,* **91:** 476–485.

Neaton JD, Wentworth D (1992) Serum cholesterol, blood pressure, cigarette smoking and death from coronary heart disease. Overall findings and differences by age for 316,099 white men. Multiple Risk Factor Intervention Trial (MRFIT) Research Group. *Archives of Internal Medicine,* **152:** 56–64.

O'Connor GT, Buring JE, Yusuf S et al (1989) An overview of randomised trials of rehabilitation with exercise after myocardial infarction. *Circulation,* **80:** 234-244.

Oliver MF (1996) Which changes in diet prevent coronary heart disease? *Acta Cardiologica,* **51:** 467.

Oliver MF (1999) Lowering cholesterol in old age. *Journal of the Royal College of Physicians,* **33:** 252–253.

Packard CJ (1999) Major statin trials: relationship between lipid changes and cardiovascular event. *European Heart Journal,* **1:** (suppl T): T2–T6.

Pfeffer MA, Braunwald E, Moyle LA et al (1992) Effect of captopril on mortality and morbidity in patients with left ventricular dysfunction after myocardial infarction: results of the survival and ventricular enlargement trial (SAVE). *New England Journal of Medicine,* **327:** 669–677.

Ramsey LE, Williams B, Johnston GD et al (1999) Guidelines for management of hypertension: report of the third working party of the British Hypertension Society. *Journal of Human Hypertension,* **13:** 569–592.

Silagy C, Mant D, Fowler G et al (1999) Nicotine replacement therapy for smoking cessation. In: Tobacco

Addiction Module of Cochrane Database of Systematic Reviews. *Cochrane Library Issue 1*. Oxford: Update Software.

Stone PH, Raabe DS, Jaffe AS (1988) Prognostic significance of location and type of myocardial infarctions: independent adverse outcome associated with anterior locations. *Journal of the American College of Cardiology*, **11:** 453–463.

Stubbs P, Collinson P, Moseley D et al (1996) Prospective study of the role of cardiac troponin T in patients admitted with unstable angina. *BMJ*, **313:** 262–264.

Tang JL, Law M, Wald N (1994) How effective is nicotine replacement therapy in helping people to stop smoking? *BMJ*, **308:** 21–26.

Thompson DR (1983) Dietary advice and heart disease: a nursing dilemma? *International Journal of Nursing Studies*, **20:** 245–253.

Thompson PL, Fletcher EE, Katavatis V (1979) Enzymatic indices of myocardial necrosis: influence on short and long term prognosis after myocardial infarction. *Circulation*, **59:** 113.

Ulbricht TLV, Southgate DAT (1991) Coronary heart disease: seven dietary factors. *Lancet*, **338:** 985–992.

Vannan MA, Taylor DJE, Webb-Peploe MW et al (1993) ACE inhibitors after myocardial infarction. *BMJ*, **306:** 531–532.

Wannamethee SG, Shaper AG, Walker M (1998) Changes in physical activity, mortality and incidence of coronary heart disease in older men. *Lancet*, **351:** 1603–1608.

Weigers SE, St John Sutton M (2000) When should ACE inhibitors or warfarin be discontinued after myocardial infarction? *Heart*, **84:** 361–362.

Wilhelmsen L (1998) Effects of cessation of smoking after myocardial infarction. *Journal of Cardiovascular Risk*, **5:** 173–176.

Wood D, Durrington P, Poulter N et al (1998) Joint British Recommendations on Prevention of Coronary Heart Disease in Clinical Practice. *Heart*, **80** (suppl 2): S1-S29.

Woodward M, Tunstall-Pedoe H (1993) Self-titration of nicotine: evidence from the Scottish Heart Health Study. *Addiction*, **88:** 821–830.

Worcester MC, Hare DL, Oliver RG et al (1993) Early programmes of high and low intensity exercise and quality of life after acute myocardial infarction. *BMJ*, **307:** 1244–1247.

Yusuf S, Peto R, Lewis J et al (1985) Beta-blockade during and after myocardial infarction: an overview of randomised trials. *Progress in Cardiovascular Diseases*, **27:** 335–371.

16

Percutaneous coronary intervention and cardiac surgery in patients with coronary artery disease

Coronary artery bypass grafting (CABG) and percutaneous transluminal coronary angioplasty (PTCA) are well-established methods of myocardial revascularisation for alleviating symptoms and improving prognosis. The term 'percutaneous coronary intervention' (PCI) describes a group of techniques that includes PTCA, stenting and athero-ablation. Other novel approaches, such as transmyocardial laser revascularisation and angioneogenesis, may provide alternatives in the future (Kornowski et al, 2000). All these forms of treatment have risks and benefits that must be considered, and revascularisation is only part of a multi-interventional strategy that includes risk factor modification, adjunctive drug therapy and rehabilitation.

The evidence relating to the efficacy of coronary revascularisation has limitations because the major randomised trials were carried out before the routine use of arterial grafts, and improved medical therapy. Initial success and rates of re-occlusion following PTCA have also changed with the introduction of new antithrombotic agents and routine deployment of stents. The published clinical trials also concentrated on interventions provided within days or a few weeks of diagnosis, a situation that does not usually occur in the UK. With long waiting lists, the benefits of revascularisation may be attenuated by the death of high-risk patients before intervention is carried out.

Despite modern advances in PCI, the best method of multivessel revascularisation remains conventional CABG, which enables a more thorough revascularisation with long-lasting symptom relief and need for re-intervention. CABG is particularly suited to those with left main stem coronary disease, those with three-vessel disease, and patients with diabetes. For many others, there is often little difference between CABG and PCI (Bourassa, 2000). However, complete relief from angina is initially only about 60% with angioplasty, but over 90% for bypass surgery. Furthermore, patients undergoing PCI do not get an arterial graft; arterial grafting of the left anterior descending coronary artery improves survival, with freedom from infarction and angina for over 10 years (Loop et al, 1986). The choice of treatment requires weighing the more invasive nature of surgery against the need for multiple further revascularisation attempts in those who initially undergo PTCA.

PERCUTANEOUS CORONARY INTERVENTION

Grüntzig first described a procedure for dilating coronary arteries in September 1977, and PTCA has since become an established and effective way of treating many serious arterial stenoses (Grüntzig, 1984; Landau et al, 1994). During the last decade, there has been a huge rise in the numbers of PCIs, challenging CABG as the preferred method for coronary revascularisation. In the period 1992–1996, the European Society of Cardiology reported an increase in revascularisation procedures of 148 000 to 327 000 PTCAs in European hospitals, compared with a smaller increase in CABG from 137 000 to 202 000. However, figures from the UK in 1998 still show an excess of bypass operations, with 28 000 CABG operations and 25 000 PTCA procedures carried out. This might suggest that waiting list delays in the UK are making many patients unsuitable for angioplasty.

PCI has obvious clinical and financial advantages over bypass surgery, since it is performed under local anaesthesia, and patients are usually fully mobile 24 h after the procedure, allowing early discharge from hospital.

Major limitations are lesions that occur in:

- Left main stem (unless protected by a graft or collaterals)
- Small and distal vessels
- Chronic occlusions
- Diffusely diseased vessels
- Old vein grafts.

INDICATIONS FOR PCI

The relative advantages and disadvantages of surgery and PCI will continue to change as improvements in both surgical and medical treatments evolve. Typical indications for PCI are shown in Box 16.1.

PERCUTANEOUS TRANSLUMINAL CORONARY ANGIOPLASTY

During PTCA, a thin double-lumen balloon is passed via a guiding catheter into the affected coronary artery. There are three types of balloon catheter – fixed-wire, over-wire and Monorail balloon catheters – the latter being the most popular in Europe. The balloon is advanced to lie within the coronary stenosis, and then inflated for about 60–120 s. This may be repeated several times, depending upon results. Improvement in patency is produced by a combination of plaque splitting, plaque compression, stretching of the arterial media and medial dissection. This is very prothrombotic, but use of glycoprotein IIb/IIIa antagonists, such as abciximab, during PCI reduces the

---

Box 16.1 Some clinical indications for percutaneous coronary intervention

- Stable angina with single- or two-vessel disease
- Primary angioplasty following acute myocardial infarction
- Rescue PCI for failed thrombolysis
- Cardiogenic shock
- Post-infarction angina
- Graft occlusion following bypass surgery
- Unstable coronary syndromes

incidence of thrombosis, myocardial infarction and death without causing excess bleeding. Heparin therapy is usual, and subacute thrombosis is now usually less than 2% under elective conditions. Long-term antiplatelet therapy substantially reduces the risk of re-occlusion.

The patency of coronary arteries continues to improve in the early weeks following PTCA due to healing and remodelling, but the main problem is restenosis that follows up to 50% of procedures, regardless of the procedure used (Epstein et al, 1994). Vessel wall recoil and thrombus formation each contribute towards early restenosis, mediated by platelet adhesion to the damaged vessel wall. Thereafter, there is an exaggerated response to the injury by vascular smooth muscle cells. These cells migrate into the intima, proliferate and secrete extracellular matrix, resulting in expansion and encroachment of the intima into the vascular lumen, producing late restenosis. Improvements in technique are reducing the need for re-intervention, and the widespread use of stents has reduced acute complications and the long-term risk of restenosis (Fischman et al, 1994; Serrays et al, 1994).

Stents

Coronary artery stents are small mesh cylinders placed in the arteries at the time of angioplasty. Other designs include coils, rings or slotted tubes. They help by increasing the vessel lumen, sealing dissections and tagging the intimal flap between the stent and the arterial wall. Recent advances in-stent technology include bifurcation and side-branch stents, and covered, coated and radioactive versions. Some are self-expanding, others require the PTCA balloon to expand them. According to design, they may offer flexibility, strength, trackability and reduced risks of in-stent stenosis.

Threatened or abrupt vessel closure following angioplasty is the best indication for stenting. Before stents were available, about 3–5% of patients sustained a myocardial infarction during PTCA, and a further 3–7% needed emergency CABG. Acute vessel closure is minimised by routine use of high inflation pressures (over 10–14 atmospheres), which allows full stent expansion and better apposition of the stent around the cir-

cumference of the vessel. This has reduced the need for emergency CABG to less than 1%.

In 1998, stents were used in approximately 70% of all PTCA procedures in the UK, and were successful in over 95% of patients undergoing elective PCI for native vessel disease and saphenous vein grafts. The National Institute for Clinical Excellence (NICE) guidelines currently advise routine stenting during PTCA of coronary arteries between 2.5 and 3.5 mm, which should increase usage to about 80–90% of all procedures.

Although stents have addressed the problem of arterial recoil, they have not prevented in-stent stenosis, which still affects 20–30% of cases. An angiographically perfectly deployed stent may be destroyed within months by this healing process, which often leads to recurrent myocardial ischaemia. The stimulus is not understood, but the most important predictors seem to be small post-procedural luminal diameters, lesion length, diabetes and use of multiple stents. Radiation emitters have been used to reduce in-stent stenosis (vascular brachytherapy), but the best hope probably lies with antiproliferative drug-eluting stents, delivering agents such as sirolimus (Rapamycin) or paclitaxel (Taxol). Drug-eluting stents will remain the focus of interest for the next few years (Gershlick, 2002).

Repeat PTCA is the most usual way of clearing in-stent stenosis, but laser angioplasty and atherectomy may also be used.

LASER-ASSISTED ANGIOPLASTY AND ATHERECTOMY

Coronary atherectomy can be used to debulk arteries with large atheromatous stenoses, and to modify plaques in preparation for PTCA and stenting. Atherectomy is particularly suited to hard, calcific lesions where the technique is used to ablate inelastic tissue.

Direction atherectomy removes atherosclerotic plaques with a cylindrical, rotating, cup-shaped blade. The catheter has a soft tapering nose cone that provides a collecting chamber for ablated tissue. The cutter is applied to different parts of the vessel wall in sequence, and is repeated several times to achieve circumferential tissue ablation. PTCA is then applied to achieve a satisfactory result. Complications include side-branch occlusion, perforation, abrupt vessel closure and distal embolisation.

Rotational atherectomy debulks plaques by drilling, using a diamond-tipped elliptical burr. Complications relate to perforation of the vessel wall, embolisation of plaque and dissections. So far, no major advantage has been shown over normal PTCA (Adelman et al, 1993; Topol et al, 1993).

Laser angioplasty uses ultraviolet, pulsed excimer light laser energy that ablates the plaque by vaporising the tissue, and providing thermo-mechanical shockwaves to disrupt the plaque. This has proved useful in completely occluded vessels that cannot be initially treated by traditional PTCA (Topaz et al, 2001). The laser is utilised to clear a path for passage of the balloon catheter. Unfortunately, vessel perforation and dissections may complicate this technique.

Atherectomy cannot be used if there is active thrombus, and Angiojet thrombectomy or transluminal thrombus extraction may be used here. The latter technique has been used to remove degenerated graft material and thrombus in saphenous vein grafts.

PRIMARY ANGIOPLASTY FOLLOWING ACUTE MYOCARDIAL INFARCTION

Acute myocardial infarction is usually caused by occlusive coronary thrombosis initiated by rupture of an atheromatous plaque. The subendocardium infarcts early after coronary occlusion, but outward extension to affect the full thickness of the ventricular wall may take several hours. Restoration of normal epicardial coronary flow to limit infarction size is the primary goal of reperfusional therapies. Pharmacological therapy with fibrinolytic agents is, for logistic reasons, the initial therapy in most patients presenting with acute myocardial infarction, but rapid transfer to an interventional centre for primary angioplasty with stent implantation may have many advantages over thrombolytic therapy.

Despite the introduction of more effective thrombolytic agents, only around 60% of patients treated with fibrinolytic therapy achieve normal TIMI grade III epicardial flow in the infarct-related artery (GUSTO Angiographic Investigators, 1993). Even if the coronary artery has been opened, there may be suboptimal tissue perfusion as a result of distal embolisation and microvascular spasm. Re-occlusion may also affect up to 30% of patients for whom fibrinolysis was initially successful.

Primary angioplasty uses balloon dilatation to disrupt the thrombus, as well as the underlying plaque, and restores normal antegrade flow in a higher proportion of patients. The procedure was first carried out in 1983 (Hartzler et al, 1983); its advantages and disadvantages are shown in Box 16.2. Primary angioplasty has been shown to be a

---

Box 16.2 Comparative advantages of primary angioplasty and thrombolysis

Primary angioplasty

Advantages

- Coronary anatomy defined; prognosis may be established
- Up to 98% of vessels recanalise immediately
- Residual stenosis cleared and stented
- Left ventricular function improves
- Intraplaque haemorrhage minimised
- Less post-infarction angina and re-infarction

Disadvantages

- Expensive
- Specialised (requires catheter laboratory and expertise 24 h/day)
- Slower to institute

Thrombolysis

Advantages

- Cheap
- Quick and simple to administer
- Avoids risks of invasive study
- Infarct-related artery opened in over half of cases

Disadvantages

- Systemic and plaque haemorrhage may occur
- Slow and unpredictable restoration of coronary blood flow
- Residual stenoses remain; post-infarction ischaemia is likely
- Coronary anatomy unknown; angiography may be required later

safe procedure, with initial patency rates in excess of 90% (Kahn et al, 1990). Patients are less likely to experience post-infarction angina, with lower rates of re-infarction, improved ventricular function, lower stroke rates, and lower mortality, compared to those treated with thrombolytic therapy (de Belder and Hall, 1999; Nunn et al, 1999). Since systemic fibrinolysis is avoided, the likelihood of bleeding complications as well as intraplaque haemorrhage is reduced. The relatively high rate of recurrent events and high rate of restenosis (Weaver et al, 1997) seem to have been helped by routine stenting that allows mechanical stabilisation of the unstable plaque (Grines et al, 1999). Primary PTCA is of particular value in patients who have had previous bypass surgery, in the elderly, and for those in cardiogenic shock, provided they are treated within the first 6 h.

Unfortunately, despite these advantages of primary PTCA, there are drawbacks. Morbidity and mortality vary with the skill of the operator, and an experienced primary angioplasty team is needed. The usual complications of elective PTCA are more frequent, and dysrhythmias are more common. Lesions in the right coronary artery are often more troublesome, the procedure often being accompanied by heart block and hypotension. The availability of an intra-aortic balloon pump and surgical back-up is desirable. The obvious drawback is that the procedure can only be performed where there are cardiac catheter facilities available, with adequate staffing to cover the 24-h period, all of which must be on-site so there are no delays. Expansion of facilities in the UK to permit primary stenting in acute myocardial infarction to deal with the 200 000 myocardial infarction admissions each year would require considerable capital investment. Even in the USA, less than 20% of hospitals are equipped with diagnostic catheter facilities. Without the infrastructure to support 24-h cover every day of the year, the provision of catheter laboratories alone may not affect either the number of cases we are able to tackle by primary angioplasty or the outcome (Rogers et al, 2000). So, although trial data support the use of primary angioplasty as the best method of revascu-

larisation in experienced and appropriately staffed interventional centres, thrombolysis will remain the initial method of restoring coronary flow in most cases. What is important is that, where fibrinolysis is contraindicated (or where thrombolysis fails), there are strategies in place for rapid transfer to an intervention centre for mechanical reperfusion by primary or rescue angioplasty (Ross et al, 1998).

CORONARY ARTERY BYPASS AND OTHER SURGICAL PROCEDURES

The main application of surgery for coronary heart disease is to improve the blood supply to the ischaemic myocardium. However, operations may also be required to repair mechanical defects that have arisen as a consequence of a myocardial infarction (e.g. mitral incompetence or ruptured interventricular septum). Surgery is most often and most safely performed electively, but is sometimes required urgently when these complications occur suddenly (Box 16.3).

Box 16.3 Some indications for surgery in coronary heart disease

Elective surgery
- Poorly controlled stable angina
- Significant left main stem coronary artery stenosis
- Three-vessel coronary artery disease
- Left main equivalent disease
- Left ventricular aneurysm producing symptoms
- Malignant dysrhythmias uncontrolled by medical therapy

Emergency surgery
- Crescendo angina uncontrolled by medical therapy
- Repair of mechanical defects
  - Mitral incompetence
  - Ventriculoseptal defect
  - Cardiac rupture
- Cardiogenic shock
- Following unsuccessful coronary angioplasty (ongoing ischaemia or threatened occlusion)

CORONARY ARTERY BYPASS GRAFTING

Sabiston first performed CABG in 1962, although the patient died in the post-operative period. The technique was quickly adopted by other cardiac surgeons with successful results (Garrett et al, 1973) and the number of operations performed has grown exponentially. As experience of this operation has improved, there has been a major fall in operative mortality and morbidity, which is attributed to better patient selection, pre-operative assessment and surgical technique.

In the early 1980s, cardiac surgeons attempted to attain a greater degree of revascularisation by bypassing most of the diseased vessels. The original 'triple bypass' then became a much longer affair, often involving five or six separate bypass vein grafts. However, results did not improve, and the typical bypass operation these days involves between two and four grafts.

The usual conduits are autogenous saphenous veins that have early patency rates of over 90%, provided aspirin is started as early as possible. Without antithrombotic therapy, 25% of grafts will be occluded at 1 year, and mortality is closely related to graft patency. Progressive intimal hyperplasia and accelerated atherosclerosis cause progressive venous graft failure, which is particularly evident beyond the fifth year. About 90% of vein grafts are occluded after 10 years (Chen et al, 1996). As a result, arterial grafts are now employed routinely to promote long-term patency.

Usual multivessel bypass surgery now uses the left internal mammary artery (LIMA) to graft the left anterior descending coronary artery (LAD), with supplemental saphenous vein grafts to other coronary lesions. At 10 years, when most saphenous vein grafts will have stenosed, over 90% of LIMA grafts are still functioning. Improved patient survival has also been confirmed with LIMA grafts, either alone, or in association with saphenous vein grafts. Use of bilateral internal mammary artery grafts (LIMA and RIMA) appears to be safe, with less post-operative angina, fewer re-operations and better long-term results (Patil et al, 2001). The right gas-troepiploic and inferior epigastric arteries may also be used in association with double internal mammary grafts, so it is possible completely to revascularise the heart arterially (Suma, 1999). The radial artery has also been used as a free graft, with 5-year patency rates of about 85% (Buxton et al, 1997).

Although arterial grafts to the LAD are associated with increased survival and long angina-free intervals, there is less convincing evidence of improved results with arterial grafts to other vessels, or for those treated with multiple arterial grafts.

Indications for CABG

The main indication for CABG is relief of symptoms, but revascularisation may be used to improve prognosis, even in asymptomatic patients (ACC/AHA, 1999). Most comparisons of the outcome of surgery and medical therapy rely on data acquired before many advances in medical, surgical and catheter-based treatments. However, a meta-analysis of seven randomised trials comparing bypass surgery with medical therapy supports the concept that the greater the amount of at-risk myocardium from extensive or proximal coronary disease, the greater the improvements in prognosis following CABG (Yusuf et al, 1994). For example, disease of the left main stem artery is associated with serious coronary events, including myocardial infarction and sudden death (Mock et al, 1982). Although disease of this artery is usually symptomatic, it may only be revealed at coronary angiography, and some centres consider that 50% occlusion of the left main stem is sufficient for urgent surgery, regardless of symptoms. Patients with mild angina or no symptoms are usually offered bypass surgery if there is significant stenosis of the left main stem, three-vessel disease or 'left main equivalent' disease (i.e. over 70% stenoses in the proximal LAD and proximal left circumflex arteries), where the European Coronary Surgery Study Group (1980) has shown that the 5-year survival rate is better for those treated surgically than for those treated medically (Table 16.1). Patients with severe

Table 16.1   5-year survival in the European Coronary Surgery Study (1980)

Group	Medical treatment	Surgical treatment
Left main stem disease	62%	93%
Three-vessel disease	85%	95%
Two-vessel disease	88%	92%

symptoms or strongly positive stress tests should undergo CABG, especially if there is impaired left ventricular function. Both symptoms and prognosis will be improved. Those with moderate angina and single- or double-artery disease (excluding left main stem or equivalent disease) are better managed by PCI in the first instance.

Patient selection

Patients vary in their reaction to anginal symptoms, and the decision to proceed to CABG needs careful consideration. Surgery for degenerative disease never cures, and bypass surgery should be postponed in those with mild to moderate coronary heart disease and good left ventricular function. Young men are often referred urgently for bypass surgery, but buying time with angioplasty is preferable, since most will develop clinically important graft atheroma within 5 years of coronary bypass. Operative risk is also greater in the elderly and for female patients, presumably because the smaller vessels and compact anatomy compromise surgical techniques and graft patency. Diabetes and hypertension also increase peri-operative risk.

Many surgeons will not consider operating on patients who have not stopped smoking because of the associated higher peri-operative risk and outcome. Ten-year survival in patients following CABG was 84% in those who stopped smoking and 68% in those who continued to smoke (Cavender et al, 1992). Post-operatively, chronic smokers are more likely to develop angina, are more often unable to return to work, and usually have more hospital admissions.

Poor operative risk factors need to be balanced against poor prognostic features of the disease itself, including low exercise tolerance and

stenoses at dangerous sites. Poor left ventricular function is an important pre-operative risk, but survival of such patients following surgery is superior to treatment with medical therapy, and it may be justified to take the risk. Occasionally, a severely reduced ejection fraction is related to myocardial ischaemia, rather than myocardial scarring, and improves with surgery.

Operative procedure

The heart is exposed through a median sternotomy. Limited grafting procedures may be carried out on the beating heart (see below), but most cases require cardioplegia with extracorporeal cardiopulmonary bypass. This is established via cannulae in the right atrium and ascending aorta, blood passing outside the body for oxygenation. The body temperature is reduced to about 26°C and cardiac arrest induced with a cardioplegic solution. The heart can be stopped for up to 2 h to allow anastomoses. The left internal mammary artery is mobilised from the chest wall and directly grafted onto the left anterior descending coronary artery. While this is going on, the long saphenous vein is stripped from the leg, flushed with heparinised blood and checked for leaks. Endarterectomy of the major coronary arteries may be needed if there is diffuse coronary disease or a complete stenosis. The distal ends of the bypass vein grafts are sutured to as many vessels as require it. The aorta is then unclamped, the patient rewarmed and normal cardiac rhythm established by defibrillation. Using special side-biting clamps, the proximal ends of the grafts are sutured to the ascending aorta, cardiopulmonary bypass is stopped, the cannulae removed and the chest closed.

Post-operative management

Patients are normally ventilated until haemodynamically stable. Arterial lines and Swan–Ganz catheters are used to monitor intracardiac pressures for the first 24 h, after which time the majority of patients can leave the intensive care unit. Patients are mobilised quickly and are often fit for discharge from hospital within 7 days. The majority of patients are able to return to work between 2 and 6 months after the operation. Aspirin must be started within 24 h of surgery (preferably within 6 h), because benefits of graft patency are lost when begun later. Aspirin should be continued for at least 12 months, and probably indefinitely to reduce the risk of graft occlusion and help prevent other major clinical vascular events, such as myocardial infarction or stroke (Antiplatelet Trialists' Collaboration, 1994). Graft patency is not prolonged by the addition of dipyridamole, or by using warfarin instead.

Problems following surgery

Early effects

Morbidity and mortality following coronary artery surgery has fallen as surgical expertise has improved. In most centres, the overall mortality is less than 3%, but much depends upon the patient group and the number of emergency operations that are undertaken. Certain variables, such as age, diabetes, left ventricular function and other co-morbidities, can be used to predict the risk of death, stroke or mediastinitis in individual cases (ACC/AHA, 1999).

The most important complications are neurological caused by hypoxia, hypoperfusion, haemorrhage or metabolic problems. Cerebral dysfunction is attributable to small atheromatous emboli being ejected from the aorta at the time of the operation (Smith et al, 1986), although other factors (e.g. inflammation and oedema) may contribute. Minimal clamping of the aorta may prevent plaque disruption, and the use of membrane as opposed to bubble oxygenators helps reduce the risk of micro-emboli. Peri-operative stroke is a sufficiently common complication that it should be discussed pre-operatively. Temporary impairment of concentration or memory is common, affecting up to half of patients in the first 6 weeks, but it may persist for many months following surgery (Newman et al, 2001; Pandit and Pigott, 2001).

The most common problem following bypass surgery is disturbance of heart rhythm, affecting up to one-third of all patients in the first 5 days. Most are benign supraventricular dysrhythmias. New-onset atrial fibrillation occurs in 30% of patients, and increases the risk of stroke. Temporary heart block occurs in 5–10% of patients.

Peri-operative myocardial infarction is a risk factor for premature death, but frequency is down to under 2.5%. Careful attention to peri-operative ischaemia is important, particularly during induction of anaesthesia and extracorporeal bypass. Global left ventricular damage is more difficult to diagnose, but is probably common. A low-output period may follow, particularly if the left ventricular function was poor to start with. Some patients need to be supported by extracorporeal bypass while the ventricular myocardium recovers.

Renal dysfunction may occur in about 8% of patients, and a fifth of these may require dialysis. This is more common in the elderly, those with heart failure, diabetes or prior renal disease. If the creatinine is over 130 mmol/l pre-operatively, the risk of acute renal failure is doubled. There may also be temporary haematological dysfunction, pulmonary disease and immunological suppression.

Pain from the sternotomy and cracked ribs can cause discomfort for a few weeks, as can pain around the long incision made for removing the saphenous vein. Mediastinitis from deep wound infections is more frequent where arterial grafts are used, and occurs in 1–4%. It carries a high mortality (25%).

Immediate and complete relief from angina is reported in about 80% of patients, and most of the remainder have marked improvement in their symptoms. Between 60% and 80% of patients are free from angina at 1 year. Left ventricular function may improve post-operatively if poor function has been due to myocardial ischaemia rather than infarction. These areas of reversibly impaired contractility are termed 'stunned' or 'hibernating' myocardium. Pre-operative scanning may be of benefit in identifying areas that may be salvageable and may be used to predict an improved operative success.

Long-term effects

The long-term benefits of CABG are determined by changes in left ventricular function, patency of the grafts and progression of generalised atherosclerosis. The 1-year survival is 95%, and the 5-year survival is 88%. An early return of angina is either due to incomplete revascularisation or premature graft occlusion. As many as 18% of vein grafts become occluded in the first month, and a quarter within 12 months. Operative technique, including the meticulous preparation of the saphenous vein graft before anastomosis, is important to minimise the risk of thrombosis. After the first year, grafts occlusion rates fall, but affect 53% within 5 years, 76% at 5–10 years, and 92% over 10 years (Chen et al, 1996).

The pathology underlying graft occlusion varies. Immediately following anastomosis, endothelial cells become oedematous and damaged, and early occlusion is usually due to platelet aggregation and thrombosis. Fibro-intimal hyperplasia of grafts first appears at 2 weeks, and is characterised by proliferation of vascular smooth muscle cells and synthesis of matrix. It is usually self-limiting, but underlies most cases of occlusion within the first year. Grafts over 3 years old show lipid-laden foam cells in the intima; beyond 5 years, rupture of atheromatous plaques is the most common initiator of graft stenosis. Preventing, retarding or reversing graft atheroma requires attention to classical risk factors, including hypertension, smoking and hypercholesterolaemia. Failure to control lipid levels results in an increased rate of graft occlusion, as well as progress of atheroma in native vessels. The Post CABG Trial suggested that the serum LDL-cholesterol should be reduced to less than 100 mg/dl, especially in those with other cardiovascular risk factors (Campeau et al, 1999).

In about a fifth of patients, angina returns acutely as an unstable coronary syndrome, about 7 years after the operation. One-third of patients experience recurrent stable angina after 10 years, although it will not necessarily be so severe. For stable patients, exercise stress testing, stress echocardiography, or myocardial perfusion scanning may confirm the diagnosis. The latter tests are more useful as more than a third will have an abnormal resting ECG. PCI with stenting is the favoured method of revascularisation if possible, because, although re-operation will produce nearly as good results (60% angina-free at 1 year), operative mortality is higher. About 4–7% of patients require a second bypass procedure in the first 10 years; most of these are young patients.

OFF-PUMP CORONARY ARTERY BYPASS

Recent surgical innovations have included greater use of arterial conduits, better methods of cardioprotection and improvements in oxygenator technology. The cardiopulmonary bypass circuit has become safer, but the risk of related stroke is still significant, rising from a rate of 0.7% for a 50-year-old man to 8% in an 80-year-old. As the average age of patients referred for CABG is increasing, the number of patients at risk is increasing. Off-pump coronary artery bypass may be a better approach to reduce morbidity, given that many peri-operative complications are actually due to extracorporeal bypass, rather than the CABG itself (Allen, 1986).

Minimally invasive direct coronary artery bypass surgery (MIDCAB) can be used for bypassing one or two coronary arteries, with anastomoses being carried out on the beating heart using stabilisers that sit astride the artery being operated on, holding the heart relatively stable. The heart rate is slowed with beta-blockers or diltiazem, to help steadiness. Suturing is done under direct vision, so the coronary artery to be bypassed must lie directly beneath the incision. Usually, the LIMA is dissected from the chest wall, using either direct vision or video guidance, and sutured directly to the LAD. Occasionally, the RIMA is used to bypass the right coronary artery. Patients with disease confined to the LAD and right coronary artery might be well served by MIDCAB using the two internal mammary arteries (Hartz, 1996).

Since there is no extracorporeal bypass, MIDCAB reduces the incidence of stroke, atrial fibrillation and requirements for post-operative transfusion and ventilation (Zenati et al, 1997), but the operation takes longer. It is not really practicable for three-vessel disease, because of lack of access to the back of the heart. The technique can equally be applied via sternotomy, still avoiding cardiopulmonary bypass.

MIDCAB is easier on the patient, and is probably less expensive than traditional CABG, but urgent conversion to conventional open-chest methods has occasionally been necessary. The hybrid procedure of MIDCAB to the LAD with angioplasty to the other vessels in those with multivessel disease may be safer and more effective than either modality alone, particularly in those with multiple co-morbidities.

Port-access coronary artery bypass surgery (PACAB) uses femoral-to-femoral cardiopulmonary bypass, with cardioplegic arrest and limited incisions. The heart is stopped and the bypasses are performed using instruments passed through the ports, rather like abdominal laparoscopic surgery. The cardiac surgeon views these operations on video monitors rather than directly. PACAB allows safe and effective surgery without sternotomy (Galloway et al, 1999), and is currently used for single-vessel bypass that is not amenable to angioplasty (about 5% of CABG cases). Single-vessel bypass is normally carried out to the LAD via a small lateral thoracotomy between the ribs. The technique can be extended to patients with three-vessel disease, but requires a larger incision, and greater surgical skill.

Percutaneous transmyocardial revascularisation applies laser energy via a cardiac catheter to create channels in the ischaemic myocardium from the endocardial side of the left ventricular wall. This is carried out to reduce anginal symptoms in patients with poorly controlled or refractory angina not amenable to CABG or PCI. It probably works by myocardial inflammation, secondary stimulation of growth factors and denervation of the myocardium (Patil et al, 2001). The intervention carries a significant morbidity, and currently is best utilised in combination with bypass surgery when laser is applied directly to the heart to improve revascularisation that cannot be achieved by CABG alone. In the future, it may be

possible to use this technique to deliver angiogenic peptides to induce further new blood vessel formation (Clarke and Schofield, 2000).

BYPASS SURGERY FOLLOWING ACUTE MYOCARDIAL INFARCTION

Although the results of CABG have improved markedly over the last 20 years, emergency surgery for acute coronary syndromes is still associated with an approximate five-fold mortality and morbidity rate. Traditionally, coronary artery surgery is delayed for several weeks following myocardial infarction as the recently infarcted heart is more susceptible to global ischaemia induced by CABG. However, it is becoming clear that it is not the time interval that is critical but the clinical state of the patient. In patients under the age of 70 years, with an ejection fraction greater than 30%, the risks do not appear to be excessive (Applebaum et al, 1991).

OPERATIONS FOR THE COMPLICATIONS OF MYOCARDIAL INFARCTION

There are three commonly performed operations for patients who have developed mechanical post-infarction complications. These are resection of left ventricular aneurysms, repair or replacement of the mitral valve and repair of the interventricular septum.

Resection of left ventricular aneurysms

After myocardial infarction, parts of the damaged left ventricle may be akinetic (i.e. do not move) or dyskinetic (i.e. move paradoxically). The latter areas, if sufficiently large, will act as a chamber that fills during diastole but does not contribute to ejection of blood during systole, since the area bulges outwards. This situation will usually improve as the infarct heals. Left ventricular aneurysms usually produce problems several weeks or even months after acute myocardial infarction and present with angina, heart failure, dysrhythmias or thromboembolic events. Surgery will usually help overall left ventricular function, but the prognosis is dependent upon how well the left ventricle performs postoperatively, as well as on the overall perfusion of the remaining myocardium. Hence, CABG is often performed at the same time as resection of the aneurysm. Surgical techniques designed to retain ventricular geometry using endoventricular patches may maintain physiological function with lower mortality than simple linear repair.

Mitral valve surgery

Left ventricular dilatation following acute myocardial infarction often associates with mitral incompetence that resolves with medical therapy. Surgery may be required if there has been acquired mitral regurgitation due to partial or complete papillary muscle rupture or major ischaemic dysfunction. The degree of valvular incompetence can vary from slight to massive. Total rupture of a papillary muscle complicates about 1% of myocardial infarctions, usually in the first week. Medical treatment of this condition is associated with 50% mortality within the first 24 h, and 94% within 8 weeks, and urgent operative intervention is required. Delay in operation appears to increase the risk of further myocardial injury, other organ injury due to hypoperfusion and death. Although operation carries a high mortality (around 30%), normal valve function may be restored by replacement with a prosthetic valve. While emergency surgery is being arranged, a sodium nitroprusside infusion can be used to help lower pulmonary capillary pressures and improve peripheral perfusion.

Repair of the mitral valve has also been reported in selected circumstances of both acute and chronic mitral regurgitation with good results. When technically possible, the supporting structure of the mitral valve is retained and helps preserve long-term cardiac function.

Repair of a ruptured interventricular septum

Rupture of the interventricular septum occurs in about 1–2% of all transmural myocardial infarcts,

usually within the first week. Rupture usually associates with anterior infarction and, untreated, will be lethal in nearly all patients within a few days. An increased frequency of acute rupture of the interventricular septum with earlier presentation has been noted since the advent of thrombolytic therapy. The clinical picture varies considerably, but patients usually present within the first 4 days following myocardial infarction with severe heart failure, and the presence of a loud pansystolic murmur at the left sternal edge. The diagnosis is confirmed by echocardiography and right heart catheterisation. Patients usually have associated multivessel disease, and will need concomitant bypass surgery (Pellerin and Bourassa, 1996). Although emergency surgical repair was formerly thought to be necessary only in patients with pulmonary oedema or cardiogenic shock, it is now recognised as equally important in haemodynamically stable patients. This is because the rupture site can expand abruptly, resulting in sudden haemodynamic collapse, even in patients who appear to be clinically stable. Immediate surgical repair is indicated when pulmonary oedema or cardiogenic shock is present, although mortality in this group is high. Initial therapy is with diuretics and vasodilators, such as sodium nitroprusside, with insertion of an intra-aortic balloon pump to augment coronary, cerebral and renal blood flow. Mortality is greatest in older patients. If the patient is stable, repair may be delayed for a short while. Mortality is about 34% in the first week after infarction compared with 11% after the first week.

Left ventricular free wall rupture

The incidence of cardiac rupture has increased since the introduction of routine thrombolysis, and usually occurs suddenly in the first week. Routine treatment with beta-blockade may help reduce this complication. Most cases present with cardiac arrest, with pulseless electrical activity seen on the ECG monitor. About 25% of cases have a subacute course because pericardial adhesions limit the speed of leakage. The presentation is then of cardiac tamponade, and can be diagnosed by echocardiography. Pericardial aspiration may be required, followed by emergency cardiac surgery, irrespective of the clinical status, as complete rupture may occur at any time. Repair of the ventricle is by direct suture or using cyanoacrylate glue to hold a patch over necrotic myocardium (Bates et al, 1997).

SURGERY FOR HEART FAILURE

Despite the fall in mortality from cardiovascular disease, the incidence and prevalence of heart failure is increasing, and now affects 2% of the population and 10% of those aged over 65 years. Although modern treatment with ACE inhibitors and beta-blockers has improved the outlook, the natural course of the disorder is progressive, and the annual mortality is 25–50%. A number of severely symptomatic patient may benefit from revascularisation or valve repair, but, for the majority, the only surgical option has been heart transplantation (see below). However, newer surgical treatments are being developed, including mechanical support, left ventricular volume reduction and cardiomyoplasty.

Partial left ventriculectomy (Batista operation) aims to reduce the left ventricular volume in dilated cardiomyopathy by removing approximately 6 cm from the circumference of the left ventricular free wall, so the heart will generate higher pressures with lower wall tensions. Batista has reported excellent results in 300 Brazilian patients to date, but published outcome data for this operation are scant.

Cardiomyoplasty involves the transposition of skeletal muscle to provide assisted contraction to the heart. Most commonly, the latissimus dorsi is elevated and transposed through the chest wall to be wrapped around the heart and is electrically stimulated to assist contractile function. The mortality at 1 year is in excess of 30% despite reported improvement in quality of life.

Left ventricular assist devices (LVADs) are implantable mechanical support devices that were developed to bridge the gap to transplantation, although, in Britain, use is currently restricted to patients denied transplantation. Evidence is accumulating that resting the heart for 3–6 months may allow recovery of the heart, allowing explantation of the devices. This raises the possibility of earlier mechanical intervention in certain forms of cardiomyopathy (e.g. viral, alcoholic), which might allow a bridge to recovery or transplantation (Tayama and Nose, 1996).

The Novacor and HeartMate are large, noisy, electrically driven LVADs available for long-term implantation. A transcutaneous driveline connects to an external power source to charge the batteries 2–3 times per day. These devices have not been submitted to randomised controlled trials. A newer concept has been adopted in the Jarvik 2000 device. A tiny axial pump sits in the apex of the left ventricle, and silently augments cardiac output with non-pulsatile flow of up to 10 litres/min. The first fully implantable artificial heart (AbioCor) was inserted in a man with end-stage heart failure in July 2001, but cardiac transplantation currently offers the best surgical treatment for end-stage heart failure.

HEART TRANSPLANTATION SURGERY

The first human heart transplant was carried out in December 1967, and cardiac transplantation is now sufficiently commonplace as not to attract public attention. More than 55 000 heart transplants have now been performed worldwide (www.ishlt.org), and there are currently nine centres in the UK performing the operation. Heart transplantation is usually carried out in patients with end-stage heart failure caused by coronary artery disease, and in the last 20 years has become the gold-standard treatment in selected cases (Dreng, 2002). Despite emerging medical and surgical treatments in advanced heart failure, transplantation offers the best survival for those at highest risk of dying. Less commonly, transplantation has been performed for non-ischaemic cardiomyopathies caused by alcohol, chemotherapy or other drugs. Transplantation may also be performed following failed valvular surgery, for intractable angina or for certain forms of congenital heart disease.

One of the greatest advances in transplant surgery has been the development of drugs that suppress rejection. The introduction of cyclosporin A (Sandimmune) in 1982 led to improved results by permitting a reduction in the high-dose steroid therapy that compromised surgical healing. Immunosuppression is now based on a triple-drug regimen of cyclosporin A, azathioprine and prednisolone. For routine first transplants, the 1-year survival is 83% and 5-year survival is 66% (NHS UK Transplant, 2001). Early morbidity is due to graft failure, acute rejection and infection. After 1 year, the most common cause of death is accelerated coronary occlusive disease, particularly in those with hypertension and who smoke. Mortality is higher in females, patients over the age of 40 years, where transplantation has been carried out for valvular disease, or where the donor heart is older than 30 years.

There seems to be little doubt of the value of cardiac transplantation in prolonging the quantity and quality of patients' lives. Cost–benefit studies show significant improvement in key aspects of life-style, and 91% of patients are able to resume normal lives (Buxton et al, 1985). The cost of a heart transplant and of the first 5 years of follow-up is approximately half the cost of 5 years of renal dialysis.

The main constraint on cardiac transplantation is the lack of donors. In the year 2000, there were only 218 heart transplants performed in the UK, and 33 heart/lung transplants. Less than half the potential recipients receive a transplant, and, of the 494 patients on the waiting list, 8% had died by the end of the year. The annual transplantation rate is likely to remain under 4500 worldwide, so the impact on treatment of advanced heart failure will remain limited. Nevertheless, it is important that transplantation programmes survive to provide a last resort for patients with end-stage heart disease while new therapies evolve, such as xenotransplantation and cell transplantation and regrowth of heart muscle.

REFERENCES

ACC/AHA (1999) Guidelines for coronary artery bypass graft surgery: executive summary and recommendations. *Circulation*, **100**: 1464–1480.

Adelman AG, Cohen EA, Kimball BP (1993) A comparison of directional atherectomy with balloon angioplasty for lesions of the left anterior descending coronary artery. *New England Journal of Medicine*, **329**: 228–233.

Allen CMC (1986) Cabbages and CABG. *BMJ*, **297**: 1485–1486.

Antiplatelet Trialists' Collaboration (1994) Overview II. Maintenance of vascular graft or arterial patency by anti-platelet therapy. *BMJ*, **308**: 159–168.

Applebaum R, House R, Rademaker A (1991) Coronary artery bypass grafting within 30 days of acute myocardial infarction. Early and late results in 406 patients. *Journal of Thoracic and Cardiovascular Surgery*, **102**: 745–752.

Bates RJ, Beutler S, Resnekov L et al (1997) Cardiac rupture: challenge in diagnosis and management. *American Journal of Cardiology*, **42**: 429–441.

Bourassa MG (2000) Clinical trials of coronary revascularisation: coronary angioplasty vs. coronary bypass grafting. *Current Opinion in Cardiology*, **15**: 281–286.

Buxton M, Acheson R, Caine N et al (1985) *Costs and Benefits of the Heart Transplantation Programmes at Harefield and Papworth Hospitals: Final Report*. London: HMSO.

Buxton B, Windsor M, Komeda M et al (1997) How good is the radial artery as a bypass graft? *Coronary Artery Disease*, **8**: 225–233.

Campeau L, Humminghake DB, Knatterud GL for the Post CABG Trial Investigators (1999) Aggressive cholesterol lowering delays saphenous vein graft atherosclerosis in women, the elderly and patients with associated risk factors. *Circulation*, **99**: 3241–3247.

Cavender JB, Rodgers WJ, Fisher LD (1992) Effects of smoking on survival and morbidity in patients randomised to medical or surgical therapy in the Coronary Artery Surgery Study (CASS). *Journal of the American College of Cardiology*, **20**: 287–294.

Chen L, Theroux P, Lesperance J et al (1996) Angiographic features of vein grafts versus ungrafted coronary arteries in patients with unstable angina and previous coronary artery bypass surgery. *Journal of the American College of Cardiology*, **28**: 1493–1499.

Clarke SC, Schofield PM (2000) Percutaneous myocardial laser revascularisation. *Heart*, **83**: 253–254.

de Belder MA, Hall JA (1999) Infarct angioplasty. *Heart*, **82**: 399–401.

Dreng MC (2002) Cardiac transplantation. *Heart*, **87**: 177–184.

Epstein SE, Speir E, Unger EF et al (1994) The basis of molecular strategies for treating coronary restenosis after angioplasty. *Journal of the American College of Cardiology* **23**: 1278–1288.

European Coronary Surgery Study Group (1980) Second interim report. *Lancet*, **ii**: 491–495.

Fischman DL, Leon MB, Baim DS et al (1994) A randomised comparison of coronary-stent placement and balloon angioplasty in the treatment of coronary artery disease. *New England Journal of Medicine,* **331:** 496–501.

Galloway AC, Shemin RJ, Glower DD et al (1999) First report of the Port Access International Registry. *Annals of Thoracic Surgery,* **67:** 51–58.

Garrett HE, Dennis EW, DeBakey ME (1973) Aortocoronary bypass with saphenous vein graft. Seven-year follow up. *JAMA,* **223:** 792–794.

Gershlick AH (2002) Intracoronary stenting: developments since the NICE report. *Heart,* **87:** 187–190.

Grines CL, Cox DA, Stone GW et al (1999) Coronary angioplasty with or without stent implantation for acute myocardial infarction. Stent-PAMI Group. *New England Journal of Medicine,* **341:** 1949–1956.

Grüntzig AR (1984) Percutaneous transluminal angioplasty: six years' experience. *American Heart Journal,* **107:** 818–819.

GUSTO Angiographic Investigators (1993) The effect of tissue plasminogen activator, streptokinase, or both on coronary artery patency, ventricular function and survival after acute myocardial infarction. *New England Journal of Medicine,* **329:** 1615–1622.

Hartz RS (1996) Minimally invasive heart surgery. Executive Committee of the Council on Cardiothoracic and Vascular Surgery. *Circulation,* **94:** 2669–2670.

Hartzler GO, Rutherford BD, McConahay DR (1983) PTCA with and without thrombolytic therapy for treatment of acute myocardial infarction. *American Heart Journal,* **106:** 965–973.

Kahn JK, Rutherford BD, McConahay DR (1990) Results of primary angioplasty for acute myocardial infarction with multi-vessel disease. *Journal of the American College of Cardiology,* **16:** 1089–1096.

Kornowski R, Fuchs S, Lean MB et al (2000) Delivery strategies to achieve therapeutic myocardial angiogenesis. *Circulation,* **101:** 454–458.

Landau C, Lange RA, Hillis LD (1994) Percutaneous transluminal coronary angioplasty. *New England Journal of Medicine,* **330:** 981–993.

Loop FD, Lyle BW, Cosgrove DM et al (1986) Influence of the internal mammary artery graft on the 10-year survival and other cardiac events. *New England Journal of Medicine,* **314:** 1–6.

Mock M, Ringqvist I, Fisher L et al (1982) The survival of medically treated patients in the Coronary Artery Surgery Study (CASS) Registry. *Circulation,* **66:** 562–568.

Newman MF, Kirchner JL, Phillips-Bute B et al (2001) Longitudinal assessment of neurocognitive function after coronary artery bypass. *New England Journal of Medicine,* **334:** 395–402.

NHS UK Transplant (2001) *Transplant Activity Report 2000* Bristol: NHS UK Transplant (www.uktransplant.org.uk)

Nunn CM, O'Neil WW, Rothbaum D et al (1999) Long-term outcome after primary angioplasty: report from the primary angioplasty in myocardial infarction (PAMI–1) trial. *Journal of the American College of Cardiology,* **33:** 1729–1736.

Pandit JJ, Pigott D (2001) Cognitive dysfunction after cardiac surgery: strategies for prevention. *British Journal of Cardiology,* **8:** 613–616.

Patil CV, Nikolsky E, Boulos M et al (2001) Multivessel coronary artery disease: current revascularisation strategies. *European Heart Journal,* **22:** 1183–1197.

Pellerin M, Bourassa MG (1996) Post-infarction ventriculo-septal rupture. *European Heart Journal,* **17:** 1778–1779.

Rogers WJ, Canto JG, Barron HV et al (2000) Treatment and outcome of myocardial infarction in hospitals with and without invasive capabilities. *Journal of the American College of Cardiology,* **35:** 371–379.

Ross AM, Lundergan CF, Rohrbeck SC et al (1998) Rescue angioplasty after failed thrombolysis: technical and clinical outcomes in a large thrombolysis trial (GUSTO–1). *Journal of the American College of Cardiology,* **31:** 1511–1517.

Serrays PW, de Jaegere P, Kiemeneji F for the BENESTENT Study Group (1994) A comparison of balloon expandable-stent implantation with balloon angioplasty in patients with coronary artery disease. *New England Journal of Medicine,* **331:** 489–495.

Smith PL, Treasure T, Newman SP et al (1986) Cerebral consequences of cardiopulmonary bypass. *Lancet,* **i:** 823–825.

Suma H (1999) Arterial grafts in coronary bypass surgery. *Annals of Thoracic and Cardiovascular Surgery,* **5:** 141–145.

Tayama E, Nose Y (1996) Can we treat dilated cardiomyopathy using a left ventricular assist device? *Artificial Organs,* **20:** 197–201.

Topaz O, Das T, Dahm J et al (2001) Excimer laser revascularisation: current indications, applications and techniques. *Lasers in Medical Science,* **16:** 72–77.

Topol EJ, Leya F, Pinkerton CA (1993) A comparison of directional atherectomy with coronary angioplasty in patients with coronary artery disease. *New England Journal of Medicine,* **329:** 221–227.

Weaver WD, Simes J, Betriu A et al (1997) Comparison of primary coronary angioplasty and intravenous thrombolytic therapy for acute myocardial infarction. A quantitative review. *JAMA,* **278:** 2093–2098.

Yusuf S, Zucker D, Peduzzi P et al (1994) Effect of coronary artery bypass graft surgery on survival: overview of 10-year results from randomised trials by the Coronary Artery Bypass Graft Surgery Trialists' Collaboration. *Lancet,* **344:** 563–570.

Zenati M, Domit TM, Saul M et al (1997) Resource utilisation for minimally invasive direct and standard coronary artery bypass grafting. *Annals of Thoracic Surgery,* **63:** 84–87.

17

Therapeutics

The following is a summary of the drugs and classes of drugs that are commonly used on the coronary care unit, together with their doses and frequent side-effects. Trade (proprietary) names are shown in parentheses. The list is not fully comprehensive or complete, and serves only as a guide. Further information should always be sought from the hospital pharmacy department, manufacturers' data sheets, the *Monthly Index of Medical Specialities* (MIMS) or the *British National Formulary* (BNF), particularly if the drug is unfamiliar. The BNF is a joint publication from the British Medical Association and the Pharmaceutical Society of Great Britain. There are useful sections on drug interactions, intravenous additives, prescribing for the elderly, cardiovascular risk factor calculation and resuscitation guidelines.

ADENOSINE (Adenocor)

Adenosine is an endogenous nucleoside that produces transient atrioventricular (AV) node block when injected intravenously. Because it has a brief half-life (1–6 s), it is very safe, but needs bolus injection for effect. It has become the treatment of choice to terminate re-entry tachycardias; additionally, it may have a diagnostic role in regular broad-complex tachycardias.

Dose   6 mg by rapid intravenous injection. If ineffective, a second bolus of 12 mg should be given, followed by a third bolus of 18 mg.

Side-effects   Transient chest pain, dyspnoea and flushing. It may cause bronchospasm, and

337

should not be used in patients with asthma. Adenosine should also not be given to patients taking dipyridamole (Persantin), as significant hypotension may result. Heart transplant patients are very sensitive to adenosine.

ADRENALINE (EPINEPHRINE)

Adrenaline (epinephrine) is the first drug recommended for all types of cardiac arrest. It has strong alpha- and beta-adrenergic agonist activity, which increases heart rate and contractility, as well as having a powerful vasoconstrictor action. Administration during cardiac arrest will result in peripheral vasoconstriction, which augments the effect of chest compression, leading to increased cerebral and coronary perfusion. The beta-agonist properties (positive chronotropic and inotropic effects) help myocardial function following attainment of sinus rhythm.

Dose   1 mg intravenously (10 ml of a 1:10 000 solution), which may be repeated every 3 min.

AMILORIDE (Amilamont)

Amiloride is a potassium-conserving diuretic that acts directly on the distal renal tubules, causing salt and water excretion. Diuresis occurs over 24 h, but full activity may be delayed for 2–3 days. It should not be used in renal failure, with potassium supplements or ACE inhibitors, unless serum potassium is closely monitored.

Dose   5–20 mg orally.

AMINOPHYLLINE

Aminophylline is a phosphodiesterase inhibitor that relieves bronchospasm, and increases the heart rate and force of myocardial contraction. More often used in the treatment of asthma, it has been used for heart failure to augment cardiac output. It may also be useful in atropine-resistant AV node block complicating inferior myocardial infarction, as this may be mediated by adenosine (Shah et al, 1987). However, aminophylline may produce serious ventricular dysrhythmias, particularly following acute myocardial infarction, and should be used with care in patients with cardiac disease.

Dose   250 mg (5 mg/kg) by very slow intravenous injection (over 20 min).

Side-effects   Dysrhythmias and convulsions. Increased toxicity in smokers.

AMIODARONE (Cordarone X)

Amiodarone is a potent class III antidysrhythmic agent, with some class II (beta-blocking) properties when given intravenously. It prolongs the duration of the action potential (similar to hypothyroidism), and increases the effective refractory period of both the atria and the ventricles. The QT interval increases. Amiodarone is of value in many different atrial and ventricular dysrhythmias, including re-entry tachycardias. The half-life is extremely long (> 28 days).

Doses

Bolus administration.   Amiodarone (150–300 mg) diluted in 10–20 ml of 5% glucose given by slow intravenous injection, over at least 3 min. Cardiac monitoring is required as acute haemodynamic effects may occur. Repeat bolus administration should not be undertaken for at least 15 min.

Amiodarone 300 mg should be considered after adrenaline (epinephrine) to treat VT/VF cardiac arrest refractory to defibrillation. A further dose of 150 mg followed by infusion can be used, to a maximum daily dose of 2 g.

Infusion.   The dose is usually 150–300 mg intravenously (5 mg/kg over 20–120 min), followed by intravenous infusion of 900 mg over 24 h (in 5% dextrose, not saline). Amiodarone may reduce the drop size in certain infusion devices, and the calculated infusion rate may be too slow. Repeated boluses or continuous infusions associate with thrombophlebitis, which may be severe. Administration by a central venous line is desirable

Oral therapy.   Oral therapy is usually started at the same time as intravenous treatment, as oral amiodarone takes about a week for maximal effect, because the half-life of the drug is very long (30–45 days). The usual oral loading dose is 200 mg three times daily for 1 week, 200 mg twice daily for 1 week and then 200 mg/per day. Some patients require a faster loading rate and higher maintenance doses. Normal maintenance is 100–200 mg/day.

Side-effects Acutely, the drug may be pro-arrhythmic. Chronic use is limited by side-effects that are mostly dose-related and time-dependent (Shukla et al, 1994). Virtually all are extracardiac:

- Reversible corneal deposits are universal, but usually not a problem. Occasionally visual haloes are caused.
- Photosensitivity is very common, and, rarely, a bluish discoloration of the skin develops.
- Thyroid dysfunction occurs in 2–3% of patients, and there may also be problems with biochemical analysis of serum thyroid hormone levels. Thyroid function tests should be carried out before treatment and then every 6 months during therapy.
- Interstitial pulmonary fibrosis or pulmonary alveolitis.
- Abnormal liver function tests.
- Peripheral neuropathy.
- Miscellaneous effects include constipation, headache, nausea, fatigue, tremor and nightmares.

Important interactions occur with warfarin and digoxin. The dose of digoxin should be halved, and the INR carefully monitored after starting therapy because of enhanced coagulant activity. Amiodarone should not be used with other drugs that increase the QT interval.

ANALGESICS

Narcotic analgesics (opiates) are used to relieve moderate to severe pain. Drugs in the group all have similar effects and side-effects, but differ in their duration of action. Although opiates are primarily analgesics, they also have sedative effects at high doses, particularly when used in combination with other centrally acting drugs (e.g. tranquillisers). They stimulate the vomiting cen-

tres in the brain so are usually given with an anti-emetic drug.

Narcotic analgesics are usually given by slow intravenous injection or infusion following acute myocardial infarction, since intramuscular absorption is unpredictable. Diamorphine is the analgesic of choice as it produces vasodilatation, thereby reducing myocardial work and oxygen consumption. It is also much more soluble and allows injection of smaller volumes of fluid.

Dose

- Diamorphine: 2.5–10.0 mg intravenously, repeated as required
- Morphine and cyclomorphine: 5–10 mg intravenously, repeated as required
- Papaveretum (Omnopon) is a mixture of the alkaloids of opium (20 mg is roughly equivalent to 12.5 mg of morphine).

Side-effects Nausea, vomiting, constipation, urinary retention, bradycardia and respiratory depression.

ANGIOTENSIN-CONVERTING ENZYME INHIBITORS

The ACE inhibitors are competitive inhibitors of the ACE kininase II. This causes reduced conversion of angiotensin I to angiotensin II, with accumulation of bradykinin, a vasodilator which is normally activated by ACE. Therapeutic effects are primarily due to vasodilatation, but aldosterone levels are also reduced (Fig. 17.1).

In patients with cardiac failure, the renin–angiotensin–aldosterone system is extremely active, resulting in angiotensin-mediated vasoconstriction with increased sodium and water retention secondary to increased aldosterone secretion. The ACE inhibitors block the conversion of angiotensin I to the potent vasoconstrictor angiotensin II, allowing vasodilatation of arteries and veins, producing a fall in blood pressure. In addition, the ACE inhibitors inhibit the breakdown of bradykinin, another potent vasodilator. Unfortunately, it is probably the high levels of bradykinin that give rise to the common ACE-inhibitor cough.

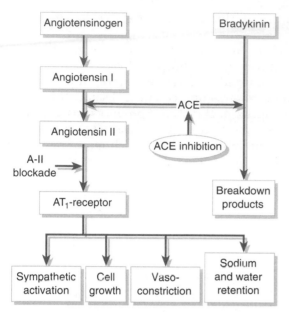

Figure 17.1 Sites of action of angiotensin-converting enzyme (ACE) inhibitors and angiotensin II (A-II) blockers.

Although used in the treatment of hypertension, the major role of ACE inhibitors is in the treatment of cardiac failure, resulting in symptomatic improvement and reduced mortality (Packer, 1992). They oppose angiotensin-induced left ventricular hypertrophy, and slow the progression to left ventricular dysfunction. Early routine use of ACE inhibitors in unselected patients following acute myocardial infarction produces a small benefit, brought about by greater benefits in high-risk patients and no effect in others. Patients with asymptomatic left ventricular dysfunction treated with ACE inhibitors may not progress to overt heart failure, although this does not necessarily affect survival rates. In those with overt cardiac failure or significant left ventricular damage, ACE inhibitors started within 1 week of myocardial infarction reduce mortality and other serious cardiovascular events (St John Sutton, 1994).

There are nine different ACE inhibitors available in the UK, of which five (captopril, enalapril, lisinopril, trandolapril and ramipril) have a good evidence base for the treatment of heart failure. Despite claims of potential advantages of one compound over another, no clinically significant differences have yet been shown in the treatment of either hypertension or heart failure.

Dose

- Captopril (Capoten, Acepril): 6.25–150 mg daily in divided doses
- Enalapril (Innovace): 2.5–40.0 mg in divided doses
- Lisinopril (Zestril, Carace): 2.5–40.0 mg daily
- Ramipril (Tritace): 5 mg twice daily
- Trandolapril (Gopten, Odrik): 4 mg once daily.

Side-effects Rash and cough are frequent (particularly in women), and are the most common reason for stopping therapy. Iron supplements may be a simple remedy for the dry cough, and should work within a week. The mechanism is not known. First-dose hypotension is rarely a problem in mild to moderate heart failure, and hospital admission for initiation of therapy is seldom required. Transient taste disturbance may occur in 5% of patients. Renal failure and hyperkalaemia are important complications of therapy, particularly in patients treated with concomitant spironolactone. Some side-effects occur with one ACE inhibitor but not another.

ANGIOTENSIN II RECEPTOR BLOCKERS

This large group of drugs are specific antagonists of the angiotensin II receptor, with many properties similar to the ACE inhibitors. However, they do not inhibit the breakdown of bradykinin (Fig. 17.1), and thus do not make patients cough or susceptible to angio-oedema. Their role beyond the treatment of hypertension is not yet clear.

Dose

- Candesartan cilexetil (Amias): 4–16 mg daily
- Eprosartan (Teveten): 300–600 mg daily
- Irbesartan (Aprovel): 150–300 mg daily
- Losartan potassium (Cozaar): 25–100 mg daily
- Telmisartan (Micardis): 20–40 mg daily
- Valsartan (Diovan): 40–160 mg daily.

Side-effects These are few, and include rhinitis, urticaria and myalgia.

ALPHA-BLOCKERS

This drugs selectively block post-synaptic alpha-1 receptors, leading to vasodilatation and a fall in systemic blood pressure. The group includes doxazosin, indoramin, prazosin and terazosin, and are used in the treatment of hypertension (and symptoms of prostatism).

Side-effects These are common and include postural hypotension, weakness and blurred vision.

ANTIDYSRHYTHMIC AGENTS

Suppression of serious dysrhythmias following acute myocardial infarction should be associated with a reduced mortality and morbidity, as well as relieving much of the anxiety in the patient with symptomatic dysrhythmias. Despite large advances in our understanding of the pathogenesis and pharmacological treatment of cardiac dysrhythmias, management is still largely unsatisfactory, and many patients are still treated empirically.

Classification of the antidysrhythmic agents

There are many ways of classifying antidysrhythmic drugs, such as the type of rhythm disturbance, the anatomical site of action, or their electrophysiological action. This latter classification, devised by Vaughan Williams in 1969, is based on actions on isolated myocardium, but is still used today (Vaughan Williams, 1984). The Vaughan Williams classification has many limitations, but does provide many theoretical and practical benefits for a rational approach in the treatment of dysrhythmias. Initial selection of a drug can often be simplified, and, should a second agent be required, selection from a different action group is frequently more successful than if an agent from the same group is employed.

There are four classes of drug in the Vaughan Williams classification, based on their *in vitro* effects on the action potentials of normal cardiac cells (Fig. 2.7).

Class I: Membrane-stabilising or local anaesthetic effect

(Examples: lidocaine (lignocaine), flecainide, propafenone)

These agents depress membrane responsiveness, and slow myocardial conduction by membrane-stabilising activity. The fast sodium current is inhibited, and the phase 0 rise is thus reduced. These drugs also depress the rate of diastolic depolarisation (phase 4), which reduces spontaneous automaticity.

The group is subdivided into classes Ia, Ib and Ic, on the basis of the overall effect on the action potential: class Ia drugs (quinidine, disopyramide, procainamide) moderately prolong it, class Ib drugs (lidocaine (lignocaine), mexiletine, phenytoin) slightly shorten it and class Ic drugs (flecainide, propafenone) have no effect, but widen the QRS complex. Class Ia drugs are more cardiodepressant.

Class II: Beta-blockers

(Examples: propranolol, metoprolol, atenolol)

These drugs block catecholamine stimulation of the myocardial cells, which may induce cardiac dysrhythmias They also produce direct membrane-stabilising effects, similar to those of class I drugs.

Class III: Drugs prolonging repolarisation

(Examples: amiodarone, sotalol)

The major action of these drugs is to prolong the duration of the action potential, with consequent lengthening of the effective refractory period. The membrane responsiveness, conduction velocity and rate of rise of the action potential in phase 0 are not affected. They suppress ventricular ectopic activity, ventricular tachycardia and ventricular fibrillation.

Class IV: Calcium-channel blockade in the SA and AV nodes

(Examples: verapamil, diltiazem)

These agents inhibit the slow inward calcium current and depress phases 2 and 3 (plateau phase) of the action potential. These actions are of particular importance in the upper part of the AV node and will block circus movements during re-entry tachycardias.

Adverse effects These are common in all antidysrhythmic drugs, and include pro-arrhythmia, bradydysrhythmias and negative inotropic effects.

Pro-arrhythmic activity may vary from increasing ectopic beats to life-threatening dysrhythmias. Most antidysrhythmic drugs may potentially cause abnormalities of cardiac rhythm (Podrib et al, 1987). Importantly the risk of pro-arrhythmia exists even when the underlying rhythm disturbance is benign. The CAST studies (Cast Investigators, 1989; Cast II Investigators, 1992) showed that post-infarction patients were more likely to die if treated with certain antidysrhythmic agents than with placebo, an effect attributed to the pro-arrhythmic effect of the agents used.

Bradydysrhythmias often occur because of effects on the AV and SA nodes, and are more common where there is underlying disease of the conducting tissue.

Negative inotropic effects occur by various mechanisms, and are most marked in patients with known left ventricular dysfunction.

ASPIRIN

Aspirin irreversibly blocks the enzyme *cyclo-oxygenase*, and reduces the synthesis of various prostanoids, including *thromboxane A_2*, a potent vasoconstrictor and platelet aggregant. The beneficial dose is in the range 75–300 mg daily. This effectively inhibits the ability of the blood platelets to synthesise thromboxane A_2 during their lifespan in the circulation of 7–10 days. Inhibition of platelet function produces an antithrombotic effect.

Following acute myocardial infarction, aspirin reduces the risk of subsequent non-fatal myocardial infarction, re-infarction, stroke and cardiovascular death by up to 25% (Anti-thrombotic Trialists' Collaboration, 2002). It is also used to reduce the risk of graft occlusion in those who have undergone coronary artery bypass grafting.

'Disprin CV' is aspirin specifically designed for cardiovascular disease. This formulation is micro-encapsulated for sustained release, and does not cause as much gastrointestinal upset, reducing blood loss by a half in comparison with standard aspirin. It is, of course, more expensive, and no more effective. The 100-mg formulation is recommended for prevention for coronary graft occlusion, whereas the 300-mg size is used for the other cardiovascular indications (transient ischaemic attack, post-myocardial infarction, unstable angina, etc.).

Aspirin should be considered for *primary prophylaxis* of myocardial infarction in men and women at high risk, and for patients with diabetes (Lowe, 2001).

Dose 75–325 mg/day. For acute myocardial infarction, an initial loading dose of at least 150 mg should be chewed rather than swallowed whole, to ensure rapid absorption. This is particularly important prior to thrombolysis.

Side-effects True aspirin allergy is rare, but hypersensitivity may cause bronchospasm. The risk of a major gastrointestinal bleed is increased by about 1 in 250 patients/year, even with low- or modified-release aspirin. The beneficial antithrombotic effects of aspirin generally outweigh adverse effects, and its use is strongly advised by the Joint British Recommendations on Prevention of Coronary Heart Disease (Wood et al, 1998).

ATROPINE

Atropine is an acetylcholine antagonist and gives rise to parasympathetic blockade. It thus reverses effects on heart rate, systemic vascular resistance and blood pressure mediated by parasympathetic (vagal) activity. Atropine may be useful for treating symptomatic sinus bradycardia and heart block that often occurs within 6 h of acute myocardial infarction related to ischaemia or reperfusion (Bezold–Jarish reflex). High or repetitive doses of atropine should be avoided following acute myocardial infarction, because increased parasympathetic tone protects against ventricular fibrillation. Small doses (0.3–0.6 mg) should be used to achieve minimally effective heart rate, to a maximum dose 3.0 mg. Doses of less than 0.3 mg occasionally elicit a paradoxical slowing of the heart rate.

Dose 0.3 mg intravenously for bradycardia. A single dose of 3 mg is currently recommended for cardiac arrest associated with asystole or pulseless electrical activity, to ensure complete vagal block.

Side-effects Dry mouth, confusion, tachycardia and urinary retention.

BETA-ADRENERGIC BLOCKING AGENTS

Beta-blockers reduce heart rate (particularly exercise-related tachycardia), myocardial contractility and systemic blood pressure. The overall effect is to reduce myocardial work and oxygen consumption (Table 17.1).

Clinical effects are mediated by antagonising the effects of catecholamines by competitively occupying both alpha- and beta-adrenergic receptors. Adrenergic activity is either excitatory or inhibitory.

- *Alpha receptors* seem to be associated with most of the usual adrenergic excitatory functions, such as vasoconstriction and dilatation of the pupils. Stimulation is excitatory in the heart, causing positive inotropic and chronotropic effects
- *Beta receptors* are usually inhibitory, resulting in vasodilatation (inhibition of vasoconstriction) and bronchodilatation (inhibition of bronchial constriction).

The heart and the bronchi have only beta receptors (beta-1 receptors are cardiac; beta-2 receptors are bronchial).

The choice of beta-blocker is usually influenced by the following.

Half-life

Unlike the plasma half-life, the pharmacological half-life depends on the dose. Most beta-blockers can be prescribed twice daily, providing a big

enough dose is given. Hydrophilic agents have longer plasma half-lives, and may usually be taken once daily.

Cardioselectivity

Beta-blockers differ in their relative affinity for beta-1 or beta-2 sites. Timolol, propranolol and nadolol act on both sites and are termed 'non-specific'. However, atenolol and metoprolol act predominantly on the beta-1 cardiac sites and are, therefore, termed 'cardioselective'. Cardioselectivity is relative and is lost at high doses. No beta-blocker is completely safe in patients with asthma.

Intrinsic sympathomimetic activity

Intrinsic sympathomimetic activity (ISA) or partial agonist activity implies that the drug partially stimulates the beta sites, and thus reduces the degree of cardiodepression. Oxprenolol, acebutolol and celiprolol all have ISA, but it is doubtful whether ISA confers any real advantages.

Lipid solubility

The pharmacokinetics of beta-blockers depends in part upon whether they are soluble in fat (lipophilic) or water (hydrophilic). Lipophilic agents (e.g. propranolol) are well absorbed orally and have a short half-life. Variation in oral bioavailability is largely influenced by 'first-pass' metabolism of lipid-soluble compounds by the liver. Lipophilic beta-blockers can cross the blood–brain barrier and may be responsible for central nervous system side-effects (e.g. nightmares). They are metabolised by the liver, and a reduction of dose is required in liver disease. Water-soluble (hydrophilic) agents such as atenolol, celiprolol, nadolol and sotalol are poorly absorbed orally and are excreted unchanged by the kidneys, they care is required in patients with renal impairment. They have a long plasma half-life, do not easily cross the blood–brain barrier, and are less likely to associate with sleep disturbance and nightmares.

Table 17.1 Properties of beta-adrenoceptor blocking drugs

Generic name	Cardioselectivity	Intrinsic sympathomimetic activity	Membrane-stabilising activity	Potency (propranolol = 1)	Elimination half-life (h)	Predominant route of elimination	Lipophilicity
Acebutolol	+	+	+	0.3	3–4	Renal	Low
Atenolol	+	0	0	1.0	6–9	Renal	Low
Labetalol	0	0	0	0.3	3–4	Hepatic	Low
Metoprolol	+	0	0	1.0	3–4	Hepatic	Moderate
Nadolol	0	0	0	1.0	14–24	Renal	Low
Oxprenolol	0	++	+	0.5–1.0	2–3	Hepatic	Moderate
Pindolol	0	+++	+	6.0	3–4	Renal (40%) Hepatic	Moderate
Propranolol	0	0	++	1.0	3–4	Hepatic	High
Sotalol	0	0	0	0.3	8–10	Renal	Low
Timolol	0	0	0	6.0–8.0	4–5	Renal (20%) Hepatic	Low

0, no effect; +, small effect; ++, moderate effect; +++, strong effect.

Vasodilating beta-blockers

Labetolol, celiprolol and carvedilol have vasodilating properties. Carvedilol is used in long-term treatment of heart failure. Labetolol is the drug of choice in the emergency medical management of aortic dissection.

Side-effects

Common side-effects include bradycardia, heart failure, bronchospasm, nightmares, insomnia, depression and peripheral coldness. Cold extremities are caused by unopposed alpha-adrenergic action and partly due to a fall in cardiac output. Central nervous system side-effects are common with beta-blockers that cross the blood–brain barrier (lipid-soluble agents), especially propranolol. These may produce sedation, depression and nightmares. Beta-blockers adversely affect serum lipid profiles, although this may not be so marked in agents with ISA (Jowett and Galton, 1987).

Sudden withdrawal of beta-blockade

Following sudden withdrawal of beta-blockade, there may be an increase in both the number and availability of beta-receptor sites. This may become discernible as an increased sensitivity to catecholamines, with an increase in myocardial work, heart rate and oxygen consumption. Angina, hypertension or even myocardial infarction may result. Patients should be warned of the dangers of suddenly stopping medication, because of this rebound effect. Beta-blockade should always be reduced slowly.

Therapeutic uses

Apart from treatment of hypertension, the major role of beta-blockers is in the treatment of stable angina, where 90% of patients will have improved exercise tolerance and reduced chest pain. Beta-blockers also have class II antidysrhythmic activity, and are also of particular value in supraventricular dysrhythmias. Sotalol has additional class III antidysrhythmic activity. Beta-blockers reduce catecholamine concentrations in ischaemic myocardium, decrease platelet stickiness and have been shown to modify type A behaviour (Sleight, 1986).

Beta-blockers and acute myocardial infarction

Overviews of the randomised controlled trails of short-term and long-term beta-blockade following acute myocardial infarction indicate major benefits (Yusuf et al, 1985; Freemantle et al, 1999).

Intravenous beta-blockade reduces pain, recurrent ischaemia and mortality in patients with acute myocardial infarction. Moreover, retrospective analysis of the ISIS-1 data indicates that intravenous beta-blockade resulted in a 2.5 times greater reduction in the risk of cardiac rupture, most of this benefit being achieved in the first 24 h. Beta-blockers are particularly valuable in those with persistent sinus tachycardia and associated hypertension (systolic blood pressures above 160 mmHg). Metoprolol and atenolol are safe to use intravenously, provided there is no asthma, marked bradycardia, advanced AV block, hypotension or advanced heart failure. Both are given by slow intravenous injection of 5 mg, followed by a further 5 mg after 5 min while monitoring the patient. The pulse rate should remain above 50 beats/min and the blood pressure above 100 mmHg systolic.

Timolol, metoprolol and propranolol all have good evidence for long-term cardioprotection following myocardial infarction, and reduce the risk of sudden death, non-fatal re-infarction and all-cause mortality by 20–30%. Patients at highest risk of further cardiac events are often denied beta-blocker therapy, but benefit most. This group includes those with large and anterior infarcts, those with heart failure, the elderly and those with diabetes. It is not known whether all beta-blockers are valuable for cardioprotection. Reduction in heart rate seems important, which is possibly why using beta-blockers with intrinsic sympathomimetic activity (e.g. pindolol and oxprenolol) does not confer benefit. Oral treatment with agents licensed for prophylaxis should be started within 24 h and continued for at least 2–3 years, if tolerated, at the following doses:

- Propranolol (Inderal): initially 40 mg four times a day, then 80 mg twice daily long-term
- Timolol maleate (Betim): initially 5 mg twice daily, then 10 mg twice daily long-term
- Metoprolol tartrate (Betaloc, Lopresor): 50 mg four times a day then 100 mg twice daily long-term.

The evidence for continuation of beta-blockers for beyond 2–3 years after myocardial infarction is not yet established, but most physicians would continue the drug indefinitely unless there were problems. Sudden cessation may cause a rebound in symptoms of worsening myocardial ischaemia.

Beta-blockers and cardiac failure

There is substantial evidence for the beneficial role of beta-blockers in heart failure. Metoprolol, bisoprolol and carvedilol all reduce mortality and morbidity in patients with stable NYHA class II and class III systolic heart failure (McMurray, 1999). They should be started at very low doses, and titrated up every 2–4 weeks to target doses, providing the heart failure is stable. (see Table 12.2)

During titration there may be transient worsening of heart failure symptoms, fluid retention, bradycardia or hypotension. Hence:

- If *heart failure symptoms* worsen, the dose of diuretics should be increased with a temporary reduction in the dose of beta-blocker if needed.
- If there is *symptomatic hypotension*, the dose of vasodilators should be reduced, and the dose of beta-blocker reduced if required.
- If *symptomatic bradycardia* occurs, the dose of beta-blocker should be reduced.

When the patient stabilises, up-titration can be attempted again. Increasing availability of the relevant beta-blockers in appropriate formulations has helped this.

BRETYLIUM TOSYLATE

Bretylium is an adrenergic neurone-blocking agent that suppresses noradrenaline (norepi-nephrine) release. It selectively concentrates in sympathetic ganglia to produce a state resembling chemical sympathectomy. It has class III antidysrhythmic properties and is useful in ventricular dysrhythmias, especially resistant ventricular fibrillation. Bretylium is often used in the USA where the choice of antidysrhythmic agents is limited, but it is not often used in the UK.

Dose 5–10 mg/kg infused intravenously over 10–30 min. This may be repeated after 1–2 h, to a total dose of 30 mg/kg. Min-I-Jet provides 500 mg in a 10-ml disposable syringe.

Side-effects Hypotension is common, and may persevere for several days; dopamine support may be required. Bretylium is excreted by the kidneys, and reduced doses are required in renal impairment.

BUMETANIDE (Burinex)

Bumetanide is a loop diuretic similar to furosemide (frusemide), that inhibits reabsorption of sodium and potassium in the ascending limb of the loop of Henle (loop diuretic). Following an intravenous injection, a diuresis starts within a few minutes, reaching a maximum within 15–30 min. Orally, the onset is usually after 30–60 min, and the diuresis continues for about 3–4 hours. 1 mg is about equivalent to 40–60 mg of furosemide (frusemide), but at high doses direct comparison of doses is not possible. Bumetanide may increase urine output in patients with renal failure who are unresponsive to furosemide (frusemide).

Dose 1–2 mg orally or intravenously, but doses over 5 mg are required in renal failure.

Side-effects Potassium depletion, myalgia and cramps, skin rashes. It is less ototoxic than furosemide (frusemide), and may not be so potassium- and magnesium-depleting.

CALCIUM CHLORIDE

Calcium ions can cause the asystolic heart to beat, as well as strengthening contractility. They may also counteract the effect of hyperkalaemia.

However, routine administration of calcium salts during cardiopulmonary resuscitation is no longer recommended, as calcium may cause coronary and cerebral vasospasm, as well as increasing ventricular irritability in patients taking digoxin.

Small doses may be useful for cardiac arrest complicated by hypocalcaemia or hyperkalaemia, or for patients on high doses of calcium channel blocking agents (e.g. nifedipine, verapamil or nicardipine). Calcium may be of value in the treatment of pulseless electrical activity, especially if the QRS complex is widened.

Dose 2–4 mg/kg intravenously (2 ml of 10% calcium chloride solution).

Side-effects Sudden death may occur if the patient is taking digoxin. Intramuscular or subcutaneous administration can cause tissue necrosis.

CALCIUM CHANNEL BLOCKING AGENTS

There are three main groups:

- Dihydropyridines (e.g. nifedipine, amlodipine, nicardipine)
- Phenylalkylamines (e.g. verapamil)
- Benzthiazepines (e.g. diltiazem).

Calcium antagonists are used predominantly in the treatment of hypertension, angina and supraventricular dysrhythmias. Verapamil may improve outcome when used as an alternative to beta-blockade in patients with good left ventricular function (DAVITT II, 1990), and diltiazem may reduce the risk of re-infarction in patients who present with non-Q wave infarction (Gibson et al, 1986).

Phenylalkylamines (verapamil) (Example: verapamil)

The most striking effect of verapamil is on AV node conduction, making it very useful for treatment of supraventricular tachycardias. Following an intravenous injection (5–10 mg), AV conduction is quickly reduced, and re-entry tachycardias at the AV node are terminated.

Orally, it is not so effective, because much is metabolised by the liver. Standard verapamil often seems to work where modified (slow-release) verapamil does not.

If given to a patient on beta-blockers, verapamil may cause profound hypotension, bradycardia or heart block, so care is needed. Verapamil is useful for controlling the ventricular rate in atrial fibrillation and atrial flutter, with or without digoxin. It is contraindicated in atrial fibrillation complicating the Wolff–Parkinson–White syndrome, as it gives rise to preferentially accessory conduction, which may result in ventricular fibrillation.

Dose The recommended dose is 5–10 mg intravenously over 2–3 min, which may be repeated after 30 min. Asystole may result if the patient is taking beta-blockers. Oral therapy is 40–120 mg three times a day. Higher doses are required for the treatment of angina (40–120 mg three times a day) and hypertension (120–240 mg twice daily).

Dihydropyridines

(Examples: nifedipine, amlodipine, nicardipine)

Nifedipine reduces peripheral and coronary vascular resistance. It has a mild negative inotropic effect, which is usually offset by increasing sympathetic activity secondary to its vasodilator effect. Amlodipine, nicardipine and isradipine are similar, although cardiodepression is not so marked.

Benzthiazepines

(Example: diltiazem)

Diltiazem inhibits transmission in cardiac conducting tissue and gives rise to a mild resting bradycardia. It vasodilates coronary arteries and peripheral arteries. Although used predominantly in the treatment of angina, it may also be used in higher doses for hypertension. In patients without cardiac failure, once-daily long-acting diltiazem can be used following acute myocardial infarction where beta-blockers are contraindicated. It may then reduce recurrent ischaemia and the need for coronary revascularisation (Purcell and Fox, 2001). Diltiazem is useful in the prophylaxis of recurrent supraventricular tachycardia, and is useful in controlling the ventricular rate in patients with atrial fibrillation, with or without digoxin.

Side-effects of calcium channel blockers

Vasodilator effects (flushing, headache and dizziness) sometimes occur at the start of therapy; they are most pronounced with nifedipine. Fluid retention is common, often resulting in ankle oedema. Verapamil can produce constipation and also reduces digoxin excretion. If these two drugs are given together, the dose of digoxin should be halved. Diltiazem appears to produce fewer side-effects than the other calcium blockers, as it has less effect on the heart than verapamil and less effect on the peripheral vessels than nifedipine.

CARVEDILOL (Eucardic)

Carvedilol is a beta-blocker with additional arterial vasodilating properties. It is licensed for the treatment of heart failure.

Dose   12.5–25 mg twice daily.

Dose in heart failure   Initially 3.125 mg twice daily, titrating at 2-week intervals to 25 mg twice daily (50 mg twice daily in patients weighing more than 85 kg).

CLOPIDOGREL (Plavix)

Clopidogrel is a potent and irreversible ADP receptor antagonist, and inhibits ADP-induced platelet aggregation. The CAPRIE trial (CAPRIE Steering Committee, 1996) showed that clopidogrel is more effective than aspirin in reducing stroke, myocardial infarction and vascular death. In unstable angina, the CURE (2001) trial indicated a beneficial effect when given in addition to aspirin, but with an increased risk of major bleeds. The benefits in this trial were observed as early as 2 h following an oral loading dose of 300 mg, and thus aspirin 300 mg plus clopidogrel 300

mg should be given immediately to all patients with chest pain suspected of being of cardiac origin. The drugs may be discontinued if subsequently the diagnosis was not cardiac. Therapy with clopidogrel should continue following an unstable coronary syndrome for at least 9 months.

Dose   75 mg daily.

Side-effects   Similar to aspirin.

COLCHICINE

Colchicine is used to terminate an attack of acute gout. Although very effective, gastrointestinal symptoms, including nausea, vomiting and especially diarrhoea, are very common. However, because gout usually complicates treatment of heart failure, non-steroidal drugs cannot be given, and colchicine is a very good drug for terminating the attack.

Dose   1 mg orally, and then 0.5 mg every 2–3 h until the pain subsides (or vomiting and diarrhoea occur). The dose should be reduced in renal failure.

Side-effects   Gastrointestinal. Rarely bone marrow suppression.

DIAZOXIDE (Eudemine)

Diazoxide is useful in lowering systemic vascular resistance, and is most effective when given with a loop diuretic. It has a very rapid action intravenously and should thus be given with care.

Doses   300 mg in 20 ml as an intravenous bolus. Orally, 400–1000 mg in two or three daily doses.

Side-effects   Hyperglycaemia is inevitable and often needs concomitant treatment with tolbutamide. Fluid retention may require diuretic therapy.

DIGOXIN (Lanoxin)

Digoxin inhibits the ATPase responsible for the sodium/potassium pump. It increases the force of myocardial contraction and exerts a slowing of conduction at the sinus and AV nodes. Therapeutic doses cause shortening of the QT interval and flattening (or inversion) of the T waves with ST segment sag. False positive ST changes may develop during exercise stress testing.

Oral digoxin is rapidly, and almost entirely, absorbed. A loading dose is required at approximately 15 μg/kg in divided doses, reducing to about 5 μg/kg in those with normal renal function. Effects are not directly correlated with blood levels of the drug because of variable protein-binding, penetration and uptake by the myocardium and other factors. It is primarily metabolised by the kidneys within 2–3 days, but may accumulate in renal impairment. In some patients, digoxin is inactivated by gut flora, necessitating large oral doses to achieve satisfactory blood levels. If these patients are given broad-spectrum antibiotics that affect the gut flora, digoxin toxicity may be precipitated.

The principal use of digoxin is for controlling the ventricular rate in atrial fibrillation, especially when it occurs with heart failure. Digoxin has an acute positive inotropic effect, although whether this is maintained chronically is debatable. It is of little value in cases of high-output failure, cor pulmonale and restrictive cardiomyopathy. Long-term use in congestive heart failure without rhythm disturbance is controversial, and many patients in sinus rhythm remain well after therapy with digoxin is discontinued. The Digitalis Investigation (DIG) Group (1997) showed that digoxin does not reduce mortality in patients with heart failure, but did reduce hospitalisation for worsening heart failure. In patients with thyrotoxicosis, very large doses, often supplemented with propranolol, may be required to slow the ventricular rate.

Digoxin following myocardial infarction

The role of digoxin in acute myocardial infarction is controversial (*Lancet*, 1989). In patients with left ventricular failure following acute myocardial infarction, digoxin is effective, but concern surrounds the increased myocardial

work caused by the positive inotropic effect of the drug, which may extend the area of myocardial necrosis. Beneficial haemodynamic effects are greatest in patients with moderate left ventricular failure, and the risk of extending myocardial damage is probably least in these patients. Post-infarction survival in patients with congestive heart failure and with multifocal ventricular ectopics may be improved by withholding or discontinuing digoxin.

Doses

Digoxin is very irritant to the tissues and should only be given orally or intravenously. A single intravenous dose of 1 mg by infusion produces an effect in about 10 min, with maximal effect at 1–2 h. The half-life is 36–48 h. By mouth, the effect is noted within 1 h and persists for 2–3 days, although some effect may still be present for a week. Digitalisation will take about 1 week if no loading dose is given, and may be achieved by giving 1.0–1.5 mg over 24 h in divided doses. Care is needed in the elderly and if there is co-existing hypokalaemia or renal impairment, when assessment of blood levels are helpful, although levels should not be measured within 6 h of the last oral dose.

Digoxin toxicity

A major drawback to the treatment with digoxin is the narrow margin between therapeutic doses and toxicity. Hence, adverse drug actions are very common, and many patients manifest toxicity at some time. Therapeutic levels are quoted as 0.5–2.5 mg/ml, but it must be remembered that the diagnosis of digoxin toxicity is clinical and too much reliance should not be placed on laboratory results. For example, digoxin toxicity can occur at normal blood levels if there are concomitant electrolyte upsets, thyroid disease, renal impairment or hypoxia. Patients with blood levels greater than 2.5 mg/ml may display no signs of toxicity.

The early symptoms of overdose are nausea, vomiting and diarrhoea. Headache and confusion, often with visual disturbances, are more serious. Classically, *xanthopsia* (yellow vision) is reported, but flickering dots, haloes and scotomata can occur. Digoxin toxicity can produce any rhythm disturbance, including ventricular fibrillation. The more common problems are ventricular ectopics (especially ventricular bigemini), sinus bradycardia, heart block and paroxysmal atrial tachycardia with block. The ECG usually shows other signs of toxicity such as ST–T wave changes or increased PR interval. Ventricular tachycardia is usually precipitated by short runs of ventricular ectopics.

Treatment of toxicity

If stopping digoxin is inadequate, potassium chloride is very effective, even in the absence of hypokalaemia. Potassium canrenoate (400 mg intravenously over 5 min) can be used for more urgent cases, but ECG monitoring is desirable during parenteral administration of any potassium supplement. Propranolol (2 mg intravenously) is especially useful for supraventricular dysrhythmias, and phenytoin, amiodarone and lidocaine (lignocaine) are effective in digitalis-induced ventricular dysrhythmias. Digibind (anti-digoxin antibody fragments) should be used in all serious cases.

In the case of digoxin-related bradydysrhythmias, potassium supplements should be stopped, because they potentiate heart block. Symptomatic bradycardias may require intravenous atropine, isoprenaline or even temporary cardiac pacing.

DIPYRIDAMOLE (Persantin)

Dipyridamole inhibits ADP-induced platelet aggregation. It is often used as an adjunct to aspirin, and to oral anticoagulation in patients with prosthetic heart valves to prevent emboli. Dipyridamole is sometimes used to increase coronary perfusion during nuclear scanning, where it diverts blood away from areas of poor perfusion.

Dose   300–600 mg/day in three to four divided doses.

A modified preparation is available (Persantin Retard): 200 mg twice daily.

Side-effects   May worsen coronary ischaemia. Interacts with adenosine to produce an enhanced effect.

DISOPYRAMIDE (Rythmodan, Dirythmin, Isomide)

Disopyramide is a class I antidysrhythmic agent, with electrophysiological properties similar to those of quinidine. It decreases automaticity in ectopic pacemaker cells and lengthens the effective refractory period in atrial and ventricular muscle. It thus has both ventricular and supraventricular activity.

Dose   The dose is 2 mg/kg by very slow intravenous injection, to a maximum of 150 mg in the first hour. An infusion of 0.4 mg/kg/h may then be employed, or oral therapy (400–800 mg in four doses). If the drug is going to work, it does so in the first 15–20 min. The usual therapeutic plasma levels are 2–4 µg/ml. Over half the drug is excreted unchanged in the urine, and dose reduction is required in patients with hepatic and renal impairment. The half-life is between 6 and 12 h.

Side-effects   Disopyramide has a marked negative inotropic effect, related to both serum levels and speed of administration. It should be used cautiously in patients with heart failure. Sinus node depression also sometimes occurs, so care is needed in heart block. Anticholinergic activity may cause glaucoma, retention of urine and constipation.

DOBUTAMINE (Dobutrex)

Dobutamine is a synthetic adrenergic agent, modified from isoprenaline. It stimulates beta-adrenergic cardiac receptors and thereby directly increases the force of myocardial contraction, with only small increases in heart rates. Unlike dopamine, there is little systemic vasoconstriction, because dopamine acts indirectly, by causing release of noradrenaline (norepinephrine), whereas dobutamine acts directly.

Dopamine is used to treat cardiogenic shock and heart failure, and is best administered when cardiovascular monitoring techniques are available.

Dose It is supplied in ampoules containing 250 mg of dobutamine. Following dilution, it is added to 250 or 500 ml of dextrose or saline, giving 1000 μg/ml or 500 μg/ml, respectively. It is infused intravenously, most patients responding to a dose of 2.5–10.0 μg/kg/min. Some patients may need 40 μg/kg/min. Dobutamine is often given in combination with low-dose dopamine, which is used to promote renal perfusion.

DOPAMINE (Intropin)

Dopamine is the natural precursor of noradrenaline (norepinephrine) and has similar alpha- and beta-stimulatory actions, particularly at beta-1 sites. Stroke volume is increased, with little effect on heart rate. It causes peripheral vasoconstriction, which raises blood pressure, but, unlike other sympathetic agents, produces selective renal and cerebral arterial vasodilatation.

At low doses, the renal effects are most marked, but, as the dose increases, vasoconstriction and positive inotropic and chronotropic effects are more marked. Dopamine is of major value in cardiogenic and other types of shock, and prolonged low-dose infusion is useful in heart failure.

Dopamine is given by continuous intravenous infusion, preferably by a central line, because profound localised tissue ischaemia may result with extravasation. Should signs of tissue necrosis develop, the area should be infiltrated with phentolamine (10 mg in 10 ml of saline).

Dose Each ampoule contains 800 mg of dopamine, which is diluted in 500 ml of dextrose or saline, yielding 1600 μg/ml.

Calculating the rate of administration. Dopamine exerts its effect by acting on different receptors at different doses (Table 17.2). The required dose is calculated in drops per minute by the formula:

Required dose (μg/kg/min) × Body weight (kg) × Total volume of infusion (ml) × Number of

Table 17.2 Effects of dopamine at different doses

Dose (μg/kg/min)	Effect
1–5	Dilates renal and mesenteric arterioles to produce increased renal blood flow and glomerular filtration rate and urine output
6–20	Direct inotropic effect on the heart, with dose-related increase in cardiac output and heart rate
>20	Direct alpha-action leads to peripheral vasoconstriction, which raises blood pressure. There are further inotropic and chronotropic effects on the heart

drops/ml dispensed by infusion pump, divided by Amount of dopamine added to infusion (mg) × 1000.

For example, for an infusion of 5 μg/kg/min in an 80-kg man given via a standard drip (20 drops/ml), the infusion rate would be:

$$(5 \times 80 \times 520 \times 20) = 4\,160\,000, \text{ divided by}$$
$$(800 \times 1000) = 800\,000$$

Hence infusion rate = 5.2 drops/min.

Dopamine is contraindicated in patients with uncontrolled dysrhythmias and those taking monoamine oxidase inhibitors. Hypovolaemia should be corrected before its use, and therapy should be withdrawn slowly.

ENOXIMONE (Perfan)

Enoximone is a selective phosphodiesterase inhibitor that slows the breakdown of myocardial cyclic AMP. The rate and force of myocardial contraction directly relates to the myocardial concentration of cyclic AMP, an effect that may be augmented by simultaneous administration of dopamine. Cyclic AMP also relaxes vascular smooth muscle, to effect vasodilatation. As a consequence, phosphodiesterase inhibitors will improve cardiac output, and there is usually no change in blood pressure, heart rate or oxygen consumption.

There is no evidence that enoximone improves survival, but it may be used for the short-term intravenous treatment of severe heart failure refractory to conventional treatment, providing the patient is monitored invasively.

Dose 90 µg/kg/min is given over 30 min to load the patient. A continuous infusion of not more than 24 mg/kg should be given over 24 h, in the range 5–20 µg/kg/min.

Side-effects Dysrhythmias, hypotension, pain in limbs.

EPINEPHRINE (see ADRENALINE)

ESMOLOL HYDROCHLORIDE (Brevibloc)

Esmolol hydrochloride is a cardiospecific beta-blocker with a very short duration of action, which may be used in the treatment of supraventricular tachycardias, sinus tachycardia and hypertension, especially post-operatively.

Dose 50–200 µg/kg/min by intravenous infusion.

FLECAINIDE (Tambocor)

Flecainide is a class Ic agent, which slows conduction through the His–Purkinje system and prevents retrograde conduction through accessory pathways. It is useful in chronic ventricular dysrhythmias and in re-entry tachycardias, especially the Wolff–Parkinson–White syndrome.

Dose It is available for intravenous and oral use, and its long half-life allows a twice-daily dosage. Intravenously it should be given by slow injection or infusion (2 mg/kg). Oral maintenance is 100–200 mg twice daily.

Side-effects Pro-arrhythmic effects are described, particularly in those with acute myocardial ischaemia and in those with cardiac pacemakers. Flecainide is contraindicated in the treatment of ventricular dysrhythmias following acute myocardial infarction (CAST Investigators, 1989). Dizziness and blurred vision may occur, and the drug is negatively inotropic.

FRUSEMIDE (see FUROSEMIDE)

FUROSEMIDE (Lasix, Dryptal)

Furosemide (frusemide) is a powerful loop diuretic, similar to bumetanide and torasemide.

When given intravenously for left ventricular failure, the relief is almost immediate and occurs before a diuresis has taken place. This suggests that the primary value in acute heart failure is due to a vascular effect, by causing increased venous capacitance, and that the diuretic effect is secondary.

Dose The usual dose is 40–80 mg orally or intravenously. Patients with refractory oedema or renal impairment may require very large doses (500–1000 mg). Rapid injection may cause deafness.

Side-effects Transient or permanent deafness may result if furosemide (frusemide) is injected too rapidly, particularly in those with renal impairment. Large doses must be diluted, and intravenous infusion is then a preferable method of administration.

GLYCOPROTEIN IIB/IIIA RECEPTOR ANTAGONISTS

These agents block the fibrinogen receptor on the surface of activated platelets, thus inhibiting platelet aggregation and reducing the risk of arterial thrombosis. They are more potent than other currently available antiplatelet drugs (e.g. aspirin), with an almost immediate onset of action when given intravenously. Abciximab, a monoclonal antibody, was the first agent in clinical use. Unfortunately, it binds irreversibly to the glycoprotein IIb/IIIa receptor, prolonging platelet aggregation, and may associate with increased bleeding risks. It is also not receptor-specific, and may affect other vascular receptors. Tirofiban and eptifibatide do not have these problems, and have shorter half-lives.

These agents are generally well tolerated, although bleeding is a major complication, usually at the puncture site. They are administered by initial bolus, followed by infusion over 12–96 h because of their short half-lives. Abciximab acts for much longer, and thus only needs a 12-h infusion. They are given in combination with aspirin and heparin.

The glycoprotein inhibitors are of benefit in high-risk acute coronary syndromes in prevention of death and myocardial infarction at 30 days, but are of greatest benefit in those undergoing percutaneous coronary intervention (PCI) (Alexander and Harrington, 1998). NICE guidance currently advises intravenous glycoprotein inhibitors with heparin and aspirin in high-risk acute coronary syndromes, as well as during emergency or elective PCI.

Doses
- Abciximab: 250 µg/kg over 1 min, then by intravenous infusion 125 ng/kg/min (maximum 10 µg/kg/min. In unstable angina, started within 24 hours of PCI, and continued for 12 h following the procedure. During elective PCI, started with an hour of PCI, and continued for 12 h.
- Eptifibatide: 180 µg/kg by slow intravenous injection, then by infusion 2 µg/kg/min for up to 72 h, or 96 h with PCI.
- Tirofiban: 400 ng/kg/min for 30 min, then 100 ng/kg/min for at least 48 h to a maximum of 108 h (12–24 h following PCI).

HEPARIN

Heparin is a naturally occurring, high molecular weight mucopolysaccharide with marked anticoagulation properties when given subcutaneously or intravenously. Intramuscular injection may produce large haematomas. Heparin is used to prevent thromboembolism and in the treatment of deep vein thrombosis and pulmonary emboli.

Heparin works by combining with antithrombin III in the coagulation cascade, preventing the formation of factor Xa. It also reduces platelet adhesion. Unlike warfarin, it does not block prothrombin formation in the liver.

The activated partial thromboplastin time (APTT) is used as an index of efficacy and should be maintained at about twice normal. Thrombocytopenia often complicates therapy, and platelet counts should be checked on alternate days.

Overdose, producing prolonged coagulation times, should be corrected by reducing the dose or stopping the drug altogether (the half-life is only 1.5 hs). More urgent cases can be treated with protamine sulphate (1 mg neutralises 100 units of heparin within 5 min). However, since protamine is a weak anticoagulant itself, doses exceeding 50 mg should not be given.

Heparin regimens (unfractionated heparin)

- *Low dose* (prophylaxis): 5000 units twice daily, subcutaneously. APTTs are not required.
- *Medium dose* (treatment of deep vein thrombosis or disseminated intravascular coagulation): 30 000–45 000 units daily by infusion or 4 hourly by intravenous injection. After 48 h, the dose is reduced by about 50% and adjusted according to APTT. Warfarin is usually started at the same time.
- *High dose* (pulmonary embolism, systemic embolisation): a bolus loading dose of 5000–10 000 units should be given, followed by intravenous infusion, but there should be no reduction in dose at 48 h as above. Warfarin is usually not started acutely.

Low molecular weight heparins (LMWHs) are obtained by modifying unfractionated heparin, reducing the molecular weight by about two-thirds. They are weaker inhibitors of thrombin (factor IIa), and essentially work by inhibiting enzyme Xa. The potency of the different LMWHs is expressed in international units (IU) for anti-Xa activity. After subcutaneous injection, they are better absorbed than unfractionated heparin, and regular monitoring of anticoagulation is not required.

Heparin following thrombolysis

Heparin is not required following thrombolysis with streptokinase; it is usual where clot-specific agents have been used (e.g. tissue plasminogen activator, tPA). Following thrombolysis with tPA we routinely use enoxaparin, 30 mg by intravenous injection, followed by 1 mg/kg 12-hourly for 72 h (Ross et al, 2001).

Heparin for unstable angina

Intravenous heparin has been standard therapy for unstable angina for many years. LMWH has a number of advantages over unfractionated heparin, particularly simplicity of administration and reliability of anticoagulation. The ESSENCE and TIMI IIB trials showed advantages of LMWH over unfractionated heparin for preventing death and ischaemic events (Cohen et al, 1997; Antman et al, 1999).

HIRUDIN AND HIRULOG

Hirudin and its derivatives are intravenous anticoagulants, with specific and potent antithrombin effects. These direct thrombin inhibitors are more predictable in action than heparin and are not associated with thrombocytopenia. Hirudin is isolated from the medicinal leech *Hirudo medicinalis*. Hirugen is a synthetic derivative, and hirulog is derived from linking hirugen to hirudin. They are more effective in inhibiting fibrin-bound thrombus and hold promise for preventing coronary re-occlusion following successful thrombolysis. Although the GUSTO IIB trial did not show significant benefits of hirudin over heparin in patients with acute myocardial infarction and unstable angina, the HERO trial showed an increased rate of TIMI-3 flow in the infarct-related artery when hirulog was used with streptokinase (White et al, 1997). Bleeding risks were not increased, and direct thrombin inhibition may improve clinical outcome.

HORMONE REPLACEMENT THERAPY

Oestrogen replacement is associated with a 35–50% lower risk of cardiovascular disease (Grady et al, 1992), but this does not seem to be the case when co-prescribed with progestogens as is usual in hormone replacement therapy (HRT). The Heart and Estrogen/progestin Replacement Study (HERS) showed no benefit of hormone replacement in post-menopausal women with coronary disease. In fact, there was a slight increase in cardiac events in the first year of therapy (perhaps due to an immediate prothrombotic effect), but a subsequent decreased risk (Hulley et al, 1998). Combined HRT is not currently recommended for cardioprotection

(Barrett-Connor et al, 1998), but decisions regarding HRT must be individualised, depending on the competing risks of coronary heart disease, osteoporosis, menopausal symptoms and endometrial and breast cancer. Current advice for post-menopausal women following acute myocardial infarction is that HRT should not be started for cardioprotection, but may be continued if they were already taking it (Grodstein et al, 2001).

HYDRALAZINE (Apresoline)

Hydralazine is an arteriolar vasodilator used in the treatment of hypertension. It increases heart rate and cardiac output by reducing afterload and also increases renal and cerebral perfusion. However, myocardial work and oxygen consumption are also increased, and angina may be precipitated unless it is co-prescribed with a beta-blocker or diltiazem.

Dose The oral dose is 25–75 mg three or four times daily.

Side-effects Due to vasodilatation, with postural hypotension, headache and flushing. Long-term therapy may cause a lupus syndrome, with positive LE cells.

INSULIN

Insulin has multiple metabolic effects. It promotes glucose uptake by cells, which also causes enhanced potassium uptake.

Hyperglycaemia in the peri-infarction period is best treated with insulin, since oral hypoglycaemic agents may cause unwanted metabolic side-effects, particularly if there is renal and hepatic hypoperfusion. Soluble insulin of human origin is probably the best choice to prevent formation of insulin antibodies, and should be given by intravenous infusion. Hypoglycaemia should be avoided, as the induced catecholamine response may lead to tachydysrhythmias. The DIGAMI trial (Malmberg, 1997) showed that insulin infusion followed by subcutaneous insulin for 3 months improved the outcome in patients with acute myocardial infarction presenting with hyperglycaemia. The use of potassium–insulin–glucose infusions for 24 h improves outcome in unselected patients following acute myocardial infarction (Diaz et al, 1998).

ISOPRENALINE

Isoprenaline is most often used to stabilise patients with profound bradycardia, heart block and hypotension, while awaiting pacemaker insertion.

Dose 4 mg in 500 ml of 5% dextrose, infused at a rate that produces a suitable pulse rate and blood pressure.

Side-effects Tremor, sweating and dysrhythmias.

LEPIRUDIN (Refludan)

Lepirudin is a recombinant hirudin used as a parenteral anticoagulant in patients with heparin-induced thrombocytopenia.

Dose 400 µg/kg bolus followed by an infusion of 150 µg/kg/h, adjusted according to the APTT.

Side-effects Bleeding, fever, hypersensitivity reactions

LIGNOCAINE (LIDOCAINE)

In addition to its local anaesthetic properties, lignocaine (lidocaine) is a class I antidysrhythmic agent, which has been used for many years for the control of ventricular dysrhythmias complicating acute myocardial infarction. Its major action during cardiac arrest is to inhibit the initiation of re-entry dysrhythmias in the ischaemic myocardium, but its use makes defibrillation more difficult. Amiodarone is now preferred, although lignocaine (lidocaine) may be considered after prolonged arrest.

Lignocaine (lidocaine) by infusion may be of value following ventricular fibrillation arrest to prevent recurrence, although the trend these days is to give smaller doses for shorter periods (up to 12 h) than in the past. The incidence of side-effects is then very much reduced, without

an apparent increase in further episodes of ventricular fibrillation.

Dose
Bolus therapy is 0.5 mg/kg every 10 min. Infusion is 1–4 mg/min (usually 25–50 µg/kg/min).

Side-effects Toxicity may result in hypotension, bradycardia, vomiting and fits. Reduced hepatic circulation may make lignocaine (lidocaine) toxicity more likely, and no more than 3 mg/kg should be administered.

LIPID-LOWERING AGENTS

Drug therapy to lower plasma lipids is increasingly common for primary and secondary prevention of cardiovascular disease (Wood et al, 1998). There are five groups of drugs that may be used.

1. *HMG-CoA inhibitors* (e.g. pravastatin, simvastatin). The hydroxymethylglutaryl co-enzyme A reductase inhibitors ('statins') competitively inhibit the rate-limiting enzyme in cholesterol synthesis. As endogenous synthesis of cholesterol is prevented, circulating cholesterol is taken up by the LDL receptor on the surface of cells. The statins are very potent, with cholesterol reductions of 40% sometimes being achieved.

Side-effects Myositis and hepatic dysfunction.

2. *Anion-exchange (bile sequestrant) resins* (e.g. cholestyramine, colestipol). These bind bile acids, preventing reabsorption. Cholesterol is diverted into making more bile acids, so is progressively excreted. LDL-cholesterol is reduced, but triglyceride levels may increase. Effects may be offset by an increase in cholesterol synthesis.

Absorption of drugs, particularly digoxin and diuretics, is sometimes impaired. They should be taken 1 h before, or 4–6 h after, the resins. Anticoagulant action may be enhanced or depressed. Fat-soluble vitamins may need supplementation (A, D, E and K).

3. *Fibrates* (e.g. bezafibrate, ciprofibrate, gemfibrozil, fenofibrate). These are isobutyric derivatives that inhibit cholesterol synthesis in the liver

and increase removal of very low density lipoprotein (VLDL) from the blood. They predominantly reduce triglycerides, but also reduce LDL-cholesterol and increase HDL-cholesterol. They also have the side-effect of myositis, and should be used with caution in those with renal impairment and those also taking statins. Fibrates potentiate the actions of warfarin.

4. *Nicotinic acid group* (e.g. nicotinic acid, acipimox). These inhibit lipolysis in adipose tissue, and predominantly reduce VLDL and thus triglyceride synthesis. Cutaneous flushing limits their use.

5. *Fish oils*. The omega-3 marine triglycerides (Maxepa) can reduce severely elevated triglyceride levels by inhibiting VLDL synthesis in the liver. However, cholesterol levels may go up. Fish oils were once advocated in the maintenance of bypass grafts and following coronary angioplasty. In most people, ingestion of oily fish (e.g. mackerel) 2–3 times a week is more appropriate.

Elevated serum concentrations of total cholesterol, LDL-cholesterol and total triglycerides are associated with an increased risk of cardiovascular disease. Hyperlipidaemia describes the elevation of either cholesterol, or triglycerides, or both. The term dyslipidaemia is sometimes used to describe adverse qualitative effects in lipids – for example, in those with diabetes who have a small dense atherogenic LDL. Patients with hypercholesterolaemia are most often treated with statins, which have largely replaced the use of the bile sequestrant resins as they are more effective and palatable. On average, the statins will reduce total cholesterol by 20% (LDL-cholesterol by 28%), while increasing the HDL-cholesterol by 5%. The degree of cholesterol-lowering is greater in those with high initial concentrations, although reduction to target levels will be more difficult. The statins may be used in combination with low-dose bile sequestrants for resistant or severe hypercholesterolaemia.

Those with mixed hyperlipidaemias are equally responsive to statin therapy; they may also be treated with fibric acid derivatives, especially if the triglyceride levels are markedly elevated.

Treatment of isolated hypertriglyceridaemia remains controversial. Nicotinic acid is sometimes very effective, but cutaneous flushing often limits its use. Fish oils may be of benefit in reducing triglyceride levels as part of the basic diet, but have not proved useful pharmacologically.

MAGNESIUM

The LIMIT-2 trial seemed to show a reduction in mortality in patients treated with intravenous magnesium following acute myocardial infarction. Unfortunately, this has not been confirmed in the much bigger ISIS-4 study, and the routine use of magnesium cannot be recommended (Baxter et al, 1997). However, it should be given in addition to potassium to hypokalaemia patients with serious dysrhythmias.

Dose   8 mmol of magnesium sulphate in 100 ml of 5% dextrose over 15 min, followed by 72 mmol over 24 h.

METOCLOPRAMIDE (Maxolon)

Metoclopramide is a centrally acting anti-emetic agent, which also promotes gastric emptying. Oesophageal reflux is reduced, and small bowel transit time is increased.

Dose   10 mg orally or intravenously.

Side-effects   Drowsiness, dizziness and dystonic movements of the head and neck.

MEXILETINE HYDROCHLORIDE (Mexitil)

Mexiletine is very similar to lignocaine (lidocaine), but can be given orally, and sometimes works in resistant dysrhythmias. It is used in the treatment of ventricular dysrhythmias in coronary heart disease and following myocardial infarction.

Dose   An intravenous loading dose of 100–250 mg is given over 5–10 min and is followed by a reducing infusion, starting at 2 mg/min for 1 h, then 1 mg/min for 2 h, down to 0.05 mg/min until no longer required or until oral therapy is instituted.

Oral loading is with 400 mg, followed by 200–250 mg three or four times daily. A slow-release preparation is available (Mexitil PL).

Side-effects These are related to blood levels, and a reduction in dose may be required for light-headedness, tremor and blurred vision. Gastrointestinal side-effects (nausea, vomiting and hiccoughs) sometimes limit its value.

MILRINONE (Primacor)

Milrinone is a phosphodiesterase inhibitor, similar to enoximone (see above) and suitable for short-term inotropic support. Despite its beneficial haemodynamic actions, long-term therapy with oral milrinone increases mortality and morbidity in patients with severe heart failure.

Dose The loading dose is 50 μg/kg over 10 min. Maintenance infusion is: 0.375–0.750 μg/kg/min (total daily dose should be less than 1.13 mg/kg).

Side-effects Dysrhythmias and hypotension. Chest and limb pain. Bronchospasm.

MINOXIDIL (Loniten)

Minoxidil is a direct-action arterial vasodilator that is useful in resistant hypertension. It causes fluid retention, and should be co-prescribed with diuretics (often high-dose loop diuretics). It may cause T wave changes on the ECG, and rarely a pericardial effusion.

Dose Initially 5 mg once daily orally, increasing to a maximum of 50 mg.

Side-effects Apart from fluid retention, increased hair growth is the most common side-effect.

NALOXONE (Narcan)

Naloxone is a specific opiate antidote and is indicated if there is coma or respiratory failure following administration of diamorphine or morphine. It has a short intravenous half-life and repeated doses are required, depending upon the respiratory pattern.

Dose 0.8–2.0 mg, repeated every 2–3 min, intravenously or by infusion.

Side-effects Dysrhythmias.

NICORANDIL (Ikorel)

Nicorandil is a potassium channel opening drug used in the prevention and treatment of angina. It increases membrane conductance to potassium ions, which hyperpolarises vascular smooth muscle to produce vasodilatation. It also has some nitrate-like properties. It thus reduces both cardiac preload and afterload, while dilating both the epicardial vessels and smaller resistance vessels. The Nicorandil in Angina (IONA) trial suggested that co-prescription of nicorandil with other usual anginal therapies might reduce coronary heart disease death and non-fatal myocardial infarctions in certain patient groups.

Dose 10–30 mg twice daily.

Side-effects Headaches, flushing, hypotension and tachycardia.

NITRATES

Organic nitrates have been the mainstay in the treatment of angina pectoris for over 100 years. The benefits arise from the combination of coronary and non-coronary actions, and different forms of coronary heart disease may respond differently. Nitrates relax vascular smooth muscle, mainly in the venous system, to increase capacitance and thus reduce preload to the heart. Arteriolar relaxation also occurs, with a fall in peripheral resistance (afterload). Although not a main action, coronary dilatation probably occurs, which may improve regional myocardial blood flow. These effects are most marked when the coronary arterial stenosis is due to spasm rather than a fixed lesion, but nitrates are less effective than calcium antagonists. Sublingual glyceryl trinitrate (GTN) is accepted as the standard treatment for acute episodes of angina, and the longer-acting variants are used as prophylaxis against attacks. Tolerance may develop rapidly after the initiation of therapy, but it disappears quickly after discontinuing the drug, and appears to be a function of constant plasma levels of nitrates. Long-acting oral nitrates should, therefore, be prescribed to allow a nitrate-free period.

Uses

Apart from the treatment and prophylaxis of angina, nitrates have been used in acute left ventricular failure, hypertension and the early phase of evolving acute myocardial infarction, with the hope of diminishing peri-infarction ischaemic zones and thus limiting the size of infarction. Bolus therapy is of major value in the emergency treatment of left ventricular failure.

Choice

The haemodynamic effects of GTN are short-lasting, and many different preparations have therefore been developed to prolong their effect and make them useful as prophylactic agents.

Sublingual GTN (0.3, 0.5 or 0.6 mg tablets, or spray)

This should be used as early as possible after the onset of angina or, prophylactically, before physical activity. If the pain persists, it may be repeated at 5-min intervals until relief is obtained. It must always be explained that the drug is neither addictive nor to be reserved only for emergencies. Headache and hypotension are common and may be avoided if the pill is swallowed or spat out as soon as relief is obtained. The tablets are deactivated by heat and light and must therefore be kept cool and in a dark bottle. The activity of the drug after opening lasts only 8 weeks, and old tablets should be discarded. Tablets are also deactivated if cotton-wool is placed in the bottle.

Oral nitrates

There is an extensive first-pass effect on nitrates when taken orally. That is, the amount of drug reaching the systemic circulation is very much reduced because of metabolism by the liver (the first major organ encountered after drug absorption from the gut). As a result, as little as 10% of the drug may reach the circulation, although prolonged action can be achieved by using higher or more frequent doses. Isosorbide dinitrate (Isordil, Sorbitrate, Cedocard) is swallowed whole in doses of 10–60 mg 4–6-hourly. The onset of action is after about 30 min, but sooner if the tablet is chewed. Isosorbide mononitrate (Ismo 20, Elantan) is thought not to be so extensively removed on first pass, which allows smaller doses to be given (20–40 mg twice daily).

Buccal nitrates

Sublingual GTN, Sorbichew and Nitrolingual sprays are rapidly acting preparations that can bypass the hepatic circulation and may, consequently, have better effect. Suscard Buccal is a form of nitrate that has been impregnated into an inert polymer matrix, allowing slow diffusion of the drug across the buccal mucosa. The pill is tucked under the top lip without chewing, and a gel-like coating forms around the drug, allowing it to adhere to the buccal mucosa. Slow absorption can then take place as long as the pill remains intact (usually 3–5 h).

Transdermal nitrates

The use of cutaneous nitrates has been known for 30 years; slow-release skin preparations that hold a reservoir of GTN are available. Cutaneous applications circumvent the first-pass metabolism of swallowed nitrates. Therapeutic blood levels are achieved within 1 h, and may last for up to 24 h if the patch is not removed. Tolerance will then develop.

The patches are applied to any clean, dry, non-hairy part of the skin, although the extremities should be avoided. Absorption depends upon site and blood flow, and large amounts are sometimes required to produce therapeutic blood levels. Skin irritation and variable absorption limit their use, but there is a high placebo effect, especially if patches are applied over the heart.

Intravenous nitrates

Intravenous GTN (Tridil) and isosorbide dinitrate (Isoket) are useful in the management of unstable angina, prolonged infarction pain and left ventricular failure. The dose required for pain relief varies widely, and the infusion rate (1–10 mg/h) must be titrated against pain and blood pressure.

Side-effects

The major side-effects of nitrates are due to vasodilatation, which may give rise to hypotension, tachycardia and headache. Alcohol will potentiate the effects. Side-effects will not be as prominent with continued use, if the patient can be persuaded to persevere. Beta-blockers given at the same time may help to slow the heart and relieve the headache.

NORADRENALINE

Noradrenaline (norepinephrine) stimulates cardiac beta-1 receptors to produce a positive inotropic effect and raise the blood pressure (especially the systolic blood pressure). Baroreceptor stimulation limits a simultaneous tachycardia. Alpha-adrenergic vasoconstriction takes place in vascular beds, except in the cerebral and coronary vessels, which dilate.

Noradrenaline (norepinephrine) may be useful in septic shock, although not for cardiogenic shock. It augments coronary perfusion and raises the blood pressure, although peripheral vasoconstriction may increase cardiac afterload and myocardial work without increasing cardiac output. Noradrenaline (norepinephrine) may also constrict renal capillary beds, leading to renal hypoperfusion.

Dose 1–2 µg/min are infused centrally until the blood pressure rises.

Side-effects Renal hypoperfusion and increased myocardial work. If the drug is allowed to run in too fast, hypertensive crises may occur, leading to stroke and myocardial infarction.

NOREPINEPHRINE (SEE NORADRENALINE)

PHENYTOIN (Epanutin)

Although primarily used as an anticonvulsant, phenytoin has class Ib antidysrhythmic action and is of particular value in ventricular dysrhythmias, especially those that are digitalis-induced. This is because it shortens prolonged QT intervals, increases AV node conduction and suppresses ventricular ectopic activity.

Dose An intravenous dose of 250 mg produces an effect in 5–20 min. Oral doses are 200–600 mg daily.

Side-effects Ventricular fibrillation, heart block and respiratory depression may result following intravenous administration. Oral therapy may be limited by ataxia, skin rashes and blood dyscrasias.

PROCAINAMIDE (Pronestyl)

Procainamide is derived from the local anaesthetic procaine and has class I antidysrhythmic properties, similar to quinidine. It is seldom an agent of first choice, but is of value in the treatment of ventricular ectopics, ventricular tachycardia and paroxysmal atrial tachycardia.

Dose Oral treatment is preferred: 250 mg four times daily. The usual effective antidysrhythmic plasma concentration is 4–8 µg/ml.

Intravenous administration should be under ECG control, 100 mg being given over 5 min or by infusion.

Side-effects Toxicity is rare at plasma levels under 12 µg/ml. Gastrointestinal side-effects are common, and a lupus syndrome has been described with long-term usage.

PROCHLORPERAZINE (Stemetil)

Prochlorperazine is a phenothiazine derivative often used in the treatment of nausea and vomiting. It may be associated with postural hypotension, and metoclopramide may therefore be a better choice in coronary care units.

Dose Can be given orally (5–10 mg), rectally (5 mg) or by deep intramuscular injection (12.5 mg). Intravenous injection is not recommended, as it is an irritant.

Side-effects Dry mouth, drowsiness and extrapyramidal signs.

PROPAFENONE HYDROCHLORIDE (Arhythmol)

Propafenone is a class I antidysrhythmic agent, used in the treatment and prophylaxis of supraventricular and ventricular dysrhythmias.

Dose 150 mg three times daily, increasing to a maximum of 300 mg three times daily.

Side-effects Atropine-like side-effects, including dry mouth, constipation and blurred vision. It is contraindicated in severe bradycardia, uncontrolled heart failure and advanced chronic respiratory disease, because of beta-blocker-like action.

QUINIDINE (Kinidin)

Quinidine is the dextro-isomer of quinine and, in addition to antipyretic properties, has class I antidysrhythmic properties, similar to procainamide. It also has anticholinergic activity, thus aiding AV conduction. It has been used in the prevention of ventricular tachycardia and fibrillation, but is not now commonly used, because it is unpleasant to take (nausea and vomiting) and can cause severe side-effects, such as ventricular fibrillation and heart block. An estimated 2–8% of patients develop marked QT prolongation which may precipitate torsade de pointes.

Dose Orally, 500 mg twice daily, adjusted as required.

Side-effects Gastrointestinal symptoms are common. Cardiodepression and heart block may occur, and the drug should be stopped if the QRS duration increases to more than 0.14 s.

SILDENAFIL (Viagra)

A drug used for erectile dysfunction. There are particular cautions for use in patients with cardiovascular disease, particularly those taking nitrate therapy, when marked hypotension can occur.

Dose 25–100 mg an hour before sexual activity.

Side-effects Dyspepsia, headache, dizziness.

SODIUM BICARBONATE

Intravenous sodium bicarbonate has been widely used in the past for correcting the metabolic acidosis that follows cardiac arrest. However, there is little evidence that this therapy improves outcome, and its use is no longer recommended, because of the frequent occurrence of deleterious side-effects, including increasing carbon dioxide levels, hyponatraemia, inactivation of concurrently administered catecholamines and tissue necrosis if accidentally given extravascularly.

Critically ill patients in hospital may warrant early therapy with sodium bicarbonate, if there is developing hyperkalaemia or acidosis that might precede a cardiac arrest, but these occasions are now the exception rather than the rule.

SODIUM NITROPRUSSIDE

Sodium nitroprusside is a potent parenteral vasodilator, which may be employed in hypertensive emergencies and severe left ventricular failure. It relaxes both arteriolar and venous smooth muscle. It acts rapidly (within 2 min) and should be given by controlled intravenous infusion. The drug is light-sensitive. Solutions are normally red/brown in colour, and deterioration is marked by a colour change to blue.

Dose The drug should be freshly prepared (in 5% dextrose) and used within 4 h. The normal adult dose for heart failure is 10–15 µg/min, adjusted as required. Doses should normally not exceed 400 µg/min. The maximum dose is 700–800 mg in 24 h, and the drug is best not given for periods exceeding 72 h, because of the build-up of plasma cyanide metabolites. If therapy is needed for more than 3 days, blood thiocyanate levels should be assayed.

Side-effects Nausea, sweating, dizziness and twitching denote toxicity. Sodium thiosulphate is an antedote if signs persist. Unexplained cyanosis may be due to formation of methaemoglobinaemia. Large doses of hydroxocobalamin (vitamin B_{12}, 1.5 mg/kg) may be used prophylactically to reduce plasma cyanide levels.

SPIRONOLACTONE (Aldactone)

Spironolactone is an aldosterone antagonist, and potassium-sparing diuretic. It works through an active metabolite, canrenone. Widely used for ascites secondary to liver disease, recent work has confirmed its role in cardiac failure (Pitt et al, 1999). Spironolactone 25 mg should be added to standard of therapy diuretic, ACE inhibitor and beta-blocker in NYHA II/III heart failure

Dose 25 mg daily.

Side-effects Gastrointestinal, hyponatraemia, headache. Beware of hyperkalaemia when co-prescribed with ACE inhibitors.

STATINS

There are currently four statins licensed in the UK (atorvastatin, fluvastatin, pravastatin and simvastatin). Cerivastatin (Lipobay) was withdrawn in 2001 because of 31 deaths associated with rhabdomyositis. Lovastatin is not available in the UK.

The statins are very effective in reducing cholesterol and triglyceride levels, but only pravastatin, simvastatin and lovastatin have robust outcome data (see Table 15.3). For primary prevention, pravastatin was used in the West of Scotland Coronary Prevention (WOSCOPS) trial (Shepherd et al, 1995), and lovastatin in the AFCAPS/TexCAPs trial (Downs et al, 1998). Simvastatin was used for secondary prevention in the Scandinavian Simvastatin Survival (4S) Study (1994), and pravastatin in the Long-term Intervention with Pravastatin in Ischaemic Disease (LIPID) study (LIPID Study Group, 1998) and CARE trial (Sacks et al, 1996). In these studies, daily treatment over a period of 5 years with pravastatin 40 mg, simvastatin 10–40 mg or lovastatin 20–40 mg reduced the risk of developing major coronary events by 34% in primary

prevention and by 30% in secondary prevention, the effects being seen as early as 6 months after starting treatment. An unexpected finding was a reduced occurrence of stroke (19–32%). Treatment benefits were for both men and women up to the age of 75 years. These results have been confirmed by the Medical Research Council/British Heart Foundation Heart Protection Study, which has shown efficacy of simvastatin 40 mg in both men and women aged 40–80 years at risk of coronary heart disease and who have a baseline total cholesterol of 3.5 mmol/l or greater. Increased risk is defined as a past history of myocardial infarction or other coronary heart disease, occlusive disease of non-coronary arteries, diabetes mellitus or treated hypertension.

Who should be treated with statins?

For primary intervention, treatment of cholesterol will depend upon global cardiovascular risk. Risk prediction charts appear at the back of the BNF. Currently, treatment is recommended for all those at an absolute cardiovascular risk of greater than 30% over 10 years. Reducing this threshold to 15% would mean therapy would be offered to about 25% of the UK adult population, which is not achievable within NHS funding. Patients should receive advice on non-drug measures before committing them to lifelong drug therapy (Jowett and Galton, 1987).

For secondary prevention, all patients with overt atherosclerotic disease should be started on a statin, with advice on diet and other risk-factor modification. The current advice is to reduce the serum cholesterol to below 5 mmol/l (LDL-cholesterol below 3 mmol/l), or by 30% of pre-treatment levels, whichever results in a lower concentration. Targets for primary prevention are the same. These treatment thresholds and targets may need reconsideration in the light of results from the Heart Protection Study, in which participants had interventional cholesterol levels as low as 3.5 mmol/l. In this at-risk group, 5 years' treatment with simvastatin 40 mg prevented heart attacks, stroke or other major vascular events in:

- 10% of those who have had a heart attack
- 8% of those with angina
- 7% of those who have had a stroke
- 7% of patients with diabetes.

Choice of statin

Currently, the best evidence supports pravastatin (Lipostat) and simvastatin (Zocor) for both primary and secondary intervention.

Doses   The dose range for pravastatin is 10–40 mg, and for simvastatin 10–80 mg, the dose being most effective taken at night. Practically, a starting dose of 40 mg is recommended for both drugs.

Side-effects   Gastrointestinal, altered liver function tests and low-grade myositis (with elevated creative phosphokinase levels) are the most common. Liver function tests should be monitored. Rhabdomyolysis is the more serious muscle-related event, and may occur with all statins, particularly if fibrates are co-prescribed. Creatine phosphokinase concentrations should be checked periodically.

THROMBOLYTIC (FIBRINOLYTIC) AGENTS

Streptokinase, alteplase and anistreplase have all been shown to break up coronary thrombus and reduce mortality following myocardial infarction (Fibrinolytic Therapy Trialists' Collaborative Group, 1994). Anistreplase has now been with drawn from the UK market, showing no real advantage over streptokinase.

Streptokinase has to combine with plasminogen to form an activator complex, which acts on other circulating plasminogen to form plasmin, which acts directly on fibrin, breaking it down. Streptokinase is not thrombus-specific, and conversion of plasminogen also takes place systemically, making haemorrhage more likely. Alteplase, tenecteplase and reteplase are genetically engineered versions of naturally occurring tissue plasminogen activator (tPA), and are much more clot-specific. They preferentially bind to the fibrin within the clot and thus do not activate circulating plasminogen (i.e. it is plasminogen-independent). This reduces the risk of systemic haemorrhage. Reteplase and tenecteplase are given by intravenous bolus, rather than by infusion. The use of fibrinolytic agents in coronary thrombosis is discussed in detail in Ch. 7.

The two major problems with thrombolysis in acute myocardial infarction that still need to be addressed are the re-occlusion rates following thrombolysis and the risks of haemorrhage, particularly stroke. New fibrinolytic agents and new protocols for drug administration are being tested.

TRANEXAMIC ACID (Cyklokapron)

Tranexamic acid inhibits plasminogen activation and fibrinolysis. It is therefore of great value in severe haemorrhage complicating thrombolytic therapy. However, fresh frozen plasma should also be given.

Dose   0.5–1.0 g by slow intravenous injection, 8-hourly.

Side-effects   Dizziness may follow rapid intravenous injection.

VERAPAMIL (Securon)

See CALCIUM-CHANNEL BLOCKERS.

WARFARIN (Marevan)

Warfarin inhibits the action of vitamin K in the liver and thus inhibits synthesis of four plasma procoagulants (II, VII, IX and X). Its effect commences at about 12 h and lasts for 2–5 days. The dose is titrated against the results of the prothrombin time. Because the prothrombin ratio of treated patients to untreated controls varies from laboratory to laboratory, the World Health Organization system for international standardisation of prothrombin times has allowed comparison of anticoagulant control regimens, based upon common systems of reporting, termed international normalised ratios (INR).

The decision to anticoagulate must take into account the benefits and potential hazards in each patient. The most worrying unwanted effect is bleeding, usually gastrointestinal, into the soft tissues or via the oropharynx. Intracranial haemorrhage is uncommon. This is highest in the first month of treatment. Factors increasing the risk of bleeding include immobility, uncontrolled hypertension and serious co-morbidities. Over-anticoagulation is treated by reducing the daily dose or stopping the drug altogether. If required, vitamin K_1 (phytomenadione) may be given (10 mg over 2–3 min).

Many factors affect the potency of warfarin:

- *Increased potency*: heart failure, liver disease, fever, alcohol, aspirin, cimetidine, diuretics, antibiotics and oral hypoglycaemic.
- *Decreased potency*: diabetes, hypothyroidism, hyperlipidaemia, sedatives, oral contraceptives, cholestyramine and antacids.

Anticoagulant therapy after acute myocardial infarction

Most trials on anticoagulation after myocardial infarction were undertaken when patients were treated by strict and prolonged bedrest when, of course, deep vein thrombosis and pulmonary embolism were frequent complications. Although the role of aspirin following acute myocardial infarction is clear, the use of anticoagulants as an alternative method of secondary prevention is still debated. Even the more recent trials were carried out before thrombolysis.

In contrast to aspirin, warfarin will interrupt the coagulation cascade and can prevent thromboembolic complications in patients with acute myocardial infarction. These include deep vein thrombosis, pulmonary emboli, and systemic emboli originating from intracardiac thrombus associated with transmural infarction, atrial fibrillation or heart failure. 70% of symptomatic systemic emboli produce stroke (Kistler, 1994), often producing significant mortality and morbidity. Most systemic embolisation occurs within 3 months, with the maximal risk being in the first 10 days. Echocardiography identifies intracardiac thrombus in 20–40% of patients with anterior infarction, especially if there is apical dyskinesis. Risk of thromboembolism is increased in the presence of atrial fibrillation and heart failure. In the absence of prophylaxis, 2–6% of patients with anterior myocardial infarction suffer a stroke within 28 days. This complication may be minimized by routine anticoagulation with subcutaneous heparin (SCATI Study group, 1989; Turpie et al, 1989). Patients with anterior Q

Table 17.3 Current INR Targets[a] for cardiovascular disorders

INR	Target	Range
Mechanical valves[b]		
First-generation (e.g. Starr–Edwards, Björk–Shiley)	3.5	2.5–3.5
Second-generation (e.g. St Jude Medical, Medtronic Hall)		
Mitral position	3.0	2.5–3.5
Aortic position	2.5	2.0–3.0
Bioprosthetic valves[c]	3.0	2.5–3.0
Valve repair	2.5	2.0–3.0
Atrial fibrillation	2.0	2.0–3.0
In rheumatic heart disease	3.0	2.5–4.5
Non-valvular	2.5	2.0–3.0
Recurrent deep vein thrombosis/emboli under good INR control	3.5	3.0–4.5 (+ aspirin)
Deep vein thrombosis/pulmonary embolism	2.5	2.0–3.0

[a]The recommendations for INR (international normalised ratio) *ranges* have changed to INR *targets* (British Society of Haematology, 1998).
[b]If the INR falls below 2.5 in patients with mechanical heart valves, there is a marked increase in the thromboembolic risk.
[c]For months, then changed to low-dose aspirin.

wave infarction should be considered for warfarin for 3 months to prevent thromboembolism. Rates of thromboembolism in heart failure vary from 2.5% in those with mild heart failure to 20% per annum in those with dilated cardiomyopathy. There is no evidence to recommend routine anticoagulation in all patients with heart failure in sinus rhythm (Hardman and Cowie, 1999). Concomitant low-dose aspirin should be considered for high-risk patients, despite the inherent dangers of bleeding. Target INRs are shown in Table 17.3.

REFERENCES

Alexander JH, Harrington RA (1998) Recent antiplatelet drug trials in the acute coronary syndromes: clinical interpretation of PRISM, PRISM-PLUS, PARAGON A and PURSUIT. *Drugs*, **56**: 965–976.

Anti-thrombotic Trialists' Collaboration (2002) Collaborative meta-analysis of randomised trials of antiplatelet therapy for prevention of death, myocardial infarction, and stroke in high risk patients. *BMJ*, **324**: 71–86.

Antman EM, Cohen M, Radley D et al (1999) Assessment of treatment effect of enoxaparin for unstable angina/non-Q-wave myocardial infarction. TIMI IIB–ESSENCE meta-analysis. *Circulation*, **100**: 1602–1608.

Barrett-Connor E, Wenger NK, Grady D et al (1998) Coronary heart disease in women, randomised trials, HERS and RUTH. *Maturitas*, **31**: 1–7.

Baxter GF, Sumeray MS, Walker JM (1997) Infarct size and magnesium: insights into LIMIT-2 and ISIS-4 from experimental studies. *Lancet*, **348**: 1424–1426.

British Society of Haematology (1998) British Committee for Standards in Haematology guidelines on oral anticoagulation (3rd edition). *British Journal of Haematology*, **101**: 374–387.

CAPRIE Steering Committee (1996) A randomised blinded trial of clopidogrel versus aspirin in patients at risk of ischaemic events – CAPRIE. *Lancet*, **348**: 1329–1339.

CAST Investigators (1989) Effect of encainide and flecainide on mortality in a randomised trial of arrhythmia suppression after myocardial infarction (the Cardiac Arrhythmia Suppression Trial). *New England Journal of Medicine*, **321**: 406–412.

Cohen M, Demers C, Gurfinkel EP et al (1997) A comparison of low molecular weight heparin with unfractionated heparin for unstable coronary disease. Efficacy and Safety of Subcutaneous Enoxaparin in non-Q-wave Coronary Events Study Group. *New England Journal of Medicine*, **337**: 447–452.

CURE (2001) Effects of clopidogrel in addition to aspirin in patients with acute coronary syndromes without ST elevation. *New England Journal of Medicine*, **345**: 494–502.

DAVITT II (1990) Danish Study Group on Verapamil in Myocardial Infarction. The effect of verapamil on mortality and major events after acute myocardial infarction. *American Journal of Cardiology*, **66**: 779–785.

Diaz R, Paolasso EA, Piegas LS et al (1998) Metabolic modulation of acute myocardial infarction. *Circulation*, **98**: 2227–2234.

Digitalis Investigation (DIG) Group (1997) The effect of digoxin on mortality and morbidity in patients with heart failure. *New England Journal of Medicine*, **336**: 525–533.

Downs JR, Clearfield M, Weis S for the AFCAPS/TexCAPS Research Group (1998) Primary prevention of acute coronary events with lovastatin in men and women with average cholesterol levels. *JAMA*, **279**: 1615–1622.

Fibrinolytic Therapy Trialists' Collaborative Group (1994) Indications for fibrinolytic therapy is suspected acute myocardial infarction: collaborative overview of early and major mortality from all randomised trials of more than 1000 patients. *Lancet*, **343**: 311–322.

Freemantle N, Cleland J, Young P et al (1999) Beta-blockade after myocardial infarction: systematic review and meta-regression analysis. *BMJ*, **318**: 1730–1737.

Gibson RS, Boden WE, Theroux P et al (1986) Diltiazem and re-infarction in patients with non-Q-wave myocardial infarction. *New England Journal of Medicine*, **315**: 423–429.

Grodstein F, Manson JE, Stampfer MJ (2001) Postmenopausal hormone use and secondary prevention of coronary events in the nurses' health study: a prospective observational study. *Annals of Internal Medicine*, **135**: 1–8.

Hardman SMC, Cowie MR (1999) Anticoagulation in heart disease. *BMJ*, **318**: 238–244.

Hulley SB, Grady D, Bush T et al (1998) Randomised trial of estrogen plus progestin for secondary prevention of coronary heart disease in post-menopausal women. *JAMA*, **280**: 605–613.

Jowett NI, Galton DJ (1987) The management of the hyperlipidaemias. In: Hamer J (ed.) *Drugs for Heart Disease*, 2nd edn. London: Chapman and Hall.

Kistler JP (1994) The risks of embolic stroke. Another piece of the puzzle. *New England Journal of Medicine*, **331**: 1517–1519.

Lancet (1989) Digoxin: new answers, new questions [editorial]. *Lancet*, **11**: 79–80.

LIPID Study Group (1998) Prevention of cardiovascular events and death with pravastatin in patients with coronary heart disease and a broad range of initial cholesterol levels. *New England Journal of Medicine*, **339**: 1349–1357.

Lowe GDO (2001) Who should take aspirin for primary prophylaxis of coronary heart disease? *Heart*, **85**: 245–246.

Malmberg K for the DIGAMI Study Group (1997) Prospective randomised study of intensive insulin treatment on long-term survival after acute myocardial infarction in patients with diabetes mellitus. *BMJ*, **314:** 1512–1515.

McMurray JJV (1999) Major beta-blocker mortality trials in chronic heart failure: a critical review. *Heart*, **82** (suppl IV): IV14–IV22.

Packer M (1992) Patho-physiology of chronic heart failure and treatment of heart failure. *Lancet*, **340:** 88–95.

Pitt B, Zannad, Remme WJ, Cody R et al for the Randomised Aldactone Evaluation Study Investigators (1999) The effects of spironolactone on morbidity and mortality in patients with severe heart failure. *New England Journal of Medicine*, **341:** 709–717.

Podrib PJ, Lampert S, Graboys TB et al (1987) Aggravation of arrhythmia by anti-arrhythmic drugs. Incidence and predictors. *American Heart Journal*, **59:** 38E–43E.

Purcell H, Fox K (2001) Diltiazem comes in from the cold. *European Heart Journal*, **22:** 185–187.

Ross AM, Molhoek P, Lundergan C et al (2001) Randomised comparison of enoxaparin, a low molecular weight heparin, with unfractionated heparin adjunctive to recombinant tissue plasminogen activator thrombolysis and aspirin. Second Trial of Heparin and Aspirin Reperfusion Therapy (HART II). *Circulation*, **104:** 648–658.

Sacks FM, Pfeffer MA, Moye LA et al (1996) The effect of pravastatin on coronary events after myocardial infarction in patients with average cholesterol levels. *New England Journal of Medicine*, **335:** 1001–1009.

Scandinavian Simvastatin Survival Study Group (1994) Randomised trial of cholesterol lowering in 4444 patients with coronary heart disease: the 4S study. Lancet **344:** 1383–1389.

SCATI Study Group (1989) Randomised controlled trial of subcutaneous calcium heparin in acute myocardial infarction. *Lancet*, **ii:** 182–186.

Shah PK, Nalos P, Peter T (1987) Atropine resistant post-infarction complete AV block: possible role of adenosine and improvement with aminophylline. *American Heart Journal*, **113:** 194–195.

Shepherd J, Cobbe SJ, Ford I for the West of Scotland Coronary Prevention Study Group (1995) Prevention of coronary heart disease with pravastatin in men with hypercholesterolaemia. *New England Journal of Medicine*, **333:** 1301–1307.

Shukla R, Jowett NI, Thompson DR et al (1994) Side effects with amiodarone therapy. *Postgraduate Medical Journal*, **70:** 492–498.

Sleight P (1986) Beta-adrenoreceptor blockade in the treatment of coronary heart disease. *European Heart Journal*, **7**(suppl C): 79–91.

St John Sutton M (1994) Should ACE inhibitors be used routinely after infarction? Perspectives from the SAVE trial. *British Heart Journal*, **71:** 115–118.

Turpie AGG, Robinson JG, Doyle DJ et al (1989) Comparison of high-dose with low-dose subcutaneous heparin in the prevention of left ventricular mural thrombosis in patients with acute anterior myocardial infarction. *New England Journal of Medicine*, **320:** 352–357.

Vaughan Williams EM (1984) A classification of anti-arrhythmic actions reassessed after a decade of new drugs. *Journal of Clinical Pharmacology*, **24:** 129–147.

White HD, Aylward PE, Frey MJ et al (1997) Randomised, double blind comparison of hirulog versus heparin in patients receiving streptokinase and aspirin for acute myocardial infarction (HERO). Hirulog Early Reperfusion/Occlusion Trial. *Circulation*, **96:** 2155–2161.

Wood D, Durrington P, Poulter N et al (1998) Joint British recommendations on prevention of coronary heart disease in clinical practice. *Heart*, **80** (suppl 2): S1–S29.

Yusuf S, Peto R, Lewis J et al (1985) Beta-blockade during and after myocardial infarction: an overview of the randomised trials. *Progress in Cardiovascular Diseases*, **27:** 335–371.

Index